HANDBOOK OF
ADOLESCENT HEALTH CARE

EDITOR-IN-CHIEF

Lawrence S. Neinstein, MD, FACP

Professor of Pediatrics and Medicine
Executive Director
USC University Park Health Center
Chief, Division of College Health
Department of Pediatrics
USC Keck School of Medicine
Associate Dean of Student Affairs
University of Southern California
Los Angeles, California

ASSOCIATE EDITORS

Catherine M. Gordon, MD, MSc
Debra K. Katzman, MD, FRCP(C)
David S. Rosen, MD, MPH
Elizabeth R. Woods, MD, MPH

 Wolters Kluwer | Lippincott Williams & Wilkins
Health

Philadelphia • Baltimore • New York • London
Buenos Aires • Hong Kong • Sydney • Tokyo

BP45

Acquisitions Editor: Sonya Seigafuse
Managing Editor: Ryan Shaw
Project Manager: Rosanne Hallowell
Manufacturing Manager: Kathleen Brown
Marketing Manager: Kimberly Schonberger
Design Coordinator: Stephen Druding
Cover Designer: Larry Didona
Production Services: Aptara®

Library of Congress Cataloging-in-Publication Data

Handbook of adolescent health care / editor-in-chief, Lawrence S. Neinstein ;
associate editors, Catherine M. Gordon ... [et al.].
      p. ; cm.
   Condensed version of: Adolescent Health Care / editor-in-chief, Lawrence S.
Neinstein ; associate editors, Catherine M. Gordon ... [et al.]. 5th ed.   c2008.
   Includes bibliographical references and index.
   ISBN-13: 978-0-7817-9020-8
   ISBN-10: 0-7817-9020-4
   1. Adolescent medicine—Handbooks, manuals, etc.   2. Teenagers—Health and
hygiene—Handbooks, manuals, etc.   I. Neinstein, Lawrence S.   II. Adolescent Health Care.
   [DNLM: 1.   Adolescent Medicine—Handbooks.   WS 39 H2341 2009]
   RJ550.H24 2009
   616.00835—dc22

                                                                      2008017783

Care has been taken to confirm the accuracy of the information presented and to describe generally accepted practices. However, the authors, editors, and publisher are not responsible for errors or omissions or for any consequences from application of the information in this book and make no warranty, expressed or implied, with respect to the currency, completeness, or accuracy of the contents of the publication. Application of this information in a particular situation remains the professional responsibility of the practitioner.

The authors, editors, and publisher have exerted every effort to ensure that drug selection and dosage set forth in this text are in accordance with current recommendations and practice at the time of publication. However, in view of ongoing research, changes in government regulations, and the constant flow of information relating to drug therapy and drug reactions, the reader is urged to check the package insert for each drug for any change in indications and dosage and for added warnings and precautions. This is particularly important when the recommended agent is a new or infrequently employed drug.

Some drugs and medical devices presented in this publication have Food and Drug Administration (FDA) clearance for limited use in restricted research settings. It is the responsibility of health care providers to ascertain the FDA status of each drug or device planned for use in their clinical practice.

The publishers have made every effort to trace copyright holders for borrowed material. If they have inadvertently overlooked any, they will be pleased to make the necessary arrangements at the first opportunity.

To purchase additional copies of this book, call our customer service department at (800) 638-3030 or fax orders to (301) 223-2320. International customers should call (301) 223-2300.

Visit Lippincott Williams & Wilkins on the Internet: at LWW.com. Lippincott Williams & Wilkins customer service representatives are available from 8:30 am to 6 pm, EST.

                                              10 9 8 7 6 5 4 3 2 1

10/07/08

To my incredible family
My wife, Debra;
My children,
Yael and Yossi, Aaron, and David;
My granddaughter, Bella;
My parents,
Shirley, Roz, and Ben;
and in memory of my father, Alvin

CONTENTS

CONTRIBUTORS

William P. Adelman, MD
Associate Professor, Department of
  Pediatrics
Uniformed Services
University of the Health Sciences;
Chief, Department of Adolescent
  Medicine
Walter Reed Army Medical Center
  and National Naval Medical
  Center
Bethesda, Maryland

Mark E. Alexander, MD
Assistant Professor of Pediatrics
Department of Pediatrics
Harvard University;
Chief, Non-invasive
  Electrophysiology
Department of Cardiology
Children's Hospital Boston
Boston, Massachusetts

**Seth D. Ammerman, MD, FAAP,
FSAM**
Clinical Associate Professor
Department of Pediatrics
Division of Adolescent Medicine
Stanford University
Mountain View, California;
Attending Physician
Department of Pediatrics
Division of Adolescent Medicine
Lucile Packard Children's Hospital
Palo Alto, California

**Martin M. Anderson, MD, MPH,
FAAP, FSAM**
Professor of Clinical Pediatrics
Department of Pediatrics
David Geffen School of Medicine at
  UCLA;
Professor of Clinical Pediatrics
Department of Pediatrics
Mattel Children's Hospital at
  UCLA
Los Angeles, California

Marvin E. Belzer, MD
Associate Professor of Pediatrics and
  Medicine
Department of Pediatrics
USC Keck School of Medicine;
Staff Physician
Division of Adolescent Medicine
Children's Hospital Los Angeles
Los Angeles, California

Robert J. Bielski, MD
Assistant Professor
Department of Surgery
Division of Orthopaedics
University of Chicago
Comer Children's Hospital
Chicago, Illinois

Margaret J. Blythe, MD
Professor of Pediatrics
Department of Pediatrics
Indiana University School of Medicine;
Director of Adolescent Clinical Services
Associate Medical Director of Indiana
  University Medical Group—
  Primary Care
Department of Pediatrics
Wishard Hospital
Indianapolis, Indiana

Terrill Bravender, MD, MPH
Associate Professor
Department of Pediatrics
Ohio State University;
Chief, Adolescent Medicine
Department of Pediatrics
Nationwide Children's Hospital
Columbus, Ohio

Paula K. Braverman, MD
Professor of Pediatrics
Department of Pediatrics
University of Cincinnati College of
  Medicine;
Director of Community Programs
Division of Adolescent Medicine
Cincinnati Children's Hospital
  Medical Center
Cincinnati, Ohio

Cora Collette Breuner, MD, MPH
Associate Professor
Department of Pediatrics
University of Washington;
Director
Adolescent Medicine Clinic
Children's Hospital and Regional
    Medical Center
Seattle, Washington

Matthew J. Bueche, MD
Clinical Associate Professor
Department of Orthopaedic Surgery
    and Rehabilitation
Loyola University Chicago
Stritch School of Medicine
Maywood, Illinois;
Attending Physician
Department of Surgery
Edward Hospital
Naperville, Illinois

Gale R. Burstein, MD, MPH, FAAP
Medical Director
Department of Epidemiology and
    Surveillance and STD and TB
    Control
Erie County Department of Health;
Clinical Assistant Professor
Department of Pediatrics
The Women and Children's Hospital
    of Buffalo
Buffalo, New York

Jeremi M. Carswell, MD
Instructor
Department of Pediatrics
Division of Endocrinology
Harvard University Medical School;
Clinical Instructor
Division of Endocrinology
Children's Hospital Boston
Boston, Massachusetts

Mariam R. Chacko, MD
Professor
Department of Pediatrics
Section of Adolescent Medicine &
    Sports Medicine
Texas Children's Hospital
Baylor College of Medicine
Houston, Texas

Heather Champion, PhD
Research Associate
Department of Social Science &
    Health Policy
Wake Forest University School of
    Medicine
Winston-Salem, North Carolina

Sonia Chehil, MD, FRCPC
Assistant Professor
Department of Psychiatry
Dalhousie University;
Staff Psychiatrist
Child and Adolescent Psychiatry
IWK Health Centre
Halifax, Nova Scotia

Michael Cirigliano, MD, FACP
Assistant Professor of Medicine
University of Pennsylvania School of
    Medicine
Philadelphia, Pennsylvania

Susan M. Coupey, MD
Professor of Pediatrics
Department of Pediatrics
Albert Einstein College of
    Medicine;
Chief
Division of Adolescent Medicine
Children's Hospital at Montefiore
Bronx, New York

Joanne E. Cox, MD
Assistant Professor
Department of Pediatrics
Harvard Medical School;
Associate Chief Division of General
    Pediatrics
Department of Medicine
Children's Hospital Boston
Medical Director
Children's Hospital Primary Care
    Center and Young Parents
    Program
Boston, Massachusetts

Lawrence J. D'Angelo, MD, MPH, FSAM
Professor
Department of Pediatrics, Medicine, Epidemiology, and Prevention and Community Health
George Washington University;
Chief
Division of Adolescent and Young Adult Medicine
Goldberg Center for Community Pediatric Health
Children's National Medical Center
Washington, DC

Ralph J. DiClemente, PhD
Charles Howard Candler Professor
Department of Behavioral Sciences & Health Education
Rollins School of Public Health
Emory University
Atlanta, Georgia

Amy D. DiVasta, MD, MMSc
Instructor of Pediatrics
Department of Pediatrics
Harvard Medical School;
Assistant in Medicine
Department of Medicine
Division of Adolescent Medicine
Children's Hospital Boston
Boston, Massachusetts

Wendi G. Ehrman, MD
Assistant Professor of Pediatrics
Director, Milwaukee Adolescent Health Program
Department of Pediatrics
Medical College of Wisconsin;
Staff Physician
Department of Pediatrics
Children's Hospital of Wisconsin
Milwaukee, Wisconsin

Lawrence F. Eichenfield, MD
Professor
Department of Pediatrics & Medicine (Dermatology)
University of California, San Diego;
Chief
Department of Pediatric & Adolescent Dermatology
Rady Children's Hospital-San Diego
San Diego, California

Jean S. Emans, MD
Professor
Department of Pediatrics
Harvard Medical School;
Chief
Division of Adolescent/Young Adult Medicine
Children's Hospital Boston
Boston, Massachusetts

Abigail English, JD
Director
Center for Adolescent Health & the Law
Chapel Hill, North Carolina

James A.H. Farrow, MD, FSAM
Professor
Department of Pediatrics & Medicine
Director
Department of Tulane Student Health Service
Tulane University
New Orleans, Louisiana

Martin Fisher, MD
Professor
Department of Pediatrics
New York University School of Medicine
New York, New York;
Chief Department of Pediatrics
Division of Adolescent Medicine
Schneider Children's Hospital
New Hyde Park, New York

Amy Fleischman, MD, MMSc
Instructor in Medicine
Department of Medicine
Harvard Medical School;
Assistant in Pediatrics Department of
  Endocrinology
Children's Hospital Boston
Boston, Massachusetts

Joseph T. Flynn, MD, MS
Professor of Pediatrics
Department of Pediatrics
University of Washington School of
  Medicine;
Director
Pediatric Hypertension Program
Division of Nephrology
Children's Hospital and Medical
  Center
Seattle, Washington

J. Dennis Fortenberry, MD, MS
Professor
Department of Pediatrics
Indiana University School of
  Medicine
Indianapolis, Indiana

Praveen S. Goday, MBBS, CNSP, BS
Assistant Professor
Department of Pediatric
  Gastroenterology
Medical College of Wisconsin
Milwaukee, Wisconsin

Melanie A. Gold, DO, FAAP, FACOP
Associate Professor of Medicine
Division of Adolescent Medicine
Department of Pediatrics
University of Pittsburgh School of
  Medicine;
Director of Adolescent Medicine
  Research
Director of Family Planning Services
Department of Pediatrics
Division of Adolescent Medicine
Children's Hospital of Pittsburgh
Pittsburgh, Pennsylvania

Neville H. Golden, MD
Professor of Clinical Pediatrics
Albert Einstein College of
  Medicine
Bronx, New York;
Director of the Eating Disorders
  Center
Division of Adolescent Medicine
Schneider Children's Hospital
New Hyde Park, New York

Catherine M. Gordon, MD, MSc
Associate Professor of Pediatrics
Department of Pediatrics
Divisions of Endocrine and
  Adolescent Medicine
Harvard Medical School, Children's
  Hospital Boston;
Associate in Medicine
Department of Medicine
Divisions of Adolescent Medicine
  and Endocrinology
Children's Hospital Boston
Boston, Massachusetts

Albert C. Hergenroeder, MD
Professor of Pediatrics
Department of Pediatrics
Baylor College of Medicine;
Chief
Adolescent Medicine & Sports
  Medicine Service
Texas Children's Hospital
Houston, Texas

Paula J. Adams Hillard, MD
Professor of Pediatrics
Department of Pediatrics
Professor of Obstetrics and
  Gynecology
Department of Obstetrics and
  Gynecology
University of Cincinnati College of
  Medicine
Director of Gynecology
Division of Adolescent Medicine
Cincinnati Children's Hospital
Cincinnati, Ohio

Stephen Albert Huang, MD
Assistant Professor
Department of Pediatrics
Harvard Medical School;
Director
Thyroid Program
Children's Hospital Boston
Boston, Massachusetts

Loris Y. Hwang, MD
Assistant Professor
Department of Pediatrics
University of California, San
    Francisco Children's Hospital
San Francisco, California

Marc S. Jacobson, MD
Professor
Department of Pediatrics, and
    Epidemiology and Social
    Medicine
Albert Einstein College of Medicine
Bronx, New York;
Director
Center for Atherosclerosis
    Prevention
Schneider Children's Hospital
New Hyde Park, New York

Mary Anne Jamieson, MD, FRCSC
Associate Professor
Department of Obstetrics &
    Gynecology
Queen's University;
Attending Staff
Department of Obstetrics &
    Gynecology
Kingston General Hospital
Kingston, Ontario

M. Susan Jay, MD
Professor of Pediatrics
Director of Adolescent Medicine
Medical College of Wisconsin;
Director of Adolescent Medicine
Children's Hospital of Wisconsin
Milwaukee, Wisconsin

Alain Joffe, MD, MPH, FAAP
Director
Department of Student Health and
    Wellness Center
Johns Hopkins University;
Associate Professor of Pediatrics
Department of Pediatrics
Johns Hopkins Medical Institutions
Baltimore, Maryland

Lisa M. Johnson, MD
Consultant
Adolescent Medicine
Department of Public Health
Nassau, Bahamas

Jessica A. Kahn, MD, MPH
Associate Professor of Pediatrics
Division of Adolescent Medicine
Department of Pediatrics
University of Cincinnati School of
    Medicine;
Associate Professor of Pediatrics
Division of Adolescent Medicine
Department of Pediatrics
Cincinnati Children's Hospital
    Medical Center
Cincinnati, Ohio

Debra K. Katzman, MD, FRCP(C)
Associate Professor of Pediatrics
Head, Division of Adolescent
    Medicine
Department of Pediatrics
The Hospital for Sick Children and
    University of Toronto
Toronto, Ontario

Sari L. Kives, MD, FRCSC
Assistant Professor
Department of Obstetrics/Gynecology
University of Toronto;
Staff Physician
Department of Obstetrics/Gynecology
St. Michaels Hospital for Sick
    Children
Toronto, Ontario

Jonathan D. Klein, MD, MPH
Associate Professor
Department of Pediatrics and
    Adolescent Medicine
University of Rochester School of
    Medicine and Dentistry;
Associate Chair for Community and
    Government Affairs
Golisano Children's Hospital at Stong
University of Rochester Medical
    Center
Rochester, New York

John R. Knight, MD
Associate Professor of Pediatrics
Department of Pediatrics
Harvard Medical School;
Director
Center for Adolescent Substance
    Abuse Research
Children's Hospital Boston
Boston, Massachusetts

Michael R. Kohn, MD, FRACP
Senior Clinical Lecturer
Faculty of Medicine
Sydney University
Camperdown, New South Wales;
Senior Staff Specialist
Division of Adolescent Medicine
The Children's Hospital at Westmead
Westmead, New South Wales

John Kulig, MD, MPH
Professor of Pediatrics
Professor of Public Health and
    Family Medicine
Tufts University School of Medicine;
Director, Adolescent Medicine
Department of Pediatrics
Tufts–New England Medical Center
Boston, Massachusetts

Stan Kutcher, MD, MA
Professor of Psychiatry
Sun Life Chair in Adolescent Mental
    Health
Department of Psychiatry
Dalhousie University;
Consultant Psychiatrist
Department of Psychiatry
IWK Health Sciences Center
Halifax, Nova Scotia

Judith A. Lacy, MD
Clinical Instructor
Department of Obstetrics and
    Gynecology
Stanford University
Lucile Packard Children's
    Hospital
Stanford, California

Sharon Levy, MD, MPH
Instructor
Department of Pediatrics
Harvard Medical School;
Assistant in Medicine
Department of Medicine
Children's Hospital Boston
Boston, Massachusetts

Peter R. Loewenson, MD, MPH
Assistant Professor
Department of Pediatrics
University of Minnesota;
Staff Physician
Teenage Medical Service
Children's Hospitals and Clinics of
    Minnesota
Medical Consultant
Minneapolis Public Schools
Minneapolis, Minnesota

Patricia A. Lohr, MD, MPH
Medical Director
British Pregnancy Advisory
    Service
Stratford-upon-Avon, United
    Kingdom

Keith J. Loud, MD, CM, MSc
Assistant Professor
Department of Pediatrics
Northeast Ohio Universities College
    of Medicine;
Medical Director
Adolescent Health Services
Akron Children's Hospital
Akron, Ohio

Heather R. Macdonald, MD
Assistant Professor of Clinical
    Obstetrics & Gynecology and
        Breast Surgery
Department of Obstetrics &
    Gynecology, Surgery
USC Keck School of Medicine;
Director
Women's Diagnostic Breast Center
Los Angeles County and USC
    Women's Hospital
Los Angeles, California

Joan M. Mansfield, MD
Assistant Professor of Pediatrics
Department of Pediatrics Divisions
    Endocrinology and
    Adolescent Young Adult Medicine
Harvard Medical School;
Associate in Medicine
Endocrinology and
    Adolescent/Young Adult Medicine,
Children's Hospital Boston
Boston, Massachusetts

Miguel Martinez, MSW, MPH
Program Manager
Division of Adolescent Medicine
Children's Hospital Los Angeles
Los Angeles, California

Eric Meininger, MD, MPH
Staff Physician
Community–University Health Care
    Center
University of Minnesota
Minneapolis, Minnesota

Jordan D. Metzl, MD
Assistant Professor
Department of Pediatrics
Weill Medical College of Cornell
    University;
Medical Director
The Sports Medicine Institute for
    Young Athletes
Hospital for Special Surgery
New York, New York

Catherine A. Miller, MD
Adolescent Medicine Fellow
Department of Pediatrics
University of California, San
    Francisco Children's Hospital
San Francisco, California

Melissa D. Mirosh, MD, FRCSC
Attending Staff
Department of Obstetrics and
    Gynecology
High River Hospital
Alberta, Canada

Laurie A.P. Mitan, MD
Associate Professor of Clinical
    Pediatrics
Department of Pediatrics
The University of Cincinnati College
    of Medicine;
Associate Professor
Department of Adolescent Medicine
Cincinnati Children's Hospital
    Medical Center
Cincinnati, Ohio

Wendy G. Mitchell, MD
Professor
Department of Neurology and
    Pediatrics
USC Keck School of Medicine;
Pediatric Neurologist
Division of Neurology
Children's Hospital Los Angeles
Los Angeles, California

Robert E. Morris, MD
Professor
Department of Pediatrics
University of California at Los
    Angeles
Los Angeles, California
Health Care Director
Division of Juvenile Justice
California Department of Corrections
    and Rehabilitation
Sacramento, California

Anna-Barbara Moscicki, MD, BS
Professor of Pediatrics
Department of Pediatrics;
Associate Director of Adolescent
    Medicine
Department of Adolescent Medicine
School of Medicine
University of California, San
    Francisco
San Francisco, California

Lawrence S. Neinstein, MD, FACP
Professor of Pediatrics and Medicine
Executive Director
USC University Park Health Center
Chief, Division of College Health
Department of Pediatrics
USC Keck School of Medicine
Associate Dean of Student Affairs
University of Southern California
Los Angeles, California

Anita L. Nelson, MD
Professor
Department of Obstetrics and
    Gynecology
David Geffen School of Medicine at
    UCLA
Los Angeles, California;
Medical Director
Women's Health Care Programs
Harbor–UCLA Medical Center
Torrance, California

Donald P. Orr, MD
Professor
Department of Pediatrics
Indiana University School of
    Medicine;
Director
Adolescent Medicine
Riley Hospital for Children
Indianapolis, Indiana

Ponrat Pakpreo, MD
Senior Instructor
Pediatrics, Division of Adolescent
    Medicine
University of Rochester
Rochester, New York

Mei-Lin T. Pang, MD
Research Fellow
Department of Pediatric and
    Adolescent Dermatology
Rady Children's Hospital San Diego;
Department of Dermatology
Division of Dermatology
University of California San Diego
    Medical Center
San Diego, California

Arthur Partikian, MD
Child Neurology Fellow
Department of Neurology
Children's Hospital Los Angeles
University of Southern California;
Assistant Professor of Clinical
    Pediatrics and Neurology
USC Keck School of Medicine
Women's and Children's Hospital
Los Angeles, California

Mari Radzik, PhD
Clinical Assistant Professor of
    Pediatrics
USC Keck School of Medicine
University of Southern California;
Clinical Psychologist
Division of Adolescent Medicine
Children's Hospital Los Angeles
Los Angeles, California

Gary Remafedi, MD, MPH
Professor
Department of Pediatrics;
Executive Director
Youth and AIDS Projects
University of Minnesota
Minneapolis, Minnesota

Vaughn I. Rickert, PsyD
Professor of Clinical Population and
    Family Health
Heilbrunn Department of Population
    and Family Health
Mailman School of Public Health at
    Columbia University
New York, New York

Arthur L. Robin, PhD
Professor of Psychiatry & Behavioral
  Neurosciences
Department of Psychiatry &
  Behavioral Neurosciences
Wayne State University School of
  Medicine;
Director of Psychology Training,
Chief of Psychology
Department of Child Psychiatry and
  Psychology Department
Children's Hospital of Michigan
Detroit, Michigan

David S. Rosen, MD, MPH
Professor
Departments of Pediatrics and
  Internal Medicine
University of Michigan Medical
  School;
Chief
Section of Teenage and Young Adult
  Health
Department of Pediatrics
University of Michigan Health
  System
Ann Arbor, Michigan

Owen Ryan, MPH, MIA
Graduate Research Assistant
Heilbrunn Department of Population
  and Family Health
Columbia University
Mailman School of Public Health
New York, New York

Kiarash Sadrieh, MD
Clinical Instructor
Loma Linda University School of
  Medicine
Loma Linda, California
Director
Pediatric Neurology
White Memorial Medical Center
Los Angeles, California

Sandra Loeb Salsberg, MD
Fellow in Endocrinology
Division of Endocrinology
Children's Hospital Boston
Boston, Massachusetts

Marcie B. Schneider, MD, FAAP, FSAM
Associate Clinical Professor of
  Pediatrics
Department of Pediatrics
Albert Einstein College of
  Medicine
Bronx, New York;
Associate Attending
Department of Pediatrics
Greenwich Hospital
Greenwich, Connecticut

Howard Schubiner, MD
Clinical Professor
Department of Pediatrics
Internal Medicine and
  Psychiatry
Wayne State University
Detroit, Michigan;
Faculty Internist
Department of Internal
  Medicine
Providence Hospital
Southfield, Michigan

Robert Sege, MD, PhD
Professor of Pediatrics
Department of Pediatrics
Boston University School of
  Medicine;
Director
Division of Ambulatory
  Pediatrics
Boston Medical Center
Boston, Massachusetts

Mary-Ann B. Shafer, MD
Professor
Department of Pediatrics
University of California, San
  Francisco;
Professor
Department of Pediatrics
University of California, San
  Francisco Medical Center
San Francisco, California

Sara Sherer, PhD
Assistant Professor of Clinical
    Pediatrics
USC Keck School of Medicine
University of Southern California;
Director, Psychology Postdoctoral
    Fellowship
USC UCEDD Mental Health
Department of Pediatrics
Division of General Pediatrics
Director, Behavioral Services
Division of Adolescent Medicine
Department of Pediatrics
Children's Hospital Los Angeles
Los Angeles, California

Lydia A. Shrier, MD, MPH
Assistant Professor
Department of Pediatrics
Harvard Medical School;
Director of Clinic-Based Research
Division of Adolescent/Young Adult
Medicine Children's Hospital Boston
Boston, Massachusetts

David M. Siegel, MD, MPH
Professor of Pediatrics and Medicine
Department of Pediatrics
University of Rochester;
Edward H. Townsend, Chief of
    Pediatrics
Department of Pediatrics
Rochester General Hospital
Rochester, New York

Gail B. Slap, MD, MS, FSAM
Rauh Professor of Pediatrics
Department of Pediatrics
Professor of Medicine
Department of Internal Medicine
University of Cincinnati College of
    Medicine;
Director, Division of Adolescent
    Medicine
Associate Chair for Adolescent
    Programs
Department of Pediatrics
Cincinnati Children's Hospital
    Medical Center
Cincinnati, Ohio

Norman P. Spack, MD
Assistant Professor of Pediatrics
Harvard Medical School;
Associate in Endocrinology
Children's Hospital Boston;
Senior Associate
Endocrine Division
Children's Hospital Boston
Boston, Massachusetts

Diane E.J. Stafford, MD
Instructor in Pediatrics
Department of Pediatric
    Endocrinology
Harvard University;
Assistant in Medicine
Division of Endocrinology
Children's Hospital Boston
Boston, Massachusetts

Paula L. Swinford, MS, MHA, CHES, MPA
Director
Health Promotion and Prevention
    Services
University of Southern California
Los Angeles, California

Diane Tanaka, MD
Assistant Professor of Clinical
    Pediatrics
Department of Pediatrics
USC Keck School of Medicine
University of Southern California;
Attending Physician
Division of Adolescent Medicine
Children's Hospital of Los Angeles
Los Angeles, California

Brigid L. Vaughan, MD
Instructor in Psychiatry
Harvard Medical School;
Medical Director
Psychopharmacology Program
Department of Psychiatry
Children's Hospital Boston
Boston, Massachusetts

Emmanuel B. Walter, MD, MPH
Associate Professor
Associate Director Duke Vaccine and
   Infectious Disease and
      Epidemiology Unit
Department of Pediatrics
Duke University Medical Center
Durham, North Carolina

Shelly K. Weiss, MD
Assistant Professor
Department of Paediatrics
University of Toronto;
Neurologist
Department of Paediatrics
Hospital for Sick Children
Toronto, Ontario

Merrill Weitzel, MD
Clinical Instructor
Obstetrics, Gynecology, and
   Reproductive Biology
Harvard Medical School;
Attending Physician
Department of Surgery
Children's Hospital Boston;
Attending Physician
Department of Obstetrics and
   Gynecology
Brigham and Women's Hospital
Boston, Massachusetts

Elizabeth R. Woods, MD, MPH
Associate Professor of Pediatrics
Department of Pediatrics
Harvard Medical School
Associate in Medicine
Associate Chief, Adolescent/Young
   Adult Medicine
Department of Adolescent/Young
   Adult Medicine
Children's Hospital Boston
Boston, Massachusetts

Alan D. Woolf, MD, MPH
Associate Professor of Pediatrics
Department of Pediatrics
Harvard Medical School;
Associate in Medicine
Children's Hospital
Director, Program in Pediatric
   Environmental Medicine
Co-Director, Fellowship Training
   Program in Pediatric
      Environmental Health
Fellow, The Academy at Harvard
   Medical School
Division of General Pediatrics
Children's Hospital Boston
Boston, Massachusetts

Kimberly A. Workowski, MD, FACP, FIDSA
Associate Professor of Medicine
Department of Medicine
Division of Infectious Diseases
Emory University;
Chief
Guidelines Unit
Epidemiology and Surveillance
   Branch
Division of STD Prevention
Centers for Disease Control and
   Prevention
Atlanta, Georgia

FOREWORD

It is our great pleasure to write the foreword to the first edition of *A Handbook of Adolescent Health Care*. Larry Neinstein and his associate editors provide a wonderful resource for practicing health professionals caring for adolescents, who will use this handy reference guide on a daily basis. This first volume of a small, concise handbook, based on the fifth edition of *Adolescent Health Care: A Practical Guide*, reflects the changing field of adolescent medicine: It incorporates new ideas and data into earlier versions while adding new perspectives in the field. Most importantly, the very practical approaches of previous editions of the textbook continue to permeate this latest version of one of the most useful guides written for the medical care of teenagers.

Many faculty members tell us of the very practical ways this book influences their teaching and delivery of care. We also know that many other physicians, nurses, and health practitioners, who see the majority of adolescents in private practice and public health settings, will also find this book of great use.

This small concise handbook will be of particular value to busy clinicians, health professionals in busy offices and clinics, and health professional students. It is also for those who are in training, the many subspecialists now in the field, and the larger health professional audience. This first edition includes material from the latest full version that has been brought up to date and new sections added to reflect the latest in management and care of adolescents and their families.

Dr. Neinstein and his associate editors have provided us with a solid base for the practice of adolescent medicine, adding new chapters in psychosomatic illness, complementary medicine, anxiety disorders, substance abuse, human papillomavirus (HPV), and anogenital warts. Sixty-six new authors and co-authors have contributed to this edition, further recognizing the many leading experts who add their skill and expertise to the field of adolescent health care. They have skillfully distilled and synthesized new knowledge and transformed it into useful and accessible information for the practitioner.

It is hard to believe that it has been more than 23 years since *Adolescent Health Care* was first conceived. During this time, dramatic changes in the field have occurred, including the establishment of adolescent medicine as a subspecialty in pediatrics, family medicine, and internal medicine. This recognition has served to codify special areas of interest and knowledge in the field. Expertise in adolescent health is found in academic health centers, college health centers, community agencies, and school services nationally and internationally.

It is certainly hard to predict where the field will go in the next 50 years. Clearly, adolescence as a period of life will continue to undergo dramatic changes as our young people seek new ways to redefine themselves and to explore new ideas and challenges. We will need to understand how they will influence other teenagers and how young people will have an impact on their families, their communities, and the world at large. Their health care may play a much larger role in understanding how health and illness will change in our society, in an increasingly smaller and smaller world.

One can only wonder how the daily care of teenagers will also change. Clearly, the developmental aspects of this challenging period of time will remain. But with enhanced communication between teenagers and their world, an expanded role of the Internet, iPods, and cell phones in our lives, the drive toward seeking and improving self-help and self-knowledge, it is hard to conceive of the many new ways by which we will be providing care for these young people.

With that in mind, we are sure that future editions of both the full text and the handbook will be around to assist us in meeting the challenges of youth and give us the opportunity to provide the highest quality of health care.

Iris F. Litt, MD
Dale C. Garell, MD

It is exciting to see the first edition of this small handbook version of the fifth edition of *Adolescent Health Care: A Practical Guide* come to life. As the bigger textbook has continued to grow in depth, coverage, and length, it has become evident that a smaller handbook version would be a highly useful text by itself or as a companion text for many practicing clinicians. It will have the advantage of portability and conciseness as compared to the full text. As I have continued to love to see heavily worn copies of the full edition in offices and clinics, I look forward to seeing even more worn handbook versions.

Adolescent health continues to expand as a field and includes pediatricians, internists, family medicine physicians, gynecologists, nurse practitioners, physician assistants, psychologists, social workers, nurses, health educators, nutritionists, and teachers among many others. The field has grown to include the health issues among college students, young adults with chronic illnesses transitioning into adult health care systems, adolescents in a variety of institutional settings, and adolescents served in school-based clinics. I thank all of you who are the providers of care to this population. I am always amazed and uplifted by the number of wonderful individuals from so many disciplines involved in the care of youth.

It is a daunting task to approach such a concise version of the full practical guide. To facilitate this task and to broader the approach, I have added associate editors. Dr. Debra Katzman, Dr. Catherine Gordon, Dr. David Rosen, and Dr. Elizabeth Woods are among the most respected names in the field of adolescent health care in North America. They provide a wide range of expertise ranging from gynecology, endocrinology, and mental health issues to prevention health issues, substance abuse, and sexually transmitted diseases. They have been an invaluable addition in continuing to raise the standards of this textbook. In addition to these four associate editors, I sincerely thank the many expert contributors who have helped make this first handbook edition so concise but complete. I hope that all readers will enjoy this first edition of *Handbook of Adolescent Health Care*. The intent is to make the material practical and easy to read, while maintaining a thorough approach that is evidence-based but in a concise format. I know that the tables, figures, statistics, references, and resources will help you in providing care to the many adolescents and young adults that you serve. As always, the hope is to make it easier for you, the reader, to perform appropriate evaluations and work-ups.

I dedicate this book to young people and to their health care providers. I hope this edition will serve as a wealth of information for those who care for youth and young adults. Importantly, I welcome and look forward to feedback on this edition so I can continue to improve this book as the most practical guide to adolescent health issues.

Lawrence S. Neinstein, MD

ACKNOWLEDGMENTS

It takes a tremendous effort to put together a book as comprehensive as *Handbook of Adolescent Health Care*. I am forever indebted to the late Adie Klotz, MD, a friend, teacher, and inspiration, who helped me realize the excitement of working with young people. I also acknowledge both Richard G. MacKenzie, MD, and Dale Garell, MD, who encouraged my interest in the field of adolescent medicine.

With this first edition of *Handbook of Adolescent Health Care,* I have gained four wonderful colleagues and friends who helped in the completion of this project—my four associate editors. Each one has been an incredible pleasure to work with, and each has added his or her unique qualities and expertise to this text. In addition, they have been responsive and eager to add their own input to this text. I sincerely thank Catherine Gordon, Debra Katzman, David Rosen, and Elizabeth Woods for their assistance as coeditors.

I also express my deepest appreciation to the many experts who served as authors on the many chapters of this book. Their knowledge, expertise, and dedication have helped to make this the most complete edition yet. I personally thank them for their time and effort in responding to our many, many requests, e-mails, and demands.

I want to thank both the wonderful and dedicated staff of the Division of Adolescent Medicine at Children's Hospital of Los Angeles and the staff and students at the USC University Park Center who have taught me so much about adolescents and college students. Many other health care professionals have also given me their assessments and helpful comments in the development of this first edition.

Special thanks go to several individuals at the University of Southern California. Lucy Vergara, at the USC University Park Health Center, was always there to assist in communicating with Lippincott Williams & Wilkins and co-authors. I also wish to thank Michael Jackson, Vice-President of Student Affairs, and Dr. Roberta Williams, Chair of Pediatrics, USC Keck School of Medicine, who continued to encourage my academic pursuits.

Lippincott Williams & Wilkins deserves recognition in the development of this edition. I thank Ryan Shaw, managing editor, for his assistance in being a kind facilitator in my many requests for edits and changes. I also thank Kimberly Schonberger, Marketing Manager, Rosanne Hallowell, Project Manager, and Sonya Seigafuse, Acquisitions Editor.

These past few years have been personally medically challenging ones. I would like to express my deepest thanks to several physicians whose helpful treatment and advice have kept me healthy. My heartfelt thanks goes to Dr. Gary Dosik, Dr. Brian Durie at Cedars-Sinai Medical Center, Dr. Steve Forman at City of Hope Medical Center, and Dr. Burt Liebross. I also want to thank the caring and supportive nursing staff at all of these facilities, and my wonderful friends and family who have been there for me. So, with all my heart, a deep thank you.

There are also individuals very close to me who deserve special recognition. My parents have shown me what appropriate, loving, and involved parenting can mean during one's tumultuous adolescent years and during adult life.

Without their guidance, I would not have had the skills and ability to have become the person I am. A second set of parents, Roz and Ben, have also provided unflagging support during the past 35 years. Loving thanks to all of you.

Lastly, I thank my loving wife, Debra, and my children, Yael and Yossi, Aaron, and David. Debbie has continued to support me despite even far more hours and late nights spent preparing this edition. Yael and Yossi, Aaron and David serve to inspire me with wonderful examples of healthy young adults. I love all of you and thank you for your understanding, support, and encouragement with this first edition.

CHAPTER 1

Normal Physical Growth and Development

Jeremi M. Carswell and Diane E.J. Stafford

The Endocrine Axes. Although there is activity and change in most hormonal systems during adolescence, most of the physical changes are attributed to three hormonal axes. These axes are introduced below.

Axis	Hormones
Hypothalamic-pituitary-gonadal (HPG) axis (see Fig. 1.1)	1. Gonadotropin-releasing hormone (GnRH), also called luteinizing hormone–releasing hormone (LHRH) 2. Luteinizing hormone (LH) 3. Follicle stimulating hormone (FSH) 4. Estrogen 5. Testosterone
Hypothalamic-pituitary-adrenal axis (HPA) (see Fig. 1.1)	1. Adrenocorticotropic hormone 2. Dehydroepiandrosterone (ACTH) 3. DHEA sulfate (DHEA-S)
Growth hormone (GH) axis	1. Growth hormone–releasing hormone (GHRH) 2. Growth hormone (GH) 3. Insulin-like growth factors (IGFs)

Although the exact triggers of puberty are poorly understood, there are three distinct changes in the hypothalamic-pituitary unit: (1) a nocturnal

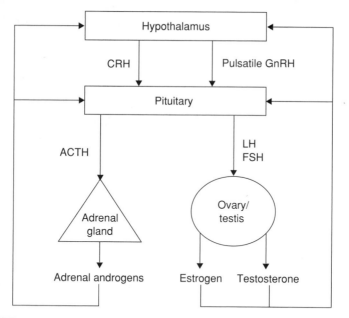

FIGURE 1.1 The hypothalamic-pituitary-gonadal and the hypothalamic-pituitary-adrenal axes.

sleep-related augmentation of pulsatile LH secretion; (2) a decrease in the sensitivity of the hypothalamus and the pituitary to estradiol and testosterone, so that the gonadotropins LH and FSH begin to increase; and (3) in the female, development of a positive feedback system, whereby critical levels of estrogen trigger a large release of GnRH, stimulating LH to initiate ovulation.

SEXUAL DEVELOPMENT IN PUBERTY

What is commonly thought of as puberty should be separated into gonadarche and adrenarche, arising from activation of the HPG axis and the HPA axis, respectively. In girls, gonadarche is represented by thelarche (the onset of breast budding); in boys, by testicular enlargement to 4 mL or above or 2.5 cm in the longest axis. Pubarche, or the growth of terminal sexual hair in girls, is mainly the result of adrenarche.

Sexual Maturity Rating Scales

The Sexual Maturity Rating (SMR) scale (also called the Tanner scale), as developed by Marshall and Tanner, allows for the accurate classification of physical pubertal maturation. For both boys and girls, there are five stages categorizing secondary sexual characteristics. These stages are shown in Figures 1.2 through 1.4. Tanner staging should be recorded yearly, as this assessment

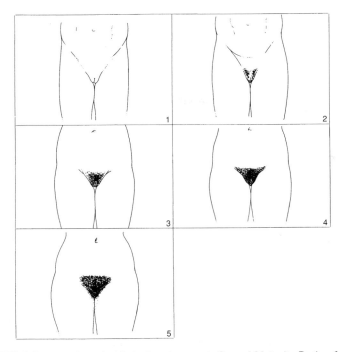

FIGURE 1.2 Female pubic hair development. *Sexual Maturity Rating 1 (SMR 1):* Prepubertal; no pubic hair. *SMR 2:* Straight hair is extending along the labia and, between ratings 2 and 3, begins on the pubis. *SMR 3:* Pubic hair has increased in quantity, is darker, and is present in the typical female triangle but in smaller quantity. *SMR 4:* Pubic hair has increased in quantity, is darker, and is more dense, curled, and adult in distribution but less abundant. *SMR 5:* Abundant, adult-type pattern; hair may extend onto the medial aspect of the thighs. (From Daniel WA, Palshock BZ. A physician's guide to sexual maturity rating. *Patient Care* 1979;30:122, with permission. Illustration by Paul Singh-Roy.)

provides critical information for identifying abnormal puberty or in assuring that puberty is progressing normally.

Girls
Events
1. *Thelarche:* Often the earliest physical sign of puberty in girls, although a minority develop pubic hair as the first sign. On average, breast development starts at age 10.0 for Caucasian girls and 8.9 years for African-American girls (Herman-Giddens et al., 1997).
2. *Growth Spurt:* Thelarche and pubarche may both be preceded by about 1 year by the growth spurt; thus the growth curve is an essential tool in the evaluation of precocious puberty.

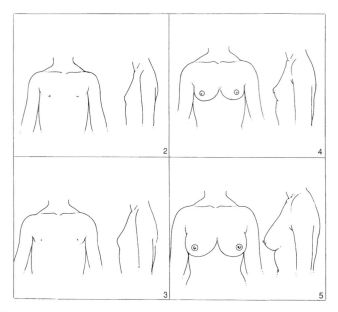

FIGURE 1.3 Female breast development. *Sexual Maturity Rating 1 (SMR 1),* not shown: Prepubertal; elevations of papilla only. *SMR 2:* Breast buds appear; areola is slightly widened and projects as small mound. *SMR 3:* Enlargement of the entire breast with protrusion of the papilla or of the nipple. *SMR 4:* Enlargement of the breast and projection of areola and papilla as a secondary mound. *SMR 5:* Adult configuration of the breast with protrusion of the nipple; areola no longer projects separately from remainder of breast. (From Daniel WA, Paulshock BZ. A physician's guide to sexual maturity rating. *Patient Care* 1979;30:122, with permission. Illustration by Paul Singh-Roy.)

3. *Menarche:* This event usually occurs during SMR B3 or B4 and about 3.3 years after the growth spurt, or roughly 2 years after breast budding.

Timing
The average length of time for completion of puberty is 4 years, but it can range from 1.5 to 8 years. The sequence of pubertal events is shown in Figures 1.5 and 1.6b.

Boys
Events
1. *Testicular Growth:* The first physical sign of puberty in the majority of boys is increased testicular volume, although the most noticeable first event of male puberty is the growth of pubic hair (Table 1.1).
2. *Growth Spurt:* Midpuberty, or the time of rising testosterone concentrations, is associated with the period of most rapid linear growth in boys, in contrast to the early growth spurt in girls. It is also at this time that the voice changes axillary hair appears, and possibly also acne. Facial hair growth typically starts about 3 years after pubic hair growth. The hair on the face, chest, back,

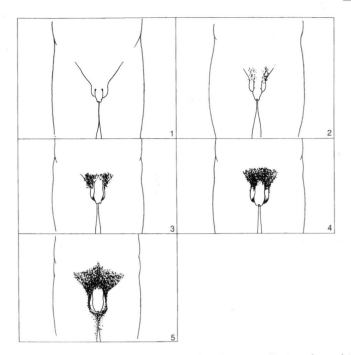

FIGURE 1.4 Male genital and pubic hair development. Ratings for pubic hair and for genital development can differ in a typical boy at any given time because pubic hair and genitalia do not necessarily develop at the same rate. *Sexual Maturity Rating 1 (SMR 1):* Prepubertal; no pubic hair. Genitalia unchanged from early childhood. *SMR 2:* Light, downy hair develops laterally and later becomes dark. Penis and testes may be slightly larger; scrotum becomes more textured. *SMR 3:* Pubic hair has extended across the pubis. Testes and scrotum are further enlarged; penis is larger, especially in length. *SMR 4:* More abundant pubic hair with curling. Genitalia resemble those of an adult; glans has become larger and broader, scrotum is darker. *SMR 5:* Adult quantity and pattern of pubic hair, with hair present along the inner borders of the thighs. The testes and the scrotum are adult in size. (From Daniel WA, Paulshock BZ. A physician's guide to sexual maturity rating. *Patient Care* 1979;30:122, with permission. Illustration by Paul Singh-Roy.)

and abdomen may continue to appear throughout and beyond puberty into adulthood, its amount and distribution being quite variable and dependent on ethnicity and family patterns.
3. *Attainment of Fertility:* Ejaculation usually occurs at SMR G3, as does the first evidence of spermarche, but fertility is not usually attained until SMR G4.

Timing
The average length of time for the completion of puberty is 3 years, but it can range from 2 to 5 years. Genital development is initiated at about 10.1 years for white boys, 9.5 years for African-American boys, and 10.4 years for

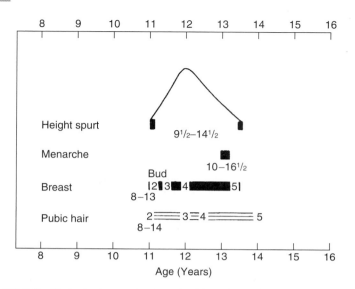

FIGURE 1.5 Biological maturity in girls. (From Tanner JM. *Growth at adolescence,* 2nd ed. Springfield, IL: Blackwell Scientific Publications, 1962, with permission. Copyright © 1962 by Blackwell Scientific Publications.)

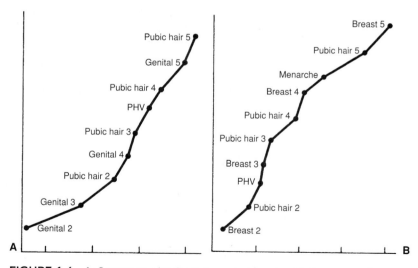

FIGURE 1.6 **A:** Sequence of pubertal events in males. **B:** Sequence of pubertal events in females. (From Root AW. Endocrinology of puberty. *J Pediatr* 1973;83:1–19, with permission.)

TABLE 1.1

Testicular Volume by Sexual Maturity Rating

Sexual Maturity Rating[a]	Volume (cm³)			
	Left Testis		Right Testis	
	Mean	SD	Mean	SD
1	4.8	2.8	5.2	3.9
2	6.4	3.2	7.1	3.9
3	14.6	6.5	14.8	6.1
4	19.8	6.2	20.4	6.8
5	28.3	8.5	30.2	9.6

[a]Mean of genital and pubic hair ratings.
Adapted from Daniel WA Jr., Feinstein RA, Howard-Peebles P, et al. Testicular volumes of adolescents. *J Pediatr* 1982;101:1010.

Mexican-American boys, with completion of puberty at 15.9 years in white boys, 15.7 years in African-American boys, and 14.9 years in Mexican-American boys. The overall trend is earlier entry into puberty with prolonged progression to maturity. While the causes of this trend are not known, boys have recently grown taller and heavier at the earlier stages of puberty than in the past. The sequence of events for an average male is shown below, in Figures 1.6a and 1.7 and Table 1.2.

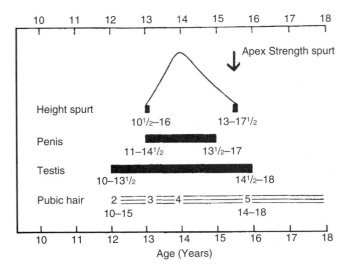

FIGURE 1.7 Biological maturity in boys. (From Tanner JM. *Growth at adolescence,* 2nd ed. Springfield, IL: Blackwell Scientific Publications, 1962, with permission. Copyright © 1962 by Blackwell Scientific Publications.)

TABLE 1.2

Means and Normal Variation in the Timing of Adolescent Secondary Sexual Characteristics (Males)

Stage	Mean Age at Onset ±2 SD (yr)	Stage	Time between Stages (yr)		
				Percentile	
			Mean	5th	95th
G2	11.6 ± 2.1	G2–3	1.1	0.4	2.2
G3	12.9 ± 2.1	PH2–3	0.5	0.1	1.0
PH2	13.4 ± 2.2[a]	G3–4	0.8	0.2	1.6
G4	13.8 ± 2.0	PH3–4	0.4	0.3	0.5
PH3	13.9 ± 2.1	G4–5	1.0	0.4	1.9
PH4	14.4 ± 2.2	PH4–5	0.7	0.2	1.5
G5	14.9 ± 2.2	G2–5	3.0	1.9	4.7
PH5	15.2 ± 2.1	PH2–5	1.6	0.8	2.7

[a]Mean is probably too high due to experimental method.
From Barnes HV. Physical growth and development during puberty. *Med Clin North Am* 1975;59:1305.

MATURATION OF THE HPG AXIS

Gonadal Steroids. The target tissues of LH and FSH are the ovaries and testes, which produce estradiol and testosterone, respectively. Testicular Leydig cells also produce androstenedione, dihydrotestosterone, and estradiol, but to a much lesser extent.

Estrogen. Estradiol from the ovary accounts for the majority of the circulating estrogens, although there is a small amount of extraovarian conversion from androstenedione and testosterone. In addition to stimulating breast growth and maturation of the vaginal mucosa, estrogen has been found to have a major impact on the skeleton, being the primary hormone responsible for epiphyseal closure.

Testosterone. The testes produce most of the circulating testosterone, but a small amount comes from extratesticular conversion of the adrenal hormone androstenedione in both males and females. Testosterone is responsible for the voice change in males and the attainment of male body habitus, while dihydrotestosterone, the product of conversion of testosterone by 5α-reductase, causes growth of the phallus and prostate.

GnRH Pulse Generator. At the time of puberty, GnRH is secreted from the GnRH pulse generator in the hypothalamus, leading to pituitary secretion of LH and FSH and subsequent secretion of estradiol from the ovaries or testosterone from the testes. The exact triggers are still incompletely understood, although new research has elucidated new potential regulators and key players in the awakening of this system. These include leptin, the genes *GPR54/KiSS-1*, as well as several neuropeptides and neurotransmitters.

ADRENARCHE

The increased secretion of androgens from the adrenal gland, called adrenarche, in the prepubertal and pubertal periods is independent of HPG changes. The two events are temporally related, with the increase in adrenal hormones preceding that of the gonadal sex steroids, although the effects are evident later. It is important to note, however, that adrenal androgens are not necessary for pubertal development or the adolescent growth spurt.

Physical Manifestations

Local conversion of DHEA-S to testosterone and then to dihydrotestosterone is responsible for hair growth in the androgen-dependent areas (face, chest, pubic area, axillae). Axillary and pubic areas are the most sensitive to the effects of androgens, which is why these areas are the first to develop sexual hair. In addition, local conversion of DHEA-S within the apocrine glands of the axillae causes body odor, and conversion within sebaceous glands is responsible for the development of acne.

PHYSICAL GROWTH DURING PUBERTY

One of the most striking changes in adolescents is their rapid growth. This height spurt is dependent primarily upon growth hormone and the insulin-like growth factors, but many other hormones may influence growth as well, especially the sex steroids. Without prompt recognition and treatment, premature or delayed puberty may have marked effects on height. Normal growth curves and stature for age are available in Figures 1.8 and 1.9 and at www.cdc.gov/growthcurves.

GH during Puberty

Most linear growth is dependent upon GH and its feedback loop. GH secretion is increased by growth hormone–releasing hormone (GHRH) and decreased by somatostatin from the hypothalamic arm of the loop. Growth hormone has been shown to double during the pubertal growth spurt. Like many hormones, GH is secreted in pulsatile fashion, with maximum rates at the onset of slow-wave sleep. It is this pulsatile secretion that renders random testing of GH unhelpful. GH exerts its effects through IGFs, mainly IGF-I (formerly somatomedin-C) and IGF-II.

Growth Velocity. Growth velocity during the pubertal growth spurt is at its highest levels outside of infancy. It should be noted that in calculating growth velocity, it is important to have an interval of 6 to 12 months, as growth is greatest in the spring and summer months. Although males and females are roughly the same height upon entry into puberty, males emerge taller by 13 cm on average. This is primarily due to boys' 2-year lag behind girls in attaining their peak height velocity, but a small amount of height may be accounted for by the higher peak velocity. Girls gain their peak height velocity of 8.3 cm/year at an average age of 11.5 years (Tanner stages B2 to B3) while boys do not reach their peak height velocity of 9.5 cm/year until the age of 13.5 years (at Tanner genital stages 3 to 4). There are also curves available for early and late maturers.

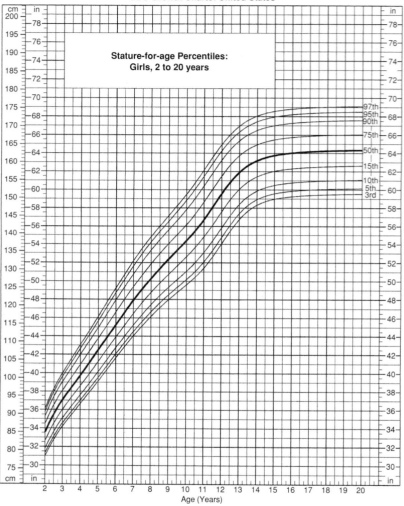

FIGURE 1.8 Stature-for-age percentiles for girls 2 to 20 years of age. (From CDC Growth Charts: United States—Advance data from Vital and Health Statistics of the Centers for Disease Control and Prevention. *Natl Ctr Health Stat* 2000;314:1–28. www.cdc.gov/nchs/pressroom/oonews/growchrt.htm)

Prediction of Final Height
Midparental "target" height:

$$\text{For girls: } \frac{(\text{father's height} - 13 \text{ cm or 5 inches}) + \text{mother's height}}{2}$$

$$\text{For boys: } \frac{(\text{father's height} + 13 \text{ cm or 5 inches}) + \text{mother's height}}{2}$$

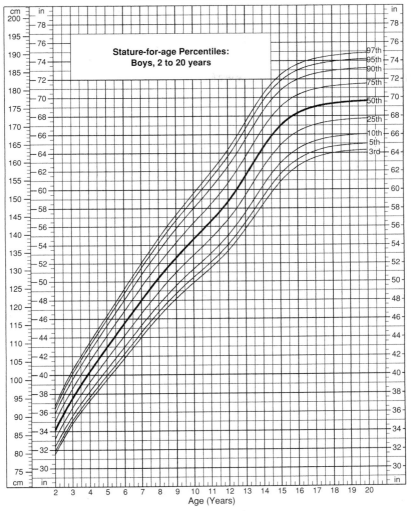

FIGURE 1.9 Stature-for-age percentiles for boys 2 to 20 years of age. (From CDC Growth Charts: United States—Advance data from Vital and Health Statistics of the Centers for Disease Control and Prevention. *Natl Ctr Health Stat* 2000;314:1–28. www.cdc.gov/nchs/pressroom/oonews/growchrt.htm)

The Bayley-Pinneau Method. This technique uses bone age to predict final height. It is based on the attainment of a bone age, on x-ray of the left hand and wrist, that is then matched to standards.

The Role of Sex Steroids. Gonadal steroids contribute to the growth spurt by inducing an increase in GH secretion and stimulating local production of IGF-1 in cartilage and bone directly. *Estrogen* is the hormone most involved with the growth spurt via its effects on bone and cartilage in men and women. Estradiol concentration correlates with the pubertal growth spurt; girls experience an increase in estradiol earlier than boys and achieve the corresponding increase in peak height velocity earlier as well. At higher doses, estrogen causes epiphyseal fusion and thus termination of linear growth. *Androgens* seem to have little direct effect on pubertal bone growth. Androgens have a role in the sexual dimorphism of the skeleton and are likely responsible for the greater increase in periosteal bone deposition and therefore bone strength in men as compared with women.

Pubertal Changes in Body Composition

During childhood, boys and girls have relatively equal proportions of lean body mass, skeletal mass, and body fat. By the end of puberty, however, men have 1.5 times more lean body mass and skeletal mass than women and women have double the fat mass.

Skeletal Mass. Changes in bone mass, or bone mineral density (BMD), parallel the alterations in lean body mass, body size, and muscle strength. Major determinants of BMD are physical activity level, heredity, nutrition, endocrine function, and other lifestyle factors. The accretion of skeletal bone mass during puberty is critical, and peak bone mass is acquired by early adulthood. This serves as the "bone bank" for the remainder of life.

1. *Age of menarche:* There is an inverse relationship between the age of menarche and the risk of osteoporosis later in life, as demonstrated by epidemiologic studies.
2. *Nutrition:* Adequate consumption of calcium and vitamin D is important for optimal accrual of bone mass. It appears that calcium intakes of between 1,200 and 1,800 mg per day result in maximal calcium absorption for children between 9 and 18 years of age.
3. *Exercise:* Weight-bearing physical activity during pre- and early puberty has been shown to improve bone strength, but results have been less promising for the effects of exercise on postmenarcheal girls.
4. *Hormonal control:* The skeletal structure also undergoes epiphyseal maturation under the influence of estradiol and testosterone, as reviewed above.

Bone Age. Skeletal maturation, or bone age, can be determined by comparing a radiograph of an adolescent's hand, wrist, or knee to standards of maturation in a normal population. Bone age is one index of physiologic maturation, providing an idea of the proportion of total growth accomplished. For example, if an adolescent is 15 years old and has a bone age of 12 years, there will be more potential growth than if the same adolescent's bone age were 15 years. The use of skeletal age is discussed further in Chapter 8.

Body Mass Index. Body mass index (BMI) increases with puberty, although it should be pointed out that BMI does not quantitate body composition. BMI varies with age, gender, and ethnicity. In children and adolescents, BMI must be compared using age-stratified standardized percentiles. Charts and tables for BMI, which should be tracked in all children, particularly teens, can be obtained from the National Center for Chronic Disease Prevention and Health Promotion of the Centers for Disease Control and Prevention (www.cdc.gov/growthcharts)

There is a strong correlation between the timing of puberty and BMI: children with a higher mean BMI mature earlier. BMI is determined as follows:

$$BMI = weight\ in\ kilograms \div [height\ in\ meters]^2$$

Or

$$BMI = [weight\ in\ kilograms \div height\ in\ cm \div height\ in\ cm] \times 10,000$$

The equivalent formula in English units is the following:

$$BMI = [weight\ in\ pounds \div height\ in\ inches \div height\ in\ inches] \times 703$$

The BMI declines from birth and reaches a minimum between 4 and 6 years of age before gradually increasing through adolescence and adulthood. The upward trend after the low point is referred to as the "adiposity rebound." Children with an earlier rebound are more likely to have an increased BMI.

WEB SITES AND REFERENCES

http://www.youngwomenshealth.org. From Young Women's Health Center at Boston Children's Hospital.

http://www.puberty101.com/. Information site on puberty and other adolescent questions.

http://www.teachingteens.com/index2.htm. Health education site on teaching teens about puberty.

http://www.cdc.gov/growthcharts. Growth charts online.

Grumbach MM. Estrogen, bone, growth and sex: a sea change in conventional wisdom. *J Pediatr Endocrinol Metab* 2000;13 Suppl 6:1439.

Herman-Giddens ME, Slora EJ, Wasserman RC, et al. Secondary sexual characteristics and menses in young girls seen in office practice: a study from the Pediatric Research in Office Settings network. *Pediatrics* 1997;99:505.

Institute of Medicine, Food and Nutrition Board: *Dietary reference intakes for calcium, phosphorus, magnesium, vitamin D, and fluoride.* Washington, DC: National Academy Press, 1997.

Marshall WA, Tanner JM. Variations in the pattern of pubertal changes associated with adolescence in girls. *Arch Dis Child* 1969;44:291.

Marshall WA, Tanner JM. Variations in the pattern of pubertal changes in boys. *Arch Dis Child* 1970;45:13.

CHAPTER 2

Psychosocial Development in Normal Adolescents

Mari Radzik, Sara Sherer, and Lawrence S. Neinstein

Adolescence is a biopsychosocial process that may start before the onset of puberty and last well beyond the termination of growth. The events and problems that arise during this period are often perplexing to parents or caregivers, health care providers, and adolescents. Understanding the adolescent psychosocial developmental process is beneficial in providing routine adolescent health care and helping adolescents and their families through problem periods (e.g., school failure and depression).

THE PROCESS OF ADOLESCENCE

Adolescents display a wide variability in biological, psychological, and emotional growth, with each adolescent responding to life's demands and opportunities in a unique way. The transition from childhood to adulthood does not occur by a continuous, synchronous process. In fact, biological, social, emotional, and intellectual growth may be totally asynchronous. About 80% of adolescents cope well with the developmental process. This ability to cope is a resiliency that is often overlooked, as the behaviors of adolescents are often the primary focus of attention. Overall, intractable and major conflict between parents and their adolescent children is not a "normal" part of adolescence.

Phases and Tasks of Adolescence

Adolescence can be divided into three psychosocial developmental phases: (1) early adolescence: approximate ages 10 to 13, or middle school years; (2) middle adolescence: approximate ages 14 to 17, or high school years; (3) late adolescence: approximate ages 17 to 21, or college or 4 years of work after high school.

Tasks that characterize the development of adolescents include (1) achieving independence from parents; (2) adopting peer codes and lifestyles; (3) assigning increased importance to body image and accepting one's body image; and (4) establishing sexual, ego, vocational, and moral identities.

EARLY ADOLESCENCE (APPROXIMATE AGES 10–13)

This period is heralded by rapid physical changes, with the onset of puberty engendering self-absorption and initiation of the adolescent's struggle for independence. Both the onset of puberty and the associated psychosocial changes occur 1 to 2 years earlier for girls than for boys.

Independence-Dependence Struggle. Common events include (1) less interest in parental activities and more reluctance to accept parental advice or criticism, occasional rudeness, more realization that the parent is not perfect; (2) an emotional void created by separation from parents and without the presence of an alternative support group can often create behavioral problems (e.g., a decline in school performance); (3) emotional lability; (4) increased ability for self-expression through speech; (5) search for new people to love in addition to parents.

Body Image Concerns. Rapid physical changes lead the adolescent to be increasingly preoccupied with body image, as characterized by (1) preoccupation with self; (2) uncertainty about appearance and attractiveness; (3) frequent comparison of own body with those of other adolescents; (4) increased interest in sexual anatomy and physiology, including anxieties and questions regarding menstruation or nocturnal emissions, masturbation, and breast or penis size.

Peer Group Involvement. The adolescent becomes more dependent on friends as a source of comfort, and this is characterized by (1) solitary friendships with a member of the same sex; (2) strongly emotional, tender feelings toward peers, which may lead to homosexual exploration, fears, and/or relationships; (3) peer contact primarily with the same sex, with some contact with the opposite sex made in groups of friends.

Identity Development. The adolescent's cognitive abilities are changing from concrete thinking to abstract thinking. During this time, the adolescent is expected to achieve academically and to prepare for the future. This period is characterized by (1) increased ability to reason abstractly, (2) frequent daydreaming, (3) setting of vocational goals, (4) testing authority, (5) a need for greater privacy, (6) emergence of sexual feelings, (7) development of the adolescent's own value system, (8) lack of impulse control and need for immediate gratification, and (9) tendency to magnify one's personal situation.

MIDDLE ADOLESCENCE (APPROXIMATE AGES 14–16)

This phase is characterized by an increased scope and intensity of feelings and by the rise in importance of peer group values.

Independence-Dependence Struggle. Conflicts become more prevalent as the adolescent exhibits less interest in parents and devotes more time to peers.

Body Image Concerns. Most middle adolescents, having experienced most of their pubertal changes, are less preoccupied with these changes. Eating disorders may become established during this developmental phase.

Peer Group Involvement. Peer groups play a powerful role and are characterized by: (1) intense involvement with the peer subculture; (2) conformity with peer values, codes, and dress in an attempt to further separate from family; (3)

increased involvement in partnering relations, manifest by dating activity, sexual experimentation, and intercourse; (4) involvement with clubs, team sports, gangs, and other groups. Friends are the primary source of influence on young people's behavior, but peer pressures are often overstated. Adolescents' reactions to peer pressure are extremely varied, and peer pressure can also involve a desire to excel in school, sports, or other positive activities.

Identity Development. The abilities to abstract and reason continue to increase, along with a new sense of individuality. Ego development is characterized by (1) increased scope and openness of feelings, (2) increased intellectual ability and creativity, (3) less idealistic vocational aspirations, and (4) a feeling of omnipotence and immortality, leading to risk-taking behavior.

LATE ADOLESCENCE (APPROXIMATE AGES 17 TO 21)

This is the final phase of the adolescent's struggle for identity and separation. A new conceptualization of the period from late adolescence through the twenties is referred to as the "emergent adult" period. These new young adults have begun to accept responsibility for their behaviors, to formulate their own decisions, and to try to be financially independent.

Independence-Dependence Struggle. This is a time of reduced restlessness and increased integration. The adolescent has become a separate entity from the family, making it possible for him or her to seek and accept parental advice and guidance. However, it is not uncommon for some adolescents to be hesitant about accepting the responsibilities of adulthood and to remain dependent on family and peers. Characteristics now include (1) a firmer identity; (2) a greater ability to delay gratification; (3) an improved ability to think ideas through and express ideas in words; (4) more stable interests; and (5) a greater ability to make independent decisions and to compromise.

Body Image Concerns. The late adolescent has completed pubertal growth and development and is typically less concerned with this process unless an abnormality has occurred.

Peer Group Involvement. Peer group values become less important and more time is spent in a relationship with one person. The selection of a partner is based more on mutual understanding and enjoyment than on peer acceptance.

Identity Development. Ego development during the late adolescence is characterized by (1) the development of a rational and realistic conscience; (2) the development of a sense of perspective, with the abilities to delay, compromise, and set limits; (3) the development of practical vocational goals and the beginning of financial independence; (4) further refinement of moral, religious, and sexual values.

CONCLUSION

Most adolescents follow the developmental tasks for each phase described above. An understanding of this general pattern will help in the evaluation of an adolescent's behavior.

WEB SITES

http://www.My.webmd.com. Web MD Health.

http://www.Connectforkids.org. For adults—parents, grandparents, educators, policymakers, and others who want to become more actively involved with youth.

http://www.apahelpcenter.org. The American Psychological Association's online resource center.

http://www.Generalpediatrics.com. The general pediatrician's view of the Internet.

http://www.Parent-teen.com. An online magazine for families with teens.

http://www.cpyu.org. Center for Parent Youth Understanding.

CHAPTER 3

Office Visit, Interview Techniques, and Recommendations to Parents

Elizabeth R. Woods and Lawrence S. Neinstein

The style and personality of the provider and his or her philosophy of medical care are particularly important in the medical care of adolescents. The provider should help to enhance family communication while assuring confidentiality when requested around personal issues. This chapter contains general guidelines for establishing better rapport with adolescents, suggested interviewing techniques, and suggestions for parents to improve communication with their teen.

GENERAL GUIDELINES FOR THE OFFICE VISIT

Liking the Adolescent
To provide effective care and establish rapport with the adolescent patient, the healthcare provider must like adolescents. If the particular condition requires more expertise than the provider has or causes personal conflicts about moral or religious issues, the adolescent should be referred elsewhere.

Meeting the Adolescent and Family: The First Session
At about the time of puberty, a transition should be made to allow more of the visit to be focused on the adolescent. One of three basic approaches may be used to start the interview; the choice may depend on the complexity of the visit, nature of the complaints, knowledge of the individual and family, and the age of the adolescent. The provider should ensure that the adolescent is seen alone for part of the visit, as during the physical examination.

Separate Time for Family and Adolescent. For new, complex patients, the provider may need an extensive history from the family and an understanding of their full agenda. This gives the parents a few minutes to relate the past history, family history, their agenda, and concerns. The adolescent should be present from the time he or she meets with the provider through to the end of the visit so that he or she does not feel that the provider is divulging confidential information to the family.

Family Together. Some healthcare providers prefer to see the family and adolescent together first. This approach can yield a great deal of information in the first few minutes regarding family dynamics and medical concerns.

Adolescent Alone. Another basic approach is to start by interviewing the adolescent alone, which is especially important for older patients. At some point, the family may be brought into the interview; however, the adolescent should be present to hear what is being said.

Summarizing. At the end of the visit, the provider should summarize the issues and plans with the adolescent. Issues that may or must be discussed with the family can be summarized with the family and the adolescent together. As the adolescent becomes a young adult, the full visit will tend to be with him or her.

Office Setup

Space. A separate waiting area or corner of the waiting room should be set aside for adolescents with information and materials appropriate for them, or separate blocks of time should be used so that age-appropriate materials can be displayed. For privacy, the examination table should be facing away from the door or an inner curtain should be added. The desk in the office should ideally be oriented so that the healthcare provider sits beside the desk, not behind it.

Appointments. Usually, the initial comprehensive visit for an adolescent should be scheduled to last 1 hour unless there are time constraints based on the practice setting. Most follow-up appointments should be scheduled for after-school hours or early in the morning to minimize missed school time. At the end of the first visit, a decision should be made with the teen and the family as to whether the adolescent can make future visits on his or her own.

Billing. When the parents are paying for services, confidentiality can be maintained by using nonconfidential or symptom-based billing codes. Alternatives include (1) confidential billing (if the insurance company allows), so that the parents are not aware of the exact nature of the visits; (2) having the adolescent pay his or her own bills on a flexible installment plan with reduced fees; (3) having the adolescent obtain Medicaid funds for conditions such as pregnancy, family planning, and substance abuse; or (4) referral to a clinic that can provide free confidential care.

Availability of Educational Materials. It is helpful to place books, pamphlets, hot-line numbers, and reliable Web site information in the waiting room or office.

Avoiding Interruptions. Constant interruptions or phone calls during the interview tend to decrease rapport.

Note Taking. The provider should take as few notes as possible during the interview.

Communicating with the Adolescent

Establishing Rapport. Establishing rapport with an adolescent, especially with a nonverbal or hostile teenager, can be difficult; therefore (1) begin the interview by introducing yourself to the teen and parents or guardians; (2) begin by chatting informally about friends, school, or hobbies; (3) let the adolescent talk for a while, even if he or she meanders; (4) treat the adolescent's comments as seriously as you would an adult's; (5) roll with resistance if the adolescent is angry about seeing you; (6) explore issues that concern the adolescent.

Ensuring Confidentiality. Establish a sense of confidentiality with the adolescent; however, the limits of this confidentiality may vary depending on the type of medical practice and current laws of a particular state. When there are concerns about safety, the provider should convey to the adolescent that this is a situation that must be shared with the parents.

Avoiding a Surrogate Parent Role. Rather than playing the role of a surrogate parent, the healthcare provider should function as a nonjudgmental extraparental adult.

Sidestepping Power Struggles. Teenagers respond better if they are allowed to arrive at their own conclusions.

Acting as an Advocate. Try to emphasize an adolescent's positive characteristics.

Importance of Listening. Listening can often be the key to developing rapport with an adolescent. Try to understand from the teen's perspective.

Gender-Neutral Terms. Use gender-neutral terms until the adolescent has indicated his or her preferences.

Instilling Responsibility. Adolescents should be made aware that they are responsible for their own care and behavior.

Displaying Interest and Concern. The adolescent must be able to feel the healthcare provider's interest and concern.

Family and Parents. The adolescent may be the primary patient, but parents cannot be overlooked and their input may be critical. Families must be consulted for the following reasons: (1) to elucidate current concerns and past medical and family history; (2) to clarify family dynamics and structure; (3) to help bring about changes in the family unit and in the adolescent; (4) to negotiate fair and consistent limits; (5) to support the adolescent in complex treatment regimens; (6) to ensure consistency of follow-up and referral care.

Hidden Agenda. Adolescents often present with chief complaints that are not representative of their true concerns. Nonverbal cues can be helpful.

Developmentally Oriented Approach. The healthcare provider should be conscious of the adolescent's developmental process and tasks. Helpful questions include those concerning (1) *body image:* "Do you have any questions or problems with the physical changes you are experiencing?" "Do you like yourself as you are?" "What would you change?" (2) *peer relationships:* "Who is your best friend?" "How many close friends do you have?" (3) *independence:* "Do you get along with your parents?" "Is your privacy respected at home?" (4) *identity:* "Are you satisfied with the way things are going for you?" "What are your plans for the future?" (5) *sexuality:* "Are you dating?" "Do you have questions or concerns about sexual activities, contraception, sexually transmitted diseases, or pregnancy?"

HEEADSS Interview. Another approach to obtain psychosocial/developmental information are the HEEADSS (*h*ome, *e*ducation/employment, *e*ating, peer group *a*ctivities, *d*rugs, *s*exuality, *s*uicide/depression, *s*afety) questions, which move from less personal issues to more personal and potentially threatening ones.

1. *Home:* Who lives with the teen? How is the teen getting along with parents, family, and siblings? Have there been any recent moves? Has the teen ever run away or been incarcerated?
2. *Education:* Is the teen in school? What is the teen good and bad at in school? What grade average does the teen maintain? Are there subjects that are more interesting, difficult or require extra help? What goals does the teen have when he or she finishes school?
3. *Eating:* What does the teen like or dislike about his or her body? Have there been recent changes in weight? Does the teen worry about gaining weight? Has the teen dieted or done other things to control weight? Does the teen feel that his or her eating is out of control?
4. *Activities:* What does the teen do after school? Community or church activities? Does the teen have friends? How much time does the teen spend watching television or playing video games?
5. *Drugs:* What types of drugs are used by the teen's peers? What types of drugs do family members use? What types of drugs does the teen use and in what amount and frequency?
6. *Sexuality:* Is the teen involved with another individual in a sexual relationship? Is the teen attracted to or prefer sex with the same, opposite, or both sexes? Has the teen had sexual intercourse? How old was the teen at the time of his or her first sexual encounter? How many partners has the teen had? Does the teen use contraception and/or condoms, and with what frequency? Is there a history of STDs, pregnancy, or abortion?
7. *Suicide and depression:* Does the teen feel sad or down or cry more than usual? Does the teen feel "bored" all the time? Has the teen made any prior suicide attempts? Does the teen have any current suicidal ideation? (Direct questions do not precipitate suicidal action.)
8. *Safety:* Does the teen use seatbelts? How much of the time? Has the teen ever ridden in the car with someone driving who was "high" or drunk? Does the teen use safety equipment for sports or other physical activities (such as a helmet for biking or skateboarding)? Is there violence in the teen's home, school, or neighborhood? Has the teen ever been physically or sexually abused? Has the teen ever had to run away to be safe?

Physical Examination

The physical examination provides an opportunity to educate the adolescent about bodily changes. The true chief complaint may be revealed during the physical examination. In general, the adolescent is examined without the presence of the guardian or parent. However, some younger or developmentally delayed adolescents prefer to have the parent present. Male providers should use a chaperone during the breast and genital examination of female patients.

Closure

Provide a brief summary of the proposed diagnosis and treatment, addressed primarily to the adolescent. Parents who accompany the adolescent to the visit should be included in a final discussion of the nonconfidential issues. Give the adolescent time to discuss final questions. Schedule follow-up appointments and encourage the adolescent to return or call with questions.

INTERVIEWING STYLE

Open-Ended Questions. The use of open-ended questions facilitates communication.

Reflection Responses. The reflection response mirrors the adolescent's feelings.

Restatement and Summation. Stopping to restate the adolescent's feelings or to summarize the interview may help to clarify the problem or encourage additional comments.

Clarification. Asking the adolescent to clarify a statement or feeling may help to crystallize the problem.

Insight Questions. Some questions may give the healthcare provider better insight into the adolescent. For example, "What do you do well?" "If you had one wish, what would it be?" "When are you the happiest? "What do you see yourself doing in 1 or in 5 years?"

Reassuring Statements. The use of reassuring statements in dealing with embarrassing subjects may often facilitate discussion.

Support and Empathy. A nonjudgmental response that recognizes and acknowledges the adolescent's feelings is often helpful during the interview.

Interview Structure

The interview should have structure, including a beginning, middle, and end: (1) the beginning of the interview should include introductions, attempts to put the adolescent at ease, and an explanation of what will be happening and why; (2) the middle part of the interview should move into defining the adolescent's problems and feelings; and (3) the end of the interview should include informing the adolescent about the results of the examination and about what will happen next. Time should be provided for the adolescent to ask questions before summarizing with the adolescent and the parents.

Written Questionnaires. If confidential questions are included, the forms should be completed privately in a confidential space (see Chapter 4).

Computer Surveys. Computerized surveys can be a nonthreatening format to some adolescents and can sometimes increase the disclosure of personal information. Paperny and colleagues have developed interactive questionnaires for teens on areas such as psychosocial risk profile, adolescent pregnancy, and family planning.

Family Considerations

To fully understand the adolescent or to effect change requires interviewing and working with the family. There are many possible family constellations, including single-parent families, stepfamilies, blended families, foster families, adoptive families, extended families, and families of choice. The dynamics of the family and the relationships within it as well as the family's and cultural and ethnic backgrounds should be understood. The following references may be helpful:

McGoldrick M, Carter B. Understanding the life cycle: the individual, the family, the culture. In F. Walsh. *Normal family processes,* 3rd ed. New York: Guilford Press, 2002.

Minuchin S. *Family healing: strategies for hope and understanding.* New York: Free Press, 1998.

Patterson GR, Forgatch MS. *Parents and adolescents living together,* 2nd ed: Part 1. *The basics.* Champaign, IL: Research Press, 2005.

Patterson GR, Forgatch MS. *Parents and adolescents living together,* 2nd ed: Part 2. *Family problem solving.* Champaign, IL: Research Press, 2005.

Optimize the Adolescent–Provider Communication

Adolescents' perceptions of their provider's behavior and assurance of confidentiality contribute to their willingness to return for follow-up visits and adherence to the treatment plans.

RECOMMENDATIONS TO PARENTS OF ADOLESCENTS

General Guidelines. (1) Listen to the teenager, and treat his or her comments seriously; (2) avoid power struggles, be flexible; (3) deliver clear messages and set clear limits; (4) show interest and concern in the adolescent's activities; (5) spend time together and time alone together; (6) show trust in the teenager; (7) encourage positive behaviors and choices; (9) strive for a good communication in the family and keep a sense of humor; and (10) resolve conflicts together.

Challenges of the Teen Years. (1) Parents must adapt to changes in their relationship with their teen; (2) parents must limit testing and *experimentation by teens;* (3) parents must *not overreact to rejection;* (4) parents must recognize that *separation is difficult for teens and their parents;* (5) adolescents are at *maximal growth velocity and change* and are more vulnerable to risks; (6) *modern* *family issues* add additional challenges; (7) excessive exploitive and violent *messages through the media* add to the challenges; (8) adolescents' *feelings of invulnerability* lead to exposure to risks; (9) parents may be more bothered and remember *conflicts* longer than their teens; and (10) a set of five to ten *"house rules"* can be helpful.

WEB SITES

http://www.ama-assn.org/ama/pub/category/1980.html. Guidelines for preventive services.

http://brightfutures.aap.org/web/. Guidelines for prevention visits for children and adolescents.

http://www.cahl.org/. Center for Adolescent Health & the Law, Abigail English, JD.

http://aap.org/. Resources and position papers of the American Academy of Pediatrics.

http://www.adolescenthealth.org/. Position papers from the Society for Adolescent Medicine.

http://www.usc.edu/adolhealth. Adolescent health online curriculum.

http://www.youngwomenshealth.org. Children's Hospital Boston Web resources.

CHAPTER 4

Preventive Health Care for Adolescents

David S. Rosen and Lawrence S. Neinstein

The goals of preventive health care for adolescents are to promote optimal physical and mental health and support healthy physical, psychological, and social growth and development. Because the most common morbidities and mortalities of adolescence today are preventable health conditions associated with behavioral, environmental, and social causes, preventive services for adolescents should reflect these shifts in etiology. Therefore visits to a health care provider should reinforce positive health behaviors, such as exercise and nutritious eating, while discouraging health-risk behaviors such as those associated with unsafe sexual behaviors, unsafe driving, and the use of tobacco or other drugs. Although the incidence of serious medical problems during adolescence is low, this is a time during which lifelong health habits are established. Furthermore, numerous issues and concerns may emerge during adolescence that affect overall health and well-being. Therefore adolescence is an ideal period for health professionals to invest time in health-promotion and preventive services. The various recommendations for adolescent preventive services are compared in Table 4.1.

There appear to be more similarities than differences. All of the recommendations support the immunization schedule of the Advisory Committee on Immunization Practices and all advocate health guidance for teens. The Guidelines for Adolescent Preventive Services (GAPS; Table 4.2 and Fig. 4.1), Bright Futures (a health promotion initiative of the Maternal and Child Health Bureau and the American Academy of Pediatrics), and The American Academy of Pediatrics (AAP) also recommend health guidance for parents as a strategy to help them support the growth, development, and changing needs of their adolescent. Screening and counseling for various health risks are also a common feature of the recommendations from each of the five organizations, although there is some variability in the specific recommendations for screening. Periodicity may be the most important distinction among the five sets of recommendations. GAPS, Bright Futures, and the AAP specifically recommend *annual* visits for preventive services, whereas the U.S. Preventative Task Force (USPSTF) and American Academy of Family Physicians (AAFP) recommend visits every 1 to 3 years based on the specific needs of the individual. However, the new Bright Futures will unify these recommendations (http://brightfutures.aap.org/web/).

Although guidelines help to standardize and provide structure to the range of preventive services offered to adolescents, service delivery remains a more challenging issue. To better serve adolescents, preventive services must be

TABLE 4.1

Comparisons among Recommendations for Adolescent
Preventive Services

Subject	AAFP	AAP	AMA	BF	USPSTF
Immunizations:					
ACIP recommendations	Yes	Yes	Yes	Yes	Yes
Health guidance for teens:					
Normal development[a,b]	Yes	Yes	Yes	Yes	No
Injury prevention[a,c]	Yes	Yes	Yes	Yes	Yes
Nutrition[a]	Yes	Yes	Yes	Yes	Yes
Physical activity[a]	Yes	Yes	Yes	Yes	Yes
Dental health[a]	Yes	Yes	No	Yes	Yes
Breast or testicular self-examination[a]	Yes	Yes	No	Yes	No
Skin protection[a]	Yes	Yes	Yes	Yes	Yes
Health guidance for parents[a]	No	Yes	Yes	Yes	No
Screening/counseling[d]:					
Obesity[a]	Yes	Yes	Yes	Yes	Yes
Contraception[e]	Yes	Yes	Yes	Yes	Yes
Tobacco use[a]	Yes	Yes	Yes	Yes	Yes
Alcohol use[a]	Yes	Yes	Yes	Yes	Yes
Substance use[a]	Yes	Yes	Yes	Yes	Yes
Hypertension[a]	Yes	Yes	Yes	Yes	Yes
Depression/suicide[a]	No	Yes	Yes	Yes	No
Eating disorders[a]	No	Yes	Yes	Yes	No
School problems[a]	No	Yes	Yes	Yes	No
Abuse[a]	No	Yes	Yes	Yes	No[f]
Hearing[a]	Yes	Yes	No	Yes	No
Vision[a]	No	Yes	No	Yes	No
Tests:					
Tuberculosis[e]	Yes	Yes	Yes	Yes	Yes
Papanicolaou test[e]	Yes	Yes	Yes	Yes	Yes
Human immuno-deficiency virus infection[e]	Yes	Yes	Yes	Yes	Yes
Sexually transmitted diseases[e]	Yes	Yes	Yes	Yes	Yes
Cholesterol[e]	Yes	Yes	Yes	Yes	No
Urinalysis[a]	No	Yes	No	No	No
Hematocrit[a]	No	Yes	No	No	No

TABLE 4.1

(Continued)

Subject	AAFP	AAP	AMA	BF	USPSTF
Periodicity of visits	Tailored	Annual	Annual	Annual	Tailored
Target age range (yr)[g]	13–18	11–21	11–21	11–21	11–24

AAFP, American Academy of Family Physicians; AAP, American Academy of Pediatrics; AMA, American Medical Association; BF, Bright Futures; USPSTF, U.S. Preventive Services Task Force; ACIP, Advisory Committee on Immunization Practices.

[a]Procedure is recommended for all adolescents/parents.

[b]This includes providing adolescents with information on normal physical, psychosocial, and sexual development.

[c]This includes activities such as promoting the use of safety belts and safety helmets, placement of home fire alarms, and reducing the risk of injury from firearms and violence. Organizations differ in the activities they include for injury prevention.

[d]The AAP recommends "developmental/behavioral assessment."

[e]Procedure is recommended for selected adolescents who are at high risk for the medical problem.

[f]Child abuse is not addressed as a separate screening topic, but is included in the general screening for family violence.

[g]The AAP, AMA, and BF make a distinction among developmental stages of adolescence.

From Elster AB. Comparison of recommendations for adolescent clinical preventive services developed by national organizations. *Arch Pediatr Adolesc Med* 1998;152:193, with permission.

available through a *wide range of health care settings*. These include private physicians' offices; managed care organizations; community-based adolescent health, family planning, and public health clinics; and as part of school-based and school-linked health services. Simple skills-based *training for clinicians in adolescent preventive services* has been convincingly shown to increase the likelihood of appropriate screening and counseling as well as provider self-efficacy in a variety of clinical settings. *Reimbursement* for these services will continue to be problematic. *National standards of care* such as those discussed in this chapter may increase the likelihood that payers will begin to provide reimbursement for adolescent preventive services. However, for such services to become routinely available to all adolescents will require a dramatic shift in both health care provider and health care consumer expectations—from a re-active, acute-care orientation to a proactive view that values health promotion and disease prevention.

PREVENTIVE CARE FOR ADOLESCENTS

Many of the most effective health promotion and disease prevention strategies aimed at adolescents are straightforward and consistent among the various recommendations and guidelines discussed earlier (GAPS, Bright Futures, USPSTF, AAP, and AAFP). Furthermore, because health-risk behaviors and health habits have their genesis in adolescence, healthy behaviors and lifestyle choices established during adolescence have the potential to persist into adult life and to

TABLE 4.2

Guidelines for Adolescent Preventive Services (GAPS) Recommendations

1. From ages 11–21, all adolescents should have an annual preventive services visit.
   a. These visits should address both biomedical and psychosocial aspects.
   b. Complete physical examinations should be done during three of these preventive visits, one each during early (11–14 years), middle (15–17 years), and late (18–21 years) adolescence.
2. Preventive services should be age and developmentally appropriate and should be sensitive to individual and sociocultural differences.
3. Physicians should establish office policies regarding confidential care for adolescents and how parents will be involved in that care. These policies should be made clear to adolescents and their parents.
4. Parents or other adult caregivers should receive health guidance at least once during their child's early adolescence, once during middle adolescence, and preferably once during late adolescence. Health guidance should include the following information:
   a. Normative adolescent development, including physical, sexual, and emotional development
   b. Signs and symptoms of disease and emotional distress
   c. Parenting behaviors that promote healthy adolescent adjustment
   d. Why parents should discuss health-related behaviors with their adolescents, plan family activities, and act as role models
   e. Methods for helping their adolescent avoid potentially harmful behaviors:
      • Monitoring and managing adolescents' use of motor vehicles
      • Avoiding having weapons in the home
      • Removing weapons and potentially lethal medications from the homes of adolescents with suicidal intent
      • Monitoring their adolescent's social and recreational activities for the use of tobacco, alcohol, and other drugs and sexual behavior
5. All adolescents should receive health guidance annually to promote a better understanding of their physical growth, psychosocial and psychosexual development, and the importance of becoming actively involved in decisions regarding their health care.
6. All adolescents should receive health guidance annually to promote the reduction of injuries. Counseling includes the following:
   a. How to avoid use of alcohol or other drugs while using motor or recreational vehicles
   b. How to use safety devices, including seat belts and bicycle helmets
   c. How to resolve interpersonal conflicts without violence
   d. How to avoid the use of weapons
   e. How to promote appropriate physical conditioning before exercise
7. All adolescents should receive health guidance annually about dietary habits, including the benefits of a healthy diet, and ways to achieve a healthy diet and safe weight management.
8. All adolescents should receive health guidance annually about the benefits of exercise and should be encouraged to engage in safe exercise on a regular basis.

TABLE 4.2

(Continued)

9. All adolescents should receive health guidance annually regarding responsible sexual behaviors, including abstinence. Latex condoms to prevent STDs, including HIV infection, and appropriate methods of birth control should be made available, as should instructions on how to use them effectively.

10. All adolescents should receive health guidance annually to promote avoidance of tobacco, alcohol, other abusable substances, and anabolic steroids.

Screening recommendations:

11. All adolescents should be screened annually for hypertension according to the protocol developed by the National Heart, Lung, and Blood Institute Second Task Force on Blood Pressure Control in Children.

12. Selected adolescents should be screened to determine their risk of developing hyperlipidemia and adult coronary heart disease, following the protocol developed by the Expert Panel on Blood Cholesterol Levels in Children and Adolescents.

13. All adolescents should be screened annually for eating disorders and obesity by determining weight and stature, and by asking about body image and dieting patterns.

14. All adolescents should be asked annually about their use of tobacco products, including cigarettes and smokeless tobacco.

15. All adolescents should be asked annually about their use of alcohol and other abusable substances and about their use of over-the-counter or prescription drugs for nonmedical purposes, including anabolic steroids.
    a. Adolescents whose substance use endangers their health should receive counseling and mental health treatment, as appropriate.
    b. Adolescents who use anabolic steroids should be counseled to stop.
    c. The use of urine toxicology for the routine screening of adolescents is not recommended.

16. All adolescents should be asked annually about involvement in sexual behaviors that may result in unintended pregnancy and STDs, including HIV infections.
    a. Sexually active adolescents should be asked about their use and motivation to use condoms and contraceptive methods, their sexual orientation, the number of sexual partners they have had in the last 6 months, if they have exchanged sex for money or drugs, and their history of prior pregnancy or STDs.
    b. Adolescents at risk for pregnancy, STDs, or sexual exploitation should be counseled on how to reduce this risk.

17. Sexually active adolescents should be screened for STDs. The frequency of screening for STDs depends on the sexual practices of the individual and the history of previous STDs. STD screening includes the following:
    a. Cervical culture (females) or urine leukocyte esterase analysis (males) to screen for gonorrhea
    b. An immunologic test of cervical fluid (female) or urine leukocyte esterase analysis (male) to screen for genital *Chlamydia*

TABLE 4.2

(Continued)

c. A serological test for syphilis if the individual has lived in an area endemic for syphilis, has had other STDs, has had more than one sexual partner within the last 6 months, has exchanged sex for drugs or money, or is a male who has engaged in sex with other male(s)

d. Evaluation for human papilloma virus by visual inspection (males and females) and by Pap test.

18. Adolescents at risk for HIV infection should be offered confidential HIV screening with the ELISA and confirmatory test. Testing should be performed only after informed consent is obtained from the adolescent and should be performed in conjunction with both pretest and posttest counseling.

19. Female adolescents who are sexually active or any female 18 years of age or older should be screened annually for cervical cancer by use of a Pap test.

20. All adolescents should be asked annually about behaviors or emotions that indicate recurrent or severe depression or risk of suicide.

21. All adolescents should be asked annually about a history of emotional, physical, or sexual abuse.

22. All adolescents should be asked annually about learning or school problems.

23. Adolescents should receive a tuberculin skin test if they have been exposed to active tuberculosis, have lived in a homeless shelter, have been incarcerated, have lived in or come from an area with a high prevalence of tuberculosis, or currently work in a health care setting. Recommendations for immunizations:

24. All adolescents should receive prophylactic immunizations according to the guidelines established by the federally convened Advisory Committee on Immunization Practices.

a. Adolescents should receive a bivalent Td vaccine 10 years after their previous DTP vaccination.

b. All adolescents should receive a second trivalent MMR vaccination, unless there is documentation of two vaccinations earlier during childhood. An MMR should not be given to adolescents who are pregnant.

c. Susceptible adolescents who engage in high-risk behaviors should be vaccinated against hepatitis B virus. Widespread use of the hepatitis B vaccine is encouraged because risk factors are often not easily identifiable among adolescents. Universal hepatitis B vaccination should be implemented in communities where intravenous drug use, adolescent pregnancy, or STD infections are common.

STD, sexually transmitted diseases; HIV, human immunodeficiency virus; ELISA, enzyme-linked immunosorbent assay; DTP, diphtheria and tetanus toxoids and pertussis; MMR, measles-mumps-rubella.

Adapted from GAPS Executive Committee, Department of Adolescent Health. *American Medical Association guidelines for adolescent preventive services*. Chicago: American Medical Association, 1992.

Guidelines for Adolescent Preventive Services

Preventive Health Services by Age and Procedure

Adolescents and young adults have a unique set of health care needs. The recommendations for Guidelines for Adolescents Services (GAPS) emphasize annual clinical preventive services visits that address both the developmental and psychosocial aspects of health, in addition to traditional biomedical conditions. These recommendations were developed by the American Medical Association with contributions from a Scientific Advisory Panel, comprised of national experts, as well as representatives of primary care medical organizations and the health insurance industry. The body of scientific evidence indicates that the periodicity and content of preventive services can be important in promoting the health and well-being of adolescents.

Procedure	Age of Adolescent										
	Early				Middle			Late			
	11	12	13	14	15	16	17	18	19	20	21
Health Guidance											
Parenting*		●				●					
Development	●	●	●	●	●	●	●	●	●	●	●
Diet and Physical Activity	●	●	●	●	●	●	●	●	●	●	●
Healthy Lifestyle**	●	●	●	●	●	●	●	●	●	●	●
Injury Prevention	●	●	●	●	●	●	●	●	●	●	●
Screening											
History											
Eating Disorders	●	●	●	●	●	●	●	●	●	●	●
Sexual Activity***	●	●	●	●	●	●	●	●	●	●	●
Alcohol and Other Drug Use	●	●	●	●	●	●	●	●	●	●	●
Tobacco Use	●	●	●	●	●	●	●	●	●	●	●
Abuse	●	●	●	●	●	●	●	●	●	●	●
School Performance	●	●	●	●	●	●	●	●	●	●	●
Depression	●	●	●	●	●	●	●	●	●	●	●
Risk for Suicide	●	●	●	●	●	●	●	●	●	●	●
Physical Assessment											
Blood Pressure	●	●	●	●	●	●	●	●	●	●	●
BMI	●	●	●	●	●	●	●	●	●	●	●
Comprehensive Exam			●			●			●		
Tests											
Cholesterol			1			1			1		
TB			2			2			2		
GC, Chlamydia, Syphilis, & HPV			3			3			3		
HIV			4			4			4		
Pop Smear			5			5			5		
Immunizations											
MMR		●									
Td		●				○					
Hep B		●				6			6		
Hep A			7			7			7		
Varicella			8			8			8		

1. Screening test performed once if family history is positive for early cardiovascular disease or hyperlipidemia.
2. Screen if positive for exposure to active TB or lives/works in high–risk situation, eg homeless shelter, jail, health care facility.
3. Screen at least annually if sexually active.
4. Screen if high risk for infection.
5. Screen annually if sexually active or if 18 years or older.
6. Vaccinate if high risk for hepatitis B infection.
7. Vaccinate if at risk for hepatitis A infection.
8. Offer vaccine if no reliable history of chicken pox or previous immunization.
* A parent health guidance visit is recommended during early and middle adolescence.
** Includes counseling regarding sexual behavior and avoidance of tobacco, alcohol, and other drug use.
*** Includes history of unintended pregnancy and STD.
○ Do not give if administered in last five years.

FIGURE 4.1 Recommended frequency of GAPS preventive services. [From *Guidelines for adolescent preventive services* (Recommendations monograph). Chicago: American Medical Association, 1995. Available at: http://www.ama. assn.org/ama/pub/category/1981.html]

have a strongly positive effect on adult health as well. In this context, the Society for Adolescent Medicine has endorsed the use of guidelines as a strategy to improve the delivery of adolescent preventive services (information available at www.adolescenthealth.org.

Healthy People 2010 provides national objectives aimed at improving health and well-being. Of its 467 objectives, 107 are relevant for adolescents and young adults and 21 have been identified as critical health objectives. Further information regarding *Healthy People 2010* is available at www.healthypeople.gov/.

Clinical Settings for Adolescent Preventive Services

Improving the delivery of adolescent preventive services depends on the integration of standards and service delivery across multiple systems and points of access, including public clinics, managed care organizations, private physicians' offices, school-based and school-linked clinics, and community-based agencies. In fact, there is evidence to suggest that traditional office-based care for teens may fall short of the care they receive in other settings. School-based and school-linked health resources have become more important in the overall landscape of health services available to adolescents (see http://www.gwu.edu/~mtg and http://www.nasbhc.org). Adolescents who use school-based health services are highly satisfied with the care they receive. Moreover, school-based and school-linked services seem to play a unique and complementary role in meeting the health needs of some teens. For example, there is evidence to suggest that teens may be more willing to access school health rather than traditional health resources to address mental health, substance use, and reproductive health concerns.

Preventive Services Visit

General Suggestions for Providing Adolescent Preventive Services. Caring for adolescents requires a different approach, format, and style than does caring for either children or adults, so it is not surprising that many health care providers report discomfort in caring for adolescents. This discomfort is exacerbated when sensitive health concerns must be discussed or treated or when providers feel poorly trained or ill equipped to manage the specific issues before them. Although there is no substitute for proper training or a teen-friendly office environment, the following general suggestions provide a framework for the delivery of adolescent health services:

1. Create a comfortable and conducive atmosphere for discussion, disclosure, and counseling by ensuring privacy and minimizing interruptions.
2. Confidentiality is of paramount importance to teens; therefore, a foundation of confidentiality should be established so that the teen feels comfortable with the provider and trusts him or her enough to discuss sensitive subjects. Especially in discussing sensitive issues, the examiner should be direct, empathetic, and nonjudgmental.
3. Most of the history should be obtained privately and directly from the teenager. Still, it is valuable to obtain additional history from parents, both to corroborate the teen's history and to gather additional information. Collateral information from others (e.g., school personnel) may be very helpful in some circumstances.

4. Screening for health-risk behaviors and providing developmentally appropriate guidance should be an integral and essential component of a preventive services visit.
5. There should be adequate time left at the end of the visit to summarize the session and answer any questions that the adolescent may have.
6. The physical examination provides an excellent opportunity to discuss concerns that the adolescent might have about a particular body region. It is especially important to discuss growth and development with younger adolescents. Teaching and encouraging breast or testicular self-examination can be done with older adolescents.

Questionnaires and Other Health Screening Tools. Questionnaires and screening forms can be efficient tools for collecting information, thereby reducing the amount of time spent with patients. Some patients also find it easier to disclose sensitive information via questionnaire than face to face. Screening questionnaires and personal interviews may therefore be considered complementary, although neither alone will be adequate in all situations. The American Medical Association's GAPS program has published a series of carefully constructed and updated questionnaires for both adolescents and their parents; it is available at http://www.ama-assn.org/ama/pub/category/1981.html.

Screening tools that have been more formally and rigorously validated can be useful in practice, particularly to screen for behavioral and mental health problems. For example, the Beck Depression Inventory is a well-validated and easily administered tool to screen for depression. A wide variety of other tools are available to screen for family function, behavioral difficulties, and other mental health problems.

History

A comprehensive history is the most important aspect of the preventive services evaluation. Essential domains include past medical history, family history, psychosocial history, and an age-appropriate review of systems. Any current health concerns should also be sought.

Past Medical History. Past medical history is best obtained from both the adolescent and the parents and should include the following: (1) childhood infections and illnesses; (2) prior hospitalizations and surgery; (3) significant injuries; (4) disabilities; (5) medications, including prescription medications, over-the-counter medications, complementary or alternative medications, vitamins, and nutritional supplements; (6) allergies; (7) immunization history; (8) developmental history, including prenatal, perinatal, and infancy history as well as history of problems with walking, talking, eating, learning, peer relations, and school functioning; and (9) mental health history, including a history of hospitalization, outpatient counseling, medications, school interventions, and other treatment.

Family History. Information about family history is most accurately obtained from the parents. It should include the following: (1) age and health status of family members; (2) significant medical illnesses in the family, such as diabetes, cancer, heart disease, tuberculosis, hypertension, and stroke; (3) history of mental illness in the family, such as mood disorders, anxiety disorders, schizophrenia, and alcoholism; and (4) vocational status of parents.

Psychosocial History. This history is obtained primarily from the adolescent while he or she is being interviewed alone. Some material will also be gathered from the parents or from interviews with the family together. Obtaining much of this information is dependent on successfully establishing trust and rapport between the practitioner and the adolescent. Many clinicians rely on the HEEADSS (or the updated HEEADSS) acronym to guide their psychosocial history:

1. *Home:* Family configuration and family members, living arrangements, relationships among the adolescent and family members
2. *Education/Employment:* Academic or vocational success, future plans, and safety at school or in the workplace
3. *Eating:* Brief nutrition history, risk factor for obesity, concerns about weight or body image, disordered eating behaviors
4. *Activities:* Friendships with peers of the same and opposite sex, recreational activities, dating activity and relationships, sexual activity
5. *Drugs:* Personal use of tobacco, alcohol, illicit drugs, anabolic steroids; peer substance use; family substance use; driving while intoxicated
6. *Sexuality:* Sexual orientation, sexual activity, sexual abuse
7. *Suicide (Mental Health):* Feelings of sadness, loneliness, depression; pervasive boredom; inappropriately high levels of anxiety; suicidal thoughts
8. *Safety:* Risk of unintentional injury, risk from violence, fighting or weapon carrying, abuse

Review of Systems. The review of systems covers the following areas:

1. *Vision:* Trouble reading or watching television, vision correction
2. *Hearing:* Infections, trouble hearing, earaches
3. *Dental:* Prior care, pain, concerns (e.g., braces)
4. *Head:* Headaches, dizziness
5. *Nose and throat:* Frequent colds or sore throats, respiratory allergies
6. *Skin:* Acne, moles, rashes, warts
7. *Cardiovascular:* Exercise intolerance, shortness of breath, chest pain, palpitations, syncope, physical activity
8. *Respiratory:* Asthma, cough, smoking, exposure to tuberculosis
9. *Gastrointestinal:* Abdominal pain, reflux, diarrhea, vomiting, bleeding
10. *Genitourinary:* Dysuria, bed-wetting, frequency, bleeding
11. *Musculoskeletal:* Limb pain, joint pain, or swelling
12. *Central nervous system (CNS):* Seizures, syncope
13. *Menstrual:* Menarche, frequency of menses, duration, menorrhagia or metrorrhagia, pain
14. *Sexual:* Sexual activity, contraception, pregnancy, abortions, sexually transmitted diseases (STDs) or STD symptoms

Physical Examination

The examination allows the clinician to assess growth and pubertal development and to instruct the adolescent in methods of self-examination and other means of health promotion. The physical examination also affords the adolescent an opportunity to ask about any specific health concerns, and it provides the clinician with the opportunity to detect unnoticed diseases. The examination should be performed in such a way as to preserve the adolescent's modesty. Main elements of the physical examination include the following.

Height, Weight, and Vital Signs. Height, weight, blood pressure, and pulse should be measured. The serial measurement of height and weight allows for monitoring of the adolescent's growth and for the earlier detection of risk factors for obesity. Body mass index (BMI) should be calculated and tracked. Blood pressure should be recorded with an appropriately sized cuff. If blood pressure is elevated, it should be rechecked on at least three separate visits before a diagnosis of hypertension is considered.

Vision Screening. Adolescents should have a vision screening on their initial evaluation and every 2 to 3 years thereafter.

Hearing Screening. There is increasing concern about threats to hearing, and every adolescent should have at least one hearing screening performed during the adolescent years.

Sexual Maturity Rating. The sexual maturity rating (SMR), discussed in Chapter 1, is the method by which pubertal development is evaluated and described. Because many "normal values" in adolescents depend more on SMR than on age, evaluation of SMR is important not only in describing pubertal milestones but also in adequately assessing many physical parameters (e.g., BMI), and laboratory values (e.g., hemoglobin).

Skin. Check for evidence of acne, warts, fungal infections, and other lesions. Carefully inspect moles, especially in patients who are at particular risk for melanoma.

Teeth and Gums. Check for evidence of dental caries or gum infection. Look for signs of smokeless tobacco use. Enamel erosions are sometimes the first clue to the vomiting associated with some eating disorders. Regular checkups with a dentist should be encouraged.

Neck. Check for thyromegaly or adenopathy.

Cardiopulmonary. Check for heart murmurs or clicks.

Abdomen. Check for evidence of hepatosplenomegaly, tenderness, or masses.

Musculoskeletal. The musculoskeletal examination is especially important in adolescent athletes, in whom instabilities or other evidence of previous injury is the best predictor of future injury. Check for signs of overuse syndromes or osteochondroses. Check for scoliosis, particularly in premenarchal females.

Breasts. Examine for symmetry and developmental variations; in girls, assess SMR. Examine for masses or discharge; in boys, identify gynecomastia (present in approximately one third of pubertal males). If breast self-examination is to be taught and encouraged, it should be done only when developmentally appropriate.

Neurologic. Test strength, reflexes, and coordination.

Genitalia (Male). Examine the penis and testicles. Assess SMR. Look for signs of STDs. Retract the foreskin in uncircumcised patients. Check for hernia.

Pelvic Examination (Female). Indicated for female adolescents who have ever been sexually active and for any female adolescent who requests an examination. In addition, pelvic examination is indicated for female adolescents with pelvic pain, an atypical or changing vaginal discharge, or an undiagnosed menstrual disorder. "Annual" pelvic examination and PAP screening, which had previously been recommended for all women beginning at approximately 18 years of age, are now recommended beginning 3 years after coitarche or age 21, whichever comes earlier. Annual screening for STDs is clearly recommended for sexually active female patients (see Chapter 48).

Rectal Examination. Rectal examination is not routinely indicated as a screening procedure.

Laboratory Tests

Laboratory tests should be kept to a minimum in the asymptomatic adolescent. Suggested screening tests include the following.

Hemoglobin or Hematocrit. A screening hemoglobin or hematocrit is recommended at the first encounter with the adolescent or at the end of puberty, or both. Although the normal levels remain stable for females throughout adolescence, the normal levels in males are dependent on age and, more importantly, on SMR.

Urinalysis. A routine urinalysis, including a dipstick test for glucose and protein and a microscopic evaluation, is recommended at the first encounter with the adolescent or at the end of puberty or both. However, up to one third of healthy adolescents have small amounts of proteinuria that is nonpathologic and requires no treatment (see Chapter 28).

Sickle Cell Screening. Screening for sickle cell anemia is recommended at the first visit with an African-American adolescent if it has not been documented already.

Sexually Active Adolescents. Suggested tests for sexually active adolescents include the following:

1. Females. Cervical gonorrhea and chlamydial culture or nonculture test and vaginal wet mount are recommended. Syphilis serology should be considered in high-risk populations or where syphilis is prevalent. Screening for the human immunodeficiency virus (HIV) should be offered to all sexually active adolescents and should be encouraged for adolescents with any history of STD. Begin annual Pap smears 3 years after coitarche or at age 21.

2. Males. A leukocyte esterase test on the first 15 mL of a random urine sample is recommended to screen for chlamydial infection. However, there is concern about the sensitivity and specificity of this test. In high-risk populations, annual urethral screening for gonorrhea and chlamydial infection by culture or nonculture test can be encouraged. Syphilis serology should be considered in high-risk populations or where syphilis is prevalent. Screening for the HIV virus should be offered to all sexually active adolescents and should be encouraged for adolescents with any history of STD.

3. Men Who Have Sex with Men. Annual syphilis serology, gonorrhea cultures (urethral, rectal, and pharyngeal), screening for *Chlamydia*, and HIV screening are recommended. Homosexual males who are not already immunized should be screened for hepatitis B as well. Those with negative surface antigen and antibody tests should receive hepatitis B vaccine.

Cholesterol and Fasting Triglyceride Testing. Targeted cholesterol and fasting triglyceride testing is indicated in adolescents with heart disease, hypertension, diabetes mellitus, or a family history of heart disease or hyperlipidemia. Targeted screening in adolescents misses one third to one half of those with elevated cholesterol concentrations, so some authorities advocate at least one screening cholesterol test during adolescence.

Human Immunodeficiency Virus Antibody Testing. Universal screening for antibody to HIV is being recommended by the CDC for adults and adolescents. At a minimum, individuals at risk should be encouraged to receive HIV testing after a discussion regarding the benefits and possible negative consequences of the results (see Chapter 32). Individuals with any STD should be screened for others, including HIV infection.

Tuberculin Testing. A purified protein derivative (PPD) tuberculin skin test should be considered at the first encounter with the adolescent based on an assessment of individual risk factors and recommendations of the local health department (in high-risk areas, screening is usually recommended yearly).

IMMUNIZATIONS

Obtaining the immunization history and completing the proper immunizations is increasingly important in the care of adolescents. This is a group that still has significant rates of nonimmunization. Because vaccination schedules remain a moving target, clinicians are well advised to keep abreast of the latest vaccine recommendations of the Advisory Committee on Immunization Practices (ACIP) of the CDC. The current immunization schedule is available at http://www.cdc.gov.

General Vaccination Information

Vaccination of adolescents is safe and should be seen as a high priority for adolescents whose previous immunizations are lacking or incomplete. Adolescents who have been partially vaccinated can have their vaccination completed without restarting the series. Likewise, adolescents who begin vaccination can complete it at any time after the vaccination process is interrupted, even if there has been a substantial delay between doses. Vaccines should not be given more frequently than at the recommended intervals. Although not every possible combination of vaccines has been explicitly tested, there are no contraindications to giving any or all of these vaccines simultaneously as long as they are given at separate and appropriate anatomic sites.

Informed Consent. The clinic or office should obtain a signature of either the patient, parent, or guardian to acknowledge having been provided with vaccine information. This should also be noted in the medical record. Appropriate documentation of vaccination includes consent for vaccination, immunization type, date of administration, injection site, manufacturer and lot number of vaccine, and name and address of the health care provider administering the vaccine.

Vaccination during Pregnancy. Because of theoretical risks to the developing fetus, live-attenuated virus vaccines are not routinely given to pregnant women or to those who are likely to become pregnant within 3 months after receiving the vaccine. There is no convincing evidence of risk to the fetus after immunization of pregnant women with inactivated virus vaccines, bacterial vaccines, or toxoids. This includes tetanus and diphtheria toxoid. There is also no risk to the fetus from passive immunization of pregnant women with immune globulin. Because measles-mumps-rubella (MMR) vaccine viruses are not transmitted from individuals receiving them, children of pregnant women may receive these vaccines.

Adolescents with Human Immunodeficiency Virus Infection. Vaccine recommendations for HIV-infected adolescents are described in the text for individual vaccines and summarized in Table 4.3.

Diphtheria, Tetanus, Pertussis

It is now well known that adolescents and adults have a higher incidence and prevalence of pertussis than children. In adolescents, pertussis infection typically presents clinically as a mild respiratory infection that goes on to produce a protracted (3 weeks or more) cough. Two new tetanus toxoids—diphtheria toxoid and acellular pertussis (Tdap)—created for use in adolescents and adults, have recently been approved for use in the United States. Both of these vaccines have been demonstrated to be safe and effective when administered as a single booster dose to adolescents. The ACIP now recommends that

TABLE 4.3

Recommendations for Immunization of Human Immunodeficiency
Virus–Infected Patients

Vaccine	Asymptomatic	Symptomatic
Tdap/Td	Yes	Yes
IPV	Yes	Yes
MMR	Yes	Yes, consider
Hepatitis B	Yes	Yes
Varicella	No	No
Pneumococcal	Yes	Yes
Meningococcal	Optional	Optional
Influenza	Optional	Yes

IPV, inactivated poliovirus vaccine; MMR, measles-mumps-rubella.

adolescents aged 11 to 18 who have completed their primary vaccination series against diphtheria, pertussis, and tetanus now receive a single dose of Tdap instead of the Td. The preferred age for Tdap is age 11 to 12 years; ideally, Tdap should be given concurrently with the new tetravalent meningococcal conjugate vaccine (Menactra; see below). Adolescents who have already received a single dose of Td should still receive a single dose of Tdap between the ages of 11 and 18 years. An interval of at least 5 years is recommended (but not required) between Td and Tdap in order to reduce the risk of reactions. After Tdap vaccination, Td boosters continue to be recommended every 10 years throughout life. The dose of Tdap is 0.5 mL administered intramuscularly in the deltoid muscle.

Hepatitis A

The hepatitis A vaccination now offers effective, long-lasting protection against this virus. The vaccines are inactivated and come in adult and pediatric formulations, with different dosages and administration schedules. Almost 100% of children, adolescents, and adults develop protective levels of antibody to hepatitis A virus after completing the vaccine series.

Hepatitis B Vaccine

Two recombinant hepatitis B vaccines (Recombivax HB and Engerix-B) are used in the United States today. Universal vaccination is now recommended in the United States, and the ACIP recommends the three-dose hepatitis B vaccine series for adolescents at age 11 to 12 years who have not previously been immunized.

Haemophilus Influenzae Type B

Haemophilus influenzae. type B vaccine is indicated for those adolescents not previously immunized who are at risk because of splenic dysfunction or other conditions. A single dose of 0.5 mL is recommended.

Human Papillomavirus

Two vaccines for prophylaxis against human papillomavirus (HPV) have been developed, a quadrivalent vaccine (Gardasil, Merck , Inc.) and a bivalent vaccine (see Chapter 66). The quadrivalent vaccine was licensed in June 2006 by the FDA; the ACIP has recommended that it be routinely given to girls at age 11 to 12. The quadrivalent vaccine targets HPV types 16 and 18 (the most common HPV types implicated in cervical cancer) as well as HPV types 6 and 11 (the most common HPV types associated with genital warts). Thus far, both vaccines have been shown to be safe, highly immunogenic, and to prevent infections with HPV 16 and/or 18 in randomized, double-blind, placebo-controlled trials. Approximately 70% of cervical cancer is related to HPV 16 and 18 and 90% of genital warts are related to types 6 and 11. Thus the potential is very high to prevent a significant number of both genital warts and cervical cancers. Vaccine-related adverse effects have been rare and no serious adverse effects have been reported. The current recommendation is that the quadrivalent vaccine (Gardasil) be given to girls at age 11 to 12, but the vaccination series of three vaccines can be started as early as age 9 at the discretion of the health care provider. Ideally vaccination should occur prior to the onset of sexual activity, as the vaccine will not be effective against any HPV subtypes that may already have been acquired. However, women between the ages of 13 and 26, even if they are already sexually active, are thought to benefit from the vaccine as well, acquiring protection from any HPV subtypes to which they have not already been exposed. "Catch-up" vaccination has also been recommended by the ACIP. The vaccine is not currently recommended for males.

Influenza

Influenza continues to cause major outbreaks of illness, usually beginning in December or January each year. Two types of vaccine are available, an inactivated vaccine and a live attenuated vaccine. Both vaccine types contain three virus strains (two type A and one type B), representing the strains most commonly found worldwide and predicted to be most likely to cause infections in the coming year. Vaccines are updated annually and are administered in the fall. Influenza in adolescents is discussed in detail in Chapter 29.

Measles

Because of the problem of waning immunity, it is now universally recommended that children and adolescents receive a second vaccination either at primary school or on entry to junior high school. If these opportunities are missed, the vaccine should be caught up whenever the teen presents for health care. Likewise, all young adults who enter college or other institutions of postsecondary education should have documentation of receiving two doses of measles vaccine; those who do not have such documentation should receive a second dose of vaccine. In practice, measles vaccine is usually administered as MMR vaccine.

Meningococcal Vaccine

Routine vaccination against meningococcal disease is now the recommendation of the ACIP and AAP, coinciding with the availability of a new tetravalent meningococcal polysaccharide-protein conjugate vaccine (MCV4) marketed as Menactra by Sanofi Pasteur. Like the meningococcal vaccine that preceded it, MCV4 provides immunity against serotypes A, C, Y, and W135. However, unlike the previous meningococcal vaccine, the new vaccine is likely to provide protection that is substantially longer-lasting. The current recommendation is for adolescents to be immunized as part of a preadolescent health supervision visit at age 11 to 12. For those not receiving the vaccine at age 11 to 12, immunization before high school entry is recommended. The vaccine is given as a single 0.5-mL dose administered intramuscularly.

Mumps

Despite a low incidence of mumps, an outbreak in 2006 highlights the importance of continued vigilance. Many of the involved individuals in this outbreak were college students, indicating the importance of this age group as susceptible individuals. Mumps vaccine has few side effects, and more than 90% of susceptible patients develop protective, long-lasting antibodies. Mumps vaccine is usually administered as MMR. Susceptible adolescents should receive a single dose of mumps vaccine alone or as MMR.

Pneumococcal Vaccine

Pneumococcal vaccine is indicated for individuals with a chronic illness, particularly of the cardiovascular or pulmonary system. It is also indicated for those who are at increased risk of pneumococcal disease, including patients with nephrotic syndrome, sickle cell disease, asplenia or functional asplenia, HIV infection, or B-cell immune deficiency, as well as patients at risk for meningitis. The duration of immunity is unclear, and revaccination is not currently recommended by the CDC; however, some centers recommend reimmunization with pneumococcal vaccine (Pneumovax 23) 3 to 5 years after primary immunization for patients who are at especially high risk.

Poliovirus

The last reported case of poliomyelitis caused by locally acquired wild-type virus in the United States occurred more than 20 years ago. Killed-virus inactivated poliovirus vaccine (IPV) is now the vaccine of choice, and oral poliovirus vaccine (OPV) is no longer recommended for use in the United States. Routine vaccination of nonimmunized adults is not required unless they are at particularly high risk because of travel to endemic areas, exposure to wild poliovirus, or occupational exposure. Immunosuppression is not a contraindication to vaccination. There is a theoretical risk during pregnancy, so vaccination of pregnant women should be avoided.

Rubella

Cases of rubella have often occurred among nonimmunized adults in outbreaks in colleges and workplaces; therefore proof of rubella and measles immunity should continue to be required for attendance from both male and female students. All students who enter institutions of postsecondary education should have documentation of having received at least one dose of rubella vaccine or other evidence of rubella immunity. Rubella vaccination is usually administered as MMR.

Varicella

Varicella results in more than 9,000 hospitalizations annually; in 2004, it accounted for 9 reported deaths. Whereas younger patients usually have uncomplicated chickenpox, older patients have more serious infections with higher rates of complications. A live-attenuated varicella vaccination for chickenpox is marketed under the name Varivax and is about 70% to 90% effective in preventing varicella. Varicella vaccination is now recommended for persons of all ages without documented chickenpox or measurable levels of protective antibody. Children and young adolescents between 1 and 13 years of age without documented varicella infection should receive a single dose of varicella vaccine. Adolescents 13 years or older should receive two doses of varicella vaccine 4 to 8 weeks apart. Varivax is a live-attenuated vaccine and should be avoided in immunosuppressed patients (including those who are immunocompromised from HIV infection) and those who are receiving immunosuppressive therapy. About 5% to 10% of vaccinated persons develop a rash, which can be contagious. Other adverse reactions include redness, hardness, and swelling at the injection site as well as fatigue, malaise, and nausea.

PREVENTIVE HEALTH INTERVENTIONS

Clinicians working with adolescent patients must feel comfortable in screening for psychosocial morbidity and assessing the level of risk in individual adolescent patients. This includes screening patients for risks associated with sensitive health issues such as sexual behavior, substance use, and mental health concerns. However, screening is insufficient if it is not followed up with appropriate and effective intervention strategies when patients screen "positive" for serious health risks. The following should be kept in mind in designing practical office interventions:

1. Health education should be targeted to the specific needs of the patient.
2. The patient and physician should agree on the goals for behavior change and the approach to be used.
3. Barriers to proposed changes should be explored, and specific strategies to overcome these barriers should be discussed.
4. Monitoring, feedback, and positive reinforcement should be an integral part of the plan.
5. Once behavioral change has occurred, a plan for maintenance should be addressed.

The G-A-P-S Algorithm

As part of the GAPS project, the AMA has attempted to develop a standardized method of assessment and intervention that embodies current health education principles but remains practical for office practice. The mnemonic G-A-P-S is used: *g*ather information, *a*ssess further, *p*roblem identification, and specific solutions (Fig. 4.2). A publication from the AMA, *GAPS: Clinical Evaluation and Management Handbook,* includes fully developed algorithms for each of the GAPS recommendations (available at http://www.ama-assn.org/ama/pub/category/1981.html).

G: Gather Initial Information. Screen for problems using simple trigger questions, such as, "Have you been feeling down and blue?" or "Do you usually wear a seat belt while riding in a car?" As has already been discussed, this initial screening step may be facilitated by use of questionnaires, computers, or nonclinician personnel.

A: Assess Further. Assess the level and nature of risk. Identify the seriousness of the problem by assessing the patient's knowledge and involvement, predisposing and protective factors, the availability of family and other support, and the consequences for the patient's health and function (e.g., school, peer relationships). The intervention offered depends on the assessed risk. Often, low risk can be successfully managed with health information, a few targeted suggestions, and positive reinforcement about the issue. If the patient is at high risk, he or she probably needs an in-depth evaluation that may be beyond the bounds of a preventive services visit. Either a return visit for more intensive intervention or referral is warranted. Patients who are at intermediate risk also require an explicit intervention.

P: Problem Identification. This step involves working with the patient toward an agreement on the problem, helping the patient decide to make a change, and working with the patient to develop a specific plan for that change. The goal is to be "patient-centered" in the approach—that is, to help the *patient* decide what is in his or her best interest, rather than forcing the patient to accept the physician's view of the problem or behavior. Problem identification is an attempt to define the problem in terms that the patient accepts. Once agreement on problem definition is reached, proceed to the next step. If the patient does not agree that there is a problem with a specified behavior, look for areas of agreement and common ground. Clinician

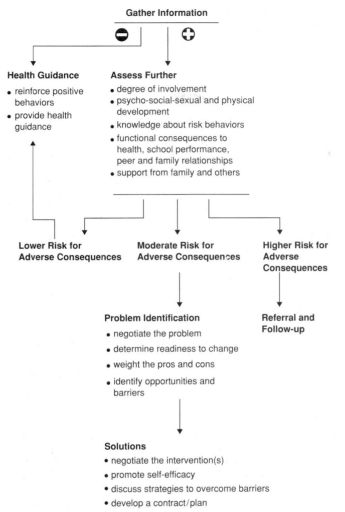

FIGURE 4.2 Algorithm for providing health screening and guidance to adolescents. [From *Guidelines for adolescent preventive services* (Recommendations monograph). Chicago: American Medical Association, 1995.]

perseveration on areas of obvious disagreement is unlikely to be productive and may negatively affect subsequent discussions. The clinician guides the adolescent to weigh the pros and cons of making a certain change. The adolescent may find several reasons to make (or not make) the change in behavior, and it is helpful to address these reasons explicitly. In beginning to develop a "plan," find out what the adolescent is willing (or not willing) to do. Make sure the plan is concrete and fully detailed. Decisions should be framed as being in the adolescent's hands. Try to avoid sweeping changes that are unrealistic, such as avoiding alcohol use for life.

S: Specific Solutions: Self-Efficacy, Support, Solving Problems, and "Shaking on a Contract." *Self-efficacy* is assessed by asking whether the adolescent thinks he or she will be able to carry out the proposed plan. If the adolescent is ambivalent, revisit perceived barriers and attempt to redefine specific solutions. Plans should be achievable so that success becomes self-reinforcing. An overly ambitious plan may need to be modified. *Support* is important, and adolescents should be encouraged to identify people who can help them carry out their plan. Hopefully, they will be able to call on resources such as trusted adults or close friends. At times, the clinician can also help adolescents to disclose information to parents or others. *Solving problems* reminds us to assess the barriers that the adolescent foresees and to work with the adolescent in developing specific strategies to overcome them. For example, if an adolescent recognizes that he or she will have difficulty not drinking at an upcoming party, it is essential to have a plan for dealing with that situation. It is usually most helpful if adolescents come up with their own solutions, but they often can be helped to recognize solutions or options they might not have considered. *"Shaking on a contract"* is a crucial step. It serves as a tangible reinforcement of the proposed plan and implies some commitment on the adolescent's part. It is important to specify the actions agreed to and the time frame in which the actions are to be taken. If you are able to involve another party in the contract, such as a friend or parent, there is likely to be better compliance. Follow-up is critical and should be arranged in some form—either a visit, telephone contact, or e-mail—in the time frame agreed to in the contract.

WEB SITES AND REFERENCES

http://odphp.osophs.dhhs.gov. Office of Disease Prevention and Health Promotion.

http://www.ama-assn.org/ama/pub/category/1947.html. Adolescent Health Online (AMA).

http://brightfutures.aap.org/web/ New web site for AAP/Bright Futures

http://www.aap.org. American Academy of Pediatrics.

http://www.aafp.org. American Academy of Family Physicians.

http://www.adolescenthealth.org. Society for Adolescent Medicine.

http://www.nasbhc.org. National Association of School-based Health Centers.

http://www.cdc.gov/nccdphp/dash. CDC Department of Adolescent and School Health.

http://www.cdc.gov. Centers for Disease Control and Prevention.

http://www.acha.org. American College Health Association.

http://www.adolescenthealthlaw.org. Center for Adolescent Health and the Law.

http://www.ama-assn.org/ama/pub/category/1980.html. GAPS AMA site.

American Academy of Pediatrics, Committee on Psychosocial Aspects of Child and Family Health. *Guidelines for health supervision III* (Updated). Elk Grove Village, IL: American Academy of Pediatrics, 2002.

American Medical Association. *AMA guidelines for adolescent preventive services (GAPS): recommendations and rationale.* Baltimore: Williams & Wilkins, 1994.

American Medical Association. *AMA guidelines for adolescent preventive services (GAPS): clinical evaluation and management handbook.* Baltimore: Williams & Wilkins, 1995.

Centers for Disease Control and Prevention. Immunization of adolescents: recommendations of the Advisory Committee on Immunization Practices, the American Academy of Pediatrics, the American Academy of Family Physicians, and the American Medical Association. *MMWR Morb Mortal Wkly Rep* 1996;45(RR-13): 1–16.

Elster AB. Comparison of recommendations for adolescent clinical preventive services developed by national organizations. *Arch Pediatr Adolesc Med* 1998;152:193.

Goldenring J, Rosen DS. Getting into adolescent heads: an essential update. *Contemp Pediatr* 2004;21:64.

Green M. *Bright futures: guidelines for the health supervision of infants, children, and adolescents.* Arlington, VA: National Center for Education in Maternal and Child Health, 1994.

Rosen DS, Elster A, Hedberg V, et al. Clinical preventive services for adolescents: position paper of the Society for Adolescent Medicine. *J Adolesc Health* 1997;21:203.

U.S. Preventive Services Task Force. *Guide to clinical preventive services: an assessment of the effectiveness of 169 interventions,* 2nd ed. Baltimore: Williams & Wilkins, 1996.

U.S. Preventive Services Task Force. *Guide to clinical preventive services: an assessment of the effectiveness of 169 interventions,* 3rd ed. 2001–2004; accessed online at http://www.ahrq.gov/clinic/gcpspu.htm

CHAPTER 5

Vital Statistics and Injuries

Ponrat Pakpreo, Jonathan D. Klein, and Lawrence S. Neinstein

Intentional and unintentional injuries are responsible for the majority of the morbidity and mortality experienced by adolescents. Injuries are preventable health problems, but the prevention of injuries poses considerable challenges to medical and public health professionals. The public health approach to injury prevention includes educational strategies, environmental modifications, and engineering techniques.

DEMOGRAPHICS

In 2005, adolescents 10 to 19 years old numbered just over 42 million or 14.2% of the U.S. population, and 20.8 million young adults 20 to 24 years old made up an additional 7.1% of the U.S. population. From 2000 to 2005, the adolescent population 10 to 14 years of age increased by 1.4%, compared with the 4.7% increase among 15- to 19-year-olds. It is projected that by 2010, the population 10 to 19 years of age will have decreased to 41.1 million, a decline of just over 2%. It is projected that the population between ages 20 and 24 will increase by 3.4%, to 21.7 million. The number of adolescents aged 10 to 19 is projected to increase through 2050; however, as a percentage of the total U.S. population, the number of adolescents, while decreasing, will likely stabilize by 2010.

Hispanic adolescents 10 to 14 years of age are among the fastest-growing segments of the U.S. population, having increased by 19.6% between 2000 and 2004. Hispanic teens between the ages of 10 and 19 represent 2.4% of the entire 2004 U.S. population and 17.2% of the U.S. Hispanic population. Hispanic youth are second in overall numbers compared to non-Hispanic whites. African-American youth between the ages of 10 and 19 are third, making up 15.7% of the 10- to 19-year age group in the United States.

DATA SOURCES

Adolescent demographics, morbidity, mortality, and health behaviors change from year to year. The most current data are available on the Internet; important sites are listed below.

Demographic and General Health Data

1. *Health, United States, 2006:* Available at: http://www.cdc.gov/nchs/hus.htm. *Health, United States* is an annual report on trends in health statistics. The

46

report consists of two main sections: a chartbook containing text and figures that illustrates major trends in the health of Americans and a trend tables section containing 147 detailed data tables.

2. *The 2006 Statistical Abstract: U.S. Census Bureau* (http://www.census.gov/compendia/statab/). Each year the Census Bureau publishes data related to U.S. demographics, health, education and a other information.

3. *NHIS: The National Health Interview Survey (NHIS)* (http://www.cdc.gov/nchs/nhis.htm). This is a multistage probability sample survey conducted annually by the National Center for Health Statistics (NCHS) during in-home interviews of the civilian noninstitutionalized U.S. population. The NHIS sample frame is also linked to several other national health survey efforts. The objectives of the NHIS surveys are to monitor the health and health care of the U.S. population by collecting and analyzing data on a broad range of health topics. Current topic include health status and limitations, utilization of health care, injuries, family resources, health insurance, access to care, selected health conditions (including chronic conditions), health behaviors, functioning, HIV/AIDS testing, and immunization.

4. *National Vital Statistics System:* (http://www.cdc.gov/nchs/nvss.htm). The National Vital Statistics System is the oldest and most successful example of intergovernmental data sharing in public health. These data include births, deaths, marriages, divorces, and fetal deaths recorded across the United States.

5. *Healthy People 2010* (http://www.healthypeople.gov/) outlines national health promotion and disease prevention objectives, which are monitored and updated over time. Of the 467 *Healthy People 2010* objectives for children and adults, 107 are relevant to adolescents and young adults. Adolescent health experts convened and identified 21 critical health objectives, which reflect some of the leading causes of morbidity and mortality among adolescents and young adults. Table 5.1 lists the 21 critical health objectives as well as baseline data and 2010 target goals.

6. *Healthy Campus 2010* (http://www.acha.org/info_resources/hc2010.cfm). This program establishes national college health objectives and serves as a basis for developing plans to improve student health. It is a parallel series of health objectives to *Healthy People 2010* but adapted for the college population.

Mortality Data

1. *Health, United States, 2006* as described above

2. *Deaths: Final Data for 2003.* This yearly publication is available at the National Center for Health Statistics website. The 2003 final report is at: http://www.cdc.gov/nchs/products/pubs/pubd/hestats/finaldeaths03/finaldeaths03.htm

3. *National Center for Injury Prevention and Control (NCIPC)* (http://www.cdc.gov/ncipc/). The NCIPC has a vast array of data and information on injuries and injury prevention in all age groups. Also at this site are two interactive data tools: WISQARS and injury maps.

  a. *WISQARS* (Web-based Injury Statistics Query and Reporting System) is available at http://www.cdc.gov/ncipc/wisqars/default.htm. This site is the Injury Center's interactive, online database, which provides customized injury-related mortality data and nonfatal injury data. Results can be stratified by age, gender, ethnicity, and region of the country.

TABLE 5.1

National Initiative to Improve Adolescent Health—21 Critical Health Objectives for Adolescents and Young Adults

Objective No.	Objective	Baseline (yr)	2010 Target
16-03 (a, b, c)	Reduce deaths of adolescents and young adults		
	10- to 14-yr-olds	21.5/100,000 (1998)	16.8/100,000
	15- to 19-yr-olds	69.5/100,000 (1998)	39.8/100,000
	20- to 24-yr-olds	92.7/100,000 (1998)	49.0/100,000
Unintentional Injury			
15-15 (a)	Reduce deaths caused by motor vehicle crashes (15- to 24-yr-olds).	25.6/100,000 (1999)	[a]
26-01 (a)	Reduce deaths and injuries caused by alcohol- and drug-related motor vehicle crashes (15- to 24-yr-olds).	13.5/100,000 (1998)	[a]
15-19	Increase use of safety belts (9th–12th grade students).	84% (1999)	92%
26-06	Reduce the proportion of adolescents who report that they rode, during the previous 30 days, with a driver who had been drinking alcohol (9th–12th grade students).	33% (1999)	30%
Violence			
18-01	Reduce the suicide rate		
	10- to 14-yr-olds	1.2/100,000 (1999)	[a]
	15- to 19-yr-olds	8.0/100,000 (1999)	[a]
18-02	Reduce the rate of suicide attempts by adolescents that require medical attention (9th–12th grade students).	2.6% (1999)	1%
15-32	Reduce homicides		
	10- to 14-yr-olds	1.2/100,000 (1999)	[a]
	15- to 19-yr-olds	10.4/100,000 (1999)	[a]
15-38	Reduce physical fighting among adolescents (9th–12th grade students).	36% (1999)	32%
15-39	Reduce weapon carrying by adolescents on school property (9th–12th grade students).	6.9% (1999)	4.9%

Substance Use and Mental Health

26-11 (d)	Reduce the proportion of persons engaging in binge drinking of alcoholic beverages (12- to 17-yr-olds).	7.7% (1998)	2%
26-10 (b)	Reduce last-month use of illicit substances (marijuana) (12- to 17-yr-olds).	8.3% (1998)	0.70%
06-02	Reduce the proportion of children and adolescents with disabilities who are reported to be sad, unhappy, or depressed (4- to 17-yr-olds).	*b*	*b*
18-07	Increase the proportion of children with mental health problems who receive treatment	59% (2001)	66%

Reproductive Health

09-07	Reduce pregnancies among adolescent females (15- to 17-yr-olds).	68/1,000 (1996)	43/1,000
13-05	(Developmental) Reduce the number of new HIV diagnoses among adolescents and adults (13- to 24-yr-olds).	16,479 (1998)*d*	*c*
25-01 (a, b, c)	Reduce the proportion of adolescents and young adults with *Chlamydia trachomatis* infections (15- to 24-yr-olds).		
	• Females attending family planning clinics	5% (1997)	3%
	• Females attending sexually transmitted disease clinics	12.2% (1997)	3%
	• Males attending sexually transmitted disease clinics	15.7% (1997)	3%
25-11	Increase the proportion of adolescents (9th–12th grade students) who:		
	• Have never had sexual intercourse	50% (1999)	56%
	• If sexually experienced, are not currently sexually active	27% (1999)	30%
	• If currently sexually active, used a condom the last time they had sexual intercourse	58% (1999)	65%

TABLE 5.1

(Continued)

Objective No.	Objective	Baseline (yr)	2010 Target
Chronic Diseases			
27-02 (a)	Reduce tobacco use by adolescents (9th–12th grade students).	40% (1999)	21%
19-03 (b)	Reduce the proportion of children and adolescents who are overweight or obese (12- to 19-yr-olds)	11% (1988–1994)	5%
22-07	Increase the proportion of adolescents who engage in vigorous physical activity that promotes cardiorespiratory fitness 3 or more d/wk for 20 or more min per occasion (9th–12th grade students).	65% (1999)	85%

HIV, human immunodeficiency virus. Bolded objectives numbers indicate critical health outcomes. Behaviors that substantially contribute to important health outcomes are in normal font.

[a] 2010 target not provided for adolescent/young adult age-group.

[b] Baseline and target inclusive of age-groups outside of adolescent/young adult age parameters.

[c] Developmental objective-baseline and 2010 target to be provided by 2005.

[d] Proposed baseline is shown but has not yet been approved by the Healthy People 2010 Steering Committee.

Adapted from the National Adolescent Health Information Center. *21 critical health objectives for adolescents and young adults. Data from the U.S. Department of Health and Human Services. Healthy People 2010,* Vol. 1 and 2. Washington, DC: U.S. Government Printing Office. Available at http://nahic.ucsf.edu/nationalinitiative. November 2000.

b. *Injury Maps.* The Injury Center's interactive mapping system, http://www.cdc.gov/ncipc/wisqars/default.htm, helps identify the impact of injury deaths in a particular county, state, region, or the entire United States.

Morbidity Data, Including Diseases, Health Risks, and Health Behaviors

1. *NHANES, The National Health and Nutrition Examination Survey* (http://www.cdc.gov/nchs/nhanes.htm), is conducted by the NCHS on overall health risks and behaviors. Data collection is unique in that it combines home interviews with objective health measures and physical examinations conducted in a mobile examination center. The goals of this survey include the following: To estimate the number and percentage of persons in the U.S. population and designated subgroups with selected diseases and risk factors; to monitor trends in prevalence, awareness, treatment, and control of selected diseases or conditions, including those unrecognized or undetected; to monitor trends in risk behaviors and environmental exposures; to analyze risk factors for selected diseases (including heart disease, diabetes, osteoporosis, and infectious diseases); to study the relationship between diet, nutrition, and health, including a focus on iron deficiency anemia and other nutritional disorders, children's growth and development, and overweight/physical fitness; to explore emerging public health issues and new technologies; and to establish a national probability sample of genetic material for future genetic testing.

2. *The National Ambulatory Medical Care Survey* and *National Hospital Ambulatory Medical Care Survey* (http://www.cdc.gov/nchs/about/major/ahcd/ahcd1.htm) focus on characteristics of patients' visits to physicians' offices, hospital outpatient settings, and emergency departments. Additionally, these surveys collect data on diagnoses and treatments, prescribing patterns, and characteristics of clinical facilities.

3. Reproductive Health. *The National Survey of Family Growth* (http://www.cdc.gov/nchs/nsfg.htm), has data on reproductive health behaviors.

4. *National Survey of Children with Special Health Care Needs* (http://www.cdc.gov/nchs/about/major/slaits/cshcn.htm). This survey assesses the prevalence and impact of special health care needs among children in all 50 states and the District of Columbia.

5. Cancer Data. *National Cancer Institute, Surveillance Epidemiology and End Results* (http://seer.cancer.gov/publicdata/). The SEER public use data include SEER incidence and population data associated by age, sex, race, year of diagnosis, and geographic area (including SEER registry and county).

6. Infectious Diseases. *The Summary of Notifiable Diseases* is available each year in the MMWR. Search at www.cdc.gov/mmwr.

7. Sports Injury Data. *The National Center for Catastrophic Sport Injury Research* (http://www.unc.edu/depts/nccsi/) collects and disseminates death and permanent disability sports injury data that involve brain and/or spinal cord injuries.

8. *Youth Risk Behavior Surveillance System (YRBSS):* (http://www.cdc.gov/HealthyYouth/yrbs/index.htm) The Youth Risk Behavior Surveillance System was developed in 1990 to monitor priority health risk behaviors that contribute to the leading causes of death, disability, and social problems among youth and adults in the United States. Behaviors studied include

tobacco use, unhealthy dietary behaviors, inadequate physical activity, alcohol and other drug use, sexual behaviors that contribute to unintended pregnancy and sexually transmitted diseases, including HIV infection, and behaviors that contribute to unintentional injuries and violence. The survey examines the prevalence of health risk behaviors, trends over time, comparable data among subgroups of adolescents, and progress toward *Healthy People 2010* objectives.

The survey includes representative samples of representative samples of ninth- through twelfth-grade students both in public and private schools. The YRBSS also includes three additional national surveys conducted by CDC:

a. *Youth Risk Behavior Survey*, conducted in 1992 as a follow on to the National Health Interview Survey among nearly 11,000 persons aged 12 to 21 years.

b. *National College Health Risk Behavior Survey*, conducted in 1995 among a representative sample of about 5,000 undergraduate students.

c. *National Alternative High School Youth Risk Behavior Survey*, conducted in 1998 among a representative sample of almost 9,000 students in alternative high schools. Some notable statistics reported by the 2003 YRBSS are presented in Table 5.2.

9. *National College Health Assessment (NCHA)* (http://www.acha-ncha.org/index.html). The ACHA-National College Health Assessment (NCHA) is a national research effort organized by ACHA to assist health care providers, health educators, counselors, and administrators in collecting data about college students' habits, behaviors, and perceptions on the most prevalent health topics. Topics include alcohol, tobacco, and other drug use, sexual health, weight, nutrition, and exercise as well as mental health and injury prevention, personal safety, and violence.

10. *Add Health* (http://www.cpc.unc.edu/addhealth) is a nationally representative study that explores the causes of health-related behaviors of adolescents in grades 7 through 12 and their outcomes in young adulthood. *Add Health* examines how social contexts (families, friends, peers, schools, neighborhoods, and communities) influence adolescents' health and risk behaviors. Wave 1 was initiated in 1994 and is the largest, most comprehensive survey of adolescents ever undertaken. Data at the individual, family, school, and community levels were collected in two waves between 1994 and 1996. In 2001 and 2002, *Add Health* respondents, 18 to 26 years old, were reinterviewed in a third wave to investigate the influence that adolescence has on young adulthood. Data are gathered from adolescents themselves, their parents, and school administrators. Already existing databases provide information about neighborhoods and communities.

11. Substance Abuse. Monitoring the Future Study (www.monitoringthefuture.org). Monitoring the Future (MTF) is an ongoing study of the behaviors, attitudes, and values of American secondary school students, college students, and young adults. Each year, approximately 50,000 eighth-, ninth-, and twelfth- grade students are surveyed. This study provides perhaps the most complete and comprehensive examination of substance use and abuse patterns both cross-sectionally and longitudinally in the United States.

Another source of national data is the Fed Stat gateway at http://www.fedstats.gov/. This site has links to over 70 federal agencies that collect national data on a wide range of areas.

TABLE 5.2

Percentage of High School Students Who Engaged in Selected Health-Risk Behaviors, by Grade—United States Youth Risk Behavior Survey, 2005

Behavior	9th Grade	10th Grade	11th Grade	12th Grade	Total
Rarely or never used safety belts[a]	10.9	8.6	10.1	10.8	10.2
Rarely or never wore motorcycle helmets[b]	36.8	31.9	38.2	39.5	36.5
Rarely or never wore bicycle helmets[c]	83.0	84.3	82.2	84.0	83.4
Rode with a drinking driver[d]	27.9	27.8	28.0	30.1	28.5
Participated in a physical fight[e]	43.5	36.6	31.6	29.1	35.9
Carried a weapon[f]	19.9	19.4	17.1	16.9	18.5
Lifetime cigarette use[g]	48.7	52.5	57.5	60.3	54.3
Current cigarette use[h]	19.7	21.4	24.3	27.6	23.0
Current smokeless tobacco use[j]	7.6	7.5	8.4	8.4	8.0
Lifetime alcohol use[k]	66.5	74.4	76.3	81.7	74.3
Current episodic heavy drinking[l]	19.0	24.6	27.6	32.8	25.5
Lifetime marijuana use[m]	29.3	37.4	42.3	47.6	38.4
Lifetime cocaine use[n]	6.0	7.2	8.7	8.9	7.6
Lifetime ecstacy use	5.8	6.0	6.5	6.7	6.3
Lifetime methamphetamine use	5.7	5.9	6.7	6.4	6.2
Ever injected drugs[o]	2.4	2.3	1.7	1.7	2.1
Ever had sexual intercourse	34.3	42.8	51.4	63.6	46.8
Sexual intercourse with four or more partners (lifetime)	9.4	11.5	16.2	21.4	14.3
Used condom during last sexual intercourse[p]	74.5	65.3	61.7	55.4	62.8
Used birth control pills before last sexual intercourse[p]	7.5	14.3	18.5	25.6	17.6
Ate fruits and vegetables[q]	21.3	21.4	18.8	18.3	20.1
Played on a sports team[r]	60.4	58.0	54.9	49.2	56.0

(continued)

TABLE 5.2

(Continued)

Behavior	9th Grade	10th Grade	11th Grade	12th Grade	Total
Engaged in moderate physical activity[s]	36.9	38.5	34.4	32.9	35.8
Made a suicide plan in last 12 mo	13.9	14.1	12.9	10.5	13.0

[a]When riding in a car or truck as a passenger.

[b]When riding on a motorcycle.

[c]When riding on a bicycle.

[d]Rode at least once during the 30 days preceding the survey in a car or other vehicle driven by someone who had been drinking alcohol.

[e]Fought at least once during the 12 months preceding the survey.

[f]Carried a gun, knife, or club at least 1 day during the 30 days preceding the survey.

[g]Ever tried smoking, even one or two puffs.

[h]Smoked cigarettes on one or more of the 30 days preceding the survey.

[j]Used chewing tobacco or snuff on one or more of the 30 days preceding the survey.

[k]Ever drank one or more drinks.

[l]Drank five or more drinks of alcohol on at least one occasion during the 30 days preceding the survey.

[m]Ever used marijuana.

[n]Ever tried any form of cocaine (i.e., powder, "crack," or "freebase").

[o]Respondents were classified as injecting-drug users only if they (a) reported injecting-drug use not prescribed by a physician and (b) answered "one or more time" to any of the following questions: "During your life, how many times have you used any form of cocaine including powder, crack, or freebase?" "During your life, how many times have you used heroin (also called *smack, junk,* or *China White*)?" "During your life, how many times have you used methamphetamines (also called *speed, crystal, crank,* or *ice*)?" or "During your life, how many times have you taken steroid pills or shots without a doctor's prescription?"

[p]Among respondents who had sexual intercourse during the 3 months preceding the survey.

[q]Ate five or more servings of fruits and vegetables (fruit, fruit juice, green salad, and cooked vegetables) during the 7 days preceding the survey.

[r]During the 12 months preceding the survey.

[s]Activities that did not cause sweating or hard breathing for at least 30 minutes at a time on five or more of the 7 days preceding the survey.

Adapted from Centers for Disease Control and Prevention. Youth risk behavior surveillance, 2005. *MMWR CDC Surveill Summ* 2006b;55(SS-5):1–108.

MORTALITY

Leading Causes of Death

The 10 leading causes of death for youth between ages 10 and 14 years vary slightly from those of older adolescents and young adults. The leading causes of mortality for each age group (per 100,000) are shown in Table 5.3. Unintentional injuries, homicides, and suicides are the top three causes of death in the 15- to 24-year-old population. In the 10- to 14-year-old-age group, both unintentional injuries and suicide are leading causes. Malignant neoplasms are the second highest cause of mortality. HIV-related deaths are sixth in young adults 25 to

TABLE 5.3

Ten Leading Causes of Death, United States, 2004, by Age Group

Rank	All Ages	Age Groups 10 to 14	15 to 24	25 to 34
Total number of deaths	2,397,615	3,946	33,421	40,868
1	Heart disease 652,486 (27.2%)	Unintentional injury 1,540 (39.9%)	Unintentional injury 15,449 (46.2%)	Unintentional injury 13,032 (31.9%)
2	Malignant neoplasms 553,888 (23.1%)	Malignant neoplasms 493 (12.5%)	Homicide 5,085 (15.2%)	Suicide 5,074 (12.4%)
3	Cerebrovascular 150,074 (6.3%)	Suicide 283 (7.2%)	Suicide 4,316 (12.9%)	Homicide 4,495(11.0%)
4	Chronic low-respiratory disease 121,987 (5.1%)	Homicide 207 (5.2%)	Malignant neoplasms 1,709 (5.1%)	Malignant neoplasms 3,633 (8.9%)
5	Unintentional injuries 112,012 (4.7%)	Congenital anomalies 184 (4.7%)	Heart disease 1,038 (3.1%)	Heart disease 3,163 (7.7%)
6	Diabetes mellitus 73,138 (3.1%)	Heart disease 162 (4.1%)	Congenital anomalies 483 (1.4%)	HIV 1,468 (3.6%)
7	Alzheimer disease 65,965 (2.8%)	Chronic low-respiratory disease 74 (1.9%)	Cerebrovascular 211 (0.6%)	Diabetes mellitus 599 (1.5%)
8	Influenza and pneumonia 59,664 (2.5%)	Influenza and pneumonia 49 (1.2%)	HIV 191 (0.6%)	Cerebrovascular 567 (1.4%)
9	Nephritis 42,480 (1.8%)	Benign neoplasms 43 (1.1%)	Influenza and pneumonia 185 (0.6%)	Congenital anomalies 420 (1.0%)
10	Septicemia 33,373 (1.7%)	Cerebrovascular events 43 (1.1%)	Chronic low-respiratory disease 179 (0.5%)	Septicemia 328 (0.8%)
All others	533,548 (22.2%)	868 (22.0%)	4,575 (13.7%)	8,089 (19.8%)

HIV, human immunodeficiency virus. Adapted from CDC. Wisqars. at www.cdc.gov/ncipc/wisqars, last accessed 12. 2006.

34 years of age and eighth in the leading causes of death during adolescence among 15- to 24-year-olds.

In general, the leading cause of death is the same among different ethnicities in all age groups except those between the ages of 15 to 44 years. Among individuals aged 15 to 34 years, unintentional injuries are the leading cause of death for all races except African Americans, where homicides are the leading

TABLE 5.4

Unintentional (Accidental) Deaths by Age and Type, United States, 2004

Age (yr)	All Types	Motor Vehicle	Drowning	Fires and Burns	Firearms	Falls	Poisoning
10–14	1,540	1,013	138	87	35	26	47
15–19	6,825	5,224	304	66	80	87	643
20–24	8,624	5,763	270	120	92	154	1,616

CDC. WISQARS. 2006, last accessed 12.4.2006.

cause of death. Homicide also ranks higher as a cause of death in this age group among Hispanics as compared with non-Hispanics.

Unintentional Injuries

Unintentional injuries are the fifth leading cause of death in the United States for the total population but the leading cause of death among 1- to 44-year-olds. The leading cause of death due to unintentional injury is motor vehicle accidents. Table 5.4 shows the unintentional deaths by age and type. The data are particularly striking for adolescent drivers. Although the 12 million adolescent drivers represent 6% of total drivers, they account for approximately 14% of the fatal accidents.

Intentional Injuries

Homicide. Homicide continues to be a major public health problem in the United States, particularly for young African-American males. Homicide remains the number two cause of death in the 15- to 24-year-old population and the number one cause of death among African-American males ages 15 to 24 years. Over 75% of homicides in older adolescents and young adults involve firearms. In 2004, African-American males 18 to 24 years old had the highest homicide victimization rate at 95.5 per 100,000, more than double the rate for black males 25 years of age (38.3 per 100,000) and older.

Suicide. Adolescent suicide rates remained stable between 1900 and 1955 and then began to rise dramatically. Currently, suicide is the third leading cause of death for adolescents and young adults ages 10 to 14 years and 15 to 24 years (CDC Wisqars, 2006). In 2004, the suicide rate was 10.35 per 100,000, accounting for 4,316 deaths within the 15- to 24-year-old population. This represents almost 13% of all suicides as well as almost 13% of all deaths within that age group. For both 15- to 19- and 20- to 24-year-olds, suicide rates are highest among Native Americans and whites. African Americans had the lowest rates among 15- to 19-year-olds and Asians had the lowest rate among 20- to 24-year-olds. The ratio of attempted to completed suicides among adolescents is estimated to be between 50:1 and 100:1, with the incidence of unsuccessful attempts being higher among females than among males. The true number of deaths from suicide may actually be much higher than indicated, because some suicide deaths are recorded as "accidental."

Ingestion of pills is the most common method among adolescents who *attempt* suicide. Firearms, used in nearly 50% of adolescent suicides, cause the greatest number of deaths for male and female adolescents who *complete* suicides. More than 90% of suicide attempts involving a firearm are fatal because there is little chance for rescue. Firearms in the home, regardless of whether they are kept unloaded or locked, are associated with a higher risk of adolescent suicide.

In a national survey of high school students in 2003, a total of 16.9% reported having seriously considered attempting suicide during the 12 months preceding the survey. Overall, female students (21.3%) were significantly more likely than male students (12.8%) to have considered suicide. More serious ideation, having made a specific plan to attempt suicide during the preceding 12 months, was reported by 16.5% of students nationwide. Female students were more likely to have made a plan than were male students (18.9% versus 14.1%). Furthermore, 8.5% of high school students reported having attempted suicide at least once within the previous 12 months. More female than male students reported having made an attempt (11.5% versus 5.4%). Hispanic and white females most often reported considering suicide, making a suicide plan, and having attempted suicide than other female and male students. Of all students who reported a history of suicide attempts, only 2.9% had been treated by a doctor or nurse for an attempted suicide-related injury, poisoning, or overdose.

Firearm Injuries. In 2004 in the United States, there were 29,569 (9.95/100,000) deaths from firearm injuries, including those related to accidents, suicides, and homicides. Most of the firearm deaths in the adolescent and young adult age group are related to suicide or homicide. Adolescent male deaths due to firearms were eight times the rate among females.

Cancer

Excluding intentional and unintentional injuries, cancer is the leading cause of death in adolescents and is the leading cause of death by disease. It is the second cause of death among younger adolescents 10 to 14 years old and ranks fourth among 15- to 24-year-olds. In 2005, an estimated 9,510 children, under 15 years of age, will be diagnosed with cancer, and 1,585 will die from the disease. On average, 1 or 2 of every 10,000 children in the country develops cancer.

The types of tumors that occur in the adolescent population, especially those 15 to 19 years old, differ significantly from those that predominate in younger children or adults. During adolescence, there are increases in incidence and mortality due to Hodgkin disease, germ cell tumors, central nervous system (CNS) tumors, non-Hodgkin lymphoma, thyroid cancer, malignant melanoma, and acute lymphoblastic leukemia. Table 5.5 lists the incidence, mortality, and 5-year survival rates of the top cancer sites among 5- to 19-year-olds. Of the 12 major types of childhood cancers, leukemias and brain and other CNS tumors account for more than one-half of new cases. Leukemias make up approximately one third of childhood cancers, and leukemia is the number one cause of death from malignancies among 15- to 24-year-olds. Overall 5-year survival rates for adolescents aged 10 to 14 with cancer have improved from 58.8% (1975 to 1977) to nearly 80% (1996 to 2002); for those between the ages of 15 to 19, the 5-year survivals rates have improved from 67.7% to 79.7%. This is reflected in a decreasing cancer mortality rate.

TABLE 5.5

Childhood Cancer, SEER Incidence, Mortality, and 5-Year Survival Rates (per 100,000) for Top Cancer Sites by Age Group 2000–2003

	Incidence	Mortality	5-yr Survival 1975–1977	5-yr Survival 1996–2002
Ages 5–9				
All sites	11.2	2.5	58.2	77.9
Brain and other nervous system	3.2	0.9	58.0	72.4
Leukemia	3.8	0.7	52.0	80.7
Acute lymphocytic	3.2	0.4	55.2	84.0
Ages 10–14				
All sites	12.5	2.5	58.8	79.7
Bone and joint	1.3	0.3	53.8	69.88
Brain and other nervous system	2.6	0.7	59.5	80.1
Hodgkin lymphoma	1.1	0	78.7	95.2
Leukemia	2.8	0.8	35.2	70.5
Acute lymphocytic	1.9	0.4	43.6	80.7
Ages 15–19				
All sites	21.0	3.6	67.7	79.7
Bone and joint	1.5	0.5	51.0	63.3
Melanoma of the skin	1.7	0	75.1	97.5
Testis	3.4	0.1	66.0	91.7
Brain and other nervous system	2.0	0.5	64.7	79.9
Thyroid	1.8	—	100	97.5
Hodgkin lymphoma	3.0	0.1	88.9	94.9
Non-Hodgkin lymphoma	1.7	0.3	45.2	75.5
Leukemia	3.0	1.1	24.4	48.9
Acute lymphocytic	1.7	0.5	29.5	52.7

Adapted from National Cancer Institute. *SEER cancer statistics review, 1975–2003.* Bethesda, MD: National Cancer Institute, Available at http://seer.cancer.gov/cgi-bin/csr/1975_2003/search.pl#results. Accessed 12.3.2006

Human Immunodeficiency Virus

HIV remains one of the 10 leading causes of death in all ages between 15 and 54 years. HIV infection ranks 14th for ages 10 to 14 years, 10th for ages 15 to 24, and 6th for ages 25 to 34. HIV mortality in the second and third decades of life often represents infection acquired during the teen years.

UNINTENTIONAL INJURIES

Unintentional injuries account for 44% of all injury deaths to children and adolescents in the United States. Among youth between the ages of 1 and 19 years, unintentional injuries are responsible for more deaths than homicide, suicide, congenital anomalies, cancer, heart disease, respiratory illness, and HIV combined. Table 5.4 is a summary of unintentional and accidental deaths by age and type in 2004. Among 10- to 19-year-olds, the majority of nonfatal injuries are due to unintentional injury (90.7%), assault (7.9%), and self-harm (1.3%).

Morbidity

Deaths only partially convey the enormous damage caused by childhood injuries. It is estimated that for every childhood death caused by injury there are approximately 34 hospitalizations, 1,000 emergency department visits, many more visits to private physicians and school nurses, and an even larger number of injuries treated at home. Approximately 21 million children in the United States are injured each year. This equates to an injury rate of 1 in 4 children, or 56,000 nonfatal injury episodes each day that require medical attention or limit children's activity.

Leading Causes of Injuries

Four types of injury—being struck by or against an object or person, falls, motor vehicle traffic–related injuries, and being cut by a sharp object—account for almost 60% of all injury-related visits to emergency departments by adolescents. Of these four causes, only motor vehicle traffic–related injuries are a significant source of mortality. Sports injuries make up more than 40% of injuries classified as "being struck by or against an object or person." At each age, the rate of such injuries among males is twice that among females.

Epidemiology

The risk of injury is clearly related to the physical, mental, and emotional developmental milestones of children or adolescents; for this reason, age is a predictable risk factor for injury. Adolescents are most likely to suffer from motor vehicle injuries and injuries resulting from firearms and other forms of violence. At 10 years of age, slightly less than half of all deaths are caused by injury; by 18 years, however, more than 80% are injury-related. For every type of injury except bicycle deaths, there are substantial rate increases between early and late adolescence.

Beginning at approximately 1 or 2 years of age and continuing until the seventh decade of life, males have higher rates of injury than females. This gender difference during childhood does not appear to be caused by differences in developmental or motor skills. In part, it may be related to greater exposure of males to hazards or to gender-based differences in behavior. For nearly all injuries in 2003, the male death rate from injuries exceeds the rate in females: 2.1 times among adolescents ages 10 to14 years old, 2.8 times for ages 15 to 19 years old, and 3.97 times for young adults 20 to 24 years old.

Injury/death rates vary substantially by race and ethnicity. The highest injury fatality rates are among African-American and Native American adolescents and the lowest rates are among Asian youth. One explanation for these racial differences appears to be related to poverty, which is another important risk factor in predicting adolescent injuries.

Factors Contributing to Adolescent Injuries

Socioeconomic Factors. Poor children are at greatest risk for injury; studies have indicated that their risk level is two to five times that of children who are not poor. This is true for pedestrian injuries, fires and burns, drownings, and intentional injuries.

Environmental Factors. These include hazards such as all-terrain vehicles (ATVs), backyard swimming pools, firearms, kerosene heaters, traffic patterns, and gang activity.

School Environment. Because children and adolescents spend much of their day at school, it follows that many of the injuries they sustain occur there; between 33% and 50% of all child and adolescent injuries happen on school grounds. Males are injured at school more often than females. Falls are the most common cause of injury in secondary schools, and they usually result in minor injury. Also frequent are burns, strains, sprains, and dislocations. The number of injuries that occur in vocational classrooms and on athletic fields increases with age and grade level. A large number of those injuries involve the improper use or malfunctioning of equipment.

Developmental Factors. Factors contributing to high injury rates in adolescents often relate to the discrepancies between an adolescent's physical development and his or her cognitive and emotional development. Adolescent health is influenced by the strengths and vulnerabilities of individuals and also by the character of the settings in which they live. These settings—the schools they attend, the neighborhoods they call home, their families, and the friends who make up their social network—play an important role in shaping adolescent health, affecting how individuals feel about themselves as well as influencing the choices they make about behaviors that can affect their health and well-being. Several developmental characteristics of the adolescent contribute to risk-taking behaviors and may lead to injuries and death: experimentation with adult roles; experimentation with risky behaviors or situations when opportunities for healthy risk taking are not available or provided; challenge of authority or rules; and desire for peer approval and a tendency to join peer activities and to follow peer norms. Placing these characteristics in an environment where there is alcohol, tobacco, violence, unprotected sex, fast cars, and drugs heightens adolescents' risk of injury and death.

Automobile Injuries

Automobile injuries are the leading cause of mortality and morbidity among all Americans ages 1 to 64 years. Crashes involving adolescent drivers are typically single-vehicle accidents, primarily run-off-the-road crashes, and involve driver error and/or speeding. Among youth 10 to 19 years of age, motor vehicle traffic–related injuries account for almost 36% of all deaths and 74% of deaths due to unintentional injuries. A 2006 review of the teen driver (AAP, 2006) reviews risk factors and recommendations for health care providers.

Risk Factors for Automobile Injuries. Teenagers are at particularly high risk for motor vehicle crashes, primarily because of their inexperience and risk-taking behaviors. Research shows that teenagers are more likely than older drivers to speed, run red lights, make illegal turns, tailgate, ride with an intoxicated driver, and drive after using alcohol or other drugs. Males are more likely than females to engage in risky driving behaviors such as drive after drinking alcohol, and they are less likely to wear seatbelts. Younger age, driving at night, having other teen passengers in the vehicle, and driving after drinking alcohol all increase the risk of motor vehicle crashes.

Alcohol. In a 2005 national survey of high school students, 28.5% of respondents said that, within the past 30 days, they had ridden in a motor vehicle driven by someone who had been drinking alcohol, and 9.9% reported having driven a motor vehicle after drinking alcohol. Data show that at all blood alcohol concentrations (BACs), the risk of being involved in a motor vehicle crash is greater for teenagers and young people than for older people. Teenage male drivers with a BAC in the 0.5% to 0.10% range are 18 times more likely and female drivers 54 times more likely than sober teenagers to be killed in single-vehicle crashes.

Graduated Licensing Programs. Motor vehicle crashes are highest in the first 2 years that drivers have their licenses. Graduated licensing programs are ideally designed to have three phases of supervision, including a supervised learning period, an intermediate restricted license, and then an unrestricted license. In the intermediate phase, new drivers have limits on higher-risk conditions such as late-night driving and transporting other adolescent passengers while unsupervised. After this phase, the restrictions are removed and the driver is fully licensed. Early data from states that have implemented graduated driving demonstrate a decrease in adolescent motor vehicle related crashes and fatalities. Almost all states have enacted some form of a graduated driver licensing law.

Nonautomobile Injuries

Drowning. Drowning was the second leading cause of unintentional death in children younger than 15 and the third cause of unintentional death in those 15 to 24 years old in 2004. Approximately 1,500 children and adolescents die of drowning each year in the United States. Drowning is unique as an injury problem because of its high case-fatality rate and because of the relative lack of impact that medical care has on outcome. Approximately 50% of children and adolescents requiring care for a submersion incident will die. Swimming pools play a role in drowning among young, school-age children and among adolescents; immersion in natural bodies of water, either while swimming or boating, also plays an increasingly important role. Males 15 to 19 years old are more than 10 times as likely as females of the same age to drown. Alcohol use is involved in about 25% to 50% of adolescent and adult deaths associated with water recreation.

Firearms. Firearms are the sixth leading cause of death due to unintentional injuries in the adolescent age group. Adolescents and young adults have the highest rate of unintentional firearm–related fatalities; males between the ages of 20 and 24 years have the highest risk. More than 75% of homicides of older adolescents and young adults are committed with a firearm. It is estimated that there are three nonfatal firearm injuries for every death associated with a firearm. In 2005, a total of 5.4% of high school students in a national survey reported having carried a gun to school within the previous 30 days.

Bicycle Accidents. Bicycle deaths are most likely to occur in the summer and fall and between the hours of 3 P.M. and 9 P.M. Nearly 70% of fatal bicycle accidents involve head injuries. In 2005, of all high school students who reported riding a bicycle within the preceding 12 months, 83.4% reported never or rarely wearing a bicycle helmet; 86% of bicycle-related deaths involved riders without helmets. Bicycle helmets decrease the risk of head injury by 85% and brain injury by 88%.

Skateboards. Most documented injuries occur in boys aged 10 and 14 years, ranging from minor cuts and abrasions to multiple fractures and, in some cases, even death. Head injuries account for approximately 3.5% to 9% and fractures of both upper and lower extremities account for 50% of all skateboarding injuries. Not surprisingly, 33% of those injured on skateboards experience some form of trauma within the first week of participating in the sport.

All-Terrain Vehicles. Children younger than 16 years of age account for 47% of ATV injuries and 36% of deaths; those younger than 12 years represent 15% of all deaths. Risk factors for injury include rider inexperience, intoxication with alcohol, excessive speed, and lack of helmet use. Head injuries account for most ATV-related deaths. Other nonfatal injuries include head and spinal trauma, abdominal injuries, abrasions, lacerations, and fractures.

Boating Accidents. Most boating fatalities from 2004 (70%) were caused by drowning; the remainder were due to trauma, hypothermia, carbon monoxide poisoning, or other causes. Among those who drowned, 90% were not wearing life jackets. Alcohol was involved in about one third of all reported boating fatalities. Personal watercraft were involved in 25%.

Poisoning. The percentage of unintentional deaths due to poisoning actually increases with age in the adolescent population. Adolescent females are more likely to die by poisoning than are males. In 2004, there were 90 reported adolescent fatalities, comprising 7.6% of all poison-related fatalities. Of these, over 50% were presumed suicides and 27% were caused by intentional abuse. Common household items are often the cause of poisonings. For young adolescents aged 10 to 14 years, about 80% of all poisoning deaths are from substances other than medications. In contrast, medications cause 58% of all poisoning deaths among adolescents aged 15 to 19 years. The most lethal substances for children of all ages are stimulants, street drugs, cardiovascular drugs, and antidepressants.

Sports Injuries. Sports participation also results in about 750,000 sports-related injuries each year that require hospital-based emergency treatment. In total, injury rates are reported to be as high as 81% of all participants, with more than 3 million injuries annually resulting in time lost from sports. Football is associated with the highest number of catastrophic injuries (causing death, permanent severe functional disability, or severe injury without permanent functional disability). Male athletes account for 84% of all adolescent sports-related injuries, despite the fact that rates are often higher among females, because fewer girls participate overall. However, the number of catastrophic injuries among female athletes has increased. According to the National Center for Catastrophic Sports Injury Research, the incorporation of gymnastic type stunts in cheerleading has lead to these sports accounting for 50% of catastrophic injuries among high school girls and 64% of such injuries among college female athletes. Within any given season, it is estimated that 48% of all adolescent athletes sustain at least one injury. Table 5.6 shows the percentages of injury types and body locations within six common high school sports.

TABLE 5.6

Injuries in Six Sports: Injury Type and Body Location, 1996–1998 (percentage with each sport)

Sport	Injury Type					Body Location			
	Head Injury	Fracture Dislocation	Open Wound	Contusion Abrasion	Sprain Strain	Head	Upper Extremity	Lower Extremity	Torso
Baseball/softball	7	24	17	20	32	37	32	26	3
Basketball	2	23	13	17	44	17	34	45	4
Bicycling	9	20	27	34	8	29	34	29	7
Football	5	29	11	23	31	16	47	28	8
Skating	4	39	9	17	25	10	50	30	9
Soccer	10	26	7	30	25	22	30	41	8

Adapted from Cheng TL, Fields CB, Brenner RA, et al. Sports injuries: an important cause of morbidity in urban youth. *Pediatrics* 2000;105:e32.

Football has the highest number and rate of mild traumatic brain injuries. Basketball causes more facial and dental injuries among adolescents than any other sport. For both boys and girls, the ankle or foot is the most common site of basketball injuries, accounting for 39.3% of injuries in boys and 36.6% in girls. Knee injuries make up 11.1% of all injuries in boys and 15.7% in girls. Of all baseball injuries, 55% involve ball or bat impact, often to the head. During baseball games, base running accounts for the largest proportion of injuries (25.7%), The injury rate for softball is 27% higher than that of baseball, with softball injuries similar to those that occur in baseball. Among all sports, soccer accounts for the highest number of injuries in girls. The most common site of soccer injury for both boys and girls is the ankle or foot. Concussive injuries during soccer often occur due to head-head or head-ground impact.

PREVENTION OF INJURIES

Most unintentional injury deaths of children can be prevented. Three key approaches to injury prevention are education, environment and product changes, and legislation or regulation. Education can serve to promote changes in individual behaviors that increase the risk of injury and/or death. Environment and product modifications can make the adolescent's physical surroundings, toys, equipment, and clothes less likely to facilitate an injury. Legislation and regulation are among the most powerful tools to reduce adolescent injury, but they also require the most energy and concentrated efforts on the part of individuals and groups. Some examples of preventive strategies that can be recommended in clinical practice include:

1. Limit access to alcohol and promote safety belt use among teenagers.
2. Have parents impose restrictions and limitations of driving privileges on their teenage children including restricting the number and age of passengers carried by teenage drivers.
3. Recommend that bicycle helmets be mandatory for all riders.
4. Suggest bicycle curfews to keep riders off the streets after dark.
5. Advise against unsafe bicycle riding, such as "riding double" or stunt riding.
6. Encourage swimming lessons at an early age.
7. Educate parents about the dangers of leaving children unattended at swimming pools.
8. Restrict adolescents younger than 16 years of age from operating personal watercraft unless accompanied by an adult.
9. Encourage training and aerobic conditioning for athletes before the start of their season.
10. Ask questions about depression, suicidal thoughts, and other risk factors associated with suicide during visits with adolescents.
11. Recommend that guns be removed from the home or, if present, that they be kept unloaded and that ammunition be stored and locked separately from guns.
12. Advise parents to limit their adolescents' viewing of violence in the media.
13. Provide counseling and other interventions/support to youth who have experienced or witnessed violence at home or in their neighborhoods.

REFERENCES AND ADDITIONAL READINGS

American Academy of Pediatrics, Committee on Injury, Violence, and Poison Prevention and Committee on Adolescence. The teen driver. *Pediatrics* 2006;118:2570.

American Academy of Pediatrics, Committee on Adolescence. Suicide and suicide attempts in adolescents. *Pediatrics* 2007;120:669.

National Center for Catastrophic Sports Injury Research. *Twenty-second Annual Report on Catastrophic Sports Injury Research: Fall 1982–Spring 2004.* Last updated June 2005. Available at: http://www.unc.edu/depts/nccsi/AllSport.htm.

National Center for Health Statistics. *Health, United States, 2006, with adolescent health chartbook.* Hyattsville, MD: 2006. Available at: http://www.cdc.gov/nchs/hus.htm.

CHAPTER 6

Nutrition

Michael R. Kohn

Growth in height and weight and changes in body composition are greater and more rapid during adolescence than at any other time in life except infancy. There is a significant change in the eating habits and food consumption of adolescents, and they have been found to have the highest prevalence of unsatisfactory nutrition.

Assessment of nutritional status and appropriate nutritional counseling should be part of health supervision visits. The MyPyramid Food Guide (www.MyPyramid.gov) is a helpful educational tool developed to promote dietary guidance and awareness of the health benefits to be gained from improvements in nutrition, physical activity and lifestyle (Fig. 6.1).

POTENTIAL NUTRITIONAL PROBLEMS

Risk Factors

Increased nutritional needs during adolescence are related to several factors: (1) adolescents gain 20% of their adult height and 50% of their adult skeletal mass. Therefore caloric and protein requirements and gender-specific nutrient needs are maximal during this period. (2) Adolescents engage in increased physical activity. (3) They tend to have poor eating habits, often including (a) missed meals; (b) high-sugar snacks of low nutritional value, (c) food choices depending on peer pressure, (d) poor eating habits and inadequate meal preparation within the family, (e) many meals and snacks obtained from vending machines or fast-food restaurants, and (f) inadequate financial resources to purchase food or prepare nutritious meals.

Other factors that influence nutritional needs during adolescence include level of activity, special diets (i.e., vegetarian), chronic illness, substance abuse, menstruation, and pregnancy and lactation.

NUTRITIONAL ASSESSMENT

Assessing the nutritional status of an adolescent should be part of a comprehensive health evaluation, especially in adolescents who are nutritionally at risk. Nutritional assessment requires repeated measurements of nutritional status over time. Methods used in this nutritional assessment include dietary and clinical evaluation, measurements of body composition, and laboratory data.

Anatomy of MyPyramid

One size doesn't fit all

USDA's new MyPyramid symbolizes a personalized approach to healthy eating and physical activity. The symbol has been designed to be simple. It has been developed to remind consumers to make healthy food choices and to be active every day. The different parts of the symbol are described below.

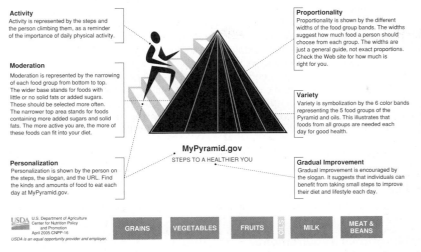

Activity
Activity is represented by the steps and the person climbing them, as a reminder of the importance of daily physical activity.

Moderation
Moderation is represented by the narrowing of each food group from bottom to top. The wider base stands for foods with little or no solid fats or added sugars. These should be selected more often. The narrower top area stands for foods containing more added sugars and solid fats. The more active you are, the more of these foods can fit into your diet.

Personalization
Personalization is shown by the person on the steps, the slogan, and the URL. Find the kinds and amounts of food to eat each day at MyPyramid.gov.

Proportionality
Proportionality is shown by the different widths of the food group bands. The widths suggest how much food a person should choose from each group. The widths are just a general guide, not exact proportions. Check the Web site for how much is right for you.

Variety
Variety is symbolization by the 6 color bands representing the 5 food groups of the Pyramid and oils. This illustrates that foods from all groups are needed each day for good health.

MyPyramid.gov
STEPS TO A HEALTHIER YOU

Gradual Improvement
Gradual improvement is encouraged by the slogan. It suggests that individuals can benefit from taking small steps to improve their diet and lifestyle each day.

USDA U.S. Department of Agriculture Center for Nutrition Policy and Promotion April 2005 CNPP-16
USDA is an equal opportunity provider and employer.

GRAINS   VEGETABLES   FRUITS   OILS   MILK   MEAT & BEANS

FIGURE 6.1   New USDA food pyramid. (From U.S. Department of Agriculture Center for Nutrition Policy and Promotion. www.mypyramid.gov. April 2005.)

Dietary Data

Dietary information can be obtained from a food record kept by the teenager, a dietary history obtained from a nutritionist, a 24-hour recall, or a diet questionnaire. Helpful screening questions include (1) How many diets have you been on in the past year? (2) Do you feel you should be dieting? (3) Do you feel dissatisfied with your body size? (4) Does your weight affect the way you feel about yourself?

Anthropometric Measurements

Weight. Weight is a short-term indicator of nutrition.

Height. Height is a long-term indicator of nutrition.

Body Mass Index (BMI). BMI is equal to the weight in kilograms divided by the square of the height in meters or BMI = kg/m^2. Weight, height, and BMI-for-age charts are available at www.cdc.gov/growthcharts/.

Skin Fold Measurements. Triceps skin fold measurement is helpful in evaluating the adipose tissue component and degree of obesity.

Waist-Hip Ratio (WHR). WHR is useful in young adults and is equal to the circumference of the waist divided by the circumference of the hips. A WHR >1.0 in adult men or 0.8 in adult women can predict complications from obesity independent of BMI.

Clinical Evaluation

1. Skin: *Pallor* (Iron deficiency), follicular hyperkeratosis (vitamin A deficiency or excess), xanthoma (hyperlipidemia), petechiae (vitamin C deficiency)
2. Eyes: Night blindness (vitamin A deficiency), angular palpebritis (riboflavin, niacin deficiencies)
3. Lips: Angular stomatitis, cheilosis (riboflavin, niacin deficiencies)
4. Tongue: Glossitis (niacin, folic acid, vitamin B12, or B6 deficiencies), papillary atrophy (riboflavin, niacin, folic acid, vitamin B12, or iron deficiencies), *loss of taste* (zinc deficiency).
5. Gums: Soft, spongy, or bleeding (vitamin C deficiency)
6. Teeth: Excessive dental caries (diet high in refined sugar)
7. Hair: Dry, dull, and brittle (protein-calorie malnutrition)
8. Nails: Brittle with frayed borders (malnutrition, iron or calcium deficiency), concave or eggshell (free edge curved sharply outward) (vitamin A deficiency)
9. Other signs of malnutrition: muscle wasting, delayed sexual maturation and growth, amenorrhea and hepatomegaly

Laboratory Tests

These should include hemoglobin, hematocrit, ferritin, serum protein and albumin.

Nutritional Requirements

Dietary Reference Intakes (DRIs) provide quantitative estimates of nutrients to plan and evaluate diets for healthy people. The DRIs consist of four nutrient reference values:

1. *Recommended Dietary Allowance (RDA)*: This is the dietary intake level that is sufficient to meet the nutrient requirements of almost all healthy individuals.
2. *Adequate Intake (AI):* This is the value based on observed or experimentally determined approximations of nutrient intake by a group—used when RDA cannot be determined.
3. *Estimated Average Requirement (EAR)*: The intake value estimated to meet the requirement defined by a specified indicator of adequacy in 50% of an age- and gender-specific group.
4. *Tolerable Upper Intake Level (UL)*: This is the maximum level of daily nutrient intake that is unlikely to pose risks of adverse health effects to most individuals.

The DRIs include these nutrients: (1) calcium, vitamin D, phosphorus, magnesium, and fluoride; (2) folate and other B vitamins; (3) antioxidants (e.g., vitamin C, vitamin E, selenium); (4) macronutrients (e.g. proteins, fats, carbohydrates); (5) trace elements (e.g., iron, zinc); (6) electrolytes and water, and (7) other food components (e.g., fiber, phytoestrogens).

Energy Requirements. Determined by basal metabolic rate, growth status, physical activity and body composition. Caloric intakes (Table 6.1) vary by body size and activity level.

Protein. Requirements are highest during peak height velocity. Most teens' diets exceed RDA for protein.

TABLE 6.1

Recommended Dietary Allowances for Adolescents

Category	Male (yr)			Female (yr)			Pregnancy	Lactating (first 6 mo)	Lactating (second 6 mo)
	11–14	15–18	19–24	11–14	15–18	19–24			
Weight (kg)	45	66	72	46	55	58			
Height (cm)	157	176	177	157	163	164			
Energy (cal)	2,500	3,000	2,900	2,200	2,200	2,200	+300	+500	+500
Protein (g)	45	59	58	46	44	46	60	65	62
Minerals									
Iron (mg/d)	12	12	10	15	15	15	30	15	15
Zinc (mg/d)	15	15	15	12	12	12	15	19	16
Iodine (μg/d)	150	150	150	150	150	150	175	200	200
Vitamins									
Vitamin A (IU)	10	10	10	10	10	10	10	10	10

Adapted from Food and Nutrition Board, National Research Council. *Recommended dietary allowances*, 10th ed. Washington, DC: National Academy Press, 1989.

Carbohydrates. the primary source of dietary energy. Carbohydrates should make up about 50% of daily caloric intake. No more than 10% to 25% of calories should come from sweeteners (sucrose/high fructose corn syrup). Alcohol provides 7 calories of energy per gram and can be a significant source of calories.

Fat. Adolescents require dietary fat and essential fatty acids for many vital functions. A teenager's diet should contain <30% of calories from fat. Most adolescents' total and saturated fat intake is greater than recommended.

Minerals
Iron. There is an increased need for iron during adolescence because of the rapid growth, increase in muscle mass, blood volume and increase iron because of menstrual losses in females.

Calcium. Calcium is important for attaining skeletal health, especially during adolescent growth and development. The DRI for calcium for 9- to 18-year-olds is 1,300 mg/day (Table 6.2). Many adolescents have inadequate calcium intakes, in part due to the substitution of carbonated beverages for milk; they may therefore need to take supplemental calcium (absorption varies from 25% to 35%). Optimal absorption of calcium supplements occurs when no more than 500 mg/dose is taken with food.

Zinc. Zinc is needed for adequate growth, sexual maturation, and wound healing. The RDA for zinc is age-dependent and ranges between 8 and 11 mg/day.

Vitamins. Vitamin requirements increase during adolescence.

GUIDELINES FOR NUTRITIONAL THERAPY

General Recommendations
1. Be aware of and sensitive to the family context, lifestyle and cultural milieu.
2. Reinforce the benefits of dietary and lifestyle changes.
3. Use the MyPyramid Food Guide (Fig. 6.1) to recommend the appropriate number of daily servings from each food group.
4. Recommend that teenagers participate in a regular exercise program.
5. Simplify good nutrition concepts.
6. Suggest that meals and snacks be eaten regularly.

Special Conditions
Vegetarians. Vegetarians (except for vegans) are likely to have an adequate nutritional intake.

Types of Vegetarians. (1) *Semivegetarians* eat milk products and limited seafood and poultry but no red meat. (2) *Lactovegetarians* consume milk products but no eggs, meat, fish, or poultry. (3) *Ovolactovegetarians* consume milk products and eggs but no meat, fish, or poultry. (4) *Vegans* consume vegetable foods only and no foods of animal origin (i.e., no eggs, milk products, meat, fish, or poultry). (5) *Fruitarians* consume raw fruit and seeds only.

TABLE 6.2

Recommended Dietary Allowances (Light Face Type) and Adequate Intake (Bold Face Type) Values, by Age

Daily Amount	Male (yr)			Female (yr)			Pregnant (yr)		Lactating (yr)	
	9–13	14–18	19–30	9–13	14–18	19–30	<19	19–30	<19	19–30
Calcium (mg)	1,300	1,300	1,000	1,300	1,300	1,000	1,300	1,000	1,300	1,000
Phosphorus (mg)	1,250	1,250	700	1,250	1,250	700	1,250	700	1,250	700
Magnesium (mg)	240	410	400	240	360	310	400	350	360	310
Fluoride (mg)	2	3	4	2	3	3	3	3	3	3
Selenium (pg)	40	55	55	40	55	55	60	60	70	70
Vitamin C (mg)	45	75	90	45	65	75	80	85	115	120
Vitamin D (μg)	5	5	5	5	5	5	5	5	5	5
Vitamin E (mg)	11	15	15	11	15	15	15	15	19	19
Thiamine (mg)	0.9	1.2	1.2	0.9	1.0	1.1	1.4	1.4	1.5	1.5
Riboflavin (mg)	0.9	1.3	1.3	0.9	1.0	1.1	1.4	1.4	1.6	1.6
Niacin (mg)	12	16	16	12	14	14	18	18	17	17
Vitamin B_6 (mg)	1.0	1.3	1.3	1.0	1.2	1.3	1.9	1.9	2.0	2.0
Folacin (μg)	300	400	400	300	400	400	600	600	500	500
Vitamin B_{12} (μg)	1.8	2.4	2.4	1.8	2.4	2.4	2.6	2.6	2.8	2.8
Pantothenic acid (B_5) (mg)	4	5	5	4	5	5	6	6	7	7
Biotin (μg)	20	25	30	20	25	30	30	30	35	35
Choline (mg)	375	550	550	375	550	550	450	450	550	550

Adapted from Food and Nutrition Board, National Academy of Sciences. U.S. Department of Agriculture. www.nalusda.gov/fnic/etext/000105.html. 1998.

Supplemental Needs of Vegetarians
Potential nutrition issues with vegetarian diets include macronutrient and micronutrient deficiencies such as protein, fat, vitamin B12, iron, zinc, calcium, and vitamin D.

Lactose Intolerance

Teens with lactose intolerance are at risk of inadequate calcium intake. Some adolescents can tolerate small amounts of milk products. Lactose-reduced dairy products and lactase enzyme replacement pills or liquid may be helpful.

Pregnancy

Energy requirements are greater for pregnant adolescents than for nonpregnant adolescents. Pregnant adolescents should not consume <2,000 kcal/day; in many cases their needs may be higher. The best gauge of adequate energy intake during pregnancy is satisfactory weight gain. Folate is essential and taking folic acid before (400 μg/day) and during (600 μg/day) early pregnancy can reduce the risk of spina bifida and other neural tube defects in infants. The calcium recommendation during pregnancy is 1,300 mg/day. A low dose vitamin-mineral supplement is recommended for pregnant adolescents. Pregnant teens should be counseled against dieting.

Athletes

Risk of Iron and Zinc Deficiency. Both male and female adolescent athletes are at risk for iron deficiency. For the athlete who is not anemic but has low iron stores (ferritin level <16 μg/L), 50 to 100 mg of elemental iron daily (ferrous gluconate 240 or 325 mg twice daily or ferrous sulfate 325 mg daily or twice daily) should be recommended. For the anemic athlete, 100 to 200 mg of elemental iron daily (ferrous gluconate 325 mg three times daily or ferrous sulfate 325 mg twice daily), should be given. Laboratory measurements should be repeated after 2 to 3 months to document response to therapy. Athletes with iron deficiency anemia may also be zinc-deficient.

Sodium and Potassium. Athletes need increased intakes of sodium and potassium. This requirement will generally be met as they increase their calorie intake.

Calories. Athletes who engage in 2 hours per day of heavy exercise need 800 to 1,700 extra calories per day.

Hydration. Attention must be given to hydration before and during activity.

Weight Restrictions. Avoid any major weight restriction during the adolescent growth spurt. Eating disorders are prevalent among athletes. The female athlete triad (amenorrhea, disordered eating, and osteoporosis) should be suspected in an athlete with secondary amenorrhea.

Carbohydrate Loading. Diets that are consistently high in carbohydrate are not recommended. An athlete may consider a high-carbohydrate, low-fat meal 3 to 6 hours before an event and an optional snack 1 to 2 hours before the event. Foods high in carbohydrates (60% to 70%) have also been recommended after competition to replace glycogen stores. However, a diet of 5,000 kcal/day that contains 45% carbohydrates is sufficient to restore muscle glycogen within 24 hours. An initial "depletion phase" consisting of vigorous workouts and low-carbohydrate eating before competition is no longer recommended.

Ergogenic Nutritional Supplements. Anecdotal reports (not proven) suggest that compounds such as bee pollen, caffeine, glycine, carnitine, lecithin, brewer's yeast, and gelatin may improve strength and endurance.

Teens should be aware that the long-term effects of using nutritional supplements have not been studied. Most athletes can maximize their performance through consistent, appropriate training and attention to adequate nutrition rather than relying on supplement use.

WEB SITES

For Health Professionals

http://www.mypyramid.gov. MyPyramid from USDA.
http://www.vrg.org. Vegetarian Resource Center.
http://www.americanheart.org. American Heart Association diets.
http://www.nutrition.org. American Society for Nutritional Sciences.
http://www.iom.edu/topic.asp?id=3708. Food and Nutrition Board home page.
http://www.drugfreesport.com/choices/supplements. Nutritional supplements, NCAA sponsored site.

CHAPTER 7

Understanding Legal Aspects of Care

Abigail English

The legal status of minors—younger than age 18 years in almost all states—differs from that of adults. For adolescents who are age 18 years or older, the governing laws are essentially the same as for other adults. The important legal issues in providing health care to adolescents who are minors are:

1. Consent: Who is authorized to give consent for the adolescent's care and whose consent is required?
2. Confidentiality: Who has the right to control the release of confidential information about the care, including medical records, and who has the right to receive such information?
3. Payment: Who is financially liable for payment and is there a source of insurance coverage or is public funding available that the adolescent can access?

LEGAL FRAMEWORK

Minors, like adults, have constitutional rights, although the scope of their respective rights differs. All states have statutes authorizing minors to give their own consent for health care in specific circumstances. Laws provide protection for the confidentiality of adolescents' health care information. The financing of health care services for all age groups and income levels affects adolescents' access to health care.

Constitutional Issues

The U.S. Supreme Court has held repeatedly that minors have constitutional rights in areas such as juvenile court due process, free speech, and privacy. The early cases established that the right of privacy protects minors as well as adults and encompasses minors' access to contraceptives and the abortion decision. Initially, the Supreme Court held that parents cannot exercise an arbitrary veto with respect to the abortion decisions of their minor daughters. However, in subsequent cases, the Court concluded that a state may enact a requirement of parental consent or notification for minors who are seeking abortions, but it must also, at minimum, establish an alternative procedure. This procedure would allow a minor to obtain authorization for an abortion without first notifying her parents by allowing her either to make her own decision if she is "mature" or to obtain a court order that an abortion would be in her best interests. As of February 2007, at least 34 states have laws in effect that require either the consent or notification of at least one parent. All of these states provides for a "judicial bypass" and several provide for consent or notification of an adult family member other than a parent. Some of these statutes are not being enforced because they have been enjoined by the courts.

State and Federal Laws

Most of the specific legal provisions that affect adolescents' access to health care are contained in state and federal statutes, regulations, and court decisions.

CONSENT

Consent of a parent is usually required before medical care can be provided to a minor. Exceptions allow someone other than a biological parent—a caretaker relative, foster parent, juvenile court, social worker, or probation officer—to give consent. In emergencies, care may be provided without prior consent to safeguard the life and health of the minor, with notice to parents as soon as possible thereafter. Numerous laws also authorize minors themselves to give consent for care, based on either the status of the minor or the services sought.

All states authorize minors to consent to one or more of the following services: pregnancy-related care; diagnosis and treatment of STDs, HIV/AIDS, and reportable or contagious diseases; examination and treatment related to sexual assault; counseling and treatment for drug or alcohol problems; and mental health treatment, particularly outpatient care. Some of the statutes contain age limits or other specific criteria.

All states also authorize one or more of the following groups of minors to give consent for their own health care: emancipated minors, those who are living apart from their parents, minors serving in the armed forces, married minors, minors who are the parents of a child, high school graduates, and minors who have attained a certain age, or "mature minors."

THE MATURE MINOR DOCTRINE AND INFORMED CONSENT

"Mature minors" may have the legal capacity to give consent for their own care. Unless a state has explicitly rejected the mature minor doctrine, there is little likelihood a practitioner will incur liability for failure to obtain parental consent provided that the minor is an older adolescent (typically at least age 15 years) who is capable of giving an informed consent and the care is not high risk, is for the minor's benefit, and is within the mainstream of established medical opinion. The basic criteria for determining whether a patient, including a minor patient, is capable of giving an informed consent are that the patient must be able to understand the risks and benefits of any proposed treatment or procedure and its alternatives and must be able to make a voluntary choice among the alternatives.

PRIVACY AND CONFIDENTIALITY

Confidentiality protections encourage adolescents to seek necessary care on a timely basis and to provide a candid and complete health history. They also support adolescents' growing sense of privacy and autonomy, keeping in mind that adolescents usually do share health information with their parents.

Laws and policies that protect confidentiality include federal and state constitutions; federal laws regarding medical privacy, Medicaid, family planning programs, and federal drug and alcohol programs; state laws regarding confidentiality, medical records, evidentiary privileges, professional licensing, and funding; court decisions; and professional ethical standards. The federal medical privacy regulations known as the Privacy Rule of the Health Insurance Portability and Accountability Act (HIPAA) are of critical importance. Confidentiality protections are rarely absolute, so practitioners should consider (1) What information *is* confidential (because it is considered private and is protected against disclosure)? (2) What information *is not* confidential (because such information is not protected)? (3) What *exceptions* are there in the confidentiality requirements? (4) What information can be released *with consent*? (5) What other mechanisms allow for *discretionary* disclosure without consent? (6) What *mandates* exist for reporting or disclosing confidential information?

In general, even confidential information may be disclosed as long as authorization is obtained from the patient or another appropriate person. Often, when minors have the legal right to consent to their own care, they also have the right to control disclosure of confidential information about that care. Sometimes, however, disclosure over the objection of the minor is required: if a specific law requires disclosure to parents; if a mandatory reporting obligation applies, as in the case of suspected physical or sexual abuse; or if the minor poses a severe danger to him or herself or to others.

When the minor does not have the legal right to consent to care or to control disclosure, the release of confidential information must generally be authorized by the minor's parent or the person (or entity) with legal custody or guardianship. Even when this is necessary, however, it is still advisable—from an ethical perspective—for the practitioner to seek the agreement of the minor to disclose confidential information and certainly, at minimum, to advise the minor at the outset of treatment of any limits to confidentiality. Confidentiality and disclosure issues often can be resolved by discussion and informal agreement between a physician, the adolescent patient, and the parents without reference to legal requirements.

The HIPAA Privacy Rule

Generally, the HIPAA Privacy Rule gives parents access to the health information of their unemancipated minor children, including adolescents. However, the rule specifies that "state and other applicable law" determines when parents may have access to protected health information for minors, who have consented to their own care and who therefore considered "individuals" under the rule.

Specifically, if state or other law explicitly requires information to be disclosed to a parent, HIPAA allows a health care provider to disclose the information. If state or other law explicitly permits but does not require information to be disclosed to a parent, HIPAA allows a health care provider to exercise discretion to disclose or not. If state or other law prohibits the disclosure of information to a parent without the consent of the minor, HIPAA does not allow a health care provider to disclose it without the minor's consent. If state or other law is silent or unclear on the question, an entity covered by the rule has discretion to determine whether or not to grant access to a parent to the protected health information as long as the determination is made by a health care professional exercising professional judgment.

PAYMENT

A source of payment is essential to ensure that adolescents have access to the health care they need. This is particularly critical for adolescents from low-income families or those who have no family to support them; it is even more critical when a young person needs confidential care.

Some of the state minor consent laws specify that if a minor is authorized to consent to care, it is the minor rather than the parent who is responsible for payment. In reality, however, few if any adolescents are able to pay for health care "out of pocket" unless there is a sliding fee scale with very minimal payments required.

Some federal and state health care funding programs enable minors to obtain confidential care with little or no cost to them. Most notable is the federal Title X Family Planning Program. However, these programs do not ensure access to comprehensive health services for teens, and health insurance coverage is therefore essential.

Adolescents are uninsured and underinsured at higher rates than other groups in the population, although young adults are uninsured at the very highest rates and those living below the poverty level are at the greatest risk for lacking health insurance. Medicaid and the State Children's Health Insurance Program (SCHIP) have been increasingly important in providing coverage for low-income adolescents and helping them obtain access to comprehensive care.

However, even when adolescents are covered by public or private insurance, they may be unable to access that coverage without the involvement of their parents. Thus, more than other age groups, they may be dependent for specific services on care that is provided at no cost or based on a sliding fee scale through federal- and state-funded programs.

It is only through a comprehensive understanding by practitioners of the legal framework for adolescent health services, including the relationships among consent, confidentiality, and payment issues, that adolescents' access to the health care they need can be ensured.

Note. A chart summarizing the minor consent provisions contained in the laws of all 50 states and the District of Columbia may be found on the website of the Center for Adolescent Health & the Law at www.cahl.org. The Alan Guttmacher Institute, (web site below), also has a chart with this information.

WEB SITES AND REFERENCES

http://www.cahl.org. Center for Adolescent Health & the Law.
http://www.healthlaw.org. National Health Law Program (NHeLP).
http://www.youthlaw.org/. National Center for Youth Law (NCYL).
http://www.healthprivacy.org. Health Privacy Project.
http://www.hhs.gov/ocr/hippa/. Office for Civil Rights (OCR) (re HIPAA Privacy Rule).

http://www.guttmacher.org. Guttmacher Institute.

http://www.familiesusa.org. Families USA.

http://www.aap.org. American Academy of Pediatrics.

http://www.adolescenthealth.org. Society for Adolescent Medicine.

English A. Financing adolescent health care: legal and policy issues for the coming decade. *J Adolesc Health* 2002:31(Suppl):334.

English A, Ford CA, The HIPAA privacy rule and adolescents: legal questions and clinical challenges. *Perspect Sexual Reprod Health* 2004;36:80.

English A, Kenney KE. *State minor consent laws: a summary,* 2nd ed. Chapel Hill, NC: Center for Adolescent Health & the Law, 2003.

Ford CA, English A. Limiting confidentiality of adolescent health services: what are the risks? *JAMA* 2002;288:752.

Morreale MC, Dowling EC, Stinnett AJ, eds. *Policy compendium on confidential health services for adolescents*, 2d ed. Chapel Hill, NC: Center for Adolescent Health & the Law, 2005.

Morreale MC, English A. Eligibility and enrollment of adolescents in Medicaid and SCHIP: recent progress, current challenges. *J Adolesc Health* 2003;32(Suppl):25.

Planned Parenthood Federation of America, Inc. Major U.S. Supreme Court Rulings on Reproductive Health and Rights (1965–2003). Available at http://www.ppfa.org/pp2/portal/files/portal/medicalinfo/abortion/fact-abortion-rulings.pdf.

Society for Adolescent Medicine. Confidential health care for adolescents: position paper. *J Adolesc Health*. 2004;35:160–167 (prepared by Ford CA, English A, Sigman G).

Disclaimer. Please note that this chapter does not represent legal advice. Health care practitioners are reminded that laws change and that statutes, regulations, and court decisions may be subject to differing interpretations. It is the responsibility of each health care professional to be familiar with the current relevant laws that affect the health care of adolescents. In difficult cases involving legal issues, advice should be sought from someone with state-specific expertise.

CHAPTER 8

Abnormal Growth and Development

Joan M. Mansfield and Lawrence S. Neinstein

Growth hormone and thyroid hormone are the primary hormonal determinants of growth during mid-childhood. This is followed by the adolescent growth spurt, which is caused by the hormones of puberty (estrogen and androgens). Growth hormone secretion increases during the pubertal growth spurt. As puberty progresses, estrogen causes epiphyseal fusion, with eventual termination of growth in height. In evaluating growth during adolescence, it is necessary to assess whether a teen has reached puberty, whether puberty is proceeding normally, and whether the epiphyses are still open.

SHORT STATURE WITHOUT DELAYED PUBERTY

Most hormonal deficiencies, chronic diseases, and malabsorptive states that slow growth will also cause some delay in or failure of normal progress through puberty. An adolescent should be considered for an evaluation of short stature (below the third percentile on a cross-sectional growth chart) if (1) the linear growth rate is <4 to 5 cm/year during the years prior to the normal age for peak linear growth velocity, (2) there is no evidence of a peak linear growth velocity by age 16 years in boys and 14 years in girls, (3) deceleration below an individual's established growth velocity occurs, (4) the adolescent's height is more than 2 standard deviations (SDs) below the calculated midparental height (see Chapter 1), or (5) the adolescent's height is more than 3 SDs below the mean.

Useful initial evaluations are:

1. A review of the growth chart
2. X-ray of the left hand and wrist for *bone age,* since this can determine whether there is potential for more growth and can be used to estimate predicted adult height.

3. Measure the parents' heights and calculate a *midparental height* (MPH). For girls,

MPH = [mother's height + (father's height − 13 cm or 5 inches)] / 2

For boys,

MPH = [(mother's height + 13 cm or 5 inches) − father's height] / 2

A height percentile consistent with the midparental height can still give a good clue that the short stature is genetic.

Intrauterine growth retardation may be associated with poor growth throughout childhood and short final height. There are some syndromes, such as Down syndrome, associated with marked short stature and normal timing of puberty. Deletion of a portion of the X chromosome can present with short stature, but normal puberty. A karyotype is sometimes useful in evaluating the extremely short child with normal puberty. Skeletal dysplasias such as hypochondroplasia also present with severe short stature and abnormally short extremities.

DELAYED PUBERTY

In general, 2 SDs above and below the mean are used to define the range of normal variability. Delayed development is defined by the absence of breast budding by age 13 in girls or lack of testicular enlargement by age 14 in boys. Alterations in the chronologic relationship of pubertal events include phallic enlargement in the absence of testicular enlargement in boys or the absence of menarche by age 16, or 4 years after the onset of breast development, in girls. If puberty is interrupted, there is a regression or failure to progress in the development of secondary sexual characteristics, accompanied by a slowing in growth. The challenge is to differentiate between constitutional delay of puberty and organic diseases such as chronic illness, nutritional insufficiency, tumor, or primary endocrinopathy associated with delayed development. Specific guidelines include the following:

MALES
1. Genital stage 1 (G1) persists >13.7 years, or pubic hair stage 1 (PH1) persists >15.1 years.
2. More than 5 years have elapsed from initiation to completion of genital growth.
3. The following SMRs persist past the listed guidelines:
   a. G2 >2.2 years PH2 >1.0 year
   b. G3 >1.6 years PH3 >0.5 year
   c. G4 >1.9 years PH4 >1.5 years

FEMALES
1. Breast stage 1 (B1) persists >13.4 years, PH1 persists >14.1 years, or there is failure to menstruate beyond the age of 16 years.
2. More than 5 years have elapsed between initiation of breast growth and menarche.
3. The following SMRs persist past the listed guidelines:

a. B2 >1.0 year PH2 >1.3 years
b. B3 >2.2 years PH3 >0.9 year
c. B4 >6.8 years PH4 >2.4 years

Delayed development occurs more commonly in boys. Most of these boys have constitutionally delayed development; however, the clinical presentation of the patient with constitutional delay may be indistinguishable from that of the patient with puberty delayed due to an organic lesion. Adolescents with constitutional delay of puberty have often been slow growers throughout childhood and have a family history of delayed development.

Functional Causes of Delayed Puberty

Secretion of gonadotropin-releasing hormone (GnRH) can be inhibited centrally by:

1. Inadequate nutrition (eating disorders, malabsorption, inflammatory bowel disease, celiac disease)
2. Chronic disease, (renal failure, renal tubular acidosis, cystic fibrosis, cyanotic congenital heart disease, thalassemia major, sickle cell disease, AIDS, severe asthma, or poorly controlled type 1 diabetes)
3. Severe environmental stress
4. Intensive athletic training
5. Hypothyroidism: Classic signs include slow growth and pubertal delay with dull, dry skin and perhaps with scalp hair loss, decrease in pulse rate and blood pressure, constipation, and cold intolerance. A goiter is not always present
6. Drugs [e.g., opiates, methylphenidate (Ritalin)]
7. Glucocorticoid excess (Cushing disease or exogenous)

Hypothalamic Causes of Delayed Puberty

The ability of the hypothalamus to secrete GnRH may be damaged by:

1. Local tumors, infiltrative lesions [e.g., central nervous system (CNS) leukemia or histiocytosis X]
2. CNS irradiation, traumatic gliosis, or mass lesions such as brain abcesses or granulomas
3. Congenital defects in the ability to secrete GnRH (idiopathic hypogonadotropic hypogonadism) may be associated with midline craniofacial defects or olfactory defects (Kallmann syndrome) and may be familial. There are several syndromes characterized by extreme obesity, short stature, and delayed puberty. These include Prader Willi and Lawrence-Moon-Bardet-Biedel syndromes.

Pituitary Causes of Delayed Puberty

Puberty may not begin or may fail to proceed if the pituitary cannot respond to GnRH stimulation with LH and FSH production. This may be due to a pituitary tumor, selective impairment of gonadotrope function by hemochromatosis, or congenital or acquired hypopituitarism. Excessive prolactin production by a prolactinoma or other tumor may interrupt or prevent puberty. Patients with prolactinomas may present with stalled puberty. Prolactinomas are more common in girls than boys. Psychotropic drugs such as antipsychotics are a frequent cause of hyperprolactinemia. Patients with significantly elevated prolactin levels should have a cranial examination by magnetic resonance imaging (MRI) with contrast. Prolactinomas can be treated medically with cabergoline or bromocriptine.

Gonadal Failure

The most common cause of gonadal failure is *gonadal dysgenesis*, which occurs in association with abnormalities of sex chromosomes. These patients are phenotypic females with immature female genitalia. The most common phenotype is *Turner syndrome,* which is caused by absence of part or all of a second sex chromosome. Pure gonadal dysgenesis presents as absent puberty in patients with a normal karyotype (46,XX or XY), normal stature, and a female phenotype. Males with *Klinefelter syndrome* (47,XXY) may present with poorly progressing puberty. In the 47,XXY patient with pubertal development, the testes become small and fibrotic. Gynecomastia and eunuchoid body habitus are often seen.

The causes of gonadal failure with normal karyotype include (1) autoimmune oophoritis or orchitis (sometimes with multiple autoimmune endocrine abnormalities); (2) radiation or chemotherapy (e.g., agents such as cyclophosphamide); (3) viral or tubercular orchitis or oophoritis; (4) resistant ovary syndrome; (5) gonadal failure associated with other diseases such as congenital galactosemia in girls, ataxia telangiectasia, or sarcoidosis (Fragile X may present as secondary amenorrhea in females with ovarian failure); and (6) enzymatic defects that render the gonad unable to produce estrogens or androgens are other rare causes of primary gonadal failure. In males who are cryptorchid, the testes may fail to function. Bilateral testicular torsion resulting in anorchia is another cause of gonadal failure in males.

Complete androgen insensitivity presents as a phenotypic female with tall stature, absence of sexual hair, normal breast development and timing of puberty, but absence of menarche. The vagina is a short pouch and there is no uterus. The karyotype is 46XY, and testosterone levels are elevated. Patients who have congenital absence of the uterus and upper vagina have normal female puberty but do not have menarche.

WORKUP OF DELAYED PUBERTY

History

A detailed history and physical examination will minimize the laboratory testing needed to evaluate the adolescent. The past medical history should focus on history of chronic disease, congenital anomalies, previous surgery, radiation exposure, chemotherapy, or drug use.

Growth charts are important in evaluating the adolescent with delayed puberty. The child whose delayed puberty is associated with a nutritional deficiency due to an eating disorder, inflammatory bowel disease, or celiac disease is usually underweight for height. In contrast, the child who has delayed puberty on the basis of an endocrinopathy, such as acquired hypothyroidism, is often mildly overweight.

In the review of systems, special attention should be paid to weight changes, dieting, environmental stress, exercise and athletics, gastrointestinal symptoms, headache, neurologic symptoms, and symptoms of hypothyroidism. Family history should include the heights and timing of puberty of family members, history of anosmia, and history of endocrine disorders.

Physical Examination

1. *Measurements of height, weight, and vital signs.* Arm span and ratio of upper to lower segment (measure symphysis pubis to floor for lower, subtract lower from total height for upper), can be useful for patients who have either short extremities (short bone syndromes, congenital short stature syndromes) or long extremities. The normal U/L ratio is 1.7 at birth, 1.0 at age 10 years, and 0.9 to 1.0 in adulthood in whites and 0.85 to 0.9 in African Americans.
2. A search should be made for *congenital anomalies*, including midline facial defects.
3. The patient should be examined for *secondary sexual development,* which may be quantified by Tanner staging of the breasts and pubic hair in girls and genitalia and pubic hair in boys. In boys, measurements of the testicular volume are useful in assessing the presence and progression of sexual development. Pubic hair may be present, although the genitalia are prepubertal in a boy who had normal adrenarche but lacks gonadal activation. Any evidence of abnormal sexual development, such as clitoromegaly or hirsutism in girls or gynecomastia in boys, should be noted.
4. *External genitalia*: The examination of the external genitalia in girls should focus on obvious congenital anomalies and assessment of estrogen effect. A pale pink vaginal mucosa with white secretions indicates the presence of estrogen. A pelvic examination is not necessary as a part of the initial evaluation of a girl with delayed pubertal development, but should be done if possible to rule out gynecologic congenital anomalies in a girl who has normal pubertal development but delayed menarche. The pelvic exam should be carried out by a practitioner who is familiar with the techniques for examining teen girls who are not sexually active.
5. *Neurologic examination* should include a fundal exam, visual fields by confrontation, and olfactory testing if appropriate.

Laboratory Tests

The most useful initial examination in delayed puberty and slow growth is often an x-ray of the left hand and wrist for *bone age assessment*. This information can be used to assess how much potential for height growth remains in the patient with short stature and delayed development. A *predicted adult height* can be obtained using the Bayley-Pinneau tables in the *Atlas of Skeletal Maturation* by Gruelich and Pyle. The bone ages of patients with growth hormone deficiency or hypothyroidism are usually delayed several years behind their chronological ages. Table 8.1 describes the typical relationships between bone age, height age, and chronological age for various causes of delayed puberty or short stature.

Laboratory evaluation should be focused according to the clinical impression. In the patient who is underweight for height, studies would include screening tests for chronic disease or malabsorptive states such as celiac disease. Initial laboratory studies to be considered in the adolescent with delayed puberty include:

TABLE 8.1

Typical Relationships between Bone Age, Height Age, and Chronological Age for Causes of Delayed Puberty or Short Stature

Cause of Delayed Puberty or Short Stature	Relationship between Bone Age (BA), Chronological Age (CA), and Height Age (HA)
Genetic	HA < BA = CA
Skeletal dysplasia	HA ≤ BA <CA or BA < HA < CA
Constitutional	HA = BA < CA
Hypopituitarism	HA ≤ BA < CA
Hypothyroidism	BA < HA < CA
Hypogonadism	BA ≤ HA < CA
Systemic illness	BA = HA < CA

1. Complete blood cell count, erythrocyte sedimentation rate, electrolytes, BUN, creatinine, and urinalysis. Evaluation for celiac disease (anti–tissue transglutaminase and total IgA, or celiac panel).
2. Thyroid function tests, prolactin, LH and FSH, dehydroepiandrosterone sulfate, testosterone or estradiol, and insulin-like growth factor 1 (IGF-1) and insulin-like growth factor–binding protein 3 (IGFBP-3). Growth hormone is secreted primarily during sleep, so daytime levels are usually low. Insulin growth factor I (IGF-1) and IGFBP-3 are used to assess growth hormone sufficiency. Patients with delayed puberty and slow growth often have temporarily decreased growth hormone secretion due to pubertal delay, which increases to normal as puberty begins. If growth hormone deficiency is suspected, the patient should be referred to a pediatric endocrinologist.
3. *Hormonal tests*: Daytime early to midpubertal (Tanner breast stage 2) LH and FSH concentrations are indistinguishable from prepubertal levels, usually with a very low LH and FSH higher than LH. In the early stages (Tanner stage 2) of puberty, breast budding and vaginal maturation in girls and penile and testicular enlargement in boys are more sensitive indicators of pubertal neuroendocrine-gonadal function than a single daytime measurement of LH and FSH levels estradiol or testosterone. Testosterone or estradiol levels may be valuable in following the patient whose puberty is not progressing normally by clinical assessment of growth and secondary sexual development.

   Elevated *LH and FSH levels* are suggestive of primary gonadal failure. If LH and FSH levels are elevated, further laboratory evaluation would include blood karyotyping. *Pelvic ultrasound* may be used to visualize the uterus and ovaries, but should be interpreted with caution, since the prepubertal uterus is small and may be missed on ultrasound.
4. MRI: If there is a suspicion of a central nervous system tumor, cranial magnetic imaging with contrast is the best way to evaluate the hypothalamus and pituitary.

The chief diagnostic challenge in the patient with pubertal delay is to distinguish between constitutional delay and true GnRH deficiency. No single test

TABLE 8.2

Criteria for Provisional Diagnosis of Constitutional Delay of Puberty

Required features
　Detailed negative review of systems
　Evidence of appropriate nutrition
　Linear growth of at least 3.7 cm/yr
　Normal findings on physical examination, including genital anatomy,
　　sense of smell, and U/L body-segment ratio
　Normal CBC, sedimentation rate, urinalysis results, adjusted T_4 concen-
　　tration, and noncastrate levels of serum LH and FSH
　Bone age delayed 1.5–4.0 yr compared with chronological age
Supportive features
　Family history of constitutional delay of puberty
　Height between 3rd and 25th percentiles for chronological age

　U/L, upper-to-lower; CBC, complete blood cell; LH, luteinizing hormone; FSH,
follicle-stimulating hormone.
　From Barnes HV. Recognizing normal and abnormal growth and development
during puberty. In: Moss AV, ed. *Pediatrics update: reviews for physicians*. New York:
Elsevier–North Holland Publishing, 1979:103, with permission.

reliably separates patients with constitutional delay from those with idiopathic
hypogonadotropic hypogonadism. This diagnosis is made by excluding the
other causes and using the guidelines in Table 8.2.

MANAGEMENT OF DELAYED PUBERTY

Prior to age 14 years in girls and age 16 years in boys, if there is no evidence
of an underlying disease or neurologic abnormality and the initial evaluation
reveals prepubertal hormone levels, the adolescent can be seen at 6 month intervals for measurements of growth, assessment of pubertal status by physical
examination, and reassurance if progression of secondary sexual development
is evident. After the first signs of testicular or breast enlargement are observed,
follow-up at regular intervals is desirable to reassure the patient and parents
that puberty is progressing.

　If the evaluation reveals *primary gonadal failure,* cyclic estrogen and progestin therapy in girls or testosterone therapy in boys will be necessary. Adolescents with *hypogonadotropic hypogonadism or hypopituitarism* will also need
estrogen or testosterone replacement, often with replacement of other hormones as well. Short courses of estrogen or testosterone can also to be used to
initiate development in *constitutional delay of puberty* if there is no sign of development by age 14 in girls or 15 in boys. Many patients with delayed puberty
have decreased bone density for age. The optimal dose of estrogen replacement for increasing bone density in adolescents is higher than in menopausal
women. The importance of appropriate calcium (1300 mg /day) intake by diet
or supplements, and provision of at least 400 IU vitamin D to support bone
calcification should be stressed.

In boys with constitutional delay of puberty, 3 to 6 month courses of testosterone 1% gel or intramuscular testosterone enanthate cypionate can be used to initiate secondary sexual development. Since sex steroids cause fusion of epiphyses, care must be taken in the timing and monitoring of these therapies so that final height is not compromised. These patients should therefore be referred to an endocrinologist . Males with gonadal failure, hypopituitarism, or hypothalamic hypogonadism are maintained on long-term testosterone replacement using testosterone gel. They should receive dietary adequate calcium and vitamin D and should have DXA scans for spinal and hip bone density measurements.

Treatment of Short Stature with Growth Hormone

Patients with growth hormone deficiency usually present with extreme short stature and slow growth (<4 cm per year) well before adolescence, although acquired growth hormone deficiency (e.g., due to head trauma) may present in adolescence. Growth hormone stimulation testing is usually done by a pediatric endocrinologist.

Growth hormone has been used to increase height velocity and increase final adult height in patients who do not have growth hormone deficiency by growth hormone stimulation tests. Growth hormone is approved for use in patients with short stature due to Turner syndrome. Growth hormone treatment should ideally be initiated early in childhood, when growth rate begins to fall off.

PRECOCIOUS PUBERTY

In boys, development under age 9 years is considered precocious and is rare. There is controversy over the definition of precocious puberty in North American girls. In girls, the cutoff has traditionally been 8 years, but recent data suggest that the age threshold for this definition should be set at a younger age: breast or pubic hair under age 7 in white and under age 6 years in African-American girls. Girls who have both pubic hair and breast development at ages 7 to 8, should have at least a measurement of bone age for height prediction, a review of growth and history, and consideration of further testing. Girls with rapid progression or unusual progression of puberty—a predicted height under 150 cm or <2 SDs below target MPH, those with neurological symptoms, or girls who are having psychological difficulty owing to early puberty should be referred for further evaluation and consideration of possible suppression of puberty with GnRH analog therapy.

The vast majority of girls with central precocious puberty have idiopathic precocious puberty. Boys are much more likely to have a specific lesion (e.g., CNS tumor, malformation, damage, or infiltration) causing their precocity. Other causes include ovarian cysts (e.g., in McCune-Albright syndrome), ovarian or adrenal estrogen-secreting tumors, severe hypothyroidism, or exposure to exogenous estrogen. In boys, in addition to the central causes listed above, causes include androgen exposure, congenital adrenal hyperplasia, gonadal and adrenal tumors secreting androgens, and familial activating mutations of the LH receptor.

Incomplete Forms of Precocious Puberty

Self-limited (transient) breast budding usually occurs in girls from age 6 and up. There is no sustained growth spurt or bone age advancement in these girls. Benign premature adrenarche presents with underarm odor, and pubic and axillary hair development in children of age 6 to 8 years. Bone age is often slightly advanced and adrenal androgens are in the pubertal range. Twenty percent of the girls with benign premature adrenarche will go on to develop polycystic ovary syndrome as teens. Virilization in girls is rare and can be due to an androgen-secreting adrenal or ovarian tumor, topical androgen exposure, or congenital adrenal hyperplasia. Signs of virilization include rapid growth and bone age advancement, deepening of the voice, clitoromegaly, or muscular development.

EVALUATION OF PRECOCIOUS PUBERTY

History. History includes a review of family history of endocrine or pubertal disorders, timing of puberty in family members, use of estrogen- or androgen-containing gels by family members, and heights of family members. The growth chart should be obtained.

Physical Examination. The physical exam includes measurement of height and weight, vital signs, skin examination for large irregular café au lait spots (suggestive of McCune-Albright syndrome), fundoscopic examination, assessment for thyroid enlargement, abdominal exam, Tanner staging (measurement of breast or testicular dimensions and pubic hair assessment). The vaginal introitus can be examined for signs of estrogen effect on the labia minora and presence of leukorrhea in the frog-leg position. Internal examination is not necessary unless unexplained vaginal bleeding is present, in which case an experienced observer can often visualize the vagina and cervix in the knee chest position without instrumentation. In boys, the testicular exam should focus on any testicular asymmetry, masses, or phallic enlargement without testicular enlargement, suggesting a source of androgens outside of the testes (e.g., congenital adrenal hyperplasia).

Laboratory Evaluation. A bone age x-ray of the left hand and wrist is useful (Fig. 8.1). If the bone age is 2 years advanced, more evaluation is usually indicated.

Laboratory evaluation might include serum LH, FSH, estradiol, DHEAS, and TSH in girls; in boys, it might include testosterone and 8 A.M. 17-OH-progesterone, DHEAS, β-hCG, LH, and FSH. LH and FSH will be in the prepubertal range (LH less than FSH) in the early stages of central puberty. By the time of Tanner 3 breast or gonadal development, LH and FSH are often pubertal. If estradiol is markedly elevated and LH and FSH are suppressed, an ovarian cyst or, rarely, tumor is suspected. A pelvic ultrasound will confirm. In boys, a β-hCG should be measured to rule out a β-hCG–producing tumor causing testosterone production. A cranial MRI scan with contrast should be ordered to rule out a CNS lesion in all boys with central precocious puberty and in girls under age 6; it should be considered in girls between 6 and 8 years of age depending on the history. An ACTH stimulation test may be needed if congenital adrenal hyperplasia is suspected.

Treatment. If the evaluation has not revealed a specific cause and the child has central precocious puberty, GnRH analog treatment such as depot

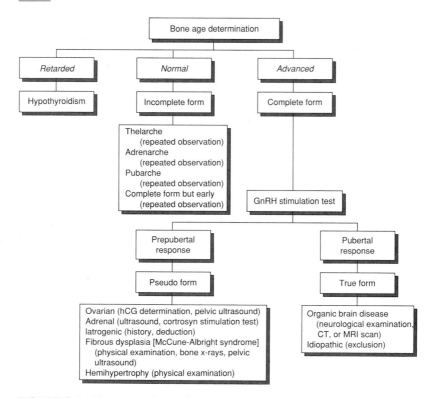

FIGURE 8.1   Flow sheet for evaluation of isosexual precocious puberty. MRI, magnetic resonance imaging. (Adapted from Brenner PE. Precocious puberty in the female. In: Mishell DR, Davajan VC, eds. *Reproductive endocrinology, infertility, and contraception.* © 1979 by FA Davis Co.)

leuprolide should be considered. Most girls in the 7- to 9-year range do not require treatment for suppression of puberty. Often parents are most worried about how they will handle menses in a grade school child. In most cases they can be reassured that menarche is not imminent and that it can be suppressed if necessary by treatment with a GnRH analog. Untreated girls should be followed at 6- to 12-month intervals. If the child has an initial predicted adult height <62 in. (157 cm), bone age measurement may have to be repeated in 6 to 12 months, since the predicted height can decline with rapid bone age advancement.

WEB SITES AND REFERENCES

http://www.magicfoundation.org. Magic Foundation with information about growth disorders and brochures about many disorders.
http://www.hgfound.org. Human Growth Foundation Web site with information and support for children and adults with growth disorders.

http://www.keepkidshealthy.com/welcome/conditions/delayed_puberty.html. Information from keepkidshealthy on delayed puberty.

http://tumers.nichd.nih.gov/ClinFrInfro.html. Information about Turner syndrome from the National Institutes of Health.

http://www.toosoon.com. Information from Lupron Association on precocious puberty.

http://humatrope.com. Information from Lilly on GH.

Bailey N, Pinneau SR. Tables for predicting adult height from skeletal age: revised for use with the Gruelich and Pyle hand standard. *J Pediatr* 1952;40:423.

Herman-Giddens ME, Slora EJ, Wasserman RD, et al. Secondary sexual characteristics and menses in young girls seen in office practice: a study from the pediatric research in office settings network. *Pediatrics* 1997;99:505.

Kaplowitz P, Oberfield S. Reexamination of the age limit for defining when puberty is precocious in girls in the United States: implications for evaluation and treatment. *Pediatrics* 1999;104:936.

Sun SS, Schubert CM, Chumlea WC, et al. National estimates of timing of sexual maturation and racial differences among US children. *Pediatrics* 2002;110:911.

Sybert VP, McCauley E. Turner's syndrome. *N Engl J Med* 2004;351:1227.

Wilson TA, Rose SR, Cohen P, et al. Update of guidelines for the use of growth hormone in children: the Lawson Wilkins Pediatric Endocrinology Society Drug And Therapeutics Committee. *J Pediatr* 2003;143:415.

Wu T, Mendola P, Buck GM. Differences in the presence of secondary sex characteristics and menarche amoung US girls: the third National Health and Nutrition examination survery, 1988–1994. *Pediatrics* 2002;110(4):752.

CHAPTER 9

Thyroid Disease in Adolescents

Stephen Albert Huang and Lawrence S. Neinstein

The prevalence of thyroid abnormalities in teens 11 to 18 years of age is about 3.7%, with more females than males affected. This chapter covers common thyroid problems in adolescence.

CLINICAL EVALUATION FOR THYROID DISEASE

History. Including (1) family history of goiter, thyroiditis, other thyroid problems, or other autoimmune disease; (2) symptoms of fever, thyroid swelling or pain; (3) drug history (use of goitrogens, including lithium, iodine excess, or anticonvulsants), (4) exposure to radiation; (5) pubertal and menstrual history; (6) change in weight; (7) growth problems; (8) change in behavior, sleep pattern, activity level, or function in school; (9) change in bowel habits

Physical Examination. Including (1) height, weight, BMI; (2) pulse, blood pressure; (3) skin texture or lesions; (4) presence of tremor; (5) eye examination (presence of exophthalmos or lid lag); (6) deep tendon reflexes—normal or delayed relaxation phase; (7) thyroid examination

Examination of the Thyroid. The normal thyroid is bilobed and connected by an isthmus that overlies the tracheal cartilages. The main lobes are usually equal in size, but the right lobe tends to enlarge to a greater degree in patients with diffuse thyromegaly. Examination of the thyroid is best performed with the patient seated and the neck in moderate extension. Inspect, and then palpate the gland and cervical and supraclavicular lymph nodes. Because the thyroid is ensheathed in the pretracheal fascia, it moves on swallowing, a critical feature in the differentiation of thyroid tissue. Provide a cup of water during palpation.

Thyroid Tests. In euthyroid individuals, 99.98% of serum thyroxine (T4) and 99.7% of serum triiodothyronine (T3) is bound to serum protein (mostly thyroxine-binding globulin, or TBG) and is biologically inactive. Total thyroid hormone concentrations can be abnormal not only in persons with thyroid dysfunction but also in individuals with abnormal binding due to factors that alter the concentration of TBGs (e.g., oral contraceptive pills, pregnancy, heredity, heroin, methadone, liver disease, androgens, nephrosis, acromegaly, high-dose steroids) or affinity of TBG (e.g., salicylates, furosemide, mefenamic acid,

TABLE 9.1

Thyroid Function Tests in Patients with Thyroid Dysfunction

	Serum TSH	Free T4 (or free T4 index)	Free T3 (or free T3 index)
Euthyroid	Normal	Normal	Normal
Primary hypothyroidism	High	Normal or low	Normal or low
Central hypothyroidism	Low/normal/ high	Low	Normal or low
Thyrotoxicosis	Low	Normal or high	Normal or high
Inappropriate TSH secretion	Normal or high	High	High

heparin, phenytoin, barbital). This issue can be resolved by measuring a serum free T4 (or free T3) or a free T4 index (FT4I). For most patients, the simultaneous measurement of serum TSH and free T4 (or FT4I) is sufficient to diagnosis thyroid dysfunction or to rule it out (Table 9.1).

Serum Thyroid Function Tests. These would include serum total T4, adjusted T4 or free T4 index, serum free T4, and serum total T3. Serum T3 can be useful in the rare thyrotoxic patient with a low serum TSH, but a normal serum free T4. In addition, serum TSH is useful, as modern TSH assays are sufficiently sensitive to detect the suppressed TSH concentrations associated with hyperthyroidism. TSH is the most sensitive test for diagnosing primary thyroid hypothyroidism (high TSH) or thyrotoxicosis (low TSH, usually <0.1 μU/mL).

Thyroid Antibodies. Titers of antithyroglobulin and anti-thyroid peroxidase (anti-TPO, sometimes also called antimicrosomal) antibodies are elevated in most patients with Hashimoto thyroiditis. Antimicrosomal antibodies have about 99% sensitivity, compared with 36% for antithyroglobulin antibodies. Titers of thyroid-stimulating immunoglobulin (TSI) and other TSH-receptor antibodies are typically elevated in Graves' disease and can be used for diagnosis and monitoring of the disease.

Thyroid Radioiodine Uptake (RAIU). A measurement of thyroidal uptake of radioactive iodine. Iodine123 is preferred because of the lower radiation dose. The chief value of this test is in the differential diagnosis of thyrotoxicosis.

Thyroid Scan. A thyroid scan evaluates thyroid anatomy and function. It can be useful in the differential diagnosis of thyroid nodules and in the identification of ectopic thyroid tissue. Iodine-123 is the preferred radionuclide.

THYROMEGALY

Causes. Diffuse thyromegaly/thyroiditis (autoimmune thyroid disease, classic Hashimoto thyroiditis, Graves disease); painless sporadic thyroiditis, postpartum thyroiditis, painful subacute); environmental goitrogens (iodine deficiency, medications such as thionamides and lithium); familial goiter, idiopathic thyromegaly, nodular thyromegaly; hypofunctioning and hyperfunctioning thyroid nodules

Clinical Presentation. Thyromegaly often occurs in combination with thyroid dysfunction, and such patients typically present with hypothyroid or thyrotoxic symptoms. Symptoms related to the compression/displacement of the trachea (stridor), esophagus (dysphagia), or recurrent laryngeal nerve (hoarseness) are unusual and generally limited to rare individuals with very large and rapidly growing goiters. Painful subacute thyroiditis can present with thyroid pain or tenderness, sometimes preceded by symptoms of fever or upper respiratory infection.

Evaluation. Although some goiters are idiopathic, thyromegaly requires an investigation for underlying pathology. Ultrasonography can accurately estimate thyroid size and can also be used to evaluate potential nodules. Because the most common causes of goiter are associated with thyroid dysfunction, thyroid function tests should be obtained with thyromegaly and monitored every 4 to 6 months.

Therapy. The management of nodular thyromegaly focuses on the evaluation for possible malignancy (hypofunctioning nodules) or hyperthyroidism (hyperfunctioning nodules). If thyroid dysfunction is present, it should be treated. Since many teenagers remain euthyroid for years and spontaneous resolution is possible, specialists are divided between close observation without treatment versus the use of exogenous levothyroxine (titrated to a low normal serum TSH concentration of 0.2 to 0.3 μU/mL).

HYPOTHYROIDISM

Causes. Most congenital hypothyroidism is permanent and requires lifelong replacement therapy. Outside of the newborn period, acquired hypothyroidism is usually due to autoimmune thyroiditis. Pediatric autoimmune thyroiditis peaks in early to midpuberty, with a female preponderance of 2 to 1. Improvements in measuring circulating autoantibodies have obviated the need for biopsy in the diagnosis of autoimmune thyroid disease. Thyroiditis is defined as evidence of "intrathyroidal lymphocytic infiltration," with or without follicular damage. Two types of chronic autoimmune thyroiditis (also known as chronic lymphocytic thyroiditis) are causes of persistent hypothyroidism: Hashimoto disease (goitrous form, type 2A) and atrophic thyroiditis (nongoitrous form, type 2B).

Clinical Presentation. The presentation of chronic autoimmune thyroiditis includes hypothyroidism, goiter, or both. Symptoms may be subtle, even with marked biochemical derangement. Growth and pubertal development may be delayed. Growth is usually compromised to a greater degree than weight gain, and the bone age is delayed.

Evaluation

1. *TSH and free T4.* Serum TSH concentration is elevated in primary hypothyroidism. If the differential diagnosis includes central hypothyroidism or if the

overall suspicion for hypothyroidism is high, a free T4 measurement should be included (Table 9.1). In mild hypothyroidism, serum T3 remains normal due to the increased peripheral conversion of T4 to T3 and the preferential secretion of T3 by the gland; therefore, measurement of serum T3 is not useful in the diagnosis or monitoring of patients with primary hypothyroidism.

2. *Antithyroid antibodies.* The presence of goiter or elevated TSH values should prompt the measurement of anti-TPO antibodies to confirm the diagnosis of chronic autoimmune thyroiditis. Anti-TPO antibodies are the most sensitive screen for chronic autoimmune thyroiditis. Anti-thyroglobulin antibodies may be added if anti-TPO titers are negative. If antithyroid antibodies are absent, less common etiologies of primary hypothyroidism—such as transient hypothyroidism (post–subacute thyroiditis), external irradiation, and consumptive hypothyroidism—should be considered.

3. *Evaluation after biochemical hypothyroidism is confirmed.* The initial history should evaluate energy level, sleep pattern, menses, cold intolerance, and school performance. In addition to palpation of the thyroid, the health care provider should assess the extraocular movements, fluid status, and deep tendon reflexes. Chronic autoimmune thyroiditis may be the initial presentation of an autoimmune polyglandular syndrome; the possibility of coexisting autoimmune diseases such as type 1 diabetes, Addison disease, and pernicious anemia must be addressed by the history.

Therapy

Initiation. Some experts advocate a graded approach to initiation of therapy. Alternatively, a starting dose can be estimated based on age and ideal body weight. Average daily requirements approximate 2 to 4 μg/kg in 10- to 15-year-olds and 1.6 μg/kg during adulthood (average maintenance is between 50 and 200 μg), but dosing must be individualized on the basis of biochemical monitoring.

Response to Levothyroxine and Monitoring. TSH normalization is the goal of replacement; aim for a target range of 0.5 to 3 μU/mL. Thyroid function tests should be obtained 6 weeks after the initiation or adjustment of dosage. Once biochemical euthyroidism has been achieved, TSH can be monitored every 4 to 6 months in the growing teen and yearly once linear growth is complete. A variety of conditions or drugs may alter levothyroxine requirements (Table 9.2).

Side Effects. Although rare, case reports have described the development of pseudotumor cerebri around the initiation of levothyroxine. A temporary reduction in the levothyroxine dose is appropriate to consider in this situation. Reactions to specific dyes or binders can be addressed by switching the levothyroxine preparation and/or manufacturer.

Subclinical Hypothyroidism. This is defined as TSH elevation with normal serum free T4. The majority of patients are asymptomatic; there is debate as to the need for treatment. Because studies in adults suggest that individuals with the combined risk factors of hyperthyrotropinemia and positive thyroid antibodies are at risk for progression to overt hypothyroidism, it is common to recommend thyroid hormone replacement in patients with persistent TSH values >10 μU/mL or with TSH values >5 μU/mL in combination with goiter or thyroid autoantibodies.

TABLE 9.2

Conditions that Increase Levothyroxine Requirements

Pregnancy

Gastrointestinal disease	Mucosal diseases of the small bowel (e.g., sprue) Jejunoileal bypass and small bowel resection Diabetic diarrhea
Drugs which impair L-T$_4$ absorption	Cholestyramine Sucralfate Aluminum hydroxide Calcium carbonate Ferrous sulfate
Drugs which may enhance CYP3A4 and thereby accelerate levothyroxine clearance	Rifampin Carbamazepine Estrogen Phenytoin Sertraline Statins
Drug which impairs T$_4$ to T$_3$ conversion	Amiodarone
Conditions which may block type 1 deiodinase	Selenium deficiency Cirrhosis

Adapted from Larsen PR. Hypothyroidisim and thyroiditis. In: Larsen PR, Melmed S, Polonsky KS, eds. *Williams textbook of endocrinology,* 10th ed. Philadelphia: WB Saunders, 2003.

Pregnancy. Levothyroxine requirements increase during gestation. Untreated maternal hypothyroidism may adversely affect the intellectual development of the fetus. A TSH should be checked if pregnancy is diagnosed and frequency of monitoring increased. Young women who are treated for hypothyroidism and are euthyroid on replacement can be advised to increase their prepregnancy dose empirically by taking two extra daily doses each week (a 29% increase) beginning the week pregnancy is confirmed. They should then undergo thyroid function testing and obtain professional guidance promptly.

HYPERTHYROIDISM AND THYROTOXICOSIS

Causes of Thyrotoxicosis and Hyperthyroidism

Common. Graves' disease is the most common cause of hyperthyroidism in the United States, with a prevalence increasing in adolescent and young adult females and peaking at about age 25 years. Graves' hyperthyroidism is caused by thyroid-stimulating antibodies that bind and activate the thyrotropin receptor, leading to thyromegaly and the hypersecretion of thyroid hormone. Lymphocytic infiltration and the accumulation of glycosaminoglycans in the orbital connective tissue and skin cause the extrathyroidal manifestations of Graves' ophthalmopathy and dermopathy.

Uncommon. Transient thyrotoxicosis due to the release of preformed thyroid hormones from a damaged gland. This includes painless sporadic thyroiditis, painless postpartum thyroiditis, and painful subacute thyroidits. These forms of thyrotoxicosis are self-limited because the thyroid gland contains a limited quantity of preformed hormone. It is hypothesized that painless postpartum thyroiditis and painless sporadic thyroiditis may result from thyroid autoimmunity. Because painful subacute thyroiditis is often preceded by a prodrome of infectious symptoms, a viral etiology has been proposed. In practice, the precipitating insult of transient thyroiditis in any individual patient is usually unknown, but care is unaffected as thyrotoxicosis is self-limited and supportive therapies are nonspecific. Also in this category is *toxic nodular goiter,* manifesting as a single adenoma or multiple nodules.

Rare. These include ectopic thyroid tissue [e.g., struma ovarii (ovarian teratoma-containing thyroid tissue)], inappropriate TSH secretion, pituitary tumor, thyrotoxicosis facticia, and thyroid cancer

Clinical Presentation. The presentation of Graves' disease during adolescence may be insidious; a careful history often reveals a several-month history of progressive symptoms. A goiter is palpable in the majority of cases, with diffuse enlargement that is smooth, rubbery, and nontender. Extrathyroidal manifestations such as ophthalmopathy and dermopathy are rarer than in adults, and tend to be less severe. In adolescents, prolonged hyperthyroidism from Graves' disease may accelerate linear growth and bone maturation.

Evaluation

TSH and Free T4. Thyrotoxicosis is recognized by an elevation of free T4 with a decreased or suppressed TSH. Free T4 may be normal in early disease or in iodine-deficient patients; a free T3 should be added if TSH is suppressed and serum free T4 is normal (Table 9.1).

Duration of Disease. If a biochemical derangement has been documented, the duration of thyrotoxicosis can facilitate the differentiation of Graves' disease from painless thyroiditis: (1) More than 8 weeks, Graves' is the most likely etiology; with the constellation of thyrotoxicosis, goiter, and orbitopathy, all suggesting Graves', no additional laboratory or imaging tests are necessary to confirm the diagnosis. (2) Less than 8 weeks and if thyromegaly is subtle and eye changes are absent, an iodine-123 uptake test should be performed to address the possibility of transient thyrotoxicosis secondary to painless sporadic thyroiditis or painful subacute thyroiditis. The RAIU in these conditions will be low, distinguishing them from the more common Graves' disease (Table 9.3). Hyperfunctioning nodules must be large to cause hyperthyroidism (about 2 to 3 cm or more); radioiodine thyroid scanning is reserved for patients in whom a discrete nodule(s) is palpable. Iodine-123 uptake will localize to the hyperfunctioning nodule(s) and radionuclide signal in the surrounding tissue will be low secondary to TSH suppression. Thyrotoxicosis factitia can be recognized by a low RAIU and serum thyroglobulin in the presence of thyrotoxicosis and a suppressed TSH.

TABLE 9.3

Differential Diagnosis of Thyrotoxicosis

Causes of Thyrotoxicosis

Thyrotoxicosis associated with sustained hormone overproduction (hyperthyroidism):
High RAIU
Graves' disease
Toxic multinodular goiter
Toxic adenoma
Increased TSH secretion

Thyrotoxicosis without associated hyperthyroidism:
Low RAIU
Thyrotoxicosis factitia
Subacute thyroiditis
Chronic thyroiditis with transient thyroiditis (painless thyroiditis, silent thyroiditis, postpartum thyroiditis)
Ectopic thyroid tissue (struma ovarii, functioning metastatic thyroid cancer)

Adapted from Davies TF. Thyrotoxicosis. In: *Williams Textbook of Endocrinology*, 10th ed. Philadelphia: WB Saunders, 2003.

Therapy

Medical Therapy (Antithyroid Drugs)

Symptomatic End-Organ Therapy with a Beta Blocker Such as Propranolol
Antithyroid Medications. The thionamide derivatives methimazole (MMI) and propylthiouracil (PTU) are the most commonly used agents. Both block thyroid hormone biosynthesis, and PTU, when used at doses over 450 to 600 mg per day, also inhibits the extrathyroidal activation of T4 to T3. The recommended starting doses in adolescents are as follows:

Free T4 (or FT4I)	Tapazole dose
<1.5 times the upper limit of normal range	10 mg qd
1.5 to 2 times the upper limit of normal range	10 mg bid
>2 times the upper limit of normal range	20 mg bid

Owing to its longer half-life, MMI can be administered daily or twice a day compared with the thrice daily dosing of PTU. Therefore, it is a first choice for initial therapy except for those patients who are pregnant and those who present with severe hyperthyroidism. For severely hyperthyroid patients, PTU is the preferred thionamide because of its ability to inhibit conversion of T4 to T3. Also used is a combination of high-dose PTU (up to 1,200 mg per day divided into doses taken every 6 hours) and inorganic iodine (SSKI, 3 drops taken orally twice daily for 5 to 10 days) will speed correction.

Response to Antithyroid Drugs and Monitoring. After the free T4 has fallen to the upper half of normal, the dose should be decreased by one half or one third. Further dose adjustments are guided by serial thyroid function tests, depending on the free T4. After pituitary TSH secretion recovers from suppression, TSH normalization is the goal of therapy. Monitor thyroid function every 3 months and 3 weeks after dose adjustment.

Side Effects. Antithyroid drugs are usually well-tolerated, but side-effects are more common in children than in adults.

1. Common: pruritus, fever, rash, urticaria; less commonly, gastrointestinal distress, change in taste sensation, and production of insulin autoantibodies (causing hypoglycemia).
2. Agranulocytosis (granulocyte count <500/μL) is a serious idiosyncratic reaction that can occur with either MMI or PTU. A baseline white count should be obtained prior to the initiation of antithyroid drugs, and teens and their parents should be counseled that fever, sore throat, or other serious infections warrant the immediate cessation of antithyroid drugs, notification of the clinician, and a white blood cell count with differential.
3. Hepatitis is another serious, but rare adverse reaction associated with the thionamides, so symptoms suspicious of hepatitis (jaundice, right-upper-quadrant abdominal pain, etc.) also warrant the immediate cessation of antithyroid drugs and notification of a clinician.

Remission. Reports of long-term remission rates in children and adolescents are variable, ranging anywhere from 30% to 60%. If a patient has a normal serum TSH concentration for 5 months to a year on a minimal dose of antithyroid medication (5 mg/day of methimazole or 50 mg/day of PTU), a trial off medication may be offered. Antithyroid drugs can be discontinued and TSH concentrations monitored at monthly intervals.

Subclinical Hyperthyroidism. "Subclinical hyperthyroidism" describes patients who have a subnormal serum TSH but normal concentrations of both free T4 and free T3. Patients are generally asymptomatic. No consensus exists as to indications for therapy in teens, but if there are no risk factors (e.g., history of cardiac disease), asymptomatic adolescents can be followed without treatment. Thyroid function tests should be monitored every few months.

Definitive Therapy. The two options for the definitive treatment of Graves' disease are radioiodine (iodine 131) and thyroidectomy. Both likely result in life-long hypothyroidism and there is disagreement in the literature as to their indications. Because a remission of Graves' disease occurs in a significant percentage of adolescents, we recommend the long-term use of antithyroid medications until young adulthood. However, if patient noncompliance prevents the successful treatment of thyrotoxicosis or both antithyroid medications must be discontinued secondary to serious drug reactions, definitive therapy is appropriate.

1. Radioiodine ablative therapy: Therapeutic administration of iodine-131 is the definitive treatment of choice in adults. Several studies support that the incidence of secondary malignancy in children or adolescents treated with iodine 131 is not increased. At some point in young adulthood, it is

appropriate to revisit the option of definitive therapy for those individuals on medical therapy. Definitive therapy results in permanent hypothyroidism but allows for a simpler regimen of medication and laboratory monitoring (daily levothyroxine and yearly TSH measurement).
2. Surgery: Thyroidectomy is rarely used electively for the definitive therapy of Graves' disease in the United States except for patients with massive thyromegaly (over eight times normal size) or for those who have coexisting cytologically abnormal thyroid nodules. The experience of the individual surgeon is the primary determinant of morbidity due to thyroidectomy. Thus, referral to a surgeon with a low personal complication rate and extensive experience with subtotal thyroidectomy is required.

THYROID NODULES

Prevalence. In comparison to the 5% to 10% cancer prevalence cited for adults, early pediatric series reported a 40% to 60% prevalence of thyroid cancer in children with nodules. More recent studies estimate the cancer prevalence of pediatric thyroid nodules to be 5% to 33%.

Causes. High doses of neck irradiation increase the risk of developing thyroid nodules. Thyroid nodules are also associated with several genetic disorders including multiple endocrine neoplasia type 2, the PTEN hamartoma tumor syndromes (Cowden syndrome, Bannayan-Riley-Ruvalcaba syndrome), and familial adenomatous polyposis.

Clinical Presentation. Thyroid nodules may be detected on physical examination, as an incidental finding on radiographic studies, or brought to medical attention by the patient or family. All nodules of significant size should be evaluated for the possibility of malignancy.

Evaluation. Because the prognosis of thyroid cancer depends in part upon tumor size, the early identification of differentiated thyroid cancer is the primary goal in the evaluation of nodular thyroid disease. The medical history should include inquiry into prior irradiation, as well as determination of whether there is a family history of thyroid cancer and if there are extrathyroidal manifestations. A complete review of systems should include symptoms of thyroid dysfunction and neck compression. Physical examination should include palpation of both the thyroid gland and the cervical lymph nodes. Nodules that are hard, large, adherent to adjacent structures, or associated with lymphadenopathy should heighten the suspicion of cancer.

Laboratory Evaluation. The initial evaluation should include thyroid function testing (serum TSH) to screen for autonomous/hyperfunctioning nodule(s). Diffuse thyromegaly and/or hyperthyrotropinemia warrant the measurement of antithyroid antibodies to diagnosis possible chronic autoimmune thyroiditis, but it is important to realize that the diagnosis of autoimmune thyroid disease does not exclude the possibility of coexisting thyroid cancer.

Imaging Studies and Ultrasound. More than 90% of thyroid nodules are cold by thyroid scanning and therefore require biopsy. The authors recommend that iodine-123 thyroid scanning/scintigraphy to detect benign hyperfunctioning nodules be reserved for patients with suppressed serum TSH concentrations. For all others, ultrasound is the most cost-effective imaging modality to confirm the presence of a thyroid nodule. Because of limitations of physical examination alone, thyroid ultrasonography should be performed in all adolescents with suspected thyroid nodules prior to any attempt at biopsy. Cytology should be obtained in all patients prior to considering surgery. Ultrasound-guided fine-needle aspiration is the procedure of choice, as it improves the diagnostic accuracy of fine-needle aspiration guided by palpation alone and reduces the likelihood of accidental penetration into the trachea or the great vessels.

Suggested Approach for the Evaluation of Thyroid Nodules

Measure serum TSH concentration prior to endocrine consultation. If it is suppressed, an iodine-123 scan should be obtained to evaluate for a hyperfunctioning nodule. If the serum TSH is normal or high, the patient should be triaged directly to a center with experience in the management of thyroid nodules and cancer, and a thyroid nodule ≥ 1 cm in diameter should be biopsied by ultrasound-guided fine-needle aspiration. If surgery is indicated, referral to a surgeon with extensive experience in pediatric thyroidectomy and a low complication rate is paramount. Children with thyroid nodules <1 cm or with benign cytology should be followed chronically by serial ultrasound every 6 to 12 months; ultrasound-guided fine-needle aspiration should be repeated if significant interval growth or concerning sonographic features develop.

WEB SITES

http://www.tsh.org. Thyroid Foundation of America information on thyroid disease; also has links to many more sites.

http://www.thyroid org. Home page of the American Thyroid Association.

http://www.endocrineweb.com/thyroid.html. From Endocrine Web page, information on many thyroid problems with information on thyroid hormone, tests, disease states, and more.

http://www.nlm.nih.gov/medlineplus/thyroiddiseases.html. The National Institutes of Health search area on thyroid diseases.

http://www.aacc.org. The National Association of Clinical Biochemists provides guidelines for laboratory supfor the diagnosis and monitoring of thyroid disease.

CHAPTER 10

Diabetes Mellitus

Donald P. Orr

CLASSIFICATION AND ETIOLOGY

Classification of diabetes is based on presumed etiology. Common types of diabetes include the following:

1. Type 1 diabetes results from beta-cell destruction, usually leading to insulin deficiency.
   a. *Immune mediation*: Type 1 diabetes is linked to the major histocompatibility genes (DQ) associated with diabetes, and believed to be mediated by T cells.
   b. *Idiopathic*: Non-immune-mediated diabetes is uncommon. Atypical diabetes mellitus (ADM) presents as acute-onset diabetes with weight loss, ketosis, and diabetic ketoacidosis; it requires insulin during the initial treatment.
2. Type 2 diabetes is predominantly insulin resistance with relative insulin deficiency.
3. Other specific types.
   a. Specific genetic defects of beta-cell function have been identified.
      • *Maturity-onset diabetes of youth (MODY)*. This is a group of defects in beta-cell function, impaired insulin secretion with minimal or no defects in insulin action, autosomal-dominant inheritance, and onset usually before the age of 25 years.
      • *Mitochondrial DNA:* This very rare genetic form of diabetes is almost always associated with other symptoms—deafness, neurologic disorders, cardiac failure, renal failure, and myopathy.
   b. Various genetic defects of insulin action include type A insulin resistance, leprechaunism, Rabson-Mendenhall syndrome, lipoatrophic diabetes, and others.
4. Diseases of the exocrine pancreas leading to destruction of endocrine function.
   a. *Cystic fibrosis (CF):* CF-related diabetes (CFRD) results from insulinopenia, often complicated by insulin resistance during periods of infection, and treatment with steroids. Insulin treatment is associated with increased body weight and improvement in pulmonary function.
   b. *Others:* Pancreatitis, trauma/pancreatectomy, neoplasia, hemochromatosis, fibrocalculous pancreatopathy.

5. Endocrinopathies including acromegaly, Cushing syndrome, hyperthyroidism, and pheochromocytoma.
6. Drugs including glucocorticoids, pentamidine, protease inhibitors, thyroid hormone, diazoxide, and thiazides.
7. Genetic syndromes sometimes associated with diabetes include Down's syndrome, Klinefelter syndrome, Turner syndrome, Wolfram syndrome, Friedreich ataxia, Huntington chorea, Laurence-Moon-Biedl syndrome, myotonic dystrophy, and Prader-Willi syndrome.
8. Gestational diabetes mellitus (GDM). The risk for subsequent development of diabetes is elevated; approximately 17% develop type 1 DM and 17% to 70% develop type 2.

DIAGNOSIS

The level of fasting plasma glucose (FPG) has been recommended for screening and diagnosing DM (Table 10.1). Impaired fasting glucose level and impaired glucose tolerance results are now considered to indicate prediabetes. Individuals with prediabetes are at increased risk for developing diabetes; therefore, the test should be repeated in 3 months.

- FPG <100 mg/dL (5.6 mmol/L)—normal fasting glucose
- FPG 100 to 125 mg/dL (5.6 to 6.9 mmol/L)—IFG (impaired fasting glucose/prediabetes)

TABLE 10.1

American Diabetes Association, 2005, Criteria for the Diagnosis of Diabetes Mellitus

1. Symptoms of diabetes plus casual plasma glucose concentration $\geq$200 mg/dL (11.1 mmol/L); casual is defined as any time or day without regard to time since last meal
   Or
2. FPG $\geq$126 mg/dL (7.0 mmol/L); fasting is defined as no caloric intake for at least 8 hr
   Or
3. 2-hr PG $\geq$200 mg/dL (11.1 mmol/L) during an OGTT; the test should be performed as described by the World Health Organization using a glucose load containing the equivalent of 75 g anhydrous glucose dissolved in water

In the absence of acute metabolic decompensation, these criteria should be confirmed by repeated testing on a different day
The third measure (OGTT) is not recommended for routine clinical use

FPG, fasting plasma glucose; PG, postprandial glucose; OGTT, oral glucose tolerance test.
From The Expert Committee on the Diagnosis and Classification of Diabetes Mellitus. Report of the expert committee on the diagnosis and classification of diabetes mellitus. *Diabetes Care* 2005;28(Suppl 1):S37, with permission.

- 2-hour postload glucose 140 to 199 mg/dL (7.8 to 11.1 mmol/L)—IGT (impaired glucose tolerance/prediabetes)
- FPG _>126 mg/dL (7.0 mmol/L) —provisional diagnosis of diabetes (the diagnosis must be confirmed, as described below)

SCREENING

1. Type 1 DM: No screening is recommended.
2. Type 2 DM: FPG testing every other year starting at 10 years or at onset of puberty
   a. In overweight patients
   b. In those who have any two of the following risk factors:
      - Family history of type 2 diabetes in first- or second-degree relative
      - Race/ethnicity Native American, African-American, Hispanic, Asian/ Pacific Islander
   c. Signs of or conditions associated with insulin resistance, such as acanthosis nigricans, hypertension, dyslipidemia, and polycystic ovary syndrome

PREVENTION

Type 1 Diabetes. There is no effective prevention at this time.

Type 2 Diabetes. Several studies of adults with IGT have shown that lifestyle changes (intensive physical activity, reduced carbohydrates, and weight loss) and metformin with standard diet and exercise recommendations reduce the risk for progression to diabetes.

EVALUATION AND TREATMENT

At initial presentation, determine the type of diabetes when possible and assess fluid and acid-base status. Measurement of autoantibodies may be useful if etiology is unclear. Type 2 DM usually has an insidious presentation and is suggested by obesity, acanthosis, hypertension, dyslipidemia, or strong family history of type 2 DM. Normal weight and mild symptoms suggest very early type 1 DM or MODY.

1. *Education:* This includes information about diabetes, blood glucose testing, hypoglycemia, hyperglycemia, and insulin administration. Periodic reeducation by a certified diabetes educator is recommended.
2. *Meals, food, and nutrition*: Diet is adjusted for the individual to provide sufficient calories and nutrients; limiting fat to 30% or less of total calories is encouraged. Weight reduction and exercise are important for those who are overweight, particularly if type 2.
3. *Accessing glycemic control:* Although normal levels of blood glucose (BG) are the goal (70 to 120 mg/dL before meals and fasting), most patients are not able to achieve consistently *normal* levels glycated hemoglobin.
   a. *Capillary BG testing:* Testing is recommended before meals and bedtime snack. Testing at 2 to 3 A.M. is useful for evaluating nighttime hypoglycemia and fasting hyperglycemia.

b. Glycated hemoglobin should be measured at each visit (generally quarterly). Glycated hemoglobin values reflect the average BG over the previous 8 to 12 weeks. It has been suggested that all glycated hemoglobin assays be standardized and reported in values equivalent to HbA$_{1c}$. Based on the Diabetes Control and Complications Trial (DCCT), the target HbA$_{1c}$ level is $\leq 7\%$.

4. *Insulin:* Rapid-acting insulin analog preparations include lispro (Humalog) and aspart (NovoLog). They have a more rapid onset and shorter duration of action. Two extended-acting analogs are available: glargine (Lantus) and detemir (Levemir). They have a time to onset of 2 to 4 hours. Glargine provides a peakless duration of >24 hours, while detemir has a somewhat shorter duration of 12 to 20 hours and may require twice-daily administration (Table 10.2).

a. *Insulin delivery devices:* Many different devices are available.

b. *Insulin syringes:* Available in 0.3-, 0.5-, and 1.0-mL sizes with needles of 28, 29, or 30 gauge and 8.0- or 12.7-mm length.

c. *Insulin pens:* These are disposable and prefilled or hold cartridges of 300 units of short-acting, rapid-acting, neutral protamine Hagedorn (NPH), 70/30 (70% NPH/30% regular), 75/25 (75% NPH/25% lispro or aspart), and glargine insulins.

d. *Continuous subcutaneous insulin infusion (CSII) (external insulin pumps):* Basal insulin rates can be preprogrammed. The patient must determine the mealtime amount of insulin to be delivered or corrective bolus and instruct the pump to deliver this amount at the correct time.

e. Inhaled insulin, in combination with injected long-acting insulin, has been demonstrated in phase 3 clinical efficacy trials to be safe and as effective.

5. *Treatment of patients who require insulin*: Insulin therapy is always necessary for type 1 DM and those with insulin deficiency.

a. *Insulin regimens:* Adding prelunch short- or rapid-acting insulin to a standard twice-daily insulin regimen will decrease presupper hyperglycemia, with less risk of hypoglycemia associated with a very large prebreakfast dose of intermediate-acting insulin.

b. Contemporary MDI insulin regimens are based on the use of a longer-acting insulin (glargine) to provide *basal* insulin requirements, and premeal *boluses* of rapid-acting insulin to cover the amount of carbohydrate consumed (food dose) and correct for fluctuations in premeal BG (corrective dose).

6. *Treatment of type 2 DM and MODY*

a. Acute management of newly diagnosed symptomatic patients: Individuals who are ketotic and those with significant hyperglycemia at diagnosis (BG >250 mg/dL) will require initially insulin therapy to reduce BG levels. Metformin therapy is generally begun when the patient is no longer ketotic. Insulin can be slowly withdrawn over the subsequent 3 to 4 months as glycemic control is achieved. Modifications in diet and exercise are the mainstay of treatment.

b. Patients with insidious onset and mild hyperglycemia can be initially managed with diet and exercise as described below.
- *Diet:* Distribute carbohydrates throughout the day to include snacks.
- Exercise will increase insulin sensitivity independent of weight loss.
- *Oral hypoglycemic therapy:* Failure to see improvement in FBG (HbA$_{1c}$ $\leq 8\%$) in the face of substantial weight loss or after 3 months

TABLE 10.2

Characteristics of Human Insulin Preparations

Informal Description	Proprietary or Other Name	Onset (hr)	Peak (hr)	Effective Duration (hr)	Maximum Duration (hr)	Technical Description
Rapid acting	Lispro, aspart, glulisine	0.25	1–2	2–3	4	Insulin analog
Short acting	Regular	0.5–1.0	2–3	3–6	4–6	Insulin
Intermediate acting	Neutral protamine hagedorn (NPH)	2–4	4–10	10–16	14–18	Insulin isophane (suspension)
Long acting	Detemir	1–2	8–11	12–20	14–22	
	Glargine	2–4	None	>24	24–36	Analog

Adapted from Orr DP. Contemporary management of adolescents with diabetes mellitus. Part 2: type 2 diabetes. *Adolesc Health Update* 2000;12(3):3, with permission.

suggests that diet and exercise alone will be insufficient to achieve satisfactory control. Initiate oral hypoglycemic agent or insulin therapy. Oral hypoglycemic agents will generally be required at some point in the treatment of type 2 DM.

- Biguanide (metformin) is the first-line oral hypoglycemic agent for obese adolescents, as it is not associated with weight gain. Major side effects are mild gastrointestinal symptoms. Lactic acidosis is rare. Discontinue and ensure adequate hydration prior to contrast studies that may impair renal function and with dehydration.
- Sulfonylurea (SU) drugs and the related meglitinides (*repaglinide* and *netaglinide*) enhance insulin release from the beta cell and may decrease insulin resistance. Use may be associated with weight gain. Potential interactions with sulfonamides, fluconazole, and ciprofloxacin may result in hypoglycemia. SU drugs generally may be given as a single morning dose.
- Glucosidase inhibitors are most useful when employed in conjunction with other hypoglycemic agents to assist in managing postprandial hyperglycemia. They must be given before each meal, not to exceed three times per day.
- Thiazolidinediones ("insulin sensitizers") increase insulin action. Liver enzymes must be monitored. These agents do not represent the initial pharmacotherapeutic agent for type 2 DM.

    Consider combining oral agents or adding insulin when a single medication has not achieved the desired degree of control. Add the second medication at the lowest dose and increase slowly, watching for hypoglycemia. If target BG levels have not been achieved in 4 to 6 months, the addition of insulin is indicated. Insulin may be used as a single nighttime dose of an intermediate-acting (NPH) or single dose of long-acting (glargine at any time of day) to lower FBG, or it may be given in divided doses. Adding a single dose to an oral regimen is advantageous because lower doses of insulin and the oral agent may be used.

COMPLICATIONS, ASSOCIATED CONDITIONS, AND FOLLOW-UP CARE

1. *Autoimmune disorders (type 1 DM only):* Some 10% to 15% of patients with type 1 diabetes develop autoimmune thyroiditis. Annual/semiannual measurement of thyroid-stimulating hormone to detect hypothyroidism are recommended.
2. *Microvascular complications*
   a. *Retinopathy:* Yearly dilated funduscopic examination
   b. *Nephropathy:* Annual screen for urinary microalbumin. Attempt to maintain BP $\leq 130/80$ mm Hg. Angiotensin converting enzyme (ACE) inhibitors have been shown to delay the progression of nephropathy.
   c. *Neuropathy* is rarely symptomatic during adolescence. Examine feet for pulses, sensation, deep tendon reflexes, hygiene, calluses, and evidence of infection. Symptomatic autonomic neuropathy (heart rate invariability and/or postural hypotension) and gastroparesis (postprandial nausea or vomiting, postprandial hypoglycemia, and diarrhea or constipation) are rare in this age group.

3. *Macrovascular complications:* These complications are rarely symptomatic during adolescence and young adulthood.
4. *Dyslipidemia:* Dyslipidemia (elevated triglycerides and decreased high-density-lipoprotein cholesterol) is common in type 2 DM and poorly controlled type 1 DM. Yearly measurement of fasting lipid profiles is recommended among those with previously abnormal profiles or ongoing poor glycemic control.
5. *Hypertension:* ACE inhibitors/receptor antagonists are the drugs of choice.
6. *Gluten sensitivity:* Evaluate with IgA antiendomysial or IgA anti–tissue transglutamase antibodies if symptoms are suggestive of malabsorption or unexplained postprandial hypoglycemia.
7. *Eating disorders:* Suspect when the HbA_{1c} is high, and weight loss or excess concerns about weight are present.
8. *Hypoglycemia:* Severe hypoglycemia is common with intensified regimens targeting euglycemia.
9. *Alcohol use:* For patients who drink, educate about its potential for severe hypoglycemia.

SPECIAL CONSIDERATIONS FOR COMPLIANCE WITH ADOLESCENTS

1. Identify the reason for poor control and develop a management strategy. Depression, serious psychopathology, and recurrent diabetic ketoacidosis (DKA) are indications for referral.
2. Identify one reasonable and measurable target behavior for action.
3. Identify short-term reinforcers relevant to the adolescent.
4. Establish a realistic time frame for accomplishment based on behavior and goal.
5. Provide frequent feedback.
6. Examine the extent of parental support and monitoring.
7. Group coping-skill training improves long-term glycemic control and quality of life.
8. Consider referral to a diabetes specialist if control has not improved within 6 months.

WEB SITES AND REFERENCES

http://www.diabetes.org. Web site of the American Diabetes Association.
http://www.jdf.org. Web site of the Juvenile Diabetes Foundation.
http://diabetes.niddk.nih.gov/ National Institute of Digestive Disease and Kidney.
http://www.aadenet.org. Association of Certified Diabetes Educators.
http://www.aace.com/clin/guidelines/diabetes_2002.pdf. Diabetes Clinical Guidelines of the American Association of Clinical Endocrinologists and the American College of Endocrinology.
http://www.joslin.org/main.shtml. Joslin Diabetes Program.
http://www.childrenwithdiabetes.com. Children with Diabetes.
http://www.childrenwithdiabetes.com/d_06_150.htm. Software to download GB meter results to computer.
http://www.childrenwithdiaetes.com/d_0i_000.htm. Information about BG meters.
http://www.fastfoodfacts.com. Nutrition in the fast lane.

American Diabetes Association. Diagnosis and classification of diabetes mellitus. 2008;31(Suppl 1):S57.

American Diabetes Association. Standards of medical care in diabetes. *Diabetes Care* 2005;28(Suppl 1):S4.

American Diabetes Association. Type 2 diabetes in children and adolescents. *Diabetes Care* 2008;31(Suppl 1):S12.

CHAPTER 11

Gynecomastia

Alain Joffe

DEFINITION

Gynecomastia refers to an increase in the glandular and stromal tissue of the male breast. When identified during puberty, it is usually a benign and transient condition but can represent a serious underlying disorder or persist long enough that the adolescent seeks treatment. With the rising prevalence in obesity over the last few decades, true gynecomastia must be distinguished from fatty tissue.

EPIDEMIOLOGY

Gynecomastia occurs in 19.6% of 10.5-year-old males, reaches a peak prevalence of 64.6% at age 14, and becomes less common thereafter. Approximately 4% of adolescents will have severe gynecomastia (>4.0 cm in diameter) that persists into adulthood.

ETIOLOGY

The balance between estrogen and testosterone levels determines the extent of breast tissue development in males; an increase in estrogen relative to testosterone can lead to gynecomastia. Mechanisms to account for an increase in estrogen or a decrease in androgen activity include (1) increase in serum estrogen concentrations (e.g., estradiol secretion from testicular or adrenal tumors, excessive extraglandular conversion of androgens to estrogens by aromatase, as in liver disease, obesity, or with medication or drug use; or exogenous intake of estrogens); (2) decrease in serum androgen concentrations (e.g., impairment of testosterone production in Leydig cells, as in primary or secondary hypogonadism or congenital enzyme defects); or (3) alterations of estrogen and androgen receptors.

CLINICAL MANIFESTATIONS

Bilateral (concurrent or sequential) involvement in 77% to 95% of cases

1. Type 1: One or more freely mobile subareolar nodules

2. Type 2: Subareolar nodules, extending beyond the areolar perimeter
3. Type 3: Significant breast enlargement (resembling female SMR 3)

DIFFERENTIAL DIAGNOSIS

Differential diagnosis includes the following (Braunstein, 1993, 2007):

1. *Physiologic:* Pubertal gynecomastia.
2. *Medication or drug use:* Sufficient evidence exists to implicate calcium-channel blockers, cancer chemotherapeutic agents, histamine$_2$-recptor blockers, ketoconazole, and spironolactone. Braunstein (1993) considers the strongest relationship to exist for those medications/drugs listed below that are marked with an asterisk (*):
   a. *Hormones:* Estrogens,* testosterone,* anabolic steroids,* hCG*
   b. *Psychoactive agents:* Phenothiazines, atypical antipsychotic agents, diazepam, haloperidol, tricyclic antidepressants
   c. *Cardiovascular drugs:* Digoxin,* verapamil, captopril, methyldopa, nifedipine, enalapril, reserpine, minoxidil
   d. *Antiandrogens or inhibitors of androgen synthesis:* Cyproterone,* spironolactone,* flutamide*
   e. *Antibiotics:* Isoniazid, metronidazole, ketoconazole*
   f. *Antiulcer medications:* Cimetidine,* ranitidine, omeprazole
   g. *Cancer chemotherapeutics:* Particularly alkylating agents*
   h. *Drugs of abuse:* Marijuana, alcohol, amphetamines, heroin, methadone
   i. *Other:* Phenytoin, penicillamine, theophylline, metoclopramide, saquinavir, indinavir (and other antiretroviral drugs)
3. *Underlying medical disorders:* Renal failure and dialysis, recovery from malnutrition primary gonadal failure, secondary hypogonadism, hyperthyroidism, liver disease (including cirrhosis and hepatoma), neoplasms, (testicular, adrenal, tumors with ectopic hCG production, particularly lung, liver, and kidney cancer), enzyme defects in testosterone biosynthesis, androgen insensitivity syndromes, excessive extraglandular aromatase activity
4. *Pseudogynecomastia*
5. *Breast mass:* Because of cancer, dermoid cyst, lipoma, hematoma, or neurofibroma

DIAGNOSIS

1. *History:* Screen for medication and drug use and clues suggesting systemic illness.
2. *Physical examination.*
   a. Differentiation of gynecomastia from pseudogynecomastia
   b. Findings of hypogonadism, hyperthyroidism, hypothyroidism, or liver disease
   c. Testicular mass or atrophy

Pubertal gynecomastia can be presumed as the etiology of the breast enlargement in adolescents who (1) present with a unilateral or bilateral, subareolar, rubbery or firm mass(es); (2) are not using any medications associated with gynecomastia; (3) have a normal testicular exam; and (4) lack any evidence of renal, hepatic, thyroid, or other endocrine disease. No further tests are necessary, but the patient should be reevaluated in 6 months. If medication or drug use is suspected, it should be discontinued and the adolescent reexamined in 1 month.

Laboratory Assessment

If an endocrine disorder is suspected, measure testosterone, estradiol (E2), LH and hCG.

1. Elevated hCG concentration: perform testicular ultrasonography
   a. Mass found: testicular germ cell tumor
   b. Normal sonogram: extragonadal germ cell tumor or hCG-secreting neoplasm likely; chest film and abdominal computed tomography (CT) indicated
2. Decreased testosterone concentration with:
   a. Elevated LH concentration: primary hypogonadism
   b. Normal or low LH concentration: measure serum prolactin
      • Elevated prolactin level: probably prolactin-secreting pituitary tumor. Obtain MRI of hypothalamic pituitary area.
      • Normal prolactin level: secondary hypogonadism
3. Elevated testosterone and LH concentrations: measure T4 and TSH concentrations
   a. Elevated T4 and low TSH concentrations: hyperthyroidism
   b. Normal T4 and TSH concentrations: androgen resistance
4. Elevated E2 with low or normal LH concentrations: perform testicular ultrasonography.
   a. Mass found: Leydig or Sertoli cell tumor
   b. Normal: perform adrenal CT or MRI
      • Mass found: adrenal neoplasm
      • No mass: increased extraglandular aromatase activity
5. Normal concentrations of hCG, LH, testosterone, and estradiol: idiopathic gynecomastia

THERAPY

1. Underlying causes should be treated as appropriate.
2. In most individuals with pubertal gynecomastia, only reassurance is needed. The condition will usually improve or resolve within 6 to 12 months.
3. Medical intervention: No drugs are approved by the U.S. Food and Drug Administration for treatment of adolescent gynecomastia. Medical therapy should be reserved for those individuals who have more than mild to moderate gynecomastia and who are significantly concerned about the condition. Tamoxifen might be used at an oral dosage of 10 to 20 mg twice daily for approximately 3 months (Ting, 2000).
4. In adolescents with moderate to severe gynecomastia associated with psychological sequelae, surgical treatment is preferred. Recent surgical advances include the use of ultrasonic liposuction.

PROGNOSIS

Pubertal gynecomastia usually resolves in 12 to 18 months. In 27% of affected adolescents, the condition lasts for more than 1 year, and in 7.7% more than 2 years. A small percentage of cases may persist into adulthood.

REFERENCES AND ADDITIONAL READINGS

Braunstein GD. Clinical practice. Gynecomastia. *N Engl J Med* 2007;357:1229.

Ting AC, Chow LW, Leung YF. Comparison of tamoxifen with danazol in the management of idiopathic gynecomastia. *Am Surg* 2000;66:38.

CHAPTER **12**

Cardiac Risk Factors and Hyperlipidemia

Marc S. Jacobson, Michael R. Kohn, and Lawrence S. Neinstein

Atherosclerosis begins in childhood and results from the interaction of environmental factors with the genetic endowment. Interventions to reduce risk factors in children and adolescents have been demonstrated. Whether there is also a reduction in subsequent cardiac disease remains to be determined. However, it is now advisable to screen for risk factors and provide appropriate interventions for those risk factors that are remediable.

CARDIAC RISK FACTORS

Nonintervenable. (1) Age ≥ 45 years for men, 65 years for women, (2) male gender, (3) family history of cardiovascular disease in first-degree relatives (≤ 55 years of age for men, <65 years for women) with atherosclerosis or its sequelae, or (4) parent with elevated cholesterol concentration (>240 mg/dL)

Intervenable. (1) Smoking; (2) Systolic or diastolic blood pressure (BP) above the 95th percentile; (3) diabetes mellitus; (4) diet high in saturated fats and cholesterol, with total fat intake accounting for $>30\%$ of daily caloric intake; (5) dyslipidemia, including:

a. Total cholesterol: >170 mg/dL and younger than 20 years, or >200 mg/dL for those older than 20 years.
b. Low-density lipoprotein (LDL) cholesterol (LDL-C): >130 mg/dL. For persons older than 20 years, see the "Screening in Young Adults" section, below, for new guidelines by the Adult Treatment Panel III (ATP III).
c. High-density lipoprotein (HDL) cholesterol (HDL-C): <40 mg/dL.
d. Triglycerides: >150 mg/dL.

e. Ratio of serum very-low-density lipoprotein (VLDL) cholesterol to triglycerides of >0.3.

Additional intervenable risk factors include (6) obesity (>30% above expected weight, or body mass index (BMI) above the 95th percentile for age); (7) insulin resistance with hyperinsulinemia; (8) homocystinemia (>10 nmol/L); (9) high serum lipoprotein Lp(a) concentration; and (10) high serum C-reactive protein (CRP) concentration.

In general, individuals are considered at low risk for atherosclerotic disease if they have zero or one cardiovascular risk factor, moderate risk with more than one risk factor other than diabetes mellitus, and high risk with a presence of diabetes or any evidence of atherosclerosis.

RISK-FACTOR INTERVENTION

It remains prudent to recommend a heart-healthy lifestyle to reduce atherosclerosis and arterial disease. This approach includes the following:

1. Promoting regular physical activity
2. Counseling on the importance of maintaining an ideal body weight
3. Advocating smoking prevention or cessation
4. Monitoring BP and treating when persistently elevated
5. Recommending a heart-healthy diet with <30% of total calories as fat and very little saturated fat for all individuals
6. Ensuring daily intake of 400 μg of folic acid whether through diet or supplementation.

CLASSIFICATION OF HYPERLIPIDEMIAS

Historically, patients with hyperlipidemia have been classified into five major groups according to plasma lipoprotein patterns (lipoprotein phenotyping). More recent classifications of hyperlipidemia are either extensions of the earlier models based on more specific data obtained from newer laboratory techniques (Table 12.1) or are based on recently described genetic and metabolic disorders. The nomenclature remains cumbersome and there is still much overlap, particularly when attempts are made to reconcile these two systems. Each of the two classification systems has clinical utility at present. As the field of molecular genetics advances, it is likely that the two systems will be fused into a single classification on the basis of pathophysiology and the degree of risk.

Although familial forms of hyperlipidemia, identifiable in the standard clinical laboratory assessment, account for only 2% of cases, they are responsible for more than 20% of premature CAD. Most cases of hyperlipidemia occur as a result of diet and lifestyle factors in association with genetic polymorphism in apoE, lecithin-cholesterol acyltransferase, lipoprotein lipase, and other lipid enzymes and cofactors. Hyperlipidemia also occurs as a result of medical conditions or the use of medications such as estrogens, isotretinoin, and beta₃-adrenergic blockers.

1. Familial hypercholesterolemia (Table 12.2)
   a. *Monogenic:* An autosomal-codominant disorder resulting from insufficient activity of the cell surface receptors for LDL. A number of different

TABLE 12.1

Phenotypic Classification

1. **Hypercholesterolemia with normal triglycerides**
   a. Elevated LDL-C, type IIa
      —Primary: Familial hypercholesterolemia
                   Familial combined hypercholesterolemia
                   Mixed genetic-environmental hypercholesterolemia
      —Secondary: Anorexia nervosa
                   Acute intermittent porphyria
                   Biliary obstruction (lipoprotein X)
   b. Elevated HDL-C
                   Familial hyperalphalipoproteinemia
                   Idiopathic

   —Secondary: Diabetes mellitus
                SLE
                Alcohol
                Nephrotic syndrome
                Pancreatitis
                Pregnancy
                Hypothyroidism
                Idiopathic hypercalcemia
                Medications: Estrogens
   b. Elevated chylomicrons, type I
      —Primary: Lipoprotein lipase deficiency
                   Familial deficiency of apolipoprotein C-II
      —Secondary: Autoimmune hyperchylomicronemia: SLE
                   Diabetes mellitus
                   Alcohol

2. **Hypercholesterolemia and hypertriglyceridemia**
   a. Elevated LDL-C and VLDL-C, type IIB
      —Primary: Familial hypercholesterolemia
                   Familial combined hypercholesterolemia
                   Familial LCAT deficiency
      —Secondary: Hypothyroidism
                   Nephrotic syndrome
                   Cushing's syndrome/glucocorticoid therapy
   b. Dysbetalipoproteinemia, type III

   c. Elevated VLDL and chylomicrons, type V
      —Primary: Familial hypertriglyceridemia
                   Familial combined hyperlipidemia
                   Apolipoprotein E (apoE-4 and apoE-2)
      —Secondary: Diabetes mellitus
                   Alcohol
                   Estrogen

3. **Hypertriglyceridemia with normal cholesterol level**
   a. Elevated VLDL only, type IV
      —Primary: Familial hypertriglyceridemia
                   Familial combined hyperlipidemia

4. **Increased risk with normal or elevated cholesterol level**
   a. Hyperbetalipoproteinemia
   b. Lp(a) hyperlipoproteinemia

LDL-C, low-density lipoprotein cholesterol; HDL-C, high-density lipoprotein cholesterol; VLDL-C, very low-density lipoprotein cholesterol; LCAT, lecithin-cholesterol acyltransferase; SLE, systemic lupus erythematosus.

From Arden MR. Primary hyperlipidemias. In: Jacobson MS, ed. *Atherosclerosis prevention: identification and treatment of the child with high cholesterol.* London: Harwood Academic Publishers, 1991:30, with permission.

TABLE 12.2

Characteristics of Inherited Hyperlipoproteinemias

Hyperlipoproteinemia	Phenotype	Cholesterol	Triglyceride	Xanthomas	Frequency (%)	Risk of CAD
Familial lipoprotein lipase deficiency	I	Normal	↑	Eruptive	Very rare	0
Familial hypercholesterolemia	IIa IIb	↑	↑	Tendon Tuberous xanthelasma	0.1–0.5	++++
Polygenic hypercholesterolemia	II	↑	Normal	Tuberous	5	++
Familial dysbetalipoproteinemia	III	↑	↑	Palmar Planar tuberous tendon	Rare	++++
Familial combined hyperlipoproteinemia	IIa IIb IV Rarely V	↑	↑	Any type	1–2	+++
Familial hypertriglyceridemia	IV Rarely V	Normal	↑	Eruptive	1	+

CAD, coronary artery disease; NL, normal.
From Arky RA, Perlman AJ. Hyperlipoproteinemia. In: Rubenstein E, Federman DD, eds. *Scientific American medicine.* New York: Scientific American, 1988, with permission.

mutations in the LDL receptor gene occur in families, all of which result in the same phenotypical disease. The mean cholesterol concentration in the heterozygous condition ranges from 250 to 500 mg/dL and in the homozygote from 500 to 1,000 mg/dL. Homozygous individuals may respond poorly to drugs and require referral to specialists for consideration of more intensive therapies. The heterozygous form has been estimated to occur in 1 of 200 to 500 individuals. A similar clinical presentation is observed in individuals with a heterozygous abnormality; however, the signs and symptoms tend to be milder and to develop later, about the fourth or fifth decade of life.

   b. *Polygenic:* A common cause of type IIa hyperlipidemia, probably associated with a combination of multiple genetic abnormalities and environmental factors. Individuals with this condition lack the typical physical features of familial hypercholesterolemia, such as xanthomas.

2. *Familial defective apoB-100:* A mutation in the apoB gene results in decreased affinity of LDL to the LDL receptor. This condition may occur in as many as 1 of 500 people, but the defect appears to account for only a small percentage (<2%) of premature coronary artery disease (CAD).

3. *Lipoprotein lipase deficiency:* A rare condition associated with very high levels of triglycerides and normal cholesterol levels. Although the risk of atherosclerosis is not elevated, the individual is at risk of having pancreatitis, particularly when the triglyceride level exceeds 500 mg/dL.

4. *Familial dysbetalipoproteinemia:* A very uncommon condition seen only rarely in adolescence. This problem should be suspected when triglyceride levels are somewhat higher than cholesterol levels in the presence of a significant cholesterol elevation. These individuals have an increased risk of premature CAD and peripheral vascular disease. They often are obese and have glucose intolerance, hyperuricemia, and tuberoeruptive and palmar xanthomas.

5. *Familial hypertriglyceridemia:* Autosomal-dominant trait. Dietary factors, obesity, and a sedentary lifestyle are additional elements involved in the degree of expression.

6. *Familial combined hyperlipidemia (FCHL):* Affected individuals have high levels of LDL-C, triglycerides, or both. This condition is usually associated with premature CAD. Affected individuals may have increases in VLDL alone, LDL alone, or VLDL plus LDL or chylomicrons. The diagnosis is made by a finding of multiple lipoprotein phenotypes in a single family when first-degree relatives are tested or when a typical pattern of modest elevation in concentrations of cholesterol and triglycerides is seen together with a low HDL-C level. FCHL occurs in about 15% of patients with CAD younger than age 60 years.

LIPID SCREENING AND MANAGEMENT

According to the National Cholesterol Education Program's (NCEP) Expert Panel, the process of screening and management differs for adolescents (age 20 years or younger) and young adults (age 20 to 35 years). In addition to classification of lipid parameters, screening involves the identification of other cardiovascular risk factors by history and physical examination (Fig. 12.1).

1. *History:* (a) Family history of premature cardiovascular diseases, (b) family history of dyslipidemia or hypertension, and (c) history of smoking

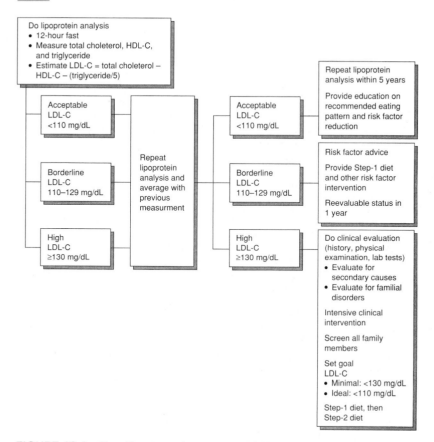

FIGURE 12.1   Classification, education, and follow-up based on LDL-C in adolescents (<20 years). [From the National Cholesterol Education Program Report of the Expert Panel on Blood Cholesterol Levels in Children and Adolescents. *Pediatrics* 1992;89 (Suppl):498.]

2. *Dietary history:* May use 24-hour recall history
3. *Physical examination:* (a) Signs of peripheral lipid deposition (xanthoma, xanthelasma, corneal arcus); (b) weight, height, BP, and sexual maturity rating; (c) body composition indexes

The NCEP Expert Panel on Blood Cholesterol Levels in Children and Adolescents and the American Academy of Pediatrics Committee on Nutrition (1998) classifies risk on the basis of *total cholesterol* levels as follows: low risk: <170 mg/dL, borderline risk: 170 to 199 mg/dL, and high risk: 200 mg/dL (95th percentile).

Providing dietary treatment for adolescents and young adults with the top 25% of cholesterol values is probably desirable, but this has not been proven to reduce CAD. Recommending drug treatment to the top 10% is even more controversial until more is known about the risk–benefit ratio for drug treatment in a younger population. At present, it seems reasonable to recommend that individuals in the borderline-risk group receive lifestyle measures, including exercise instruction, nutritional advice such as the NCEP Step 1 prudent diet, and nonsmoking advice. Those in the high-risk group should receive all these measures plus dietary counseling by a dietitian and more frequent follow-up. If possible, all adolescents should be screened once during this age period, especially (a) teens whose parents or relatives have had premature CAD or stroke or if male members of the family have had clinical evidence of atherosclerosis before the age of 55 years or female members before the age of 65 years; (b) teens whose parents have elevated concentrations of lipoproteins; (c) teens with hypertension, obesity, diabetes, or other significant cardiac risk factors; and (d) teens who are smokers.

Serum lipids are best measured after a 12- to 14-hour fast; however, the total cholesterol level can be determined in a nonfasting sample because chylomicrons from dietary fat contribute essentially no cholesterol. If a nonfasting cholesterol level is borderline or above, a fasting sample should be obtained and analyzed for triglycerides, total cholesterol, and HDL-C with a calculation of LDL-C. Risk on the basis of LDL-C is classified as "acceptable" (<110 mg/dL), "borderline" (110 to 129 mg/dL), or "high" (>130 mg/dL).

Screening in Young Adults

The Adult Treatment Panel III (ATP III) of the NCEP issued an evidence-based set of guidelines on cholesterol management in 2001. Since the publication of ATP III, several major clinical trials of statin therapy with clinical end points have been published (Grundy et al., 2004).

1. ATP III recommendations for young adults between the ages of 20 and 35 years are as follows:
   a. Fasting lipid profile is the preferred method of assessing lipid risk and should be determined in every young adult regardless of family history at least once every 5 years. The lipid profile is interpreted by the following guidelines:
   - LDL-C

Optimal	< 100 mg/dL
Near optimal	100 to 129 mg/dL
Borderline high	130 to 159 mg/dL
High	160 to 189 mg/dL
Very high	190 mg/dL

   - Total cholesterol

Desirable	<200 mg/dL
Borderline	200 to 239 mg/dL
High	>240 mg/dL

   - HDL-C

Low	<40 mg/dL
High	>60 mg/dL

   b. In those without CAD, the following LDL-C goals and treatments apply: LDL-C goal is <160 mg/dL, at which point therapeutic lifestyle changes

(TLC) are indicated. At LDL-C >190 mg/dL, lipid-lowering medications should be considered. At 160 to 189 mg/dL, LDL-C use of lipid-lowering drugs is based on clinical judgment, taking into account two additional factors: *life habits* (e.g., obesity, sedentary lifestyle, and atherogenic diet) and *emerging risk factors* (e.g., Lp(a), homocysteine, prothrombotic and proinflammatory plasma factors, as well as impaired glucose tolerance).

2. Results from recent trials have resulted in updated ATP III recommendations for adults as follows:

   a. Therapeutic lifestyle changes (TLC) remain essential.

   b. The trials confirm the benefit of cholesterol-lowering therapy in high-risk patients and support the ATP III treatment goal of LDL-C <100 mg/dL.

   c. Patients with diabetes are included in the high-risk category and benefit from LDL-lowering therapy.

   d. New footnotes to the ATP III treatment algorithm include:

   • In high-risk persons, the recommended LDL-C goal is <100 mg/dL, but when risk is very high, an LDL-C goal of <70 mg/dL is a reasonable clinical strategy, based on the available clinical evidence.

   • When a high-risk patient has high triglycerides or low high-density lipoprotein cholesterol (HDL-C), consideration can be given to combining a fibrate or nicotinic acid with an LDL-lowering drug.

   • For moderately high-risk persons (2+ risk factors), the recommended LDL-C goal is <130 mg/dL, but an LDL-C goal <100 mg/dL is a therapeutic option.

   • When LDL-lowering drug therapy is employed in high-risk or moderately high-risk persons, therapy should achieve at least a 30% to 40% reduction in LDL-C levels.

   • Any person at high risk or moderately high risk who has lifestyle-related risk factors (eg, obesity, physical inactivity) should make lifestyle changes (TLC) to modify these risk factors regardless of LDL-C level.

A complete report with helpful clinical tools is available online at http://www.nhlbi.nih.gov/guidelines/cholesterol/index.htm

HYPERTRIGLYCERIDEMIA

Moderate hypertriglyceridemia alone is not independently correlated with CAD. Severe hypertriglyceridemia (≥1,000 mg/dL) is associated with an increased incidence of acute life-threatening pancreatitis and must be aggressively treated with diet, weight loss, and pharmacotherapy. The Framingham study has found that a triglyceride concentration of >150 mg/dL in combination with an HDL level of <35 mg/dL is as good a predictor of CAD as LDL elevation. Thus, in the presence of an elevated triglyceride and a low HDL concentration, treatment with the TLC diet and exercise intervention is recommended. The ATP III now defines hypertriglyceridemia more strictly than previously: Normal triglycerides, <150 mg/dL; borderline-high triglycerides, 150 to 199 mg/dL; high triglycerides 200 to 499 mg/dL; and very high triglycerides, >500 mg/dL.

For adolescents, the 90th percentile should be used as the upper limit of normal for age and sex.

NONLIPID RISK-FACTOR ASSESSMENT

Insulin/Glucose Ratio. Insulin resistance is indicated by an elevated ratio. It is associated with the metabolic syndrome (syndrome X), which consists of at least three of the following five: central adiposity, hypertension, elevated triglyceride levels, decreased HDL-C levels, impaired glucose tolerance. In adolescents, the metabolic syndrome is best managed with lifestyle changes aimed at overweight and obesity. ATP III recognizes metabolic syndrome as a secondary target of cardiovascular-risk reduction after LDL lowering. Routine screening of fasting insulin is not indicated but is reserved for individuals with risk factors for type 2 diabetes (such as family history, obesity, or acanthosis nigricans).

Homocysteine. Elevated plasma total homocysteine is an independent risk factor for atherosclerotic vascular disease and has been linked to an increased risk of thrombosis. Risk increases continuously across the spectrum of homocysteine concentrations and may become appreciable at levels $>10 \, \mu$mol/L. Folic acid is the mainstay of treatment, because homocysteine levels can be reduced with folic acid supplementation, but vitamins B12 and B6 may have added benefit in selected patients.

THERAPY FOR HYPERLIPIDEMIA

General Principles

1. Diagnose and treat secondary causes.
2. Reduce risk factors. Intervene with those risk factors that can be altered, including smoking, hypertension, and diabetes.
3. Start a heart-healthy diet. The principal treatment of hyperlipidemia in adolescents and adults is a diet with modified amounts of fat, saturated fat, and cholesterol without increased simple carbohydrates. The goals of dietary therapy are to lower total cholesterol and LDL-C concentration to below the 90th percentile—preferably below the 75th percentile. Nutritional management is described in two steps as recommended by the NCEP Expert Panel on Blood Cholesterol Levels in Children and Adolescents. If adherence to the NCEP Step 1 diet fails to achieve the minimal goals of therapy, the Step 2 diet should be prescribed.

   The Step I diet from the American Heart Association (AHA) is very similar to the diet recommended by the AHA for the general public with the exception that the Step I diet is followed in a medical setting. The Step II diet has further reductions in cholesterol and saturated fat for those already on a Step I diet or for those with a higher level of cholesterol or more risk factors. Step I and Step II diets should be combined with regular physical activity in all patients and weight reduction in the overweight.

   The pediatric recommendations differ from those for adults in that careful consideration and monitoring of energy and micronutrient consumption are needed for support of normal growth and development. This is particularly important during the adolescent growth years, when energy, protein, mineral, and vitamin requirements are increased. Nutritional counseling focusing on meeting fat and cholesterol recommendations while ensuring adequate macronutrient and micronutrient intake is needed.

Step I and Step II diets are outlined at the AHA Web site (http://www. americanheart.org).

Vitamin Therapy

The ATP III acknowledges the importance of meeting the daily recommended intake (DRI) of vitamins and minerals but does not recommend megavitamin therapy beyond the DRI because of the negative data from clinical trials of beta-carotene and antioxidant vitamins. We recommend all adolescents take an over-the-counter multivitamin with 100% of the DRI for folic acid (400 μg).

Stanols and Plant Sterols

As adjunctive LDL-C-lowering therapy, the ATP III recommends the addition of plant-derived cholesterol absorption-inhibiting compounds such as esters of cholestanol or other nonabsorbed sterols available as margarine or salad dressing (at two to three servings per day). Studies, mainly from Europe, have shown an additional 10% to 15% LDL-C reduction with daily use of these compounds in persons consuming a low-saturated-fat, low-cholesterol diet.

Drug Therapy

The risk-benefit ratio for lipid-lowering drug therapy is unknown in adolescents. However, pharmacotherapy is considered when:

1. Xanthomas are present on physical examination or *all of the following four criteria are met:*
2. Supervised diet modification fails to lower LDL-C to acceptable levels or by at least 15% below baseline.
3. A parent has died or had severe atherosclerotic sequelae in his or her forties or younger.
4. The adolescent's LDL-C concentration is >190 mg/dL in the absence of other risk factors or >160 mg/dL in the presence of any of the following: smoking, hypertension, diabetes, and clinical signs of atherosclerosis.
5. In individuals older than 20 years, base treatment on the ATP III LDL goals outlined previously in the section entitled "Screening in Young Adults."

Tables 12.3 and 12.4 summarizes mechanisms of action and major effects and lists recommended doses and side effects of the drugs used for hyperlipidemic conditions.

Adherence to Drug Therapy

1. Drug therapy should be considered an adjunct not a replacement for therapeutic lifestyle change (TLC). Many teens, once they are able to make healthier food choices and get regular vigorous physical activity, can get their LDL-C into the target range without medications.
2. The teen must be well informed about the goals of drug treatment and the side effects,
3. It is important to start with small doses of drugs, particularly with sequestrants or nicotinic acid.
4. The frequency of use of the medication and the impact on lifestyle must be discussed.
5. It is important to maintain regularly scheduled follow-ups with the teen.

TABLE 12.3

Drug Therapy for Hyperlipidemia

Type of Drug	Mechanism of Action	Major Effects	Example	Starting Dose	Adverse Reactions
Statin	Inhibits cholesterol synthesis in hepatic cells, resulting in increased LDL-receptor activity	Lowers LDL cholesterol and triglyceride, raises HDL-C	Atorvastatin, lovastatin, pravastatin, simvastatin, rosuvastatin	5–20 mg depending on which drug is used	Raised hepatic enzymes, muscle soreness possibly progressing to myolysis
Bile acid sequestrants	Binds intestinal bile acids interrupting enterohepatic recirculation, which in turn results in LDL-receptor up regulation	Lowers LDL-C Raises triglycerides	Cholestyramine, colesevelam	One to two packs of powder or four tablets (1 g) daily, with 8 oz water	Limited to GI tract; gas, bloating constipation, cramps, fat-soluble vitamin deficiency
Fibric acid	Probably inhibits hepatic synthesis of VLDL	Mainly lowers triglycerides and raises HDL-C, with less effect on LDL-C	Gemfibrozil, fenofibrate	Varies with preparation	Dyspepsia, constipation, raised liver enzymes, myositis, rhabdomyolisis, anemia
Nicotinic acid	Upregulates hepatic LDL receptors, decreases hepatic LDL and VLDL production	Lowers triglycerides LDL-C and Lp(a), raises HDL-C	Niaspan	500 mg begin slowly to minimize side effects	Flushing, hepatic toxicity, hyperglycemia
Cholesterol absorption inhibitor	Inhibits cholesterol absorption in small intestine, interferes with enterohepatic recirculation	Lowers LDL-C	Ezetimibe	10 mg	Hepatitis, pancreatitis, cholecystitis, diarrhea, abdominal pain, arthralgia

LDL, low-density lipoprotein; HDL-C, high-density lipoprotein cholesterol; LDL-C, low-density lipoprotein cholesterol; VLDL, very low-density lipoprotein; GI, gastrointestinal.

TABLE 12.4

Characteristics of Statin Drugs

Characteristic	Lovastatin	Pravastatin	Simvastatin	Atorvastatin	Fluvastatin
Maximum dose (mg/d)	80	40	80	80	80
Maximal LDL cholesterol reduction (%)	40	34	47	60	24
Serum triglyceride reduction produced (%)	16	24	18	29	10
Serum HDL cholesterol increase produced (%)	8.6	12	12	6	8
Plasma half-life (hr)	2	1–2	1–2	14	1.2
Optimal time of administration	With meals (morning and evening)	Bedtime	Evening	Evening	Bedtime
CNS penetration	Yes	No	Yes	No	No
Hepatic metabolic mechanism	Cytochrome P-450 3A4	Sulfation	Cytochrome P-450 3A4	Cytochrome P-450 3A4	Cytochrome P-450 2C9

LDL, low-density lipoprotein; HDL, high-density lipoprotein; CNS, central nervous system.
Adapted from Knopp RH. Drug treatment of lipid disorders. *N Engl J Med* 1999;341:498, with permission.

REFERENCES AND ADDITIONAL READINGS

The full ATP III report is available at http://www.nhlbi.nih.gov/guidelines/cholesterol/index.htm.

Grundy SM, Cleeman JI, Merz CN, et al. Coordinating Committee of the National Cholesterol Education Program. Implications of recent clinical trials for the National Cholesterol Education Program Adult Treatment Panel III Guidelines. *J Am Coll Cardiol* 2004;44:720.

National Cholesterol Education Program Expert Panel. Executive summary of the third report of the National Cholesterol Education Program Expert Panel on Detection, Evaluation, and Treatment of High Blood Cholesterol in Adults (ATP III). *JAMA* 2001;285:2486–2497.

Information for patients is available from the AHA Web site at: http://www.americanheart.org/).

CHAPTER 13

Systemic Hypertension

Joseph T. Flynn

About 1% to 2% of children and adolescents have hypertension, although the prevalence may be nearly 5% in obese minority adolescents. Most adolescents with hypertension have primary hypertension—that is, no underlying cause can be identified. Since most hypertensive adolescents are asymptomatic, BP should be measured whenever an adolescent is seen for health care to help prevent development of cardiovascular disease later in life.

DEFINITION OF HYPERTENSION IN ADOLESCENCE

BP values derived from analysis of a large database of BPs obtained in healthy children are used to define hypertension in children and adolescents ≤17 years old (Tables 13.1 and 13.2). First determine the child's height percentile, then the appropriate gender chart should be used to determine the BP percentile. The cut points used to classify hypertension in adolescents of all ages are summarized in Table 13.3.

Common to both the pediatric and adult BP classification schemes is the concept of "prehypertension," designated by a BP value of >120/80, to serve as a warning of the potential for later development of hypertension and of the need for proactive lifestyle changes that might prevent this from occurring. Staging the severity of hypertension helps to determine how rapidly a hypertensive adolescent should be evaluated and when antihypertensive drug therapy should be instituted.

ETIOLOGY

In contrast to younger children, at least 80% of hypertensive adolescents have no known cause for their BP elevation and are labeled as having primary or essential hypertension. Primary hypertension in adolescents is frequently characterized by isolated systolic BP elevation, whereas diastolic BP elevation is more likely to be present in secondary hypertension. Obesity and a positive family history of hypertension are also common in adolescents with primary hypertension. As in younger children, renal parenchymal diseases are the most common secondary cause in adolescents.

TABLE 13.1

Blood Pressure Values for Adolescent Boys 17 Years or Younger

Age (yr)	BP Percentile	Systolic BP (mm Hg) ← Percentile of Height →							Diastolic BP (mm Hg) ← Percentile of Height →						
		5th	10th	25th	50th	75th	90th	95th	5th	10th	25th	50th	75th	90th	95th
10	50th	97	98	100	102	103	105	106	58	59	60	61	61	62	63
	90th	111	112	114	115	117	119	119	73	73	74	75	76	77	78
	95th	115	116	117	119	121	122	123	77	78	79	80	81	81	82
	99th	122	123	125	127	128	130	130	85	86	86	88	88	89	90
11	50th	99	100	102	104	105	107	107	59	59	60	61	62	63	63
	90th	113	114	115	117	119	120	121	74	74	75	76	77	78	78
	95th	117	118	119	121	123	124	125	78	78	79	80	81	82	82
	99th	124	125	127	129	130	132	132	86	86	87	88	89	90	90
12	50th	101	102	104	106	108	109	110	59	60	61	62	63	63	64
	90th	115	116	118	120	121	123	123	74	75	75	76	77	78	79
	95th	119	120	122	123	125	127	127	78	79	80	81	82	82	83
	99th	126	127	129	131	133	134	135	86	87	88	89	90	90	91
13	50th	104	105	106	108	110	111	112	60	60	61	62	63	64	64
	90th	117	118	120	122	124	125	126	75	75	76	77	78	79	79
	95th	121	122	124	126	128	129	130	79	79	80	81	82	83	83
	99th	128	130	131	133	135	136	137	87	87	88	89	90	91	91
14	50th	106	107	109	111	113	114	115	60	61	62	63	64	65	65
	90th	120	121	123	125	126	128	128	75	76	77	78	79	79	80
	95th	124	125	127	128	130	132	132	80	80	81	82	83	84	84
	99th	131	132	134	136	138	139	140	87	88	89	90	91	92	92

(continued)

TABLE 13.1

(Continued)

Age (yr)	BP Percentile	Systolic BP (mm Hg) ← Percentile of Height →							Diastolic BP (mm Hg) ← Percentile of Height →						
		5th	10th	25th	50th	75th	90th	95th	5th	10th	25th	50th	75th	90th	95th
15	50th	109	110	112	113	115	117	117	61	62	63	64	65	66	66
	90th	122	124	125	127	129	130	131	76	77	78	79	80	80	81
	95th	126	127	129	131	133	134	135	81	81	82	83	84	85	85
	99th	134	135	136	138	140	142	142	88	89	90	91	92	93	93
16	50th	111	112	114	116	118	119	120	63	63	64	65	66	67	67
	90th	125	126	128	130	131	133	134	78	78	79	80	81	82	82
	95th	129	130	132	134	135	137	137	82	83	83	84	85	86	87
	99th	136	137	139	141	143	144	145	90	90	91	92	93	94	94
17	50th	114	115	116	118	120	121	122	65	66	66	67	68	69	70
	90th	127	128	130	132	134	135	136	80	80	81	82	83	84	84
	95th	131	132	134	136	138	139	140	84	85	86	87	87	88	89
	99th	139	140	141	143	145	146	147	92	93	93	94	95	96	97

BP, blood pressure.

To use the table, first plot the child's height on a standard growth curve (www.cdc.gov/growthcharts). The child's measured systolic blood pressure and diastolic blood pressure are compared with the numbers provided in the table according to the child's age and height percentile.

National High Blood Pressure Education Program Working Group on High Blood Pressure in Children and Adolescents. The fourth report on the diagnosis, evaluation, and treatment of high blood pressure in children and adolescents. National Heart, Lung, and Blood Institute, Bethesda, Maryland. NIH Publication 05-5267, 2005.

TABLE 13.2

Blood Pressure Values for Adolescent Girls 17 Years or Younger

Age (yr)	BP Percentile	Systolic BP (mm Hg) ← Percentile of Height →							Diastolic BP (mm Hg) ← Percentile of Height →						
		5th	10th	25th	50th	75th	90th	95th	5th	10th	25th	50th	75th	90th	95th
10	50th	98	99	100	102	103	104	105	59	59	59	60	61	62	62
	90th	112	112	114	115	116	118	118	73	73	73	74	75	76	76
	95th	116	116	117	119	120	121	122	77	77	77	78	79	80	80
	99th	123	123	125	126	127	129	129	84	84	85	86	86	87	88
11	50th	100	101	102	103	105	106	107	60	60	60	61	62	63	63
	90th	114	114	116	117	118	119	120	74	74	74	75	76	77	77
	95th	118	118	119	121	122	123	124	78	78	78	79	80	81	81
	99th	125	125	126	128	129	130	131	85	85	86	87	88	88	89
12	50th	102	103	104	105	107	108	109	61	61	61	62	63	64	64
	90th	116	116	117	119	120	121	122	75	75	75	76	77	78	78
	95th	119	120	121	123	124	125	126	79	79	79	80	81	82	82
	99th	127	127	128	130	131	132	133	86	86	87	88	88	89	90
13	50th	104	105	106	107	109	110	110	62	62	62	63	64	65	65
	90th	117	118	119	121	122	123	124	76	76	76	77	78	79	79
	95th	121	122	123	124	126	127	128	80	80	80	81	82	83	83
	99th	128	129	130	132	133	134	135	87	87	88	89	89	90	91
14	50th	106	106	107	109	110	111	112	63	63	63	64	65	66	66
	90th	119	120	121	122	124	125	125	77	77	77	78	79	80	80
	95th	123	123	125	126	127	129	129	81	81	81	82	83	84	84
	99th	130	131	132	133	135	136	136	88	88	89	90	90	91	92

(continued)

TABLE 13.2

(Continued)

Age (yr)	BP Percentile	Systolic BP (mm Hg) ← Percentile of Height →							Diastolic BP (mm Hg) ← Percentile of Height →						
		5th	10th	25th	50th	75th	90th	95th	5th	10th	25th	50th	75th	90th	95th
15	50th	107	108	109	110	111	113	113	64	64	64	65	66	67	67
	90th	120	121	122	123	125	126	127	78	78	78	79	80	81	81
	95th	124	125	126	127	129	130	131	82	82	82	83	84	85	85
	99th	131	132	133	134	136	137	138	89	89	90	91	92	92	93
16	50th	108	108	110	111	112	114	114	64	64	65	66	66	67	68
	90th	121	122	123	124	126	127	128	78	78	79	80	81	81	82
	95th	125	126	127	128	130	131	132	82	82	83	84	85	85	86
	99th	132	133	134	135	137	138	139	90	90	90	91	92	93	93
17	50th	108	109	110	111	113	114	115	64	65	65	66	67	67	68
	90th	122	122	123	125	126	127	128	78	79	79	80	81	81	82
	95th	125	126	127	129	130	131	132	82	83	83	84	85	85	86
	99th	133	133	134	136	137	138	139	90	90	91	91	92	93	93

BP, blood pressure.

To use the table, first plot the child's height on a standard growth curve (www.cdc.gov/growthcharts). The child's measured systolic blood pressure and diastolic blood pressure are compared with the numbers provided in the table according to the child's age and height percentile.

From National High Blood Pressure Education Program Working Group on High Blood Pressure in Children and Adolescents. The fourth report on the diagnosis, evaluation, and treatment of high blood pressure in children and adolescents. National Heart, Lung, and Blood Institute, Bethesda, Maryland. NIH Publication 05-5267, 2005.

TABLE 13.3

Classification of Hypertension in Children, Adolescents, and Adults

Blood Pressure Classification	Children and Adolescents ≤17 Years of Age	Adults (≥18 years of age)
Normal	SBP and DBP <90th percentile	SBP <120 mm Hg and DBP <80 mm Hg
Prehypertension	SBP or DBP 90–95th percentile; or if BP is >120/80 even if <90th percentile	SBP 120–139 mm Hg or DBP 80–89 mm Hg
Stage 1 hypertension	SBP or DBP ≥95th–99th percentile plus 5 mm Hg	SBP 140–159 mm Hg or DBP 90–99 mm Hg
Stage 2 hypertension	>99th percentile plus 5 mm Hg	SBP ≥160 mm Hg or DBP ≥100 mm Hg

DBP, diastolic blood pressure; SBP, systolic blood pressure.
Adapted from Chobanian et al., 2003; and National High Blood Pressure Education Program Working Group, 2004.

DIAGNOSIS

About 10% of adolescents may have a high initial BP (≥95th percentile) at an office visit. They should be labeled as having an elevated BP and not given a diagnosis of hypertension. Before a diagnosis of hypertension can be made, at least three BP determinations on different days must show a high systolic or diastolic pressure or both. Except in the obese, only 1% to 2% of adolescents will fulfill these criteria and, by definition, have hypertension.

Accurate diagnosis of hypertension depends on accurate BP measurement:

1. Auscultation remains the most accurate technique and is the method of choice.
2. BP in the young is labile; therefore, hypertension should not be diagnosed until three elevated readings on separate occasions are obtained.
3. The length of the cuff bladder should be at least 80% of the middle arm circumference. Use the largest cuff that fits the arm while leaving the antecubital fossa free for auscultation. It is better to choose a cuff slightly too big than one too small.
4. BP measurements should be done with the adolescent in the sitting position and the sphygmomanometer at heart level.
5. For apprehensive patients, BP measurements obtained outside of the office setting, such as by a school nurse or at home, may be helpful to confirm elevated office readings.
6. Given the high prevalence of "white coat hypertension," ambulatory BP monitoring, in which BPs are obtained over a 24-hour period with an automated

device, may be a helpful part of the evaluation of an adolescent with elevated office BPs.

Diagnostic Evaluation

The diagnostic evaluation must be tailored to the individual patient, taking into account the age, sex, race, family history, and severity of hypertension.

1. *History:* The history should aim at eliciting clues to possible secondary causes, target-organ damage, and other cardiovascular risk factors. Look for symptoms of urinary tract infection or renal disease and for a family history of hypertension or other cardiovascular disease. Activity, diet, and other habits should be reviewed, especially with respect to substance use. Many substances may elevate BP (Table 13.4).
2. *Physical examination:* The examination should search for evidence of a secondary cause of hypertension or of end-organ damage and include evaluation of (a) height, weight, and calculated body mass index; (b) BP in both arms and a lower extremity; (c) femoral pulses; (d) carotid bruits or an enlarged thyroid gland; (e) funduscopic exam for arteriolar narrowing, arteriovenous nicking, hemorrhages, or exudates; (f) abdominal—bruits, hepatosplenomegaly, or flank masses; (g) heart rate, precordial heave, clicks, murmurs, or arrhythmias; (h) peripheral pulses and edema; and (i) evaluation of the skin for striae, acanthosis nigricans, café au lait spots, or neurofibromas.
3. *Laboratory testing:*
   a. Screening tests should be done in all patients: electrolytes, BUN/Cr, urinalysis, fasting lipid profile. Urine culture and CBC should be done as

TABLE 13.4

Substances That May Elevate Blood Pressure in Adolescents

Prescription Medications	Nonprescription Medications	Others
Calcineurin inhibitors (cyclosporine, tacrolimus)	Ephedrine	Caffeine
	Nonsteroidal antiinflammatory drugs[a]	Cocaine
Dexedrine[a]		Ethanol
Erythropoietin	Pseudoephedrine	Heavy metals (lead, mercury)
Glucocorticoids		MDMA ("Ecstasy")
Methylphenidate[a]		Tobacco
Oral contraceptives		Herbal preparations
Phenylpropanolamine		(*Ephedra, Glycyrrhiza*)
Pseudoephedrine		
Tricyclic antidepressants[a]		

[a]These cause elevated blood pressure relatively infrequently compared with the other agents in the table.

---

appropriate. In obese adolescents, screen for impaired glucose tolerance with fasting serum glucose.

b. Additional laboratory tests should be done as appropriate to follow up on clues from the history and physical or from the screening test results. These might include screening for connective tissue or thyroid disease.

c. Echocardiograms are now recommended by the National High Blood Pressure Education Program Working Group for all adolescents with confirmed hypertension to detect left ventricular hypertrophy.

d. Specific testing should be done only to confirm suspected secondary causes of hypertension.

e. Imaging studies such as renal ultrasounds are useful in only a very small percentage of hypertensive adolescents and should usually be obtained only in those with stage 2 hypertension or in those with stage 1 hypertension and signs or symptoms of secondary hypertension.

THERAPY

Nonpharmacologic Interventions

Since weight loss, aerobic exercise, and dietary modifications have all been shown to successfully reduce blood pressure in children and adolescents, these measures should be incorporated into the treatment plan for any hypertensive adolescent. Weight reduction: In studies where a 10% reduction in BMI was achieved, short-term reductions in blood pressure were in the range of 8 to 12 mm Hg. The "DASH diet," which is lower in sodium content and enhanced in potassium and calcium intake, has been demonstrated to be of benefit in hypertensive adults and should probably be recommended for hypertensive adolescents. Aerobic physical activity ($\geq$30 minutes per session 4 to 5 days per week) can reduce systolic BP by approximately 10 mm Hg. Patients should be advised to quit smoking, avoid excessive alcohol intake, and discontinue the use of substances that increase BP.

Pharmacologic Treatment

1. Antihypertensive medications are indicated for those who have the following: (a) any symptoms of hypertension, (b) Stage 2 hypertension, (c) evidence of hypertensive end-organ damage, (d) type 1 or type 2 diabetes, (e) secondary hypertension, or (f) persistent hypertension despite lifestyle changes.

2. If none of the above indications are present, drug treatment can be withheld in favor of lifestyle modifications. If these measures fail to lower BP after a reasonable period of time, medication should be prescribed.

3. Initial therapeutic regimens are debated. Since all classes of antihypertensive agents have now been studied in adolescents, either a diuretic, beta blocker, angiotensin converting enzyme (ACE) inhibitor, or calcium channel blocker may be chosen as the initial agent.

4. An individualized stepped-care approach (Fig. 13.1) is recommended by the National High Blood Pressure Education Program Working Group.

5. Suggested initial and maximum doses of various antihypertensive agents are given in Table 13.5. Comprehensive references should be consulted for more complete prescribing information and the potential adverse effects of these medications.

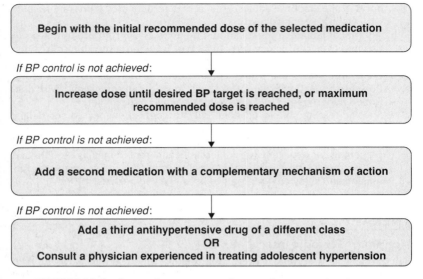

FIGURE 13.1 Stepped-care approach to antihypertensive therapy.

6. For adolescents <18 years old with uncomplicated primary hypertension, target BP should be the 95th percentile for age, gender, and height; for those with secondary hypertension, diabetes, or chronic kidney disease, target BP should be in the 90th percentile. For those ≥18 years old, BP targets should be <140/90 for those with uncomplicated primary hypertension, and <130/80 for those with secondary hypertension, diabetes, or chronic kidney disease.

7. Step-down therapy: After an extended course of drug therapy, successful lifestyle modification, and sustained BP control, a gradual reduction in or withdrawal of medication can be attempted. BP should be closely observed and nonpharmacologic measures continued.

SPECIAL POPULATIONS

1. African Americans: Hypertension develops at an earlier age and is more severe in African Americans than in whites. Although all classes of antihypertensive medications can be used, diuretics have beneficial effects on morbidity and mortality rates and should, therefore, be considered for use as initial therapy.

2. Females who take oral contraceptives: Most females who take oral contraceptives have small increases in systolic and diastolic BP and a few may develop overt hypertension.

3. Adolescents with asthma: nonselective beta-blocking drugs can worsen bronchoconstriction and, therefore, are relatively contraindicated.

4. Diabetes: ACE inhibitors or angiotensin receptor blockers should be used as the initial agent owing to their potential benefit in slowing the progression of diabetic nephropathy or even preventing it.

TABLE 13.5

Antihypertensive Agents for Use in Chronic Treatment of Hypertension in Adolescents

Class	Drug	Starting Dose	Interval	Maximum Dose[a]
Angiotensin-converting enzyme (ACE) inhibitors	Benazepril	0.2 mg/kg/d up to 10 mg/d	q.d.	0.6 mg/kg/d up to 40 mg q.d.
	Captopril	0.3–0.5 mg/kg/dose	b.i.d.–t.i.d.	6 mg/kg/d up to 450 mg/d
	Enalapril	0.08 mg/kg/d	q.d.	0.6 mg/kg/d up to 40 mg/d
	Fosinopril	0.1 mg/kg/d up to 10 mg/d	q.d.	0.6 mg/kg/d up to 40 mg/d
	Lisinopril	0.07 mg/kg/d up to 5 mg/d	q.d.	0.61 mg/kg/d up to 40 mg/d
	Quinapril	5–10 mg/d	q.d.	80 mg/d
	Ramipril	2.5 mg/d	q.d.	20 mg/d
Angiotensin-receptor blockers	Candesartan	4 mg/d	q.d.	32 mg q.d.
	Irbesartan	75–150 mg/d	q.d.	300 mg/d
α- and β-Antagonists	Losartan	0.75 mg/kg/d up to 50 mg/d	q.d.–b.i.d.	1.44 mg/kg/d up to 100 mg/d
	Labetalol	2–3 mg/kg/d	b.i.d.	10–12 mg/kg/d up to 2.4 g/d
	Carvedilol	0.1 mg/kg/dose up to 12.5 mg b.i.d.	b.i.d.	0.5 mg/kg/dose up to 25 mg b.i.d.
β-Antagonists	Atenolol	0.5–1 mg/kg/d	q.d.–b.i.d.	2 mg/kg/d up to 100 mg/d
	Bisoprolol/HCTZ	0.04 mg/kg/d up to 2.5/6.25 mg/d	q.d.	10/6.25 mg q.d.
	Metoprolol	1–2 mg/kg/d	b.i.d.	6 mg/kg/d up to 200 mg/d
	Propranolol	1 mg/kg/d	b.i.d.–t.i.d.	16 mg/kg/d
Calcium channel blockers	Amlodipine	0.06 mg/kg/d	q.d.	0.6 mg/kg/d up to 10 mg/d
	Felodipine	2.5 mg/d	q.d.	10 mg/d
	Isradipine	0.05–0.15 mg/kg/dose	t.i.d.–q.i.d.	0.8 mg/kg/d up to 20 mg/d
	Extended-release nifedipine	0.25–0.5 mg/kg/d	q.d.–b.i.d.	3 mg/kg/d up to 120 mg/d

(continued)

TABLE 13.5

(Continued)

Class	Drug	Starting Dose	Interval	Maximum Dose[a]
Central α-agonists	Clonidine	5–10 μg/kg/d	b.i.d.–t.i.d.	25 μg/kg/d up to 0.9 mg/d
	Methyldopa	5 mg/kg/d	b.i.d.–q.i.d.	40 mg/kg/d up to 3 g/d
Diuretics	Amiloride	5–10 mg/d	q.d.	20 mg/d
	Chlorthalidone	0.3 mg/kg/d	q.d.	2 mg/kg/d up to 50 mg/d
	Furosemide	0.5–2.0 mg/kg/dose	q.d.–b.i.d.	6 mg/kg/d
	HCTZ	1 mg/kg/d	b.i.d.	3 mg/kg/d up to 50 mg/d
	Spironolactone	1 mg/kg/d	q.d.–b.i.d.	3.3 mg/kg/d up to 100 mg/d
	Triamterene	1–2 mg/kg/d	b.i.d.	3–4 mg/kg/d up to 300 mg/d
Peripheral α-antagonists	Doxazosin	1 mg/d	q.d.	4 mg/d
	Prazosin	0.05–0.1 mg/kg/d	t.i.d.	0.5 mg/kg/d
	Terazosin	1 mg/d	q.d.	20 mg/d
Vasodilators	Hydralazine	0.25 mg/kg/dose	t.i.d.–q.i.d.	7.5 mg/kg/d up to 200 mg/d
	Minoxidil	0.1–0.2 mg/kg/d	b.i.d.–t.i.d.	1 mg/kg/d up to 50 mg/d

q.d., once-daily; b.i.d., twice-daily; t.i.d., three times daily; q.i.d., four times daily; HCTZ, hydrochlorothiazide.
[a]The maximum recommended adult dose should never be exceeded.

SUMMARY

Increasing numbers of adolescents may be found to be hypertensive because of the increasing prevalence of obesity. Most will have primary hypertension, but—after appropriate evaluation—a few will be found to have underlying causes. When pressures are found to be repeatedly elevated, nonpharmacologic antihypertensive measures should be started. Drug therapy is indicated only for selected individuals. The individualized stepped-care approach developed by the National High Blood Pressure Education Program Working Group is recommended. When hypertension is resistant to initial drug therapies, consultation with an expert on hypertension in adolescents should be sought.

REFERENCE

National High Blood Pressure Education Program Working Group on High Blood Pressure in Children and Adolescents. *The Fourth Report on the Diagnosis, Evaluation, and Treatment of High Blood Pressure in Children and Adolescents.* National Heart, Lung, and Blood Institute, Bethesda, Maryland. *Pediatrics* 2004;114:555–576. Also available online at http://www.nhlbi.nih.gov/health/prof/heart/hbp/hbp_ped. htm. Includes link to downloadable PDA application.

CHAPTER 14

Heart Murmurs and Mitral Valve Prolapse

Amy D. DiVasta and Mark E. Alexander

Cardiac murmurs occur in at least 50% of all normal children and are the most frequent reason for referral to a cardiologist. The vast majority are considered to be "innocent" or "physiologic" in origin. In most patients with cardiac murmurs, a careful history and physical examination establish the diagnosis and/or guide further referral and evaluation.

HISTORY

Murmurs first heard in childhood or adolescence are more likely to be innocent murmurs. Complaints of fatigue, decreased exercise tolerance, exertional chest pain, or palpitations are suggestive of pathologic heart disease. Any patient with syncope or near-syncope during exercise merits cardiac evaluation. A thorough family history should also be obtained, including a history of sudden death or a structural cardiac abnormality in a first-degree relative.

PHYSICAL EXAMINATION

A careful, stepwise examination is crucial, including performance of a dynamic cardiac exam.

1. General appearance, including assessment of growth and maturation
2. Pulses in upper and lower extremities
3. Blood pressures in arm and leg with properly sized blood pressure cuff
4. Palpation: (a) Thrill, heave, or lift over the precordium or suprasternal notch is usually pathologic; (b) Increased intensity and/or lateral displacement of the point of maximal impulse (PMI) suggests left ventricular (LV) enlargement.
5. Auscultation (see individual diagnoses for details):
   a. Splitting of S_1 can be a normal finding, but another sound close to S_1 is usually either a fourth heart sound (S_4) or an ejection click. The first and second components of S_2 should be of equal intensity and demonstrate respiratory variation. Wide, fixed splitting suggests right ventricular (RV) volume overload such as seen in an atrial septal defect. A single S_2 is also abnormal. A third heart sound (S_3) may be a normal finding in adolescents.

A fourth heart sound (S_4) may be normal in older adults but is almost always pathologic in adolescents.

  b. *Clicks:* Sharp, high-frequency sounds that are important clues to organic disease.

  c. *Murmurs:* Assess timing, loudness, length, tonal quality, and location.

DIAGNOSTIC CLUES FOR INNOCENT MURMURS

1. *History:* Asymptomatic, no family history of cardiac disease.
2. *Physical Examination:* Normal other than the presence of the murmur.
3. The timing of murmur is early systolic; almost never holosystolic or diastolic. Location may vary, but it is frequently at the lower or upper left sternal border (LSB); it does not radiate extensively. Intensity is usually grade 1-3/6 and often changes with position, louder in the supine position and quieter with sitting or standing. The murmur is vibratory in quality. There is physiologic splitting of S_2 and no clicks.

TYPES OF NORMAL MURMURS

Still's Murmur. Grade 1-3/6 low- to medium-pitched midsystolic murmur with vibratory or musical quality at the lower LSB. Murmur decreases with sitting or standing. Differentiated from hypertrophic cardiomyopathy because the murmur decreases with standing. Less harsh than a murmur associated with a ventricular septal defect.

Pulmonary Flow Murmur. Grade 1-3/6 short crescendo-decrescendo midsystolic murmur heard at the upper LSB. Murmur decreased by inspiration and sitting, increased in supine position. Differentiated from valvular pulmonary stenosis by absence of a click; differentiated from an atrial septal defect because S_2 splits normally.

Cervical Venous Hum. Medium-pitched, soft, blowing, continuous murmur heard best above the clavicle. Murmur increased by rotating the head away from the side of the murmur. Murmur decreased by jugular venous compression or supine position (unique for a normal murmur).

Supraclavicular (Carotid) Bruit. Short, high-pitched early systolic murmur, usually grade 2/6, heard above the clavicles with radiation to the neck while patient is sitting. Murmur decreased by hyperextending the shoulders (bringing the elbows behind the back).

DIAGNOSTIC CLUES FOR PATHOLOGIC MURMURS

1. *Significant History:* Growth failure, decreased exercise tolerance, exertional syncope or near-syncope, exertional chest pain
2. *Physical Examination:* Clubbing, cyanosis, decreased or delayed femoral pulses, apical heave, palpable thrill, tachypnea, inappropriate tachycardia

TABLE 14.1

Types of Pathological Murmurs

Murmur Type	Characteristics	Common Defects
Systolic ejection	Crescendo–decrescendo Begins after S_1; ends before S_2 Best heard with diaphragm	Aortic stenosis Pulmonary stenosis Coarctation of the aorta ASD
Holosystolic	Begins with and obscures S_1 Ends at S_2 Heard at LSB or apex	VSD Mitral regurgitation
Early diastolic	Decrescendo Begins immediately after S_2 High–medium pitch	Aortic insufficiency Pulmonary insufficiency
Mid-diastolic	Low pitch Rumble Best heard with bell	ASD VSD Mitral stenosis
Continuous	Extend up to and through S_2 Continue through all/part of diastole Best heard with diaphragm	PDA

ASD, atrial septal defect; LSB, left sternal border; VSD, ventricular septal defect; PDA, patent ductus arteriosus.

3. *Murmur:* Diastolic, holosystolic, loud or harsh, extensive radiation, increases with standing, associated with a thrill, abnormal S_2. See Table 14.1.

MURMURS ASSOCIATED WITH STRUCTURAL HEART DISEASE

Mild congenital heart disease, which is less common, may not present until adolescence.

Atrial Septal Defect.

1. *Physical Examination:* Signs and symptoms depend on shunt size. (a) Hyperdynamic precordium and RV lift with sizable shunt, no thrill; (b) widely split and fixed S_2; (c) pulmonary flow murmur, grade 2-3/6 systolic ejection murmur at upper LSB; (d) middiastolic rumble at lower LSB.
2. *Further Evaluation:* (a) Electrocardiogram (ECG) shows right axis deviation, right ventricular (RV) conduction delay (rSR′ pattern), right atrial enlargement, or RV hypertrophy; (b) chest x-ray shows mild to moderate cardiomegaly; increased pulmonary vascularity; (c) echocardiogram is diagnostic

with visualization of location and size of defect; (d) cardiac MRI provides excellent imaging of the atrial septum and RV volume.
3. *Management:* Both surgical closure and closure with a transcatheter device are safe, effective, and popular management choices.

Ventricular Septal Defect

1. *Physical Examination:* Shunt volume determines findings. (a) Hyperdynamic precordium with large shunt—a thrill may be present with either a large or small shunt; (b) S_2, normal with small shunts, accentuated with larger shunts. An S_3 may be present; (c) grade 2-3/6 holosystolic murmur at lower LSB; (d) middiastolic rumble at the apex with large shunts.
2. *Further Evaluation:* (a) ECG is normal, there is LV hypertrophy with large defects; (b) chest x-ray is usually normal, there is cardiomegaly and increased pulmonary vascularity in large defects; (c) echocardiogram provides anatomic detail of location and size of defect. Color Doppler permits visualization of very small defects.
3. *Management:* This is dependent on right ventricular (RV) pressure and may require cardiac catheterization to make appropriate therapeutic decisions. It is important to note that prophylaxis for bacterial endocarditis is no longer recommended for VSD.

Patent Ductus Arteriosus

1. *Physical Examination:* Shunt volume determines findings. (a) Normal precordium with small shunt, hyperdynamic with a thrill with large shunt; (b) grade 2-4/6 continuous murmur at upper LSB; (c) wide pulse pressure and bounding pulses with large shunt.
2. *Further Evaluation:* (a) ECG is normal, LV hypertrophy if left-to-right shunting is significant; (b) chest x-ray shows cardiomegaly and increased pulmonary vascularity with large shunts; (c) echocardiogram, visualization with two-dimensional and color Doppler imaging; (d) cardiac catheterization is rarely required for diagnosis but is commonly done for coil or device occlusion.

Valvular Pulmonary Stenosis

1. *Physical Examination:* Severity of obstruction determines findings. (a) RV lift with systolic thrill at upper LSB in more severe forms; (b) systolic ejection click at upper LSB that is louder with expiration (more difficult to hear in severe stenosis); (c) S_2 normal or widely split, depending on severity of stenosis; (d) Grade 2-4/6 harsh systolic ejection murmur at upper LSB, may radiate to the lung fields and back.
2. *Further Evaluation:* (a) ECG is normal, with progression to RV hypertrophy (upright T wave in lead V1) as stenosis increases; (b) chest x-ray shows prominent pulmonary artery segment with normal vascularity; (c) echocardiogram permits evaluation of valve morphology; (d) cardiac catheterization rarely required for diagnosis.
3. *Management:* Treatment of choice is balloon pulmonary valvuloplasty.

Valvular Aortic Stenosis (AS)

1. *Physical Examination:* Severity of obstruction determines findings. (a) Prominent apical impulse and systolic thrill (at upper RSB or suprasternal notch);

(b) intensity of S_1 may be diminished due to poor ventricular compliance; (c) systolic ejection click at lower LSB/apex that radiates to aortic area at upper RSB, no respiratory variation; (d) grade 2-4/6 long, harsh systolic crescendo-decrescendo ejection murmur at upper RSB; (e) high-frequency early diastolic decrescendo murmur of aortic regurgitation; (f) look carefully for features of associated Turner or Williams syndrome.

2. *Further Evaluation:* (a) ECG, normal to LV hypertrophy with strain pattern (ST-segment depression and T-wave inversion in left precordium) indicating severe stenosis; (b) chest x-ray shows prominent ascending aorta, normal vascularity; (c) echocardiogram permits evaluation of valve morphology and determination of level of stenosis—70% to 85% of stenotic valves are bicuspid; (d) cardiac catheterization is rarely required for diagnosis.

3. *Management:* In selected cases, aortic balloon valvuloplasty may be an initial palliative procedure.

Hypertrophic Cardiomyopathy

1. *Physical Examination:* (a) Normal to hyperdynamic precordium with increased LV impulse, dynamic thrill; (b) auscultation may be normal, dynamic examination is necessary and demonstrates systolic ejection murmur at the lower LSB with increasing intensity in standing position and decreasing intensity with squatting or Valsalva maneuver; (c) dynamic murmur of mitral insufficiency; (d) assess carefully for features of skeletal myopathy.

2. *Further Evaluation:* (a) ECG shows LV and/or septal hypertrophy and ST-T wave changes as well as atrial enlargement may be seen; (b) chest x-ray may show cardiomegaly; (c) echocardiogram is diagnostic, with excessive LV wall thickness, impaired ventricular filling, variable degrees of LV outflow tract obstruction, and variable systolic anterior motion of the mitral valve.

3. *Management:* Remains controversial but may include implantable defibrillators, surgical or catheter treatment, or drug therapy. Patients are restricted from competitive sports.

MITRAL VALVE PROLAPSE

Mitral valve prolapse (MVP) is a heterogeneous disorder with a wide spectrum of pathologic, clinical, and echocardiographic manifestations. Prevalence of MVP in the population is estimated to be 2% to 3% with equal gender distribution. MVP may be diagnosed at any age; symptomatic patients tend to be late adolescents or young adults. Although the diagnosis of MVP is common, clinically significant MVP is infrequent. Many cardiac symptoms (including palpitations, atypical chest pain, exercise intolerance, and syncope) that were historically attributed to the presence of MVP are no more common than in the general population and are probably unrelated to MVP. Patients whose MVP is associated with connective tissue disease are at increased risk for the development of mitral regurgitation, bacterial endocarditis, cerebral embolism, life-threatening arrhythmia, and sudden death.

1. *Physical Examination:* (a) Dynamic mid- to late-systolic click that moves later into systole with supine position or squatting and earlier into systole with standing or Valsalva; (b) high-pitched late-systolic murmur heard best at the apex of the heart—some patients have no click and only a late systolic

murmur; (c) associated physical abnormalities include scoliosis, pectus excavatum, decreased anteroposterior diameter, and stigmata of commonly associated connective tissue disorders.

2. *Further Evaluation:* (a) ECG is normal; (b) chest x-ray is normal; (c) ambulatory ECGs (Holter or event monitoring) may be indicated to evaluate for arrhythmia if the patient has palpitations that disrupt activities of daily living or cause serious symptoms (syncope, dizziness); (d) echocardiogram allows visualization of the mitral valve, assessment for mitral regurgitation, and confirmation of the diagnosis of MVP. Mild bowing of a mitral leaflet, a normal variant, should not be misdiagnosed as frank prolapse.

3. *Management:* (a) Asymptomatic patients without mitral regurgitation need reassurance but do not need activity restriction, antibiotic prophylaxis, or follow-up echocardiography; (b) patients with mitral insufficiency, ventricular arrhythmias, history of cardiac syncope, or family history of premature sudden death may require activity restrictions and careful consideration of athletic choices; (c) new recommendations from the American Heart Association significantly reduce the indications for antibiotic prophylaxis of bacterial endocarditis (Fig. 14.1).

   Routine prophylaxis for bacterial endocarditis is no longer recommended for MVP. The complete guidelines are available at: http://www.americanheart.org/presenter.jhtml?identifier=3004539 and a wallet card (Fig. 14.1) is available at: http://www.americanheart.org/presenter.jhtml?identifier=11086. (d) beta-blocking agents may be indicated for either symptomatic relief or to target a specific arrhythmia—there is no evidence that beta-blockade decreases the already low risk of sudden death; (e) mild mitral regurgitation is generally well tolerated during pregnancy; (f) first-degree relatives of patients with myxomatous MVP should be screened with echocardiography owing to the high prevalence of the diagnosis within families.

4. *Complications:* Complications of MVP are rare unless significant disease is present. (a) Arrhythmias are the most frequent complication, including premature ventricular contractions, supraventricular tachyarrhythmia, ventricular tachycardia, and bradyarrhythmia; (b) increased risk of bacterial endocarditis in patients with MVP and mitral regurgitation; (c) progressive mitral regurgitation is rare in otherwise healthy adolescents; (d) very low risk of sudden death, but the incidence is still greater than that in the general population, likely due to ventricular arrhythmia; (e) association of MVP and stroke is controversial.

MITRAL VALVE REGURGITATION

1. *Physical Examination:* Findings depend on severity of regurgitation. (a) Normal to hyperdynamic precordium; (b) grade 2-4/6 high-frequency holosystolic apical murmur; may radiate toward the base (upper LSB); (c) low-frequency apical middiastolic rumble with severe regurgitation.

2. *Further Evaluation:* (a) ECG: bifid P wave of left atrial enlargement if regurgitation is chronic and severe; (b) chest x-ray is normal or shows cardiomegaly; (c) echocardiogram demonstrates cause and severity of regurgitation; (d) patients with significant mitral insufficiency no longer require bacterial endocarditis prophylaxis. Patients are followed to identify need for afterload-decreasing agents or surgery.

PREVENTION OF BACTERIAL ENDOCARDITIS
Wallet Card

This wallet card is to be given to patients (or parents) by their physician. Healthcare professionals Please see back of card for reference to the complete statement.

Name: _____

needs protection from **BACTERIAL ENDOCARDITIS**
because of an existing heart condition.

Diagnosis: _____
Prescribed by: _____
Date: _____

You received this wallet card because you are at increased risk for developing adverse outcomes from infective endocarditis, also known as bacterial endocarditis (BE). The guidelines for prevention of BE shown in this card are substantially different from previously published guidelines. This card replaces the previous card that was based on guidelines published in 1997.

The American Heart Association's Endocarditis Committee together with national and international experts on BE extensively reviewed published studies in order to determine whether dental, gastrointestinal (GI), or genitourinary (GU) tract procedures are possible causes of BE. These experts determined that there is no conclusive evidence that links dental, GI, or GU tract procedures with the development of BE.

The current practice of giving patients antibiotics prior to a dental procedure is no longer recommended **EXCEPT** for patients with the highest risk of adverse outcomes resulting from BE (see below on this card). The Committee cannot exclude the possibility that an exceedingly small number of cases, if any, of BE may be prevented by antibiotic prophylaxis prior to a dental procedure. If such benefit from prophylaxis exists, it should be reserved **ONLY** for those patients listed below. The Committee recognizes the importance of good oral and dental health and regular visits to the dentist for patients at risk of BE.

The Committee no longer recommends administering antibiotics solely to prevent BE in patients who undergo a GI or GU tract procedure.

Changes in these guidelines do not change the fact that your cardiac condition put you at increased risk for developing endocarditis. If you develop signs or symptoms of endocarditis – such as unexplained fever – see your doctor right away. If blood cultures are necessary (to determine if endocarditis is present), it is important for your doctor to obtain these cultures and other relevant tests **BEFORE** antibiotics are started.

Antibiotic prophylaxis with dental procedures is recommended only for patients with cardiac conditions associated with the highest risk of adverse outcomes from endocarditis, including:

• Prosthetic cardiac valve

• Previous endocarditis

• Congenital heart disease only in the following categories:

  –Unrepaired cyanotic congenital heart disease, including those with palliative shunts and conduits

  –Completely repaired congenital heart disease with prosthetic material or device, whether placed by surgery or catheter intervention, during the first six months after the procedudre*

  –Repaired congenital heart disease with residual defects at the site or adjacent to the site of a prosthetic patch or prosthetic device (which inhibit endothelialization)

• Cardiac transplantation recipients with cardiac valvular disease

*Prophylaxis is recommended because endothelialization of prosthetic material occurs within six months after the procedure.

Dental procedures for which prophylaxis is recommended in patients with cardiac conditions listed above.

FIGURE 14.1 American Heart Association wallet card with recommendations for antibiotic prophylaxis of endocarditis. Available at http://www.americanheart.org/presenter.jhtml?identifier=11086. Adapted from Prevention of Infective Endocarditis: Guidelines From the American Heart Association, by the Committee on Rheumatic Fever, Endocarditis, and Kawasaki Disease. Circulation, e-published April 19, 2007. Accessible at www.americanheart.org/presenter.jhtml?identifier=3004539.

All dental procedures that involve manipulation of gingival tissue or the periapical region of teeth, or perforation of the oral mucosa*

*Antibiotic prophylaxis is NOT recommended for the following dental procedures or events: routine anesthetic injections through noninfected tissue; taking dental radiographs; placement of removable prosthodontic or orthodontic appliances; adjustment of orthodontic appliances; placement of orthodontic brackets; and shedding of deciduous teeth and bleeding from trauma to the lips or oral mucosa.

Antibiotic Prophylactic Regimens Recommended for Dental Procedures

Situation	Agent	Regimen – Single Dose 30-60 minutes before procedure	
		Adults	Children
Oral	Amoxicillin	2 g	50 mg/kg
Unable to take oral medication	Ampicillin **OR**	2 g IM or IV*	50 mg/kg IM or IV
	Cefazolin or ceftriaxone	1 g IM or IV	50 mg/kg IM or IV
Allergic to penicillins or ampicillin – Oral regimen	Cephalexin**† **OR** Clindamycin **OR**	2 g 600 mg	50 mg/kg 20 mg/kg
	Azithromycin or clarithromycin	500 mg	15 mg/kg
Allergic to penicillins or ampicillin and unable to take oral medication	Cefazolin or ceftriaxone† **OR** Clindamycin	1 g IM or IV 600 mg IM or IV	50 mg/kg IM or IV 20 mg/kg IM or IV

*IM – intramuscular; IV – intravenous
**Or other first or second generation oral cephalosporin in equivalent adult or pediatric dosage.
†Cephalosporins should not be used in an individual with a history of anaphylaxis, angioedema or urticaria with penicillins or ampicillin.

Gastrointestinal/Genitourinary Procedures: Antibiotic prophylaxix solely to prevent BE is no longer recommended for patients who under-go a GI or GU tract procedure, including patients with the highest risk of adverse outcomes due to BE.

Other Procedures: BE prophylaxis for procedures of the respiratory tract or infected skin, tissues just under the skin, or musculoskeletal tissue is recommended **ONLY** for patients with the underlying cardiac conditions shown above.

Adapted from *Prevention of Infective Endocarditis: Guidelines From the American Heart Association,* by the Committee on Rheumatic Fever, Endocarditis, and Kawasaki Disease. *Circulation*, e-published April 19, 2007. Accessible at www.americanheart.org/presenter.jhtml?identifier=3004539.

Healthcare Professionals – Please refer to these recommendations for more complete information as to which patients and which procedures need prophylaxis.

American Heart | **American Stroke**
Association₀ | **Association**₀
*Learn and Live*₁₂₀

The Council on Scientific Affairs of the American Dental Association has approved this statement as it relates to dentistry.

National Center
7272 Greenville Avenue
Dallas, Texas 75231 -4596
americanheart.org

50-1605 0705

FIGURE 14.1 *(Continued)*

SYSTEMIC CONNECTIVE TISSUE DISEASE AND THE HEART

Marfan Syndrome: An autosomal dominant global connective tissue disorder with ocular, musculoskeletal, and cardiac involvement. Cardiac management in these patients is done based on the aortic root dilation. Beta blockers are used as prophylaxis to try to slow dilation, which may progress rapidly during pregnancy. Patients with Marfan's syndrome are generally restricted from high-intensity and collision sports.

Ehlers-Danlos Syndromes (EDS): A range of disorders characterized by abnormalities in collagen and musculoskeletal involvement. MVP is relatively common. Aortic root dilation is less severe and less frequent than in Marfan's syndrome. Patients with EDS may demonstrate symptoms of palpitations, presyncope, and syncope associated with the autonomic dysregulation and neurally mediated hypotension of postural orthostatic tachycardia.

REFERENCES AND ADDITIONAL READINGS

American Heart Association. Patient information on endocarditis prophylaxis, accessed at http://www.americanheart.org/downloadable/heart/1023826501754 walletcard.pdf

Wilson W, Taubert KA, Gewitz M, et al. Prevention of infective endocarditis: guidelines from the American Heart Association: a guideline from the American Heart Association Rheumatic Fever, Endocarditis, and Kawasaki Disease Committee, Council on Cardiovascular Disease in the Young, and the Council on Clinical Cardiology, Council on Cardiovascular Surgery and Anesthesia, and the Quality of Care and Outcomes Research Interdisiplinary Working Group. *Circulation* 2007;116(15):1736.

Maron BJ, Zipes DP. 31st Bethesda Conference: Eligibility Recommendations for Competitive Athletes with Cardiovascular Abnormalities. *J Am Coll Cardiol* 2005; 45:1313.

Maron BJ, Chaitman BR, Ackerman MJ, et al. Recommendations for physical activity and recreational sports participation for young patients with genetic cardiovascular diseases. *Circulation* 2004;109:2807.

CHAPTER **15**

Scoliosis and Kyphosis

Matthew J. Bueche

Scoliosis is a lateral curvature of the spine (10 degrees or greater by the Cobb method) usually associated with rotational deformity of the spine and trunk. The majority of adolescents have adolescent idiopathic scoliosis, a condition with no apparent cause. Scoliosis may be associated with neuromuscular diseases. Congenital scoliosis is deformity secondary to vertebral malformations. Nonstructural or functional scoliosis may result from leg-length discrepancy or back pain. Numerous syndromes—including Marfan, neurofibromatosis, and myelodysplasia—involve spinal deformity.

IDIOPATHIC SCOLIOSIS

Types
Infantile, onset from birth to 3 years of age; *Juvenile,* between 3 and 9 years; *Adolescent,* usually seen in females between 10 years of age and the time of skeletal maturity.

Prevalence
Approximately 2% to 3% of adolescents have a curve >10 degrees and 0.5% have a curve >20 degrees. Curves severe enough to require treatment are over seven times more frequent in females.

Natural History
Long-term complications of continued curve progression include cosmetic effects, back pain, neurologic compromise, and restrictive pulmonary disease leading to cor pulmonale and death. Severe problems are uncommon.

TABLE 15.1

Risk of Progression of Idiopathic Scoliosis

| Initial Curve (degrees) | Age at Presentation | | | |
	Girls, 10–12 yr (%)	Girls, 13–15 yr (%)	Girls, >15 yr (%)	Boys (%)
<19	25	1	<1	3
20–29	60	40	10	6
30–59	90	70	30	—
>60	100	90	—	—

From Nachemson A, Lonstein JE, Weinstein SL. Prevalence and natural history committee report. *Read at the Annual Meeting Scoliosis Research Society*. Denver, CO: Scoliosis Research Society, Sept. 25, 1982.

Risk Factors for Progression

The following factors can predict up to 80% of progressive curves: (1) age at onset and gender (Table 15.1); (2) magnitude of the curve—a 20-degree curve being associated with a 20% risk of progression whereas a 50-degree curve is associated with a 90% chance of progression; (3) skeletal maturity—Risser stage 0 curves progress 36% to 68% of the time compared to 11% to 18% of Risser stage 3 or 4 curves.

Scoliosis Screening

The American Academy of Orthopedic Surgeons advocate screening girls twice at ages 10 and 12 (grades 5 and 7) and boys once, at age 13 or 14 (grade 8 or 9) (AAOS, 1992). In contrast, the U.S. Preventive Services Task Force concluded that the harms (unnecessary brace use and unnecessary consultations) of screening for idiopathic scoliosis exceed the potential benefits. Some state laws mandate school screening for scoliosis.

Clinical Evaluation

History. This should include age and menarchal status, presence of pain, neurologic symptoms, and family history of scoliosis and spine disorders.

Physical Examination. This should include (1) height with serial measurements; (2) neurologic examination; (3) skin, including café-au-lait spots and hairy patches over the spine; (4) pelvic obliquity (e.g., leg-length inequality); (5) sexual maturity rating to evaluate risk of progression; (6) spinal examination—performed with the patient standing, wearing underwear, and a gown open in the back—including (a) side-to-side symmetry, (b) shoulder height, (c) iliac crest symmetry and palpation to ascertain leg-length equality; (d) forward bending—the Adams forward bend test is performed with the adolescent bending forward with arms extended and knees straight while the examiner looks for asymmetry of the trunk and rib hump or paralumbar prominence, which should be measured with an inclinometer; (e) lateral exam—evaluation for sagittal plane deformity is performed with the examiner at the patient's side

TABLE 15.2

Signs of Nonidiopathic Scoliosis

Region	Finding	Possible Significance
Skin	Hairy patch over spine	Congenital spinal anomaly
	Café-au-lait spots	Neurofibromatosis
Joints	Hyperelasticity	Marfan syndrome/Ehlers-Danlos syndrome
Reflexes (including abdominal)	Abnormal	Neuromuscular disease
Extremities	Excessively long	Marfan syndrome
	Excessively short	Skeletal dysplasias
Pelvis (standing)	Obliquity	Leg length discrepancy

while the forward bend test is repeated to note the smoothness of the thoracic kyphosis (see Scheuermann kyphosis, below).

Physical examination signs indicative of nonidiopathic scoliosis are listed in Table 15.2.

Imaging

Radiographs for Suspected Scoliosis. Recommended for adolescents with an angle of trunk rotation >7 degrees as measured by an inclinometer; includes standing posteroanterior and lateral spinal radiographs using 36-in. films taken at 6-ft distance. Radiographic signs include sharply angular curve (neurofibromatosis), fused ribs (congenital scoliosis), widened intrapedicular distance (syringomyelia), left thoracic curvature (neuromuscular etiologies).

Magnetic Resonance Imaging. MRI of the full spine is recommended for adolescents with the following findings: (1) neurologic findings on physical examination; (2) unusual pain; (3) left major thoracic curve: These are associated (in 10% of cases otherwise thought to be idiopathic) with occult syrinx, Arnold-Chiari malformation, spinal cord tumor, and neuromuscular disorder. Only 2% of adolescent idiopathic thoracic curves are convex to the left.

Criteria for Referral to an Orthopedic Surgeon

These include (1) skeletally immature patients with a Cobb angle >20 degrees and (2) skeletally mature patients with a Cobb angle >40 degrees.

Treatment

Treatment of nonidiopathic scoliosis is outlined in Table 15.3.

Brace Therapy. Brace therapy should be considered in the skeletally immature adolescent whose curve measures from 25 to 40 degrees. The primary goal of brace management is to halt curve progression. This modality should not be expected to improve curvature permanently, but outcomes are better than would be expected from natural history alone. Skeletal maturation, defined as

TABLE 15.3

Management of Adolescent Idiopathic Scoliosis

Curve Size (degrees)	Therapy
0–25	Serial observation if immature
25–30 (with progression of 5–10 degrees)	Brace
30–40	Brace
>40	Surgery if immature
>50	Surgery (adult)

no further changes in height and a Risser stage IV, is usually considered the endpoint for brace use.

Surgery. Recommended for skeletally immature patients who have a curve >40 to 45 degrees or in skeletally mature patients with curves >50 degrees, particularly if curve progression has been documented. Surgery fuses the vertebrae in the curve, preventing further progression. Rods are implanted to allow for reliable fusion and curve correction.

Other Treatments. Neither exercise programs or electrical stimulation have been shown to be effective in altering the natural history of idiopathic scoliosis.

INCREASED KYPHOSIS

Normal sagittal plane posture includes rounded shoulders (thoracic kyphosis) and swayback (lumbar lordosis). Increased kyphosis in adolescents is commonly caused by juvenile postural roundback and less commonly by Scheuermann kyphosis.

Adolescent Roundback (Juvenile Postural Roundback). Many adolescents manifest an excessively kyphotic posture. The spine is flexible enough that they can stand straighter if they desire. On forward bending, the spine shows a smooth curvature when viewed from the side. Lateral radiographs may show the increased thoracic kyphosis, but the individual vertebrae and disc spaces will appear normal. A physical therapy program may be helpful for pain or appearance issues.

Scheuermann Kyphosis. Scheuermann is a relatively rigid, abnormally increased kyphosis of the thoracic and thoracolumbar spine that does not correct with hyperextension. The kyphosis results from anterior vertebral wedging. Vertebral endplate irregularities and Schmorl nodes (protrusion of disc material into the vertebral bodies) are also seen.

Natural History. Most patients with <75 degrees of kyphosis have a benign course in adulthood with some deformity, back pain, and fatigue.

Treatment. (1) Exercise programs to strengthen the lower back and improve hamstring and pectoral flexibility may be used for patients with smaller curves (<50 degrees). Exercise may improve comfort and appearance but has not been shown to improve vertebral wedging or the degree of kyphosis. (2) Bracing treatment has been used for immature patients with significant deformity. (3) Operative correction (spinal fusion) is rarely indicated and reserved for patients with marked deformity or severe pain.

WEB SITES AND REFERENCES

http://www.scoliosis-assoc.org/. Scoliosis Association, Inc., an international information and support organization.

http://www.scoliosis.org/, National Scoliosis Foundation. Patient advocacy and information.

http://orthoinfo.aaos.org/fact/thr_report.cfm?Thread_ID=262&topcategory=Children. American Association of Orthopedic Surgeons brochure on Childhood Scoliosis.

http://www.srs.org. The Scoliosis Research Society.

http://www.nlm.nih.gov/medlineplus/scoliosis.html. Medline plus health information.

Miller NH. Cause and natural history of adolescent idiopathic scoliosis. *Orthop Clin North Am* 1999;30:343.

Weinstein SL, ed. The *pediatric spine: principles and practice*, 2nd ed. Philadelphia: Lippincott, 2001.

CHAPTER 16

Common Orthopedic Problems

Keith J. Loud and Robert J. Bielski

A GENERAL APPROACH TO MANAGEMENT

1. Plain radiographs (x-rays) should be considered for any unilateral complaint, with greater urgency for pain that wakes a patient from sleep or any unexplained or persistent bilateral complaints.
2. In acute trauma, there are general criteria for immediate consultation with an orthopedic surgeon regardless of the injury site. These criteria include (a) obvious deformity; (b) acute locking (joint cannot be moved actively or passively past a certain point); (c) penetrating wound of major joint, muscle, or tendon; (d) neurologic deficit; (e) joint instability perceived by athlete or elicited by physician; (f) bony crepitus.
3. The prevention of long-term sequelae of injury depends on complete rehabilitation, which is characterized by full, pain-free range of motion (ROM) and normal strength, endurance, and proprioception. To prevent disappointment, avoid predicting time frames for return to participation, because individuals progress at different rates.

Phase 1: Limit Further Injury and Control Pain and Swelling
1. The affected part must be rested and protected.
2. Rest, ice, compression, and elevation (RICE) as often as possible during waking hours.
3. Analgesic medication (e.g., acetaminophen, NSAIDs), if prescribed, should be dosed regularly to achieve therapeutic steady-state levels, not "as needed."
4. Uninjured structures should be exercised to maintain cardiovascular fitness.

Phase 2: Improve Strength and ROM of Injured Structures
1. Relative rest is the cardinal principle.
2. Specific exercises should be done within a pain-free ROM.
3. Analgesic medication and ice should be continued, not to mask the pain and allow premature return to play but to interrupt the cycle of pain, muscle spasm, inflexibility, weakness, and decreased endurance.
4. General fitness maintenance should continue.

Phase 3: Achieve Near-Normal Strength, ROM, Endurance, and Proprioception of Injured Structures

1. Exercise is progressed following the relative rest principle.
2. Healing of ligaments and tendons treated nonoperatively manifests as minimal laxity with provocative testing, normal ROM, no tenderness or pain with stretching, and progressively less pain with activities of daily living.

Phase 4: Return to Exercise or Sport, Free of Symptoms

1. Successful rehabilitation minimizes the risk of re-injury and returns the injured structures to baseline ROM, strength, endurance, and proprioception.
2. Premature return is likely to result in further injury or another injury.
3. Functional rehabilitation should be sport-specific.
4. Supervision of the exercise progression by a rehabilitation professional such as a physical therapist or certified athletic trainer is *strongly* recommended.

COMMON INJURIES AND CONDITIONS

Large Muscle Contusions

The prototype injury in this category is the quadriceps contusion, as from a direct blow to the thigh. The pathophysiology of the injury is bleeding in and around the muscle as a result of the contusion. The muscle immediately goes into spasm, resulting in pain and disability. The key is to stop further bleeding by applying ice for 20 minutes. Apply a tight compression wrap and have the patient elevate the affected part. NSAIDs should not be given because they might promote decreased clotting. Acetaminophen can be given for pain.

The patient should start isometric contractions as soon as possible. In moderate to severe injuries, treatment by a sports-trained physical therapist is essential. The use of ultrasound can promote rapid recovery from this injury. If the bleeding is extensive and the athlete is reinjured before the hematoma has resolved, he or she is at risk for development of myositis ossificans, which can be career-threatening and may require surgical excision.

Knee Injuries

History. This is focused on the mechanism of injury, the events after the injury, and the factors that worsen or improve the pain.

1. Knee pain that occurs while running straight, without direct trauma or fall.
   a. *Chronic pain:* Likely to be patellofemoral dysfunction or syndrome (PFS).
   b. *Acute pain:* Consider osteochondritis dissecans (OCD) and pathologic fracture.
2. Knee injury that occurs during weight bearing, cutting while running, or an unplanned fall: Consider internal derangement including ligamentous and meniscal tears fracture. A player who injures the knee while cutting without being hit or having direct trauma has a torn anterior cruciate ligament tear until proven otherwise.
3. A valgus injury to the knee (i.e., a force delivered to the outside of the knee, directed toward the midline) is likely to tear the medial collateral ligament, possibly the anterior cruciate ligament, and either the medial or lateral meniscus.

4. Chronic anterior knee pain that is worse when going up stairs, after sitting for prolonged periods, or after squatting or running, is likely to be due to patellofemoral dysfunction.
5. If there is hemarthrosis within 24 hours after the injury, internal derangement is present and a diagnosis must be sought.

Physical Examination. This should include the following: (1) observation of gait; (2) inspection for swelling and discoloration; (3) observation of the vastus medialis obliquus (VMO), looking for reduced bulk and tone; (4) peripatellar palpation (tenderness over the tibial tuberosity is diagnostic of Osgood-Schlatter disease; peripatellar pain is characteristic of PFS); (5) quadriceps and hamstring flexibility; (6) signs of meniscal tears (McMurray and modified McMurray tests); (7) signs of ligamentous instability; (8) Lachman test and pivot shift test (anterior cruciate ligament); and (9) sag sign and posterior drawer test (posterior cruciate ligament).

Radiographic Evaluation. Any teen with knee pain, no history of trauma, but an equivocal examination that does not pinpoint the diagnosis must have a radiographic examination of the knee. If the hip examination is abnormal, radiographs of the hip are also needed to rule out slipped capital femoral epiphysis. Osgood-Schlatter disease and patellofemoral dysfunction do not require radiographs to establish a diagnosis. Anteroposterior and lateral views are standard. The sunrise view details the patellofemoral joint and should be ordered if patellar dislocation is suspected, while the tunnel view should be ordered if there is suspicion of osteochondritis dessicans, ACL injury, or other internal derangement. MRI evaluation in the acute or chronically injured knee should not be routine.

Management. After establishing a working diagnosis, ensure relative rest. Prescribe use of crutches if the patient cannot bear weight without pain. Knee immobilizers have a limited role in the management of acute knee injuries because they are awkward and offer minimal structural support. Apply ice for 20 minutes three or four times a day. Elevate the leg as much as possible and use a compression wrap. Prescribe analgesic medication if necessary. Start isometric quadriceps contractions on the first day if possible. If the patient cannot contract the quadriceps, consider an electrical stimulation unit until the patient is able to do so. Refer the patient for physical therapy (PT).

Subluxation and Dislocation of the Patella

Subluxation and lateral dislocation of the patella are prevalent in the second and third decades of life, with a slightly higher prevalence in females. Symptoms include pain, giving way of the knee, a popping or grinding sensation, and swelling. Subluxation of the patella can mimic the clinical picture of a torn meniscus. Complete dislocation is usually a dramatic event with the patella displaced to the lateral side of the joint, although it often reduces spontaneously.

Subluxation of the Patella. (1) Temporarily restrict or modify activity; (2) prescribe PT for a quadriceps strengthening program; (3) use a patellar sleeve or taping to stabilize the patella; (4) refer for surgery only if all other therapy fails.

Dislocation of the Patella. (1) Reduction often occurs spontaneously; (2) gentle straightening of the knee by lifting the foot may allow the patella to slide into place; (3) radiographs should be obtained because fractures are seen in up to 10% of cases; (4) immobilize the knee in a knee immobilizer for 3 weeks, followed by PT for ROM and quadriceps strengthening exercises.

Recurrent Dislocation. In some cases, therapy and bracing are successful. When the patient has more than one dislocation, however, surgical intervention may be needed.

Osgood-Schlatter Disease

Osgood-Schlatter disease is a painful enlargement of the tibial tubercle caused by traction stress at the insertion of the patellar tendon. It is a common problem, especially among active adolescent males during rapid linear growth.

Clinical Manifestations. (1) Pain and soft tissue swelling over the tibial tubercle, which is exacerbated by activity; (2) normal knee joint with full ROM; (3) unilateral involvement is more common than bilateral involvement; (4) duration is usually several months, it but can be longer.

Diagnosis. Physical examination demonstrates tenderness, swelling, and warmth of the tibial tubercle. Radiographs are not essential for diagnosis.

Therapy. (1) Reassure the adolescent and his or her parents; (2) if symptoms are mild, the patient may continue to be active. Limit activity for 2 to 4 weeks if symptoms are moderate; (3) if symptoms are severe or fail to respond to restriction of activity, immobilization with a knee immobilizer for a few weeks is effective; (4) nonsteroidal anti-inflammatory drugs and ice may provide symptomatic pain relief; (5) knee pads should be used for activities in which kneeling or direct knee contact might occur; (6) surgery is rarely indicated.

Prognosis. This is excellent, but adolescents should be informed that the process might recur if they engage in too much activity. The problem usually resolves when growth is completed.

Patellofemoral Syndrome (PFS)

Patellofemoral syndrome, or patellofemoral dysfunction, is a result of abnormal biomechanical forces that occur across the patella; it is a frequent cause of knee pain among adolescents, accounting for as much as 70% to 80% of knee pain problems in females and 30% of those in males.

Clinical Manifestations. (1) Pain is peripatellar or retropatellar and increases with activity; (2) prolonged sitting with flexed knee is uncomfortable; (3) pain is often severe on ascending or descending stairs; (4) knees may buckle or give out, especially when going up or down stairs; (5) crepitus or a grating sensation may be felt, especially when climbing stairs; (6) history of injury to the patellar area may or may not be present; (7) symptoms are bilateral in one third of adolescents; (8) two thirds of patients have at least a 6-month history of pain.

Physical Examination. (1) Inspection reveals patellar malalignment, external tibial torsion, or genu valgum ("knock knees"), which increases the Q angle; (2) there is tenderness of the articular surface of the patella; (3) retropatellar crepitation may be elicited; (4) the dynamic patellar compression test, or "grind sign," is positive if there is pain by compressing the superior aspect of the patella between thumb and index finger as the adolescent actively tightens the quadriceps in 10 degrees of flexion; (5) ROM is usually normal; (6) hamstrings are often tight; (7) joint effusion is usually absent; (8) decreased bulk of the vastus medialis may be present.

Diagnosis. The diagnosis is usually made by compatible history and physical examination. Radiographs are not indicated except to exclude other conditions.

Treatment. (1) Relative rest and NSAIDs initially; (2) most patients benefit from formal PT evaluation with progression to a home program for muscle strengthening; (3) after symptoms are controlled, a graduated running program can be instituted; (4) a maintenance program of quadriceps and hamstring exercises should be done two to three times a week; (5) bracing and taping of the knee is controversial; (6) over-the-counter arch supports can be helpful to some patients; (7) most adolescents respond to nonoperative management; (8) surgery is considered a last resort for patellofemoral pain.

Osteochondritis Dissecans

Osteochondritis dissecans is a condition of focal avascular necrosis of unclear etiology in which bone and overlying articular cartilage separate from the medial or lateral femoral condyle. The clinical course and treatment vary according to the age at onset, with children and young adolescents having a better prognosis than older adolescents and adults (Table 16.1).

Clinical Manifestations. With onset in childhood and early adolescence, the history is of intermittent, nonspecific knee pain usually related to activity. In

TABLE 16.1

Juvenile Versus Adult Osteochondritis

Characteristic	Juvenile	Adult
Age	5–15 yr	15–30 yr
Epiphyses	Open	Closed
Bilateral	30% of cases	10% of cases
Onset	Insidious	Acute
Injury	Minor factor	Major factor
Prognosis	Excellent	Fair
Complications	Seldom	Occasionally

later adolescence or young adulthood, onset is insidious or may be associated with sudden pain and swelling after an acute injury. Localized tenderness over the site of the lesion is best detected with the knee in 90 degrees of flexion for palpation of the femoral condyles, since most lesions are in the posterior femoral condyle. Bilateral involvement and synovial effusion are more common in younger than in older patients.

Radiographic Findings. The lesion may not be seen on a standard antero-posterior view and is best appreciated on the tunnel view.

Treatment. (1) Restrict symptom-producing activities; (2) immobilize with cast or knee immobilizer if symptoms are severe; (3) recommend quadri-ceps strengthening exercises; (4) NSAIDs may be useful if pain or effusion are present; (5) management is typically nonoperative in younger patients, although orthopedic or sports medicine referral is recommended for appro-priate staging and follow-up; (6) surgical consultation is required if there is a free fragment, progressive fragment formation, increasing bony sclerosis, or articular changes.

The Lower Leg: Shin Splints and Stress Fractures

Patients with these conditions experience lower extremity pain, commonly in the medial shin, that initially appears toward the end of exercise. Eventually, pain will occur earlier and persist longer. It can occur in any weight-bearing athlete but is most common in runners. Other diagnostic possibilities include compartment syndromes and vascular abnormalities.

Clinical Manifestations. The pain of shin splints is more diffuse and tender-ness is typically at the muscle–bone interface along the medial tibia. In stress fractures of the medial tibia, the pain is more pinpoint and over bone, not muscle.

Radiographic Findings. Further diagnostic studies may be indicated, since the injury spectrum from shin splints to stress reaction to stress fracture can be difficult to distinguish clinically. Plain radiographs of patients with tibial stress fractures may demonstrate callus formation a few weeks after the injury, but the most sensitive test to diagnose stress fractures has been bone scan. This is being challenged but has not yet been replaced by MRI. Consider bone density evaluation by DXA in female adolescents with stress fracture, especially those with risk factors for osteoporosis.

Treatment. Treatment includes the following: (1) relative rest and a func-tional progressive rehabilitation program; (2) analgesics or NSAIDs for 7 to 10 days, but they should not be used to mask pain and allow the athlete to return to activity prematurely; (3) ice each day for 20 minutes directly to the site; (4) shoe inserts to control overpronation if indicated; (5) increased shock absorption of the patient's shoes; (6) stretching and strengthening of the dor-siflexors, plantarflexors, and everters.

Acute Ankle Injuries

The mechanism of acute ankle injury in 85% of the cases is inversion (turning the ankle under or in). Injuries resulting from eversion are generally more serious because of the higher risk of syndesmosis injury and fracture.

Clinical Manifestations. Patients commonly present with diffuse swelling, tenderness, and decreased ROM hours to days after the injury. At a minimum the examination should include inspection for gross abnormalities, asymmetry, and vascular integrity; palpation for bony tenderness, specifically at the medial and lateral malleoli, proximal fibula, anterior joint line, navicular, and base of the fifth metatarsal; and assessment of weight bearing. The physical examination may be more informative at 3 to 4 days after injury, where examination should also include assessment of active and passive ROM, talar tilt and anterior drawer tests, and assessment for pain-free weight bearing and gait. Up to 15% of all complete ligament tears have an associated fracture. The most common sites are the talus, fifth metatarsal, fibula, and tibia. If there is bony tenderness in patients with open epiphyses, assume that a fracture is present even if radiographs are negative.

Radiographic Findings and the Ottawa Ankle Rules. A plain radiograph of the ankle or foot is indicated if there is bone tenderness at the distal/posterior 6 cm of the tibia or fibula (ankle series) or at the navicular or base of the fifth metatarsal (foot series) or if the patient is unable to take four steps both immediately after the injury and during the examination regardless of limping (Steill et al., 1996b).

Treatment. Successful treatment is defined not only by the absence of pain but also by return to full ROM, strength, and proprioception. (1) Relative rest; (2) ice; (3) elevation for the first 2 to 3 days; (4) NSAIDs or acetaminophen for pain relief; (5) compression and stability can be provided by an air stirrup, which should be used for all acute sprains not complicated by fracture; (6) casting is not indicated for ankle sprains not complicated by fracture.

Rehabilitation. This begins on the first day of evaluation. Recommend: (1) relative rest; (2) stretching, primarily soleus and gastrocnemius; (3) strengthening (e.g., band exercises); (4) proprioceptive retraining; (5) functional progression of exercise as tolerated; (6) the air stirrup should be worn in competition for 6 months after the injury.

Tarsal Coalition

Tarsal coalition is a congenital abnormality, with a prevalence of approximately 1%, that results in a partial or complete fusion between two bones of the foot. The condition may be unilateral or bilateral. It is the most common cause of a painful, stiff, flat foot after the age of 8 years.

Clinical Manifestations. Pain does not begin until the coalition begins to ossify at 8 to 12 years of age for calcaneonavicular coalitions and 12 to 15 years for talocalcaneal coalitions. Patients often complain of a recurring "ankle sprain." On examination, the patient has a rigid, flat foot and almost complete lack of inversion and eversion of the subtalar joint.

Diagnosis. If a coalition is suspected, anteroposterior, lateral, 45-degree oblique, and axial views of the calcaneus should be obtained. If the clinical picture is consistent with coalition but it is not seen on plain films, CT or MRI may demonstrate the lesion.

Treatment. Patients who have minimal symptoms or who have only incidental radiographic findings do not require treatment. When patients have significant symptoms, a short-leg walking cast for 3 to 4 weeks followed by the use of an orthosis may eliminate the symptoms. If conservative treatment fails, resection is indicated.

Slipped Capital Femoral Epiphysis

Slipped capital femoral epiphysis occurs when the femoral head slips posteriorly, inferiorly, and medially on the femoral metaphysis due to a disruption of the epiphyseal plate. The condition tends to occur in adolescents as weight increases the stress on bones that have not yet reached maturity.

Epidemiology. A chronic, gradual slip accounts for 80% or more of cases of slipped capital epiphysis during adolescence and is usually related to the combination of obesity and slow maturation. Acute slips occur secondary to severe trauma, such as a fall or an automobile accident, and are more common in younger children than in adolescents.

1. The prevalence is two to four times greater in males than in females.
2. More common in African American adolescents
3. Usually presents shortly before or during the period of accelerated growth
4. Approximately 20% of patients present with a bilateral slip.
5. Approximately 88% of patients are obese.

Clinical Manifestations. Pain is localized to hip or groin in 80% of patients. However, pain may be only in the thigh or knee. The family often notices a change in gait. A limp is present in 50% of patients; the adolescent with acute slippage may not be able to bear weight on the affected extremity. The affected leg often is held in slight external rotation and abduction. Internal rotation is diminished, adduction of hip is decreased, and there is decreased flexion of the hip.

Diagnosis. Anteroposterior and frog-leg lateral roentgenograms of the pelvis should be done. The vast majority of cases of slipped capital femoral epiphysis can be diagnosed with plain radiographs. Bone scan and MRI are rarely needed. Earlier and more subtle slips are seen on the frog-leg lateral views better than on the anteroposterior views.

Treatment. Orthopedic referral is required because surgery is the only reliable treatment. Further slippage, which leads to a worse prognosis, can be prevented by the introduction of threaded screws across the epiphyseal plate in situ. Avascular necrosis can occur with acute, large slips. Premature degenerative joint disease is a frequent late development in many patients with severe, chronic slips even after fixation.

"Growing Pains"

Pain in the lower limbs is common among children and younger adolescents, with peaks coinciding with maximal height velocity, at age 13 in boys and age 11 in girls. Intermittent bilateral pain or aching may often occur late in the day, in the evening, or at night and is usually localized to the muscles of the legs and thighs. Examination, laboratory studies, and radiographs are all normal. Treatment is conservative, with reassurance, heat, stretching, massage, and judicious use of NSAIDs.

REFERENCES AND ADDITIONAL READINGS

Steill IG, Greenberg GH, Wells GA, et al. Prospective validation of a decision rule for the use of radiography in acute knee injuries. *JAMA* 1996a;275:611.

Steill IG, Greenberg GH, McKnight RD, et al. The "real" Ottawa Ankle Rules. *Ann Emerg Med* 1996b;27:103.

CHAPTER 17

Back Pain in the Adolescent

Jordan D. Metzl and Lawrence S. Neinstein

Back pain is more common in older adolescents than it is in prepubertal and young adolescent patients. It may also be more common among adolescent athletes, especially young gymnasts, ballet dancers, and figure skaters.

ETIOLOGY

The etiology of back pain varies with age. The younger the individual, the more likely that back pain is *not* related to simple musculoskeletal strain. Back pain can be classified as:

1. *Mechanical disorders:* (a) Overuse syndromes (including muscle strain); (b) herniated nucleus pulposus; (c) slipped vertebral apophysis; (d) postural disorders; (e) vertebral compression fractures; and (f) spondylolysis and spondylolisthesis (acquired).
2. *Developmental disorders:* (a) Spondylolysis and spondylolisthesis (developmental) and (b) Scheuermann disease.
3. *Inflammation and infections:* (a) Discitis and vertebral osteomyelitis; (b) disc calcification; (c) rheumatologic conditions including ankylosing spondylitis and reactive spondyloarthropathies such as Reiter syndrome; (d) sickle cell disease and sickle cell pain crisis; and (e) epidural abscess.
4. Neoplastic processes.
5. Psychogenic causes.

EVALUATION

In most individuals with acute back pain the cause is never precisely known, but the course is usually benign and self-limited. For diagnostic purposes, back pain may also be divided into muscular, bone-related, or discogenic causes. Table 17.1 differentiates these causes using clues from the history, physical examination, and radiologic tests.

History
Key components of the history include the mechanism of injury (if any) and types of movement and activities associated with pain. Characterize the pain—including location, radiation, severity, onset, and duration, prior treatment, limitations, and exacerbating and alleviating factors. Ask about

TABLE 17.1

Common Causes of Back Pain: Differentiation and Management of Muscular, Bone-Related, and Discogenic Causes Using Clinical Clues

Clues to Pathophysiology	Muscular	Bone-Related	Discogenic
Site of pain	Localized to paraspinous muscles	Localized to center of spine	
Pain during activity	X	X	X
Pain after activity	X	X	X
Pain bending forward		X	X
Pain bending backward		X	
Straight raised leg test elicits pain			X
Pain with twisting	X		
Radiating pain		May occur if there is spondylolisthesis and the degree of slip is sufficient to impinge on the nerve root	X
Strength testing			Strength tests involving the great toe, inverted foot, thigh, and hip flexor may show weakness

Neurosensory examination	Unremarkable	Reflex deficiencies may signal spondylolisthesis that has progressed to compress spinal nerve roots	Reflex deficiencies may signal disk herniation; tingling toes may suggest spinal cord compression
Radiologic tests	Consider x-ray if pain persists >6 weeks, occult fracture is suspected, or scoliosis is present	X-rays: one AP, one lateral, and two oblique views. Consider MRI if concerned about fracture. If spondylolysis is suspected but not clear on x-ray, MRI will reveal edema	X-rays: one AP and one lateral; MRI considered gold standard; rarely CT if MRI not clear
Activity modification	Patients should be encouraged to return to play as soon as they can, using their judgment and taking nonsteroidal antiinflammatory drugs as needed.	Sports hiatus for younger patients with spondylolysis that may heal with rest. Older patients can play with or without a brace once they are pain free, but must postpone return to play until nerve-related symptoms resolve	Bed rest is not recommended

(continued)

TABLE 17.1

(Continued)

Clues to Pathophysiology	Muscular	Bone-Related	Discogenic
Indications for referral	Associated scoliosis	Spondylolysis, spondylolisthesis, or pain that persists for more than a month despite physical therapy, regardless of x-ray findings	Always
Treatment plan	Physical therapy, which may include referral to a sports-oriented physical therapist	Referral to a physical therapist and may include referral to a sports-oriented physical therapist and a sports medicine specialist if the individual is an athlete or injury is sports related	Referral to a physical therapist and orthopedist May include sports-oriented specialist if the adolescent is an athlete Options may include bracing, steroid injection and, if all else fails, microdiscectomy

Modified from Metzel JD. Back pain in the adolescent: a user-friendly guide. *Adolesc Health Update* 2005;17:5

prior injuries or periods of back pain. Ask about systemic symptoms suggestive of infection, neoplasm, or a collagen vascular disease. Ask about any family history of rheumatologic disease.

Specific History. Back pain occurring at rest, especially at night, is a common feature of vertebral involvement with a neoplastic process. Constant back pain, associated neurologic deficits, and rigidity of the spine on attempted movement may be associated with tumor or infection. History of hyperextension activities of the spine—such as gymnastics or ballet, or back pain radiating to buttocks or thighs—suggests spondylolysis or spondylolisthesis. Back pain from spondyloarthropathies is associated with insidious onset, worsening of symptoms in the morning and with rest, decrease in symptoms with activity, onset before 30 years of age, and pain that persists >3 months.

Physical Examination

This should include observation of gait and posture followed by testing of motion and strength and neurosensory testing. The back should also be evaluated in the standing, sitting, and supine positions.

1. *Standing position:* (a) Observe the patient from behind for pelvic or leg-length asymmetry; (b) check for kyphosis or scoliosis and perform forward-bending examination; (c) percuss and palpate spine for local tenderness; (d) palpate the iliac crest, specifically cartilaginous apophysis or growth plates; (e) assess range of motion. Pain on backward bending may suggest spondylolysis or a stress fracture. Pain with twisting is consistent with muscle spasm or muscle pain.
2. *Sitting position:* (a) Test muscle strength and reflexes in the lower extremities; (b) ask the patient to straighten his or her leg while seated. Patients with a disc problem arch backward in tripod position to take pressure off the sciatic nerve.
3. *Supine position:* (a) Measure leg length; (b) check for muscle atrophy; (c) do sensory examination and (d) straight leg-raising test; (e) rectal exam to identify decreased sphincter tone may be indicated in patients with chronic back pain.

Physical Examination in Specific Conditions

1. *Spondylolysis and spondylolisthesis:* The teen may have hyperlordosis. Localized tenderness may occur at L5 to S1. Neurologic deficits may be present.
2. *Infections:* Tenderness may be well localized over affected vertebrae.
3. *Tests for nonorganic causes:* e.g., holding teen's wrists next to his or her hips, turn the teen's body from side to side. Because this maneuver does not cause stress on the muscles or nerve roots, it should not cause any significant pain.

Imaging Studies

A radiologic examination should be performed for any adolescent with chronic back pain (>3 months). Other indications for radiologic examination include a history of serious trauma; known history of neoplasia; pain at rest; unexplained weight loss; drug or alcohol abuse; point tenderness; treatment with corticosteroids; temperature >38°C; and clinical manifestations of scoliosis, kyphosis, spondylolisthesis, or ankylosing spondylitis, or any neuromotor deficit. In obtaining radiographs of the lumbar spine, include anteroposterior, lateral, and oblique views. Consider an MRI if there is suspicion of a fracture, if spondylolysis is suspected but not seen on x-ray, or if there are clinical signs suggestive of significant discogenic disease.

DIAGNOSIS AND MANAGEMENT OF SPECIFIC CONDITIONS

Muscular Back Pain

First, carefully rule out other pathology, especially in the child and young adolescent. In selected cases, the evaluation may require additional imaging studies and/or laboratory tests. Keys to the diagnosis of muscular pain include: history of overuse injury, more pain on spinal rotation than with bending forward or backward, and absence of radicular symptoms. Muscular back pain is often the result of a sports-related injury. Once a diagnosis is established, create a treatment plan tailored to the athlete. Address issues such as lack of strength and flexibility or any specific athletic maneuvers that might cause pain. Treatment includes mobilization, nonsteroidal anti-inflammatory medications, and sometimes a change in activities. Cryotherapy is helpful initially. It can be applied for 15 to 20 minutes four times a day for at least the first 3 days. After that time, cold can be replaced with heat. Some adolescents may benefit from referral to a physical therapist. Usually the pain resolves within 4 to 6 weeks.

Bone-Related Back Pain

This is especially common in those who perform repetitive extension maneuvers, such as gymnasts, figure skaters, ballerinas, or volleyball players. The common presentation is lumbar pain with extension. Pain on bending backward should be considered bone-related pain until proven otherwise. Back pain that awakens teen from sleep or worsens with sleep is suspicious for a bony neoplasm, most commonly a benign osteoid osteoma.

Spondylolysis and Spondylolisthesis. In overuse or repetitive stress injury, bone-related pain is related to edema in the bone and is a sign that could progress to an overt stress facture—spondylolysis—a crack in the pars interarticularis.

1. *Etiology:* Spondylolysis is a defect of the pars interarticularis. Spondylolysis can be either acquired or developmental. Spondylolisthesis is the forward slippage of one vertebra on another, almost always L5 on S1. These two conditions often occur together; they represent the most common cause of chronic low back pain in the adolescent. Adolescents who participate in athletic activities involving large extension forces across the low back are at highest risk. These include gymnasts, ballet dancers, wrestlers, and down linemen.
2. *Clinical symptoms:* Pain localizes in the low back, sometimes radiating into the buttocks. Pain is aggravated with sporting activities or heavy lifting. Hamstring tightness is a hallmark of both of these conditions. A noticeable lordosis may be seen with spondylolisthesis.
3. *Diagnosis:* On physical examination, pain with extension (bending backward) is the hallmark feature of the examination. Point tenderness is often present.

Standing lateral films, especially the "spot lateral" film, centered on the L5–S1 junction, demonstrates the slip of spondylolisthesis. Spondylolysis is best demonstrated on oblique films that bring out the profile of the pars interarticularis. Single photon emission computed tomography (SPECT) is the most sensitive study for spondylolysis and demonstrates the early stages of a stress fracture before the pars interarticularis actually breaks. Increasingly, MRI is being used as well.

4. *Treatment:* Treatment of spondylolysis in the adolescent is largely nonoperative. Modification of activities, especially avoiding hyperextension, along with NSAIDs, physical therapy, and possibly a lumbosacral orthosis have high rates of success. Treatment of spondylolisthesis depends on the percentage of the slip.

Bone Tumors. Most spinal neoplasms in the adolescent are benign. Osteoid osteoma and osteoblastoma are most common. Patients may present with back pain that improves dramatically with NSAIDs. Pain often occurs at the same time every day. The neurologic examination is usually normal. Because of their small size, osteoid osteomas may be difficult to see on plain films. They show intense uptake on bone scans, and CT scanning helps delineate the exact location of the tumor. These tumors usually resolve spontaneously after skeletal maturity is reached. The tumor can also be surgically excised, but sometimes location makes excision difficult. Acute leukemia and spinal cord tumors are rare neoplastic causes of back pain.

Discogenic (Nerve-Related) Back Pain

Pain of this kind occurs due to herniation of an intervertebral disk and subsequent impingement on a central or peripheral nerve. Disc herniation in an adolescent is most likely to result from an acute event and is characterized by acute onset of back pain, typically with pain radiating into the legs. Findings suggestive of discogenic pain include lumbar spine pain that worsens with bending forward, radiating pain into the hip or thigh, positive straight-leg raising test, and decreased reflexes. Discogenic pain may be chronic and have a tendency to wax and wane. MRI is the study of choice for diagnosis. Nonoperative treatment is often successful and includes activity restriction (but not bed rest), NSAIDs, and physical therapy. Disc excision is reserved for those patients with persistent neurologic deficit or failure of nonoperative therapy to relieve pain.

Other Causes of Back Pain

Discitis and Vertebral Osteomyelitis. These two conditions are probably part of the same disease spectrum. Patients present with back pain, malaise, and fever. The physical examination is remarkable for localized tenderness and spine rigidity. Complete blood count with differential (often normal), erythrocyte sedimentation rate (usually elevated), and blood culture (which reveals an organism in only 41% of cases) should be obtained. Plain radiographs may reveal disc space narrowing and irregularities of the vertebral body. Technetium bone scanning shows increased uptake in the endplates. MRI is not only diagnostic, but can also delineate the degree of vertebral involvement. Because the great majority of these infections are caused by *Staphylococcus aureus*, the need for vertebral or disc aspiration is controversial. Most patients respond to bed rest and intravenous antibiotics followed by oral antibiotics and mobilization with a thoracolumbosacral orthosis. Decompression of these infections is required only if there is neurologic compromise or a failure to respond to nonoperative management. The possibility of tuberculosis infection should not be overlooked.

Rheumatologic Disease. This should certainly be considered when the onset is insidious, when there is no history of trauma, and if systemic symptoms such as fever or fatigue are present. If the history is consistent with a spondyloarthropathy or other arthritic condition, evaluation should include a CBC, sedimentation rate, and HLA B27.

Scheuermann Kyphosis. This rigid kyphosis of the thoracic spine is described in Chapter 15.

Psychogenic Pain. This is an important cause of back pain; however, its consideration should not preclude an appropriate investigation for other potential diagnoses. Back pain referred from other anatomic locations (e.g., pyelonephritis, endometriosis) should also be considered. Extensive evaluation may be required in some teens, including radiographic and/or laboratory evaluation. However, not all patients need all of these tests, particularly if the history and examination are consistent with psychogenic pain and the mental health history is consistent.

CHAPTER 18

Guidelines for Physical Activity and Sports Participation

Keith J. Loud and Albert C. Hergenroeder

All health care professionals caring for adolescents should be prepared to promote physical activity for all adolescents, assess the risks associated with athletic participation for individual adolescents, advise on prevention strategies for athletic injury and illness, and diagnose and manage activity-related morbidities and conditions. Although there has been concern about affecting adult stature with excessive sports activities during the prepubertal and pubertal years, the preponderance of evidence suggests that intense training with gymnastics, runners, figure skaters and ballet dancers does not affect adult stature.

PHYSICAL FITNESS AND CONDITIONING

Fitness has four principal components: (1) Body composition; (2) cardiovascular fitness; (3) strength; and (4) flexibility.

Body Composition. The only component of fitness that has declined in the past three decades is body composition: obesity has increased in both teens and young adults. To reduce obesity, adolescents need both reduced caloric intake and increased energy expenditure. However, more adolescents choose to diet rather than to exercise in an attempt to lose weight.

Cardiovascular Fitness. To improve cardiovascular fitness, a recommended training program would include aerobic exercise for 20 to 25 minutes three or four times per week. The Centers for Disease Control and Prevention and the American College of Sports Medicine guidelines recommend moderate-intensity physical activity on most days—either in a single session of 60 minutes or in accumulated multiple bouts, i.e., lasting at least 8 to 10 minutes.

Strength. It is established that prepubescent and pubescent subjects, like adults, can increase strength safely by resistance training. The training program should include close adult supervision, a preparticipation examination, and the use of well-maintained equipment. The American Academy of Pediatrics endorses strength training for children and adolescents if done properly.

Flexibility. There is no study demonstrating that stretching in healthy, previously uninjured subjects prevents injuries. However, improving flexibility and strength in previously injured athletes decreases the likelihood of subsequent injuries.

THE PREPARTICIPATION EVALUATION

Five major medical organizations (the American Academy of Family Physicians, American Academy of Pediatrics, American Medical Society for Sports Medicine, American Orthopedic Society for Sports Medicine, and American Osteopathic Academy of Sports Medicine) endorse a preparticipation evaluation (PPE) that is described in the third edition of the *Preparticipation Physical Evaluation* monograph (2005).

Ideally, adolescent athletes would have an annual comprehensive health evaluation performed by their primary care physicians (PCP), with additional sport-specific PPEs performed by a team physician responsible to the sponsoring athletic body and knowledgeable about the sport in question. In reality, the PPE is often the only interaction that many adolescents (particularly male) have with the health care system. Therefore, it is recommended that the PPE be incorporated into a more general health supervision visit with an established PCP. Mass screenings in large rooms such as gymnasiums are no longer considered appropriate.

The specific objectives of the PPE, as stated in the monograph, include screening for conditions that may be life-threatening or disabling, screening for conditions that may predispose to injury or illness, and meeting administrative requirements. Ideally the PPE should occur at least 6 weeks before preseason practice begins, to allow time for evaluation, treatment, and rehabilitation of identified problems *prior to* the first weeks of practice.

Medical History. The sports-specific history should assess for the following: (1) past injuries that caused the athlete to miss a game or practice; (2) any loss of consciousness or memory occurring after a head injury; (3) previous exclusion from sports for any reason; (4) allergies, asthma, or exercise-induced bronchospasm; (5) medications and supplements used currently or in the past 6 months; (6) menstrual history in females; (7) history of rapid changes in body weight and the athlete's perception of current body weight. In addition, the AHA recommends the following questions for cardiovascular screening: (8) family history of premature death; (9) family history of heart disease in close relatives or specific knowledge of certain conditions (hypertrophic cardiomyopathy, long-QT syndrome, Marfan syndrome, or arrhythmias); (10) personal history of heart murmur, hypertension, or excessive fatigue; and (11) personal history of syncope, excessive or progressive shortness of breath, or chest pain or discomfort, particularly with exertion.

Physical Examination. The PPE is a directed examination to identify medical problems or deficits that could worsen the athlete's performance or conditions that might be worsened by athletic participation. The most commonly detected abnormalities on PPEs are previously undetected or unrehabilitated musculoskeletal injuries. With this in mind, the physical examination should include assessment of the following:

1. *Height, weight, and body mass index (BMI):* Obesity by itself is not a reason for exclusion.
2. *Blood pressure and pulse:* Athletes with hypertension should be evaluated further but not excluded from participation unless the hypertension is severe. A pulse in the 40- to 50-bpm range is routine and does not need evaluation if the athlete is asymptomatic.
3. *Visual acuity and pupil equality:* Teens with corrected visual acuity below 20/40 in one or both eyes should be referred for further evaluation but are not excluded from participation if protective eyewear is worn. It is important that anisocoria be noted before any closed head injury occurs.
4. *Skin:* Infections that are highly contagious (e.g., varicella, impetigo) should be sought. Players with these infections need to be noninfectious before returning to sports in which skin-to-skin contact is possible (Table 18.1).
5. *Cardiac examination:* AHA recommendations for PPE cardiac examination include the following (Maron, 1996):
   a. Precordial auscultation in supine and standing positions to identify heart murmurs consistent with dynamic left ventricular (LV) outflow tract obstruction.
   b. Femoral artery or lower extremity pulses to exclude coarctation of the aorta.
   c. Recognize the physical stigmata of Marfan syndrome; refer for further evaluation if found.
   d. Assess brachial artery blood pressure in the sitting position.
   e. Document the presence of murmurs, clicks, or rubs.
6. *Abdomen:* Organomegaly is a disqualifying condition for collision/contact or limited contact sports until definitive evaluation and individual assessment for clearance.
7. *Genitalia:* An undescended testis is not a contraindication to participation in contact sports; however, the player should wear a protective cup to protect the other, descended testis. An evaluation for the unidentified testis is necessary.
8. General musculoskeletal screening should include muscle strength, range-of-motion and joint stability testing, and evaluation for structural abnormalities of major joints (e.g., ankle, knee, shoulder, elbow, back). More in-depth examination of the specific body parts should be pursued if there are concerns from the history or general screening exam.

Laboratory Tests. These are not recommended as routine screening tests for athletic participation.

CLEARANCE FOR SPORT PARTICIPATION

Table 18.1 lists disqualifying medical conditions for sports participation recommended by the AAP. These are guidelines only; they may not apply in specific cases. However, it is notable that all except three (carditis, diarrhea, and fever) allow for individualized or modified athletic participation after further

TABLE 18.1

Medical Conditions and Sports Participation[a]

Condition	May Participate?
Atlantoaxial instability (instability of the joint between cervical vertebrae 1 and 2) *Explanation*: Athlete needs evaluation to assess risk of spinal cord injury during sports participation.	Qualified yes
Bleeding disorder *Explanation*: Athlete needs evaluation.	Qualified yes
Cardiovascular diseases	
Carditis (inflammation of the heart) *Explanation*: Carditis may result in sudden death with exertion.	No
Hypertension (high blood pressure) *Explanation*: Those with significant essential (unexplained) hypertension should avoid weight and power lifting, body building, and strength training; those with secondary hypertension (hypertension caused by a previously identified disease) or severe essential hypertension need evaluation. The National High Blood Pressure Education Working group defined significant and severe hypertension.	Qualified yes
Congenital heart disease (structural heart defects present at birth) *Explanation*: Those with mild forms may participate fully; those with moderate or severe forms and those who have undergone surgery need evaluation. The 36th Bethesda Conference defined mild, moderate, and severe disease for common cardiac lesions.	Qualified yes
Dysrhythmia (irregular heart rhythm) *Explanation*: Those with symptoms (chest pain, syncope, dizziness, shortness of breath, or other symptoms of possible dysrhythmia) or evidence of mitral regurgitation (leaking) on physical examination need evaluation. All others may participate fully.	Qualified yes
Heart murmur *Explanation*: If the murmur is innocent (does not indicate heart disease), full participation is permitted; otherwise the athlete needs evaluation (see Congenital heart disease and Mitral valve prolapse discussed earlier).	Qualified yes
Cerebral palsy *Explanation*: Athlete needs evaluation.	Qualified yes

TABLE 18.1

(Continued)

Condition	May Participate?
Diabetes mellitus	Yes
Explanation: All sports can be played with proper attention to diet, blood glucose concentration, hydration, and insulin therapy. Blood glucose concentration should be monitored every 30 min during continuous exercise and 15 min after completion of exercise.	
Diarrhea	Qualified no
Explanation: Unless disease is mild, no participation is permitted, because diarrhea may increase the risk of dehydration and heat illness (see "Fever" in this table).	
Eating disorders	Qualified yes
Anorexia nervosa	
Bulimia nervosa	
Explanation: These patients need both medical and psychiatric assessment before participation.	
Eyes	
Functionally one-eyed athlete	Qualified yes
Loss of an eye	
Detached retina	
Previous eye surgery or serious eye injury	
Explanation: A functionally one-eyed athlete has a best corrected visual acuity of <20/40 in the eye with worse activity. These athletes would suffer significant disability if the better eye were seriously injured, as would those with loss of an eye. Some athletes who have previously undergone eye surgery or had a serious eye injury may have an increased risk of injury because of weakened eye tissue. Availability of eye guards approved by the American Society for Testing Materials (ASTM) and other protective equipment may allow participation in most sports, but this must be judged on an individual basis.	
Fever	No
Explanation: Fever can increase cardiopulmonary effort, reduce maximum exercise capacity, make heat illness more likely, and increase orthostatic hypotension during exercise; fever may rarely accompany myocarditis or other infections that may make exercise dangerous.	

(continued)

TABLE 18.1

(Continued)

Condition	May Participate?
Heat illness, history of *Explanation*: Because of the increased likelihood of recurrence, the athlete needs individual assessment to determine the presence of predisposing conditions and to arrange a prevention strategy.	Qualified yes
Hepatitis *Explanation*: Because of the apparent minimal risk to others, all sports may be played that the athlete's state of health allows. In all athletes, skin lesions should be covered properly and athletic personnel should use universal precautions when handling blood or body fluids with visible blood.	Yes
Human immunodeficiency virus infection *Explanation*: Because of the apparent minimal risk to others, all sports may be played as allowed by the athlete's state of health; in all athletes, skin lesions should be covered properly, and athletic personnel should use universal precautions when handling blood or body fluids with visible blood.	Yes
Kidney, absence of one *Explanation*: Athlete needs individual assessment for contact/collision and limited-contact sports.	Qualified yes
Liver, enlarged *Explanation*: If the liver is acutely enlarged, participation should be avoided because of risk of rupture; if the liver is chronically enlarged, individual assessment is needed before collision/contact or limited-contact sports are played.	Qualified yes
Malignant neoplasm *Explanation*: Athlete needs individual assessment.	Qualified yes
Musculoskeletal disorders *Explanation*: Athlete needs individual assessment.	Qualified yes
Neurological disorders History of serious head or spine trauma, severe or repeated concussions, or craniotomy *Explanation*: Athlete needs individual assessment for collision, contact or limited-contacted sports, and also for noncontact sports if deficits in judgment or cognition are present; research supports a conservative approach to management of concussion.	Qualified yes

TABLE 18.1

(Continued)

Condition	May Participate?
Seizure disorder, well controlled *Explanation*: Risk of seizure during participation is minimal.	Yes
Seizure disorder, poorly controlled *Explanation*: Athlete needs individual assessment for collision/contact or limited-contact sports. The following noncontact sports should be avoided: archery, riflery, swimming, weight or power lifting, strength training, and sports involving heights. In these sports, occurrence of a seizure may be a risk to self or others.	Qualified yes
Obesity *Explanation*: Because of the risk of heat illness, obese persons need careful acclimatization and hydration.	Qualified yes
Organ transplant recipient *Explanation*: Athlete needs individual assessment.	Qualified yes
Ovary, absence of one *Explanation*: Risk of severe injury to the remaining ovary is minimal.	Yes
Respiratory conditions Pulmonary compromise including cystic fibrosis *Explanation*: Athlete needs individual assessment, but generally all sports may be played if oxygenation remains satisfactory during a graded exercise test. Patients with cystic fibrosis need acclimatization and good hydration to reduce the risk of heat illness.	Qualified yes
Asthma *Explanation*: With proper medication and education, only athletes with the most severe asthma will have to modify their participation.	Yes
Acute upper respiratory infection *Explanation*: Upper respiratory obstruction may affect pulmonary function; athlete needs individual assessment for all but mild disease (see "Fever" in this table).	Qualified yes
Sickle cell disease *Explanation*: Athlete needs individual assessment. In general, if status of the illness permits, all but high-exertion, collision, or contact sports may be played. Overheating, dehydration, and chilling must be avoided.	Qualified yes

(continued)

TABLE 18.1

(Continued)

Condition	May Participate?
Sickle cell trait	Yes
Explanation: It is unlikely that individuals with sickle cell trait have an increased risk of sudden death or other medical problems during athletic participation except under the most extreme conditions of heat, humidity, and possibly increased altitude. These individuals, like all athletes, should be carefully conditioned, acclimatized, and hydrated to reduce any possible risk.	
Skin disorders: boils, herpes simplex, impetigo, scabies, molluscum contagiosum	Qualified yes
Explanation: While the patient is contagious, participation in gymnastics with mats, martial arts, wrestling, or other collision, contact, or limited-contact sports is not allowed.	
Spleen, enlarged	Qualified yes
Explanation: Patients with acutely enlarged spleens should avoid all sports because of risk of rupture; those with chronically enlarged spleens need individual assessment before playing collision, contact, or limited-contact sports.	
Testicle, absent or undescended	Yes
Explanation: Certain sports may require a protective cup.	

[a]This table is designed for use by medical and nonmedical personnel.

"Needs evaluation" means a physician with appropriate knowledge and experience should assess the safety of a given sport for an athlete with the listed medical condition. Unless otherwise noted, this is because of the variability of the severity of the disease, the risk of injury for the specific sports listed in the preceding text, or both.

From Committee on Sports Medicine and Fitness. Medical conditions affecting sports participation. *Pediatrics* 2001;107:1205, with permission.

evaluation. The goal of the PPE, once again, is promotion of *safe* physical activity for all adolescents.

After the PPE, the patient should be given one of the following recommendations:

1. Cleared without restriction
2. Cleared with recommendations for further evaluation or treatment
3. Clearance withheld pending further evaluation, treatment, or rehabilitation
4. Not cleared for certain types of sports or for all sports

If there are restrictions on participation, these should be discussed with the athlete and a parent or guardian, with clearly documented recommendations transmitted to a certified athletic trainer or coach. Otherwise, the message to the athlete may be misinterpreted.

Medical-Legal Issues and Exclusion from Sports Participation

Athletes and their parents may seek to participate in a sport against medical advice, citing section 504(a) of the Rehabilitation Act of 1973, which prohibits discrimination against an athlete who is disabled if that person has the capabilities and skills required to play a competitive sport, or the Americans with Disabilities Act of 1990. Physicians must still clear athletes for participation according to generally agreed-on guidelines for participation with known medical conditions. As Table 18.1 indicates, many such decisions must be made on an individual basis, and there may not be expert panel guidelines for all conditions. Such guidelines do exist in many instances, however, an example being the 36th Bethesda Conference guidelines (see later discussion).

Clearance for Specific Cardiac Conditions

Mortality during athletic participation is extraordinarily rare. The majority of young athletes who die during sports participation die from sudden cardiac events; most of these are asymptomatic before the event. Thus, a major focus of the PPE screening is cardiovascular risk conditions. *Any athlete complaining of true angina, syncope, presyncope, or palpitations while exercising, independent of the physical examination, should be excluded from participation until further evaluation.* Full evaluation could include, in consultation with a cardiovascular specialist, a 12-lead electrocardiogram, a continuous ambulatory (Holter) or event capture monitor, a maximal stress test, and a two-dimensional echocardiogram.

The best guidance for individual athletes with known cardiac conditions is the report of the 36th Bethesda Conference: *Eligibility Recommendations for Competitive Athletes With Cardiovascular Abnormalities,* available at http://www.acc.org/clinical/bethesda/beth36/index.pdf.

1. *Mitral valve prolapse:* This is generally a benign, asymptomatic condition. Patients can have palpitations, dizziness, supraventricular and ventricular arrhythmias, and chest pain, in which case they should be excluded from sports until fully evaluated. Sudden cardiac death in patients with mitral valve prolapse who die while exercising is rare.
   a. A midsystolic click, with or without a late systolic murmur, is the auscultatory hallmark of this condition. Mitral valve prolapse is a clinical diagnosis not requiring echocardiography unless a murmur is present, in which case an echocardiogram is indicated to assess for mitral insufficiency.
   b. Patients with mitral valve prolapse can participate in all competitive sports unless the following exist: A history of syncope documented to be arrhythmogenic in origin; family history of sudden death associated with mitral valve prolapse; repetitive forms of supraventricular and ventricular arrhythmias, particularly if exaggerated by exercise; moderate to marked mitral regurgitation; prior embolic event; or a LV systolic ejection fraction <50%.

		A. Low (<40% Max O₂)	B. Moderate (40%–70% Max O₂)	C. High (>70% Max O₂)
Increasing static component	**III. High (>50% MVC)**	Bobsledding/luge*†, field events (throwing), gymnastics*†, martial arts*, sailing, sport climbing, water skiing*†, weight lifting*†, windsurfing*†	Body building*†, downhill skiing*†, skateboarding*†, snowboarding*†, wrestling*	Boxing*, canoeing/kayaking, cycling*†, decathlon, rowing, speed-skating*†, triathlon*†
	II. Moderate (20%–50% MVC)	Archery, auto racing*†, diving*†, equestrian*†, motorcycling*†	American football*, field events (jumping), figure skating*, rodeoing*†, rugby*, running (sprint), surfing*†, synchronized swimming†	Basketball*, ice hockey*, cross-country skiing (skating technique), lacrosse*, running (middle distance), swimming, team handball
	I. Low (<20% MVC)	Billiards, bowling, cricket, curling, golf, riflery	Baseball/softball*, fencing, table tennis, volleyball	Badminton, cross-country skiing (classic technique), field hockey*, orienteering, race walking, racquetball/Squash, running (long distance), soccer*, tennis

Increasing dynamic component ⟶

FIGURE 18.1 Classification of sports. This classification is based on peak static and dynamic components achieved during competition. It should be noted, however, that higher values may be reached during training. *Danger of bodily collision; †increased risk if syncope occurs. (From Mitchell JH, Haskel W, Snell P, et al. Task Force 8: Classification of Sports, *J Am Coll Cardiol* 2005;45:1364, with permission.)

    c. Athletes with mitral valve prolapse *and* any of the symptoms just listed may participate only in low-intensity sports (i.e., low static, low dynamic—see Fig. 18.1, class I.A.).

2. *Hypertrophic cardiomyopathy:* Also known as asymmetric septal hypertrophy, is a primary abnormality of the myocardium manifest as an asymmetrically hypertrophied, nondilated left ventricle in the absence of a cardiac or systemic disease that causes LV hypertrophy. The mechanism of sudden death is not established but may be related to arrhythmia or myocardial ischemia. When present, symptoms include exertional dyspnea, angina pectoris, fatigue, and/or syncope. In many cases there are no symptoms before the sudden death. Athletes with hypertrophic cardiomyopathy must be evaluated by a cardiologist before participation.

    a. There may be a family history of sudden death, particularly related to exercise.

    b. The diagnosis is made by demonstrating LV wall thickness >15 mm, although some highly trained athletes can have a LV thickness of up to 16 mm, and some patients with hypertrophic cardiomyopathy—especially young, growing adolescents—can have a thickness <15 mm.

    c. Athletes with the unequivocal diagnosis of hypertrophic cardiomyopathy (HCM) should not participate in most competitive sports with the possible exception of low-intensity sports (Fig. 18.1, Category I.A.). This applies to athletes with and without evidence of LV outflow obstruction. There is currently no compelling evidence to preclude athletes with genotype positive for HCM who do not have phenotypic manifestations (i.e., normal echocardiogram), family history of sudden death, or any cardiac symptoms on history.

3. *Coronary artery anomalies* are rare overall. They may lead to sudden death; however, identification before death is difficult because many patients are asymptomatic before the sudden death event. The cardiac examination is normal. Cardiac consultation before participation is mandatory if this condition is suspected. If coronary artery anomalies are identified, there is complete exclusion from sports participation.

4. *Myocarditis* is a process characterized by an inflammatory infiltrate of the myocardium with necrosis and/or degeneration of myocytes. The disease progresses through active, healing, and healed phases, and arrhythmias may occur at any time.
   a. Athletes in whom a presumptive diagnosis has been made should be excluded from all competitive sports for 6 months and then have their ventricular function evaluated at rest and with exercise before being allowed to return to sports.
   b. Athletes can return to sports when their ventricular function and dimensions are normal and clinically relevant arrhythmias are absent on ambulatory monitoring.

5. *Systemic hypertension:* Although hypertension is associated with an increased risk for sudden death and complex ventricular arrhythmias, to date it has not been incriminated as a cause of sudden cardiac death in young, competitive athletes.
   a. Athletes with stage 1 hypertension in the absence of end-organ damage, including LVH, and heart disease have no restrictions, but should have BP measured every 2 to 4 months to assess the impact of exercise.
   b. Those with stage 2 hypertension should be restricted, especially from high-static sports (Fig. 18.1, Classes IIIA-C.), until their blood pressure is controlled.
   c. If athletes have true LVH (in distinction from "athlete's heart") on screening, they should be restricted from participation in high static sports (Fig. 18.1, Classes IIIA to IIIC) until the hypertension is controlled.

CAN WE PREVENT ATHLETIC INJURY AND ILLNESS?

Injury Prevention

The most important function of the PPE may be as a quality control point for injuries and rehabilitation during the past year. In general, athletes should not be allowed to return to participation in sports until the following criteria have been satisfied:

1. The injury has been accurately diagnosed.
2. The examiner is reasonably certain that the injury will not significantly worsen with continued play.
3. The examiner is reasonably certain that continued participation (with the injury) will not result in a secondary injury.
4. The athlete has achieved full range of motion (ROM) and strength in the injured joint.
5. The athlete wants to return to play.

DIAGNOSIS AND MANAGEMENT OF SPORTS-RELATED CONDITIONS

Concussion

Sports concussion is now defined as "a complex pathophysiologic process affecting the brain, induced by traumatic biomechanical forces." Current recommendations favor individual assessment and guidance based on combined measures of recovery rather than concussion grading scales. Concussion in sport may either be simple or complex, but this classification is made *retrospectively*. In simple concussion, an athlete suffers an injury that progressively resolves without complication over 7 to 10 days. In complex concussion, athletes suffer persistent symptoms, any other sequelae (such as seizure), prolonged loss of consciousness (>1 minute), or prolonged cognitive impairment after the injury. Recurrent concussions, especially those triggered by progressively less impact force, fall into this category as well.

Diagnosis and Management. Essentially *any* athlete who complains of *any* neurologic symptoms or demonstrates *any* neurologic signs (Fig. 18.2) or memory loss after *any* bodily contact (not just the head) with another athlete, the ground or other playing surface, or a projectile such as a ball or puck should be managed as having an acute concussion.

The Sport Concussion Assessment Tool (SCAT) Card (Fig. 18.2) is a handheld standardized method to evaluate the concussed athlete. It also provides a suggested approach to management, which can be summarized as "When in doubt, sit them out!" In more detail:

1. The athlete should not be allowed to return to play in the current game or practice session.
2. The athlete should not be left alone, and regular monitoring for deterioration is essential over the initial few hours after injury.
3. The player should be medically evaluated after the injury.

Return to play follows a stepwise process, with advance of no more than one step per day. If any postconcussion symptoms occur at any step, the athlete must wait until he or she is asymptomatic for at least 24 hours before resuming the progression at the previous level. The minimum time in which such a progression can be completed is a week, but it may take much longer depending on the individual case. Lack of progression should prompt referral to a neurologist, neurosurgeon, or sports medicine physician comfortable with the management of sports concussion. Neuroimaging or formal neuropsychological testing may be indicated.

Second Impact Syndrome. One of the goals of the above guidelines is to prevent diffuse cerebral swelling with delayed catastrophic deterioration, a known complication of brain trauma. This has been postulated to occur after repeated concussive brain injury in sports and is known as the *second impact syndrome* (SIS). All cases of SIS to date have been diagnosed in adolescent boys. Still, it appears most prudent to limit contact sports in all adolescent athletes until all postconcussive symptoms have disappeared, regardless of which concussion management protocol is followed.

Sport Concussion Assessment Tool
This tool represents a standardized method of evaluating people after concussion in sport. This tool has been produced as part of the Summary and Agreement Statement of the Second International Symposium on Concussion in Sport, Prague 2004

For more information see the "Summary and Agreement Statement of the Second International Symposium on Concussion in Sport" in the: Clinical Journal of Sport Medicine 2005; British Journal of Sports Medicine 2005; Neurosurgery 2005; Physician and Sportsmedicine 2005; this tool may be copied for distribution to teams, groups and organizations.

Sports concussion is defined as a complex pathophysiological process affecting the brain, induced by traumatic biomechanical forces. Several common features that incorporate clinical, pathological and biomechanical injury constructs that may be utilized in defining the nature of a concussive head injury include:

1. Concussion may be caused either by a direct blow to the head, face, neck or elsewhere on the body with an 'impulsive' force transmitted to the head.
2. Concussion typically results in the rapid onset of short-lived impairment or neurological function that resolves spontaneously.
3. Concussion may result in neuropathological changes but the acute clinical symptoms largely reflect a functional disturbance rather than structural injury.
4. Concussion results in a graded set of clinical syndromes that may or may not involve loss of consciousness. Resolution of the clinical and cognitive symptoms typically follows a sequential course.
5. Concussion is typically associated with grossly normal structural neuroimaging studies.

Post Concussion Symptoms
Ask the athlete to score themselves based on how they feel now. It is recognized that a low score may be normal for some athletes, but clinical judgment should be exercised to determine if a change in symptoms has occurred following the suspected concussion event.

It should be recognized that the reporting of symptoms may not be entirely reliable. This may be due to the effects of a concussion or because the athlete's passionate desire to return to competition outweighs their natural inclination to give an honest response.

If possible, ask someone who knows the athlete well about changes in affect, personality, behavior, etc.

Remember, concussion should be suspected in the presence of ANY ONE or more of the following:
- Symptoms (such as headache), or
- Signs (such as loss of consciousness), or
- Memory problems

Any athlete with a suspected concussion should be monitored for deterioration (i.e., should not be left alone) and should not drive a motor vehicle.

The SCAT Card (Sport Concussion Assessment Tool)
What is a concussion? A concussion is a disturbance in the function of the brain caused by a direct or indirect force to the head. It results in a variety of symptoms (like those listed below) and may, or may not, involve memory problems or loss of consciousness.
How do you feel? You should score yourself on the following symptoms, based on how you feel now.

Post Concussion Symptom Scale

	None	Moderate			Severe		
Headache	0	1	2	3	4	5	6
"Pressure in head"	0	1	2	3	4	5	6
Neck Pain	0	1	2	3	4	5	6
Balance problems/dizzy	0	1	2	3	4	5	6
Nausea or vomiting	0	1	2	3	4	5	6
Vision problems	0	1	2	3	4	5	6
Hearing problems/ringing	0	1	2	3	4	5	6
"Don't feel right"	0	1	2	3	4	5	6
Feeling "dinged"/"dazed"	0	1	2	3	4	5	6
Confusion	0	1	2	3	4	5	6
Feeling slowed down	0	1	2	3	4	5	6
Feeling like "in a fog"	0	1	2	3	4	5	6
Drowsiness	0	1	2	3	4	5	6
Fatigue or low energy	0	1	2	3	4	5	6
More than emotional	0	1	2	3	4	5	6
Irritability	0	1	2	3	4	5	6
Difficulty concentrating	0	1	2	3	4	5	6
Difficulty remembering	0	1	2	3	4	5	6
(follow up symptoms only)							
Sadness	0	1	2	3	4	5	6
Nervous or anxious	0	1	2	3	4	5	6
Trouble falling asleep	0	1	2	3	4	5	6
Sleeping more than usual	0	1	2	3	4	5	6
Sensitivity to light	0	1	2	3	4	5	6
Sensitivity to noise	0	1	2	3	4	5	6
Other:	0	1	2	3	4	5	6

What should I do?
Any athlete suspected of having a concussion should be removed from play, and told to seek medical evaluation.
Signs to watch for:
Problems could arise over the first 24-48 hours. You should not be left alone and must go to a hospital at once if you:
- Have a headache that gets worse
- Are very drowsy or can't be awakened (woken up)
- Can't recognize people or places
- Have repeated vomiting
- Behave unusually or seem confused; are very irritable
- Have seizures (arms and legs jerk uncontrollably)
- Have weak or numb arms or legs
- Are unsteady on your feet; have slurred speech
Remember, it is better to be safe. **Consult your doctor after a suspected concussion.**
What can I expect?
Concussion typically results in the rapid onset of short-lived impairment that resolves spontaneously over time. You can expect that you will be told to rest until you are fully recovered (that means resting your body and your mind). Then, your doctor will likely advise that you go through a gradual increase in exercise over several days (or longer) before returning to sport.

FIGURE 18.2 SCAT card. (From Clinical Journal of Sports Medicine 2005, with permission.)

Sequelae of Chronic Head Trauma. There is evidence that traumatic brain injury occurring over an extended period (i.e., months or years) can result in cumulative neurologic and cognitive deficits. Neuropsychiatric abnormalities can persist for up to 6 months after a concussion (not only in sports). This has led to the definition of the *postconcussional disorder* described in the *Diagnostic and Statistical Manual of Mental Disorders,* 4th edition. Dementia (decreased cognition, memory, or any of the above symptoms) resulting from a single head injury is usually not progressive. If the dementia or behavior grows progressively worse, consider another diagnosis, such as hydrocephalus or major depressive disorder.

The SCAT Card (Sport Concussion Assessment Tool) Medical Evaluation

Name: _____ Date: _____

Sport/Team: _____ Mouth guard? Y N

1) SIGNS
Was there loss of consciousness/unresponsiveness? Y N
Was there seizure or convulsive activity? Y N
Was there a balance problem / unsteadiness? Y N

2) MEMORY
Modified Maddocks questions (check if athlete answers correctly)
- At what venue are we? ____ Which half is it? ____
  Who scored last? ____
- What team did we play last? ____ ; Did we win last game? ____

3) SYMPTOM SCORE
Total number of positive symptoms (from reverse side of the card) = ____

4) COGNITIVE ASSESSMENT (5 word recall)

	(Examples)	Immediate	Delayed
Word 1 ____	cat	_____	_____
Word 2 ____	pen	_____	_____
Word 3 ____	shoe	_____	_____
Word 4 ____	book	_____	_____
Word 5 ____	car	_____	_____

Months in reverse order:
Jun-May-Apr-Mar-Feb-Jan-Dec-Nov-Oct-Sep-Aug-Jul

Digits Backwards (check correct)
5-2-8   3-9-1
6-2-9-4   4-3-7-1   ____
8-3-2-7-9   1-4-9-3-6   ____
7-3-9-1-4-2 5-1-8-4-6-8 ____

Ask delayed 5-word recall now

5) NEUROLOGIC SCREENING

	Pass	Fail
Speech	____	____
Eye Motion and Pupils	____	____
Pronator Drift	____	____
Gait Assessment	____	____

Any neurologic screen abnormality necessitates formal neurologic or hospital assessment

RETURN TO PLAY
Athletes should not be returned to play the same day of injury. When returning athletes to play they should follow a stepwise symptom-limited program, with stages of progression. For example:
1. rest until asymptomatic (physical and mental rest)
2. light aerobic exercise (e.g stationary cycle)
3. sport-specific training
4. non-contact training drills (start light resistance training)
5. full contact training after medical clearance
6. return to competition (game play)
There should be approximately 24 hours (or longer) for each stage and the athlete should return to stage 1 if symptoms recur. Resistance training should only be added in the later stages. Medical clearance should be given before return to play.

Instructions:
The side of the card is for the use of medical doctors, physical therapists, or athletic therapists. In order to maximize the information gathered from the card, it is strongly suggested that all athletes participating in contact sports complete a baseline evaluation prior to the beginning of their competitive season. This card is a suggested guide only for sports concussion and is not meant to assess more severe forms of brain injury. Please give a COPY of this card to the athlete for their information and to guide follow up assessment.

Signs:
Assess for each of these items and circle Y (yes) or N (no).

Memory:
Select any 5 words (an example is given). Avoid choosing related words such as "dark" and "moon" which can be recalled by means of word association. Read each word at a rate of one word per second. The athlete should not be informed of the delayed testing of memory (to be done after the reverse months and/or digits). Choose a different set of words each time you perform a follow-up exam with the same candidate.

Concentration / Attention:
Ask the athlete to recite the months of the year in reverse order, starting with a random month. Do not start with December or January. Circle any months not recited in the correct sequence. For digits backwards, if correct, go to the next string length. If correct, read trial 2. Stop after incorrect on both trials.

Neurologic Screening:
Trained medical personnel must administer this examination. These individuals might include medical doctors, physiotherapists or athletic therapists. Speech should be assessed for fluency and lack slurring. Eye motion should reveal no diplopia in any of the 4 planes of movement (vertical, horizontal and both diagonal planes). The pronator drift is performed by asking the patient to hold both arms in front of them, palms up, with eyes closed. A positive test is pronating the forearm, dropping the arm, or drift away from midline. For gait assessment ask the patient to walk away from you, turn and walk back.

Return to Play:
A structured, graded exertion protocol should be developed, individualized on the basis of sport, age, and the concussion history of the athlete. Exercise or training should be commenced only after the athlete is clearly asymptomatic with physical and cognitive rest. Final decision for clearance to return to competition should ideally be made by a medical doctor.

Notes:
_____
_____
_____
_____
_____

FIGURE 18.2 (*Continued*)

Cervical Spinal Injuries

The majority of catastrophic sports injuries involve the head and neck. Initially, when a player's head or neck is injured, a spinal cord injury must be assumed to be present. The patient should not be moved until a diagnosis is established that would allow cervical movement. If a cervical spine injury is suspected, the first priority is to assess the patient's cardiopulmonary status. The second priority is to do no harm. For a potential unstable cervical spine fracture or dislocation, this means allowing no one to move the athlete, including not taking off the helmet or rolling the patient over, until the appropriate emergency personnel are present. After personnel are present who can prepare the patient for transport, the cervical spine should be stabilized and the patient transported.

If the patient is unconscious, has neck pain and/or radiating pain to an extremity, or has paresis or paresthesia, it should be assumed that a cervical spine injury is present. The athlete should be immobilized on a board and transported to an emergency room. If there is no motor or sensory abnormality of the extremities, the patient is conscious, and there is no neck pain, the patient can be allowed to walk off the field for further evaluation. If at any time the patient complains of radiating pain, paresthesia, or neck pain, the physician should consider that a cervical spine fracture is present and initiate appropriate procedures.

Cervical Muscle Strain

Cervical muscle strains are common and can be painful. The mechanisms of injury include rapid acceleration or deceleration of a muscle or muscle group or repetitive contractions causing muscle fatigue and eventually muscle tearing. There should be no motor or sensory deficits on examination. The athlete will complain of pain typically in the trapezius area. There will be tenderness over the muscle body, with limitation of ROM and pain with resistance. Ice, analgesic medication, and physical therapy should be initiated immediately. Clearance for return to contact sport requires a normal range of cervical motion and strength. Midline pain and tenderness are consistent with a cervical fracture and should be treated as such in the acute setting. Any player without full ROM and strength is excluded from further contact.

"Stingers" or "Burners"

A "stinger" is a common injury in American football and is the result of trauma to the brachial plexus that occurs when a player hits another opponent with the head or shoulder. The player describes a burning pain or weakness, or both, in the distribution of a branch of the brachial plexus. Think first about the possibility that the paresthesia is secondary to a spinal cord injury. If the cervical spine is cleared (i.e., unilateral signs and symptoms, no midline cervical tenderness, and full cervical ROM), the diagnosis of brachial plexopathy can be made. Typically, these injuries are mild and the player recovers in minutes or less. The athlete may return to full participation if motor and sensory examination of the extremity is normal. However, some patients have dysesthesia and/or weakness that can last days to weeks. We suggest that patients with symptoms persisting >12 hours or weakness documented to be 3/5 or less should be referred for further evaluation.

SPECIAL CONSIDERATIONS

Female Athlete Triad

This describes the interrelationship between disordered eating, amenorrhea, and osteoporosis in female athletes participating in sports, particularly those that emphasize a lean physique. Female athletes with amenorrhea or oligomenorrhea have lower bone mineral density (BMD) and higher rates of stress fracture than eumenorrheic athletes. A long-term consequence of amenorrhea and osteopenia during the second decade may be increased risk of postmenopausal osteoporosis.

Evaluation and Treatment. The first step in addressing primary or secondary amenorrhea is to make a correct diagnosis. Hypothalamic amenorrhea associated with exercise and inadequate caloric intake is a diagnosis of exclusion. The diagnosis is made on the basis of the menstrual history, the diet history, the exercise history, and the physical examination. The menstrual history includes age at menarche, frequency and duration of menstrual period, last menstrual period, longest time period without menstruation, physical signs of ovulation, such as dysmenorrhea, and prior hormonal therapy. The diet history includes 3-day diet recall, restrictive eating habits, highest and lowest weights since menarche, satisfaction with current weight and ideal weight according to teen, bingeing and purging behaviors, and use of laxatives, diuretics, diet pills, or other supplements. The exercise history includes exercise patterns and training intensity levels, exercise done outside of required training, history of previous fractures, and overuse injuries.

Management and Follow-up. Assuming that the diagnosis of hypothalamic amenorrhea or oligomenorrhea associated with exercise and inadequate caloric intake is made, reductions in training volume and enhanced caloric intake need to occur. Amenorrheic athletes who gain weight through reduced training and improved diet may resume menses spontaneously and increase their BMD, although weight gain is not always associated with improved BMD and when BMD is improved it still tends to be below normal. If the athlete weighs 85% to 90% of estimated ideal body weight (IBW) and is exercising daily, we would recommend more aggressive changes: reduce exercise by half and add 500 kcal (two dietary supplemental drinks or snacks) per day. We do not recommend exercise if the body weight is <85% of estimated IBW unless the athlete is >80% of estimated IBW, is eumenorrheic, and her weight is increasing weekly. If the athlete has a diagnosable eating disorder, treatment must include medical, nutritional, and psychological therapy in a coordinated fashion.

The athlete should be monitored weekly until weight increases consistently. Thereafter, visits can be reduced to once every 2 weeks assuming that the teen's weight progresses toward 90% of estimated IBW and the coach is supportive of the plan. We give a written plan to the athlete and encourage her to show it to her coach.

Measurement of Bone Mineral Density. Measurement of the BMD of the lumbar spine and hip by dual-energy x-ray absorptiometry (DXA) should be considered if the patient has been amenorrheic for >6 months or oligomenorrheic, with fewer than four menses in the previous year. If the subject has been amenorrheic for >1 year and is malnourished, the DXA scan is more strongly recommended. If DXA scanning is done, it should not be repeated at an interval of <12 months.

Osteoporosis is a clinical, not densitometric, diagnosis in pediatrics. The World Health Organization (WHO) definitions of osteopenia and osteoporosis based on T-scores have little prognostic significance for adolescents. The International Society for Clinical Densitometry (ISCD, www.iscd.org) recommends utilizing only Z-scores (age, gender, and ethnicity-matched standard deviations from the mean) for patients under age 20. Since the fracture threshold in children and adolescents has not been established, terminology such as "below the expected range for age" is preferred for Z-scores ≤2.0. The physician should exercise caution in interpreting Z-scores in patients with short stature because DXA tends to underestimate BMD in short subjects and overestimate BMD in tall subjects.

Hormonal Therapy. Hypoestrogenemia, reduced serum levels of insulin-like growth factor I (IGF-I), and hypercortisolemia in anorexia nervosa contribute to BMD loss. These factors improve with weight gain but may not respond to estrogen/progestin therapy. It has not been established that estrogen/progestin in the form of oral contraceptive pills (OCPs) or other forms of replacement increases BMD or prevents stress fractures. In the absence of an established standard for the use of estrogen to prevent low bone density in adolescent and young adult females with secondary or primary amenorrhea related to overtraining and caloric restriction, the decision to treat with estrogen/progestin should be individualized. The effects of estrogen receptor modulators, bisphosphonates, recombinant insulin-like growth factor, and recombinant parathyroid hormone derivatives on the skeletons of adolescent and young adult females are not known. *Therefore, they must all be considered investigational, to be used only in research settings or by specialized skeletal centers.*

The use of combination OCPs could be considered for those female athletes who have been amenorrheic for >6 months, especially if they are malnourished, as manifested by weight <85% of their estimated IBW. In addition, since between 60% and 80% of the variance in BMD is likely attributable to heritable factors, a family history of osteoporosis should lower the threshold for treating. If the athlete has been amenorrheic for >12 months, a stronger recommendation can be made to begin OCP treatment, in addition to effecting lifestyle changes discussed earlier.

ERGOGENIC AIDS AND DRUG USE IN ATHLETES

The major categories of drugs used to improve performance by athletes include stimulants, pain relievers, and anabolic steroids. In addition, over the past decade there has been increased recognition of the use of dietary supplements as ergogenic aids. These supplements include creatine, androstenedione and dehydroepiandrosterone (DHEA), *gamma*-hydroxybutyrate, and protein powders.

Over-the-counter analgesics, decongestants, antihistamines, laxatives, antidiarrheal agents, and weight loss medications are commonly used by athletes. Athletes should be asked specifically about use of these medications during office or training room visits, because they may not perceive them to be as important as prescription drugs and may not report their use. In addition, these medications have important side effects that can affect performance, and some are banned by sports governing bodies (NCAA and United States Olympic Committee). Physicians are encouraged to consult the United States (www.usantidoping.org) and World Anti-Doping Agencies (www.wada-ama.org) when advising athletes, especially college and elite athletes, about medication and prescription drug use.

Performance-Enhancing Drugs

1. *Stimulants:* Stimulants have been used extensively to combat psychological and muscular fatigue. These substances are banned by the International

Olympic Committee (IOC) and can be detected by urine tests. They may include amphetamines, cocaine, and caffeine. Caffeine is banned by the IOC in amounts >12 μg/mL (approximately equivalent to 4 to 8 cups of coffee or 8 to 16 cups of cola).

2. *Anabolic steroids:* Anabolic steroid use is associated with increased muscle size and strength, especially in athletes who are weight training when the steroid use is initiated and who are consuming a high-calorie diet. Injected steroids are detectable in the urine for 6 months or longer. Orally administered anabolic steroids disappear from the urine after days to weeks. More information on anabolic steroids can be obtained at the NIDA Web site on steroid use: www.steroidabuse.org. Serious side effects of anabolic steroids include the following:

   a. Alteration of myocardial textural properties (as detected by echocardiogram) and function
   b. Risk of hepatic damage (manifested as elevated liver-specific enzymes)
   c. Decreased high-density lipoprotein (HDL) and increased low-density lipoprotein (LDL) cholesterol levels
   d. Oligospermia and azoospermia with decreased testicular size
   e. Premature epiphyseal closure in pubertal athletes
   f. Acne
   g. Masculinization in women manifest as deepening of the voice, acne, and hair loss
   h. Feminization in men, manifested as gynecomastia and a high voice
   i. Adverse psychological effects, including increased aggressiveness and rage in some athletes
   j. Increased use of other illicit drugs

3. *Dietary supplements as ergogenic aids:* Common characteristics of dietary supplements are that their long-term effects are not known, their benefits are minimal at best, and that the potency and purity of commercial products varies. Reputable information about dietary supplements can be found at http://dietary-supplements.info.nih.gov, but our awareness of the "latest" agents likely lags far behind their actual use by our patients. None of the following common supplements are recommended for use by adolescents: (a) androstenedione; (b) creatine; (c) dehydroepiandrosterone; or (d) γ-hydroxybutyrate, γ-hydroxybutyrolactone, and 1,4-butanediol.

Testing for Performance-Enhancing and Other Drugs. Information is available from the NCAA (www.ncaa.gov, telephone 1-913-339-1906), the U.S. Olympic Committee (1-800-233-0393, Drug Control Hotline), www.usantidoping.org, or the American College Health Association (1994) (http://acha.org/info_resources/guidelines.cfm).

WEB SITES AND REFERENCES

http://www.sportsmedicine.com/. Site connecting individuals interested in sports medicine.
http://www.acsm.org/. American College of Sports Medicine.
http://www.sportsmed.org/. American Orthopaedic Society for Sports Medicine.
http://www.unc.edu/depts/nccsi/. National Center for Catastrophic Sports Injury Research, data on sports injuries and fatalities.

http://www.cdc.gov/doc.do/id/0900f3ec80017619. U.S. Centers for Disease Control and Prevention Heads Up! Tool Kit on Concussion.

36th Bethesda Conference. Eligibility recommendations for competitive athletes with cardiovascular abnormalities. *JACC.* 2005;45:1313.

American Academy of Family Physicians, American Academy of Pediatrics, American College of Sports Medicine, et al. Preparticipation physical evaluation, 3rd ed. Minneapolis, MN: McGraw-Hill Healthcare Information, 2005.

Maron BJ, Thompson PD, Puffer JC, et al. Cardiovascular preparticipation screening of competitive athletes. A statement for health professionals from the Sudden Death Committee and Congenital Cardiac Defects Committee, American Heart Association. *Circulation* 1996;94:850 (Addendum appears in *Circulation* 1998;97:2294).

McGrory PR, Johnston K, Meeuwisse W, et. al. Summary and agreement statement of the 2nd International Conference on Concussion in Sport, Prague 2004. *Br J Sports Med* 2005;39:196.

National High Blood Pressure Education Program, Working Group on Hypertension Control in Children and Adolescents. Fourth Report on the Diagnosis, Evaluation, and Treatment of High Blood Pressure in Children and Adolescents, *Pediatrics* 2004;114:555.

CHAPTER 19

Acne

Mei-Lin T. Pang and Lawrence F. Eichenfield

Acne vulgaris is one of the most prevalent skin diseases in adolescents. Acne has important psychological consequences, and quality of life is often affected in many individuals.

ETIOLOGY

Acne develops in pilosebaceous units, typically on the face, upper chest, and upper back. The key pathogenic factors of acne vulgaris are (1) androgen-induced increased sebum production; (2) abnormal keratinization of sebaceous and follicular epithelium; (3) proliferation of *Propionibacterium acnes*; (4) inflammation.

EPIDEMIOLOGY

Acne affects 80% to 95% of people between the ages of 11 and 30 years.

CLINICAL DISEASE

Comedones. The earliest sign of acne, which often appear 1 to 2 years before puberty.

1. *Microcomedo:* Subclinical impactions of keratin, lipids, bacteria, and rudimentary hairs within the sebaceous follicle.
2. *Open comedo (blackhead):* Consists of an open, epithelium-lined sac filled with keratin and lipids. The black coloration comes from melanin pigment.

3. *Closed comedo (whitehead):* An occluded follicle typically 1 to 3 mm in size. Rupture of these lesions forms inflamed pustules, with deeper inflammation resulting in papules or nodules.

Papules. Inflammatory lesions measuring < 5 mm in diameter. They may result in postinflammatory hyperpigmentation in patients with dark complexions.

Pustules. Lesions with a visible central core of purulent material.

Nodules. Inflammatory lesions measuring 5 mm or larger that last for weeks to months and may heal with scarring.

Cysts. Deeper lesions filled with pus and serosanguineous fluid.

Scars. Types of scarring include: (1) focal depressed or "ice pick" scars; (2) perifollicular fibrosis; and (3) hypertrophic scars and keloids, which tend to form on the chest, back, jaw line, and ears and are more common in dark-skinned individuals.

Location. The face, chest, and back are the areas most prominently affected.

Grading. Acne may be classified by predominant lesion type (comedonal, papulopustular, nodular, cystic) and severity (mild, moderate, severe).

Timing. Acne can appear as early as 5 to 8 years of age. Prevalence and severity increases during puberty and peaks between the ages of 14 and 17 years in females and 16 and 19 years of age in males. Acne varies from a short, mild course to a severe disease lasting several years, often beyond 20 years of age.

DIFFERENTIAL DIAGNOSIS

Nonacne Lesions. (1) keratosis pilaris, (2) adenoma sebaceum, (3) flat warts, (4) perioral dermatitis, (5) hidradenitis suppurativa, (6) pityrosporum folliculitis

Subtypes of Acne. (1) neonatal acne, (2) gram-negative folliculitis, (3) cosmetic acne, (4) occupational acne, (5) drug-induced acne, (6) acne conglobata, (7) acne fulminans, (8) acne mechanica, (9) acne excoriée.

THERAPY

General

Several considerations are important in treating adolescents with acne:

1. Perform a thorough history and physical examination. Obtain menstrual history and use of oral contraceptive pills (OCPs) in females. The female patient should be examined for hirsutism, alopecia, and obesity.
2. Treat according to severity: (a) begin with agents that are easiest to use with the fewest side effects, advancing as needed in a stepwise fashion to stronger medications; (b) mild acne responds well to topical antibiotic or comedolytic

agents—Table 19.1 lists common over-the-counter preparations; (c) combination therapy may allow medications to work synergistically; (d) moderate-severe to severe inflammatory acne may require systemic antibiotics in addition to retinoids; (e) nodular or nodulocystic acne refractory to oral antibiotics or topical retinoids should be treated with systemic isotretinoin (Accutane); (f) combined OCPs may be useful therapy in female patients.

3. General measures and misconceptions about acne should be discussed with the patient and family: (a) a healthy diet is recommended and dietary restrictions (e.g., carbonated beverages, chocolate) are usually unnecessary; (b) being unhygienic does not cause acne. Mild soaps or cleansers should be used to wash the face two times a day. Noncomedogenic (those that do not clog pores) moisturizers and cosmetics may be used; (c) stress can worsen acne and, in turn, increase the adolescent's anxiety levels and impact on self-image; (d) neither sexual fantasies nor sexual activity causes acne; (e) premenstrual acne flares can occur.

Topical Agents
Table 19.1 summarizes available topical retinoids and antibiotics.

Benzoyl Peroxide
1. *Mechanism of action:* Bacteriocidal against *P. acnes*, mild comedolytic action
2. *Dosing:* 2.5% to 10% prescription and nonprescription gels, lotions, creams, soaps, or washes applied every other day to twice a day. Aqueous gels are better tolerated than alcohol-based compounds.
3. *Adverse side effects:* Peeling, irritation and dryness, contact dermatitis (1% to 2%), bleaching of hair and colored fabrics

Retinoids (Tretinoin-Retin-A, Avita, Altinac)
1. *Mechanism of action:* normalizes keratinization
2. *Dosing:* 0.025%, 0.05%, 0.1% cream; 0.01% or 0.025% gel applied every other night to every night.
3. *Adverse side effects:* Peeling, drying, and irritation; hyperpigmentation or hypopigmentation particularly in dark-skinned patients, and photosensitivity. A pustular eruption might occur after 3 to 4 weeks of use, indicating dislodging of microcomedos, not a new flare. Patients should be instructed to continue treatment.

Newer Retinoid Preparations
1. Tretinoin gel microspheres (Retin-A Micro 0.04% and 0.1% gel)
2. Tretinoin polymer cream (Avita)
3. Adapalene (Differin 0.1% and 0.3% Gel, Cream, Pledgets, and Solution)
4. Tazarotene (Tazorac 0.1% and 0.05% Gel and Cream)
5. Azelaic acid (Azelex 20% cream)
6. Retinoid Combinations: These include tretinoin/clindamycin gel (Ziana) and tretinoin/benzoyl peroxide (in development). These once a day topicals combine antibacterial actions as well as normalizing keratinization. Side effects are those of the respective ingredients.

Topical Antibiotics
Topical antibiotics have negligible systemic side effects, but resistance is frequently seen.

TABLE 19.1

Topical Therapeutic Options for Acne

Drug	Action	Frequency	Side Effects
Anticomedonal agents	**Topical agents**		
Tretinoin (Retin-A) cream 0.025%, 0.05%, 0.1% gel 0.01%, 0.025%, solution 0.05% Retin-A micro 0.04%, 0.1% gel Avita 0.025% cream/gel Generic tretinoin 0.025%, 0.05%, 0.1% cream, 0.01%, 0.025% gel	Normalizes keratinocyte differentiation Some anti-inflammatory effect	q.p.m.	Photosensitivity, drying
Differin (Adapalene) Gel 0.1%, 0.3%, cream 0.1%, solution 0.1%, pledgets 0.1%	Normalizes keratinocyte differentiation Some anti-inflammatory effect	q.d.	Less irritating than Retin-A
Tazorac (tazarotene) 0.05%, 0.1% gel; 0.05%, 0.1% cream	Normalizes differentiation Some anti-inflammatory effect	q.d.	
Azelex Cream 20%, Azelaic acid	Normalizes differentiation Antimicrobial	b.i.d.	Less irritating than Retin-A, also appears less effective
Salicylic acid[a]	Mild comedolytic	b.i.d.	Drying
Retinoid combinations Tretinoin/clindamycin gel (Ziana)	Normalizes differtiation	q.d.	Same as antibacterial retinoids, clindamycin
Tretinoin/benzoyl peroxide (in development at time of publication)	Normalizes differentiation	q.d.	Same as antibacterial retinoids, benzoyl peroxide
Topical antibiotic			
Benzoyl peroxide (BP)[a]: Many forms: 2%–20%, gel, lotion, wash	Comedolytic, antimicrobial, decreases antimicrobial resistance	q.d.–b.i.d.	Irritation, contact allergy, bleaches clothing
Benzamycin (5% B.P./ 3% Erythromycin) Benzaclin (5% BP/ Clindamycin 1%) (Duac)	Same as above + anti-inflammatory	q.d.–b.i.d.	Same as above
Erythromycin (Erycette, T-stat, Emgel) Clindamycin (Cleocin T) Sodium sulfacetamide (Klaron, Novacet, Sulfacet-R) Topical sulfur[a]: (Fostex, Rezamid, SAStid)	Antimicrobial Anti-inflammatory	q.d.–b.i.d.	Development of resistance, drying, odor

[a]Topical therapeutic options available as over-the-counter preparations.

1. *Erythromycin 2% (e.g., A/T/S solution, T-Stat solution, Erygel, Emgel, Aknemycin)*: Available in solutions, gels, pads, and ointment; applied twice daily.
2. *Clindamycin 1% (Cleocin T solution, C/T/S, Clindets, Clindagel, Evoclin)*: Available in a solution, lotion, foam, gel, or pledget; applied twice daily.
3. *Sodium sulfacetamide (Klaron, Sulfacet-R, Novacet, and Plexion cleanser)*: May be more effective for rosacea than for acne. They should be avoided in sulfa-allergic patients.
4. *Benzoyl peroxide 5% with 3% erythromycin (Benzamycin gel) and clindamycin 1%–benzoyl peroxide 5% gel (BenzaClin and Duac topical gel)*: Bacterial resistance has not been seen. They may be used as monotherapy or in combination with topical retinoids and/or oral antibiotics.

Other Agents

1. *Keratolytic washes and lotions (salicylic acid, sulfur, resorcinol)*: Not as effective as other monotherapy but may act synergistically when used in combination regimens.
2. *Sunlight or ultraviolet light:* Risks of photoaging and carcinogenesis outweigh benefits.
3. *Lasers and light systems:* An evolving therapeutic area, with few studies evaluating safety and efficacy.

Systemic Therapy

Table 19.2 summarizes therapeutic options for systemic therapy.

Oral Antibiotics

Oral antibiotics decrease the *P. acnes* population, reduce free fatty acids, and may decrease the inflammatory response. Approximately 3 to 6 months of treatment may be required.

1. Tetracycline
   a. *Dosing:* 250 to 500 mg once or twice daily
   b. *Side effects:* Gastrointestinal upset
   c. *Other considerations:* Inexpensive, needs to be taken on an empty stomach
2. Doxycycline
   a. *Dosing:* 50 to 100 mg once or twice daily
   b. *Side effects:* Dose-dependent phototoxicity, gastrointestinal upset, light-headedness
3. Minocycline
   a. *Dosing:* 50 to 100 mg once or twice daily; 45, 90, 135 mg once daily
   b. *Side effects:* Hyperpigmentation of teeth, oral mucosa, and skin; gastrointestinal upset, light-headedness, lupus-like reactions or hepatitis with long-term treatment
4. Trimethoprim-sulfamethoxazole
   a. *Dosing:* 160 mg trimethoprim/800 mg sulfamethoxazole once daily
   b. *Side effects:* Toxic epidermal necrolysis and allergic eruptions
5. Erythromycin
   a. *Dosing:* 250 to 500 mg two to four times daily
   b. *Side effects:* Gastrointestinal upset
6. *13-cis-Retinoic acid or isotretinoin (Accutane):* 13-*cis*-retinoic acid is reserved for treatment of severe nodular or recalcitrant acne by practitioners

TABLE 19.2

Systemic Therapeutic Options for Acne

Systemic Medication	Action	Dosage	Side Effects
Tetracycline	Antimicrobial Anti-inflammatory	250–500 b.i.d. on empty stomach	HA, GI, pseudotumor, yeast infection, OCP interaction, esophagitis, photosensitivity, tooth teratogen
Doxycycline	Same above	50–100 q.d., b.i.d. Can be taken with food	Same as above + increased photosensitivity
Minocycline	Same above	50–100 q.d., b.i.d. 45, 90, 135 q.d.	Pigment deposition, dizziness, hypersensitivity, hepatitis, lupus-like reaction
Erythromycin	Antimicrobial, anti-inflammatory	250 q.i.d.	GI distress, drug interactions— Theophylline, Carbamazepine
Oral Contraceptives: norgestimate-ethinyl estradiol (Ortho Tri-Cyclen), norethindrone-ethinyl estradiol (Estrostep), drospirenone-ethinyl estradiol (Yasmin, Yaz), levonorgestrel-ethinyl estradiol (Alesse)	Antiandrogenic Decreased sebum production		Risk of thromboembolism
Intralesional Steroids	Decrease inflammation	1–5% triamcinolone intralesional	Scarring (usually transient)
Other Antiandrogens (e.g., Spironolactone)		50–100 mg q.d.	Irregular menses, gynecomastia, hypercalcemia, teratogenic

TABLE 19.2

(Continued)

Systemic Medication	Action	Dosage	Side Effects
Accutane (Isotretinoin)	Decreases sebum production, normalizes keratinization, decreases inflammation, decreases *Propionibacterium acnes* concentrations	0.5–1.0 mg/kg/ d × 16–24 weeks	Many !!! Strong teratogen, drying, cheilitis, hypercholesterolemia, hypertriglyceridemia, paronychia, eczema, alopecia, arthralgia, depression, decreased night vision

HA, headache; GI, gastrointestinal; OCP, oral contraceptive pills.

experienced with its use and involved with government mandated registry programs.

a. *Mechanism of action:* Decreases keratinization and sebum production, diminishing *P. acnes* growth and host inflammatory response.

b. *Dosing:* 0.5 to 1 mg/kg taken daily with food to achieve a total cumulative dose of 120 mg/kg of body weight (typically 16 to 24 weeks). Isotretinoin is teratogenic; female patients must utilize two forms of contraception.

c. Laboratory monitoring
   • Complete blood count (CBC), liver function tests, cholesterol, triglycerides.
   • A government-mandated registry program requires baseline and monthly pregnancy tests in females of childbearing age.

d. Side effects
   • *Dermatologic:* Cheilitis (90%), xerosis (78%), epistaxis (46%), conjunctivitis (40%), desquamation (16%), hair thinning (9%), photosensitivity (5% to 10%), occasional pyogenic granuloma-like lesions (hypergranulation tissue), *Staphylococcus aureus* skin colonization and infections
   • *Musculoskeletal:* Arthralgias and myalgias (16%)
   • *Ophthalmologic:* Decreased night vision
   • *Gastrointestinal:* Hypercholesterolemia (7%), hypertriglyceridemia (25%), elevated liver function tests (15%)
   • *Hematologic:* Elevated erythrocyte sedimentation rate (40%), leukopenia, elevated platelets (10% to 20%)
   • *Genitourinary:* Proteinuria, hematuria, vaginal dryness, urethritis
   • *Neurologic:* Headaches (5%), pseudotumor cerebri (rare)
   • *Psychiatric:* Depression. A recent literature review did not find any studies to support a causal association between isotretinoin use and

increased risk of depression or suicidal behavior; however, a weak association could not be ruled out. Patients should be monitored for signs and symptoms of depression or other psychiatric disturbance.

Hormonal Therapy

Women with signs of hyperandrogenism (acne resistant to conventional treatment) who quickly relapse after finishing a course of isotretinoin or who have a sudden onset of severe acne should be evaluated for hyperandrogenism.

Combined Oral Contraceptives. Norgestimate-ethinyl estradiol (Ortho Tri-Cyclen) and norethindrone acetate-ethinyl estradiol (Estrostep) are approved by the FDA for the treatment of acne. Drospirenone-ethinyl estradiol (Yasmin, Yaz) and levonorgestrel-ethinyl estradiol (Alesse) are also effective. Duration of treatment is usually 6 to 9 months. The effect of injectables and patch systems on acne has not been evaluated. Progesterone-only contraceptives generally worsen acne. Potential side effects include thromboembolism. A more complete list of side effects may be found in the discussion on OCPs in Chapter 43.

Antiandrogens. Spironolactone 50 to 100 mg daily may be added to the patient's regimen if oral contraceptives alone are ineffective. Higher doses are more effective but associated with more adverse effects, including menstrual irregularities and breast tenderness. Spironolactone must be used in combination with contraception owing to potential teratogenicity.

Corticosteroids. High-dose corticosteroids (prednisone 5.0 to 7.5 mg or dexamethasone 0.25 to 0.5 mg) should be reserved for treating acne conglobata, acne fulminans, and acute flares of acne precipitated by initiating isotretinoin therapy. Intralesional corticosteroids may be useful for inflammatory cysts and nodules.

ACNE Surgery

1. *Comedone extraction:* Open comedones can be easily removed with a comedo extractor. Closed comedones require puncture with a needle or lancet *first.*
2. *Incision and drainage:* Not recommended because of possible scarring.
3. *Intralesional corticosteroids:* Injection of 0.05 to 0.1 mL per lesion of triamcinolone acetate suspension (1.0 to 2.5 mg/mL) can rapidly improve isolated inflammatory cysts or nodules. Atrophy may occur at the injection site, which usually resolves in 4 to 6 months but can be permanent.
4. *Rehabilitation:* Surgical options for scars include punch excision and grafting, chemical peels, dermal fillers, dermabrasion, and laser surgery. Avoid any cosmetic procedures for at least 6 months to 1 year after discontinuing isotretinoin.

TABLE 19.3

Step Therapy for Acne

Acne Severity	Lesion Type	Initial Treatment	If Inadequate Response*
Mild	Comedonal	BP alone q.d.–b.i.d. OR BP/topical antibiotic combo q.d.–b.i.d. OR topical retinoid QHS	Add topical retinoid OR topical antibiotic OR substitute BP/topical antibiotic combination
	Inflammatory/ Mixed	BP alone q.d.–b.i.d. OR BP/topical antibiotic combo q.d.–b.i.d OR topical retinoid QHS	Add topical retinoid or topical antibiotic OR substitute BP/topical antibiotic combination
Moderate	Comedonal	Topical retinoid +/– BP or BP/topical antibiotic combination	Increase strength or change type of topical retinoid OR add BP or BP/topical antibiotic combination to topical retinoid
	Inflammatory/ Mixed	BP or BP/combo +/topical retinoid +/– oral antibiotic	Add retinoid or oral antibiotic. Consider oral contraceptive for females. Consider referral to dermatologist
		Oral antibiotic + topical retinoid	Increase strength or change type of topical retinoid. Consider oral contraceptive in females. Add BP or BP/topical antibiotic combination. Consider referral to dermatologist

(continued)

TABLE 19.3

(Continued)

Acne Severity	Lesion Type	Initial Treatment	If Inadequate Response*
Severe	Comedonal	Consider referral OR oral antibiotic and topical retinoid OR +/− BP or BP/topical antibiotic combination OR +/− oral contraceptive for female patients	Consider isotretinoin Referral to dermatologist
	Inflammatory/ Mixed	Same as above	Same as above

*Determined by physician assessment and patient satisfaction.

BP, Benzoyl peroxide; BP combo, BP–clindamycin (Benzaclin); BP–erythromycin (Benzamycin).

Other topical antibiotic (clindamycin, erythromycin, sodium sulfacetamide) may be substituted if there is irritation, dermatitis, etc. with BP-products.

+Azelaic acid may be substituted.

Low strength retinoid can include Retin-A 0.025% cream, Retin-A Gel Micro 0.04%, Differin 0.1% Cream/Gel or Avita or generic Tretinoin 0.025% cream.

SUMMARY

In general, patient education regarding basic skin care should be provided. Treatment regimens using topical and/or systemic therapy should be tailored to the needs of the individual. Mild acne can be treated effectively with topical benzoyl peroxide alone or in combination with a topical retinoid. Moderate or inflammatory acne may require oral antibiotics in addition to a topical retinoid. Isotretinoin should be considered for patients with severe nodulocystic acne or acne refractory to systemic antibiotics. Finally, hormonal therapy may be used in females with signs or symptoms of hyperandrogenism. Table 19.3 provides a stepwise approach to treating acne.

WEB SITES

http://www.skincarephysicians.com/acnenet/. Acne Net: About acne from Roche and American Academy of Dermatology.

http://www.aad.org/pamphlets/acnepamp.html. American Academy of Dermatology pamphlet on acne.

http://www.niams.nih.gov/hi/topics/acne/acne.htm. National Institutes of Health questions and answers about acne.

http://www.ipledgeprogram.com. Registration program for patients on isotretinoin and prescribing physicians.

CHAPTER 20

Miscellaneous Dermatologic Disorders

Mei-Lin T. Pang and Lawrence F. Eichenfield

ECZEMATOUS DERMATITIS

Eczematous dermatitis is an inflammatory response of the skin to multiple factors. Both contact dermatitis and atopic dermatitis are discussed in this section.

Contact Dermatitis

Clinical Manifestations

Distribution. Areas exposed to the inciting agent, typically hands, eyelids, genitalia, and legs.

Morphology. Well-demarcated areas of pruritic, vesicular, erythematous and/or edematous lesions corresponding to the distribution of contact. If chronic, lichenification, scaling, and pigmentary changes are also seen.

Etiology

About 80% of contact dermatitis is irritant and 20% allergic. Contact and irritant dermatitis may be indistinguishable clinically. Patch testing may be helpful.

1. *Irritant dermatitis:* A non-immunologically mediated dermatitis occurring in individuals when exposed to adequate doses of the offending agent. Prior exposure is not required.
2. *Allergic contact dermatitis*: A type IV, delayed-type hypersensitivity reaction occurring in patients sensitive to a specific agent. Prior exposure is required.

Differential Diagnosis

Cellulitis, atopic dermatitis, tinea corporis, seborrheic dermatitis, scabies, psoriasis, keratosis pilaris, ichthyosis vulgaris.

Treatment

1. Identify and avoid the offending agent
2. moderate- to high-potency topical steroids applied twice daily
3. antihistamines
4. widespread, severe contact dermatitis may require systemic corticosteroids (40 to 60 mg/d for 7 days, tapered over 2 to 3 weeks)

Atopic Dermatitis

Atopic dermatitis is a common, chronic pruritic dermatitis that typically occurs in childhood (17% of children) and may improve or continue in adolescence.

Clinical Manifestations

1. *Essential features—must be present:* (a) pruritus; (b) eczematous dermatitis (acute, subacute, or chronic); (c) typical morphology (pruritic, slightly elevated flat-topped papules coalescing into lichenified, scaly plaques) and age-specific patterns (flexural areas, face, neck, and hands) (d) chronic or relapsing history
2. *Important features—support diagnosis:* (a) early age of onset; (b) atopy (i.e., personal and/or family history and IgE reactivity), and (c) xerosis
3. *Associated features—too nonspecific for diagnosis:* (a) atypical vascular responses (e.g., facial pallor); (b) keratosis pilaris/hyperlinear palms/ichthyosis; (c) ocular/periorbital changes (e.g., Denny Morgan lines); (d) other regional findings (e.g., perioral changes/periauricular lesions, pityriasis alba); (e) perifollicular accentuation/lichenification/prurigo lesions

Complications

1. *Infections:* Increased susceptibility to herpes simplex virus, *Staphylococcus aureus, Trichophyton rubrum,* warts, and molluscum contagiosum
2. *Eye:* keratoconus, recurrent conjunctivitis, periorbital darkening
3. *Skin:* exfoliative dermatitis

Differential Diagnosis

Seborrheic dermatitis, contact dermatitis, tinea corporis or pedis, scabies, psoriasis, keratosis pilaris

Treatment

1. Patient education
2. Limit bathing to 10 to 20 minutes using lukewarm to warm water and a gentle cleanser.
3. A bland moisturizer applied twice daily
4. Loose-fitting, noncoarse clothing is recommended.
5. Avoidance of airborne triggers
6. Eczematous flares caused by specific foods occur in only a minority of children.
7. Topical corticosteroids may be applied twice daily to affected areas for acute flares (see Table 20.1).
8. Topical calcineurin inhibitors may prove helpful [Tacrolimus (Protopic) 0.03% ointment is approved for use in patients 2 to 15 years of age; the 0.03% and 0.1% dosage forms are approved for short-term and intermittent long-term use in adults with moderate to severe atopic dermatitis. Pimecrolimus (Elidel) 1% cream is approved for patients at least 2 years of age with mild-moderate atopic dermatitis].
9. Systemic antibiotics (e.g., cephalexin 25 to 50 mg/kg/day divided bid/tid) for 7 to 10 days. Localized infections can be treated with topical antibiotics (e.g., mupirocin) applied tid for 7 to 10 days. Patients with eczema herpeticum should be admitted for intravenous acyclovir. Bleach baths (1/4 to 1/2 cup bleach per full tub two to three times a week) may be useful in patients with recurrent staphylococcal infections.

TABLE 20.1

Classification of Commonly Used Topical Corticosteroids According to Potency[a]

Group	Generic Name (Vehicle, Concentration)
Group 1 (most potent[b])	Clobetasol propionate (cream, foam, ointment, lotion: 0.05%) Betamethasone dipropionate (foam, ointment 0.05%) Halobetasol propionate (Ultravate, cream, ointment 0.05%) Diflorasone diacetate (Psorcon, ointment 0.05%)
Group 2	Fluocinonide (cream, ointment, gel, solution: 0.05%) Mometasone furoate (ointment 0.1%) Betamethasone dipropionate (ointment 0.05%) Amcinonide (ointment 0.1%) Desoximetasone (cream, ointment 0.25%, gel 0.5%)
Group 3	Triamcinolone acetonide (ointment 0.1%) Amcinonide (cream, lotion 0.1%) Betamethasone dipropionate (cream 0.05%) Betamethasone valerate (ointment 0.1%) Fluticasone propionate (ointment 0.005%) Diflorasone diacetate (cream 0.05%)
Group 4	Mometasone furoate (cream, lotion 0.1%) Triamcinolone acetonide (cream 0.1%) Fluocinolone acetonide (ointment 0.025%) Hydrocortisone valerate (ointment 0.2%)
Group 5	Fluticasone propionate (cream 0.05%) Fluocinolone acetonide (cream 0.025%) Betamethasone valerate (cream 0.1%) Hydrocortisone valerate (cream 0.2%) Betamethasone dipropionate (lotion 0.05%) Prednicarbate (cream 0.1%)
Group 6	Fluocinolone acetonide (oil 0.01%, solution 0.01%) Betamethasone valerate (lotion 0.05%) Triamcinolone acetonide (cream 0.1%) Desonide (cream, ointment 0.05%) Alclometasone dipropionate (cream, ointment 0.05%)
Group 7 (least potent)	Hydrocortisone (cream, ointment, lotion 1.0%, 2.5%) Dexamethasone Prednisolone Methylprednisolone Pramoxine hydrochloride (1.0%, 2.5%)

[a]Potency varies according to the corticosteroids, concentration, and vehicle. Ointments are generally more potent than creams.

[b]Use of superpotent steroids should be limited to 2 wk or less.

From Eichenfield LF, Leung DYM. *The eczemas*. New York: Summit Communications, 2004 with permission.

10. Sedating antihistamines (diphenhydramine and hydroxyzine) may be given nightly for pruritus. Doxepin is a tricyclic antidepressant with histamine-blocking properties that should be reserved for patients with severe eczema.

Pyoderma
Folliculitis
1. *Etiology:* Superficial infection of hair follicles usually caused by *Staphylococcus aureus* and streptococcus, fungi, and viruses
2. *Morphology:* Pustules with surrounding erythema near hair follicles
3. *Distribution:* Scalp, extremities, buttocks, perioral or perinasal areas, and groin or pubic area in patients who shave or wax
4. *Differential diagnosis:* Culture-negative folliculitis, eosinophilic folliculitis, acne vulgaris, rosacea, keratosis pilaris, and pseudofolliculitis barbae
5. *Treatment:* Local treatment with antibacterial cleansers and a topical antibiotic agent (e.g., clindamycin) to cover *S. aureus* and streptococcus

Impetigo
1. *Etiology:* Secondary bacterial infection usually caused by group A beta-hemolytic streptococci or *S. aureus*
2. *Morphology:* Discrete and coalescent vesicles or pustules with yellow crusting
3. *Treatment:* Topical mupirocin (Bactroban) for localized infection, systemic antibiotics for extensive or recurrent disease

Furuncles
1. *Morphology:* Staphylococcal abscesses develop around hair follicles, typically in areas of friction.
2. *Treatment:* warm compresses, antistaphylococcal antibiotics, and incision and drainage of fluctuant lesions. Consider methicillin-resistant *S. aureus* if the patient fails standard antibiotic therapy.

PAPULOSQUAMOUS ERUPTIONS

Eruptions consisting of scaly patches and plaques include psoriasis, pityriasis rosea, seborrheic dermatitis, fungal infections, drug eruptions, and secondary syphilis (see Chapter 64).

Psoriasis
Psoriasis is a chronic, genetically influenced, and immunologically based inflammatory disease of the skin and joints that affects between 1% and 3% of the population.

Etiology. Unknown.

Precipitating Factors. (1) Certain infections (streptococcal pharyngitis), (2) trauma (Koebner phenomenon), (3) stress, (4) cold weather and low humidity, and (5) administration of certain medications.

Clinical Manifestations

1. *Morphology:* Round, well-demarcated circumscribed erythematous plaques with a silvery "micaceous" scale that demonstrates pinpoint bleeding when scale is removed (Auspitz sign). Small, teardrop-size or guttate lesions are associated with streptococcal pharyngitis. Nails may show pitting, onycholysis, and oil spots.
2. *Distribution:* Scalp, trunk, elbows, and knees. Inverse psoriasis affects umbilical and intertriginous areas.
3. *Psoriatic arthritis:* Acute seronegative oligoarthritis that typically presents during childhood and rarely during adolescence.

Diagnosis. Diagnosed clinically or by biopsy if diagnosis is unclear.

Treatment. There is no cure for psoriasis. The goal of treatment is to suppress or ameliorate the disease. Many individuals will need maintenance therapy.

1. Evaluation and avoidance of precipitating factors
2. Topical corticosteroids
   a. *Indications:* Monotherapy for localized psoriasis
   b. *Dosing:* High-potency corticosteroids applied twice a day for 2 weeks, avoiding the groin and face. Transition to mid- to low-potency corticosteroids and less frequent application as plaques resolve.
   c. *Adverse effects:* Pituitary-adrenal axis suppression with potent corticosteroids, epidermal atrophy (reversible), dermal atrophy, perioral dermatitis, allergic contact dermatitis, and rosacea.
3. Calcipotriene (Dovonex) cream
   a. *Indication:* First- or second-line topical agent for mild-moderate plaque psoriasis.
   b. *Dosing:* Calcipotriene 0.005% cream applied twice a day
   c. *Adverse effects:* Irritant dermatitis
4. Tazarotene (Tazorac) gel or cream
   a. *Indication:* Second-line therapy alone or in combination for mild to moderate psoriasis
   b. *Dosing:* Applied to affected areas once daily. Efficacy may be increased when combined with a mid- to high-potency topical corticosteroid.
   c. *Adverse effects:* Pruritus, burning, erythema
   d. *Contraindications:* Unstable plaque psoriasis in progress, erythrodermic psoriasis, patients with a history of allergic contact dermatitis to tazarotene, and pregnant or lactating females.
5. Patients with severe, refractory disease should be referred to a specialist. Systemic treatment may involve the following:
   a. *Phototherapy:* Ultraviolet B (UVB) and psoralen plus ultraviolet A (UVA). UVA combined with oral or topical psoralens is reserved for severe, recalcitrant psoriasis.
   b. *Systemic therapy:* This includes methotrexate, acitretin, cyclosporine, and biological agents such as inhibitors of tumor necrosis factor alpha.

Pityriasis Rosea

Pityriasis rosea is a self-limited disorder of unknown cause frequently occurring during adolescence.

Clinical Manifestations

1. *Lesions:* Presence of a herald patch, a large, 2- to 6-cm single lesion that typically precedes the rash by 2 to 21 days. The remaining rash consists of 1- to 2-cm oval, salmon-colored macules and papules with fine overlying peripheral scale.
2. *Distribution:* Symmetric, along the body's lines of cleavage in a "Christmas tree" distribution on the trunk, upper arms, and lower neck.
3. *Other symptoms:* Mild to severe pruritus.

Differential Diagnosis. Tinea corporis, secondary syphilis, seborrheic dermatitis

Treatment

1. Resolves spontaneously within 6 to 8 weeks
2. Antihistamines or topical corticosteroids

Seborrheic Dermatitis

Seborrheic dermatitis is a chronic recurring inflammatory disease of the skin limited to areas of excessive sebaceous gland activity.

Clinical Manifestations

1. *Distribution:* Scalp, eyebrows, forehead, lips, ears, nasolabial creases, axillae, chest, inframammary folds, umbilicus, and groin
2. *Morphology:* Dry, moist, or greasy scales often crusted with yellow patches of various sizes.

Differential Diagnosis. Psoriasis, tinea corporis, pityriasis rosea, atopic and contact dermatitis

Treatment

1. Tar, selenium sulfide, sulfur, zinc, ketoconazole 2% shampoo, or combination scalp treatments applied two to three times weekly.
2. Hydrocortisone 1% to 2.5% used sparingly for short periods on the face. Ketoconazole 2% cream may be worthwhile. Many topical corticosteroids are available in solutions, shampoos, or foams for the scalp.

Fungal Infections

The dermatophytoses are the most common fungal diseases of the skin and include tinea capitis, tinea pedis, tinea cruris, and tinea unguium (onychomycosis).

Dermatophytoses

Tinea Capitis

1. *Etiology:* Most commonly caused in the United States by *Trichophyton tonsurans.*
2. *Morphology:* An enlarging scaly patch of alopecia with broken hairs present. May also present with dandruff-like scale, minimal pruritus and subtle hair loss. A granulomatous mass, or kerion, can develop.
3. Diagnosis: Wood's lamp exam, potassium hydroxide (KOH) exam, or culture

4. *Treatment:*
   a. Griseofulvin microsize 20 to 25 mg/kg/d or ultramicrosize 10–15 mg/kg/d for 6–8 weeks up to 12 to 16 weeks for clinical or mycologic cure.
   b. Terbinafine 250 mg/d for 2–4 weeks for resistant cases or patients who cannot tolerate griseofulvin.
   c. Table 20.2 reviews antifungal agents.

Tinea Corporis
1. *Epidemiology:* Commonly seen in wrestlers.
2. *Morphology:* Pruritic, annular lesions that spread centrifugally with central clearing. Hair, nails, palms, and soles are spared. Scales and pruritic vesicles may be present.
3. *Diagnosis:* KOH exam or fungal culture.
4. *Differential diagnosis:* Nummular eczema, atopic dermatitis, contact dermatitis, pityriasis versicolor, annular psoriasis, granuloma annulare, and pityriasis rosea.
5. *Treatment:* Use topical therapy for localized infections. Treat widespread or resistant lesions with griseofulvin. Systemic fluconazole, itraconazole, and terbinafine are alternatives but are not approved for the treatment of dermatophytosis.

Tinea Cruris
1. *Epidemiology:* Male adolescents, particularly during summer months
2. *Morphology:* Bilateral or unilateral crescent-shaped, reddish, scaly plaques with sharply defined, raised borders on the upper and inner surfaces of the groin and thighs with scrotal sparing.
3. *Diagnosis:* Physical exam, negative Wood's lamp examination, branching hyphae on KOH exam, or culture.
4. *Differential diagnosis:* Candidiasis, erythrasma, psoriasis, intertrigo, seborrheic dermatitis, neurodermatitis, irritant dermatitis, other pruritic groin rashes including scabies, pediculosis pubis, miliaria
5. *Treatment:* Loose clothing, thorough drying of skin, weight reduction if obese, laundering of contaminated clothing and linens, and topical powders. Topical antifungal creams or oral griseofulvin are effective regimens.

Tinea Pedis
1. *Etiology:* Contact with contaminated surfaces. Occlusive footwear and warm humid weather are predisposing factors.
2. *Morphology:* Scaling, maceration and fissuring of the toe webs that may extend to the soles of the feet.
3. *Diagnosis:* Clinical. KOH positive for branching hyphae.
4. *Differential diagnosis:* Pitted keratolysis, juvenile plantar dermatosis, dyshidrosis, psoriasis, and contact dermatitis
5. *Treatment:* (a) Use topical antifungal agents for mild infections. Treat severe or unresponsive infections with griseofulvin microsize 500 mg/d or ultramicrosize 660 to 750 mg/day for 6 to 8 weeks. Consider oral antifungals for diabetic or immunocompromised patients or for cases of moccasin tinea pedis. (b) If there is a severe inflammatory response or an "id" reaction, a short 1-week course of topical or systemic steroids is helpful. (c) Keep feet dry and well aerated.

TABLE 20.2

Antifungal Agents Available for the Treatment of Common Superficial Fungal Infections

Indications	Antifungal (Trade Name)	Formulation	Frequency
Onychomycosis	Ketoconazole (Nizoral)	Oral	200 mg/d for 2–3 mo
	Terbinafine (Lamisil)	Oral	250 mg/d for 6 wk for fingernails and 12 wk for toenails
Tinea infections	Butenafine (Mentax)	1% Cream	Once or twice daily
	Ciclopirox (Loprox, Penlac)	1% Lacquer, lotion, cream	Twice daily
	Clotrimazole (Lotrimin)	1% Solution, lotion, cream	Twice daily
	Econazole (Spectazole)	1% Cream	Once daily
	Griseofulvin (Fulvicin, Grifulvin, Gris-PEG, Grisactin, Gristatin)	Oral	500 mg/d for 4–6 wk in adults for tinea capitis, corporis, cruris, or pedis; and 10–20 mg/kg/d for 6–8 wk in children for tinea capitis, 2–4 wk for corporis, and 4–8 wk for pedis
	Haloprogin (Halotex)	Solution, cream	Twice daily
	Ketoconazole (Nizoral)	2% Shampoo, 1% cream	Twice weekly, once daily
	Miconazole (Micatin)	2% Solution, lotion, cream, powder	Twice daily
	Naftifine (Naftin)	1% Cream, 1% gel	Once daily
	Oxiconazole (Oxistat)	1% Lotion, cream	Once or twice daily
	Sulconazole (Exelderm)	1% Lotion, cream	Once or twice daily
	Terbinafine (Lamisil)	1% Solution, 1% cream	Once or twice daily
	Tolnaftate (Tinactin)	1% Solution, lotion, cream, or powder	Twice daily

Oral candidiasis	Nystatin (Mycostatin)	Solution	4–6 mL swish and swallow solution four times daily for 2 wk
	Amphotericin B (Fungizone)	Solution	1 mL oral suspension swish and swallow four times daily for 2 wk
	Anidulafungin (LY303366, VER-002)	Intravenous	Unknown
	Fluconazole (Diflucan)	Oral	In non-AIDS patients, 200 mg single dose
	Itraconazole (Sporanox) Micafungin (FK463)	Oral or intravenous	In AIDS patients, 200 mg the first day, then 100 mg for 2 wk 200 mg/d for 2 wk 50 mg/d for 10 d
	Voriconazole (Vfend)	Oral or intravenous	Intravenous: Loading dose 6 mg/kg every 12 hr for 1 d, then maintenance dose at 4mg/kg every 12 hr. Oral: >40 kg body weight: 400 mg orally every 12 hr for 1 d, then 200 mg orally every 12 hr; <40 kg body weight: 200 mg orally every 12 hr for 1 d, then 100 mg orally every 12 hr

AIDS, acquired immunodeficiency syndrome.

Tinea Unguium
Onychomycosis describes any fungal nail infection, whereas tinea unguium is specific to infection of the nail plate.

1. *Morphology:* White or yellow discoloration of the distal part of the nail with subsequent dystrophy (thickening, elevation, deformity, subungual debris).
2. *Diagnosis:* Fungal culture of subungual debris
3. *Treatment:* (a) Terbinafine 250 mg/day for 3 months for toenail infections, 6 weeks for fingernail infections; (b) itraconazole continuous therapy (100 mg twice daily for 3 months) or pulse therapy (200 mg twice daily for 1 week/month for 3 months); (c) other treatments: topical ciclopirox 8% topical solution (Penlac nail lacquer) or avulsion of the nail plate followed by topical therapy.

Dermatophytid
1. *Etiology:* A cutaneous or systemic reaction to hematogenously spread fungal antigen, commonly seen with tinea corporis and tinea pedis. Rare systemic problems including fever, anorexia, adenopathy, and leukocytosis.
2. *Morphology:* Widespread follicular scaly eruption or a vesiculobullous or scaly eruption limited to the hands.

Tinea (Pityriasis) Versicolor
1. *Predisposing factors:* Humidity, hyperhidrosis, heredity, diabetes, and systemic corticosteroids
2. *Morphology:* Scaly tan, brown, or hypopigmented macules or patches on the upper trunk and armsand occasionally the face and neck caused by *Pityrosporum orbiculare.*
3. *Diagnosis:* Presence of hyphae and spores ("spaghetti and meatballs") on KOH exam. Yellowish or brownish fluorescence on Wood's lamp exam.
4. *Differential diagnosis:* Pityriasis alba, vitiligo, pityriasis rosea, seborrheic dermatitis, syphilis
5. *Treatment*
   a. *Topicals:* Ketoconazole shampoo used as a single application or applied daily for 3 days. Other agents (selenium sulfide ketoconazole, zinc pyrithione, sulfosalicylic acid, or terbinafine) may be applied daily in the shower or overnight as tolerated for 2 weeks, then several times a month for maintenance.
   b. *Systemic treatment:* Fluconazole (400 mg as a single dose) or itraconazole (200 mg/day for 5 to 7 days) are not approved for use by the FDA in the treatment of tinea versicolor.

SKIN GROWTHS

Warts (Verrucae)
1. *Etiology:* Human papillomavirus (HPV), a DNA virus of the Papovaviridae family
   a. *Epidemiology:* 7% to 10% of the general population; 10% of children 2 to 12 years old
   b. *Transmission:* skin-to-skin contact, contact with contaminated surfaces
2. *Clinical manifestations:*
   a. *Verrucae vulgaris:* Single or multiple firm, well-demarcated hyperkeratotic papules 1 to 5 mm or larger in diameter, usually on the hands or fingers or

under nails. Filiform warts (those with projecting, thread-like structures) may be seen on the face or neck.

b. *Verrucae plana (flat warts):* 1- to 3-mm single or coalescing flat-topped, flesh-colored, or pink papules on the face, dorsal hands, wrists, or knees.

c. *Verrucae plantaris (plantar warts):* Hyperkeratotic papules on the plantar surface of the feet.

d. *Condylomata acuminata (venereal warts):* Moist, polypoid warts located in the genital area, transmitted by sexual contact (see Chapter 66).

3. *Treatment:* Approximately 70% of all warts resolve spontaneously within 2 years. There are no specific antiviral therapies for curing HPV infection, although vaccines for genital herpesviruses are available.

a. *Home therapy:* Effective in treating one half to two-thirds of patients. Warts are soaked in hot water for 10 to 20 minutes and then filed. Salicylic acid 17% is applied and covered with an occlusive dressing (e.g., duct tape). This process should be repeated nightly for up to 12 weeks. If skin irritation occurs, the patient may discontinue treatment for 1 to 2 days.

b. *Cryotherapy:* Over-the-counter cryotherapy products are not as strong as liquid nitrogen. Liquid nitrogen may be administered with spray units (cryostats) or with cotton-tipped applicators. Multiple treatments may be necessary. Liquid nitrogen should be applied to the wart tissue long enough (usually about 10 to 15 seconds) to create a white rim of 1 to 2 mm.

c. Topical tretinoin may be used for flat warts.

d. Imiquimod 5% (Aldara) has been approved to treat genital warts.

Molluscum Contagiosum

Molluscum contagiosum is a common condition caused by a poxvirus infection (see Chapter 66).

Parasitic Skin Infections

1. Pediculosis (see Chapter 67).
2. Scabies (see Chapter 67).

MISCELLANEOUS SKIN CONDITIONS

Vitiligo

1. *Epidemiology:* Vitiligo occurs in approximately 1%–2% of the population. Fifty percent of cases present before age 20. It may be associated with autoantibodies, thyroid disease, and leukotrichia (depigmentation of the hair).

2. *Etiology:* Depigmentation caused by melanocyte destruction, thought to be autoimmune-mediated.

3. *Morphology:* Depigmented, well-circumscribed macules, several millimeters to several centimeters in size. In lighter-skinned individuals, this may be first noticed during the summer.

4. *Distribution:* Usually bilateral and symmetric, but may be segmental. The face and extremities as well as areas of trauma are most commonly affected. Segmental vitiligo is usually not associated with other autoimmune diseases.

5. *Diagnosis:* Wood's lamp examination is helpful in identifying early lesions.

6. *Differential Diagnosis:* Morphea (localized scleroderma), post-inflammatory hypopigmentation, pityriasis alba, and tinea versicolor.

TABLE 20.3

Sunscreens and Protective Spectrum

	Spectrum
Chemical	
PABA	UVB
Cinnamates	UVB
Benzophenones	UVB (some UVA)
Parsol 1789 (butylmethoxy-dibenzoylmethane)	UVA
Avobenzone + Oxybenzone Ecamsule	UVA/UVB
Physical	UVA/UVB
Zinc oxide	UVA/UVB
Titanium dioxide	UVA/UVB

PABA, *p*-aminobenzoic acid; UVA, ultraviolet A; UVB, ultraviolet B.

7. *Treatment:* It is only partially satisfactory. Spontaneous repigmentation rarely occurs.
   a. Sunscreen and sun avoidance.
   b. Cover-up cosmetic such as Dermablend or Covermark.
   c. Mid to high-potency topical corticosteroid or topical calcineurin inhibitor (tacrolimus, pimecrolimus).
   d. Ultraviolet B radiation or narrow-band UVB.
   e. Topical or oral psoralens followed by long wavelength ultraviolet radiation (UVA).
   f. Autologous skin grafts.

Sunburn

Both tanning and sunburn cause DNA damage and may increase one's risk of developing non-melanoma and melanoma skin cancer, as well as photo aging. Recommendations include the following:

1. Avoid unprotected exposure from 10 a.m. to 3 p.m. Seek shade when appropriate.
2. Wear protective clothing and a hat when possible.
3. Sunscreens may lessen burning. A sunscreen with a sun protection factor (SPF) of 15 or greater with a broad spectrum of coverage (UVA and UVB) should be used regularly (Table 20.3).
4. Certain medications can increase photosensitivity. These include tetracycline, NSAIDs, and oral contraceptives.
5. Tanning beds and sunlamps should be avoided.

Prevention of sunburn is more effective than treatment. Treatment of sunburn includes soothing moisturizers and an oral NSAID as indicated.

Urticaria

Also known as hives, this is an extremely common problem, occurring in 15% of all individuals. It may be acute (<6 weeks,) or chronic (>6 weeks.)

Appearance. Pruritic, erythematous edematous papules and plaques, or "wheals," occurring anywhere on the body. Lesions usually blanch with pressure, though a dusky appearance or areas of central pallor may be seen. Individual lesions typically resolve in <24 hours, though a course of urticaria can last weeks to months. Simple urticaria involves superficial layers of the skin, whereas angioedema involves the deeper subcutaneous and submucosal tissues, particularly palms, soles, head and neck. Angioedema of the throat may cause respiratory obstruction in severe cases.

Classifications/Triggers. Usually multifactorial, however etiology is unknown in up to 50% of cases. Triggers or causes include medications, foods, infections, physical factors, and autoimmune diseases.

Evaluation. Acute transient urticarias do not need further evaluation. Chronic urticaria can be a serious disabling condition and the cause difficult to determine. Autoimmune diseases such as systemic lupus erythematosus may present with urticaria and should be considered in the differential diagnosis of chronic urticaria. Further tests should be ordered only after thorough history and physical examination looking for underlying etiologies.

Treatment. (1) Identify and avoid the inciting factor; (2) antihistamines; (3) cold baths or showers; (4) epinephrine; (5) systemic steroids.

Hair Loss

Hair loss can be extremely frightening to an adolescent. A thorough history and physical examination should be obtained.

Types of Hair Conditions

1. Male pattern alopecia: Loss of scalp hair usually in the late 20s to 30s secondary to androgenic hormones.
2. Telogen effluvium: Acute generalized hair loss 2 to 4 months after a stressful event (e.g., illness, surgery, "crash dieting," and parturition.)
3. Anagen effluvium: Hair loss caused by disruption of hair during the growth phase (e.g., antimitotic chemotherapy).
4. Alopecia areata: Sharply demarcated patches involving loss of terminal hair. Spontaneous remission is possible, but prognosis is poorer with more extensive involvement. In 25% of cases, the condition is permanent.
   a. *Etiology:* Most likely autoimmune
   b. *Diagnosis:* Clinical presentation
   c. *Differential diagnosis:* Tinea capitis, early discoid or systemic lupus erythematosus, and trichotillomania
   d. *Treatment:* Focal alopecia areata often regrows, but the course of the disease is variable and unpredictable. Potent topical, intralesional or oral corticosteroids have been used but are not curative. Other treatments include anthralin; topical immunotherapy including dinitrochlorobenzene, squaric acid dibutyl ester, diphencyprone; or minoxidil solution. Treatment may take months or years.

5. Hair loss secondary to physical factors: a) traction alopecia; b) hot comb alopecia; c) trichotillomania
6. Secondary Scalp disease: Psoriasis, fungal disease, seborrhea, or eczema
7. Metabolic disorders: Iron deficiency, hypothyroidism, hyperthyroidism, diabetes mellitus, or hypopituitarism
8. Systemic diseases: Systemic lupus erythematosus
9. Scarring alopecia: Irreversible hair loss secondary to inflammatory processes (discoid lupus erythematosus, scleroderma, lichen planus), or trauma.
10. Hair-shaft structural defects: Often associated with systemic disease. These conditions include pili torti, monilethrix, trichorrhexis, pili annulati, and Menkes' kinky-hair syndrome.

Evaluation
1. *History:* Including onset and duration, drug use, skin or scalp disease, and recent stress, surgery, illness, or dietary changes.
2. *Physical examination:* Evaluate for seborrhea, scalp disease, or an endocrine disorder.
3. *Pull test:* Lightly grasp about 20 hairs and pull gently. Normally one or two hairs will come out. If many hairs pull out, microscopic examination of the hairs will determine whether anagen or telogen hair loss is present.
4. KOH exam or fungal culture of scale may be helpful. Other tests may be ordered as indicated.
5. Referral to a dermatologist may be necessary for further evaluation and scalp biopsy if diagnosis is in question.

Therapy
Depending on etiology:
1. *Male pattern alopecia:* Oral finasteride (1 mg/day) and minoxidil solution 1% and 2% are approved in the United States for hair growth. In general, treatment for 6 to 12 months is needed to improve scalp coverage, and continuous treatment is used to retain a clinical improvement.
2. *Telogen effluvium:* Reassurance, self-limited
3. *Alopecia areata:* See previous discussion
4. *Scalp disease:* Treat underlying condition

Tattoos and Body Piercing
These have become more common among adolescents and young adults and may occur in relation to gang activity or peer pressure. In most states, minors cannot consent for body piercing and tattoos without parental consent, although this is not always followed. It is important to promote regulatory control over tattooing and body-piercing establishments to ensure sanitary conditions. Complications include pigment hypersensitivity, infections (hepatitis, tuberculosis, syphilis, and HIV), scarring (keloids can form) and milk ducts may be damaged when piercing a woman's nipple. New laser systems can effectively remove many tattoos but may be expensive, require multiple sessions, or result in pigmentary changes.

Primary Syphilis and Herpes Simplex. (See Chapters 60, 64, and 65, respectively.)

Hyperhidrosis

This condition involves excessive sweating in response to heat or emotional stimuli. Treatment with topical aluminum chloride preparations such as Certain-Dri, Xerac AC, or Drysol is often beneficial. Systemic anticholinergic agents, glutaraldehyde, and iontophoresis have also been used with varying degrees of success. Referral for botulism toxin type A (Botox) injection may be warranted in more severe cases. Rarely should surgical intervention be considered.

Pink Pearly Penile Papules

These are a normal occurrence in about 15% of postpubertal males. The lesions appear as elongated pearly white papules in one to five rows of uniform size (1 to 3 mm) and shape on the coronal margin of the penis, particularly the anterior border. They may be mistaken for condylomata acuminata. No treatment is necessary.

Acanthosis Nigricans

A condition that manifests itself as symmetric, velvety, papillomatous plaques, with increased skin-fold markings on the base of the neck and in the axillae, groin, and antecubital fossa. They may also occur on the dorsum of the hand and on the elbow, periumbilical skin and mucous membranes. Acanthosis nigricans may be commonly found during a routine physical examination in an otherwise healthy obese adolescent. Occasionally a parent is concerned about the "dirty" appearance. Most acanthosis nigricans lesions in adolescents are associated with insulin resistance secondary to obesity. These individuals may have type 2 diabetes or are at increased risk for type 2 diabetes and hyperlipidemia. Acanthosis nigricans can also be associated with hyperandrogenism and rarely with malignant conditions. Weight loss is the treatment of choice for obesity-related acanthosis nigricans.

WEB SITES AND REFERENCE

http://www.psoriasis.org/National Psoriasis Association.
http://www.aad.org/pamphlets.
http://www.nlm.nih.gov/medlineplus.
http://www.alopeciaareata.com/National Alopecia Areata Foundation.
http://www.nvfi.org/National Vitiligo Foundation.
http://www.eczema.org/National Eczema Society.
Schachner LA, Hansen RC. *Pediatric Dermatology*, 3rd ed. Edinburgh; New York: Mosby, 2003.

CHAPTER **21**

Epilepsy

Wendy G. Mitchell, Arthur Partikian, and Lawrence S. Neinstein

Epilepsy, the most common chronic neurologic condition in adolescents, is defined as recurrent unprovoked seizures. Seizures caused by specific precipitants or of non-CNS origin are considered provoked and thus not epilepsy. Adolescents with epilepsy are often well controlled with medication. New medications and surgical techniques have improved the outcome of severe, intractable epilepsy. The goals of management of epilepsy include proper diagnosis, evaluation, treatment of underlying etiologies, appropriate use of anticonvulsants, and management of associated psychosocial issues.

ETIOLOGY

Seizures represent manifestations of abnormal electrical activity in the brain, with location and pattern of spread determining clinical expression. Epilepsy may be genetic, idiopathic, or secondary to remote CNS insult. Seizures that occur *only* with acute provocation are not epilepsy, although specific stimuli or situations provoke seizures in some epileptics. Seizures may be provoked by infection, trauma, metabolic disturbances, drugs, drug withdrawal, syncope, or fever.

EPIDEMIOLOGY

1. *Prevalence:* 1 of 200 in the general population, with a higher prevalence in children
2. *Onset:* Peak ages of onset of idiopathic and age-related primary epilepsies are early school years and adolescence. Secondary epilepsy onset may occur at any age; it is occurs most often in infants and the elderly.
3. *Gender:* Slightly more common in males (RR 1.2 to 2.4)

4. *Socioeconomic status (SES), race, and ethnicity:* Slightly more common in low-SES groups and in developing countries, particularly in Latin America and Asia owing to neurocysticercosis.
5. *Mental retardation and cerebral palsy:* These increase the prevalence of epilepsy and lower the rate of remission.

CLINICAL MANIFESTATIONS

Table 21.1 lists international classifications of seizures.

SEIZURE COMPONENTS

The progression of a seizure is characterized by several variable temporal components including prodrome, aura, ictus, and postictal state, as follows:

1. Prodrome: altered behavior/mood occurring hours to days before the actual seizure—infrequent
2. Aura: sensory phenomena that are part of the seizure, representing a simple partial seizure
3. Ictus: the observed seizure event, usually with motor activity
4. Postictal state: altered neurologic function lasting minutes to 24 hours

Generalized Tonic, Clonic (GTC), or Tonic-Clonic Seizures
1. Tonic: forceful muscle contractions in flexion or extension
2. Clonic: bilateral, generally symmetric, brisk, phasic jerking movements
3. Immediately postictal: usually brief period of flaccidity, with or without incontinence
4. Postictal state: variable length of unconsciousness, stupor, confusion, headache, lethargy

Nonconvulsive Generalized Seizures (Absence or "Petit Mal")
1. No aura or prodrome
2. Ictus: brief period (few seconds to 30 seconds) of blank staring, with or without facial twitching, automatisms, loss of consciousness
3. Postictal: none, amnesia for event
4. Juvenile myoclonic epilepsy (JME) combines absence + myoclonic seizures ± GTC
5. Photosensitive epilepsy: absence + myoclonic seizures provoked by strobe conditions are a genetic epilepsy syndrome (e.g., "video game"–related seizures are seen in these patients)

Myoclonic Epilepsies
1. Myoclonus: brisk, irregular jerks involving trunk or extremities, symmetrically or asymmetrically—may be small in amplitude or massive
2. Patients are generally aware of the jerks
3. Similar movements may be tics or nonepileptic myoclonus
4. Degenerative conditions presenting with myoclonus in adolescence include progressive myoclonic epilepsies, storage disorders, subacute sclerosing panencephalitis (SSPE), and juvenile Huntington disease

Partial Seizures
1. Partial seizures begin in a localized portion of the brain and may spread. Simple partial seizures are not associated with alteration of consciousness,

TABLE 21.1

Classifications of Seizures

Generalized seizures: Bilaterally symmetrical, both in clinical and electroencephalographical manifestations, without focal features.
1. Tonic-clonic, generalized convulsive, grand mal
2. Tonic seizures
3. Clonic seizures
4. Absence seizures
   a. *Simple (impaired consciousness only):* Classic petit mal
   b. *Atypical:* Disturbed consciousness plus myoclonic component, automatisms, autonomic component, or abnormality of postural tone
5. Akinetic (atonic) seizures
6. Myoclonic seizures

Partial seizures: Clinical and electroencephalographical onset is localized to one part of the brain (focal). Simple partial seizures: No impairment of consciousness
1. Motor symptoms
2. Sensory symptoms
3. Autonomic symptoms
4. Special sensory (visual, auditory, olfactory, gustatory)
5. Psychic symptoms (fear, déjà vu, jamais vu, euphoria)

Complex partial seizures: Partial seizure with impairment of consciousness, includes most seizures described as *"psychomotor."* Seizure may begin with impairment of consciousness or as a simple partial seizure and progress to impaired consciousness.

Partial seizures with secondary generalization: Either partial simple or complex partial seizures may secondarily generalize, producing a tonic-clonic or clonic convulsion similar to a primary generalized convulsion. A partial simple seizure may progress through a complex partial seizure or directly to a secondarily generalized seizure.
1. Simple partial seizures progressing to generalized seizures
2. Complex partial seizures progressing to generalized seizures
3. Simple partial seizures progressing to complex partial seizures, progressing to generalized seizures

---

unlike complex partial seizures, which are marked by at least partial impairment of consciousness
2. Simple partial seizures with onset in infancy, adolescence, or adulthood may be associated with structural pathology (e.g., tumor, arteriovenous malformation, head injury, malformation, and stroke). Partial seizures with onset in mid-childhood are most often benign rolandic epilepsy and remit by adolescence.

Simple Partial Seizures
1. Partial seizures may include sensory, motor, special sensory, or psychic phenomena. Most partial simple seizures are motor. Clonic jerking may

remain localized, or spread up an extremity or to other extremities or the face. Speech arrest may occur and drooling is common

2. Postictal hemiparesis (Todd paralysis) may occur after any partial motor seizure
3. The electroencephalogram (EEG) typically shows focal spikes. Sleep may increase EEG yield.

Complex Partial Seizures (CPS). Older terms are *psychomotor seizure* or *temporal lobe seizure.* Structural pathology is more common here than in generalized epilepsies. Mesial temporal sclerosis may cause CPS, which consists of the following components:

1. Aura: initial sensory, autonomic, or psychic symptoms (seconds to minutes): fear, déjà vu, "rising feeling" in abdomen, tingling, and visual, auditory, olfactory, or gustatory hallucination. Consciousness and recall is retained during aura
2. Blank stare, impaired responsiveness, and minimal memory of this phase
3. Automatisms: hand wringing, picking, lip smacking, walking aimlessly, grunting, gagging, or swallowing. Directed, deliberate violence does not occur. Consciousness is lost and memory impaired. Frontal lobe CPS may produce extensor posturing, thrashing, agitated movements, bicycling leg movements, or pelvic thrusting
4. Postictal state: confusion, stupor, headache, and lethargy (seconds to hours)

DIFFERENTIAL DIAGNOSIS

Seizures

1. *Symptomatic or provoked seizures (due to acute systemic disturbance or trauma):* (a) metabolic disturbance (e.g., hypoglycemia, hyponatremia, and hypocalcemia); (b) CNS infection (e.g., encephalitis and meningitis); (c) intoxication (e.g., cocaine, alcohol, stimulants, "ecstasy," phencyclidine (PCP), ketamine, and inhalants); (d) drug or alcohol withdrawal (e.g., barbiturates, sedatives, and benzodiazepines); (e) acute head trauma (impact seizure and seizures in first few days after significant head trauma); (f) syncopal seizure: brief tonic or clonic seizure occurring after primary syncope; (g) acute stroke.
2. *Acquired (symptomatic or secondary) epilepsies due to remote CNS insult:* (a) cerebral malformations: macroscopic or microscopic (cortical dysgenesis), tuberous sclerosis; (b) intrauterine infections (e.g., cytomegalovirus and toxoplasmosis); (c) perinatal insults; (d) postneonatal infections (e.g., meningitis, encephalitis, and brain abscess); (e) posttraumatic epilepsy; (f) brain tumors and other mass lesions; (g) vascular: malformations, infarctions; (h) neurocysticercosis.
3. *Genetic changes due to progressive or degenerative conditions:* Unknown but presumed symptomatic due to epileptic encephalopathies; specific progressive myoclonic epilepsis
4. *Idiopathic and genetic epilepsy syndromes:* (a) primary generalized epilepsies; (b) childhood or juvenile absence epilepsy; (c) juvenile myoclonic epilepsy; and (d) benign focal epilepsies of childhood (benign rolandic epilepsy).

See Table 21.2 for other paroxysmal events that may suggest seizures.

TABLE 21.2

Differential between Nonepileptic Paroxysmal Events and Seizures

Paroxysmal Event	Typical Features Distinct from Seizures
Syncope (vasovagal)	Prodrome: pallor, light-headedness; visual changes: loss of color, field constriction
Migraine	Typical migraine auras (scintillating scotomata, tingling) followed by headache are unlikely to be confused with seizures. Acute confusional or hemiplegic migraine may be hard to distinguish.
Cardiac disease	Documented brady- or tachyarrhythmia; low-output state.
Hyperventilation and anxiety states	Perceived panic or fright; observed overbreathing; improvement with breathing into bag.
Orthostatic hypotension	Precipitation of loss of consciousness with positional change.
Sleep disturbances	Narcolepsy: cataplexy, sleep attacks, sleep paralysis, and hypnagogic hallucinations.
	Excessive daytime drowsiness due to sleep apnea.
	Parasomnias: sleepwalking, REM sleep disturbance.
	Night terrors: common in younger children; usually abate by adolescence.
	Periodic leg movements in sleep: generally familial; kicking or rhythmic movements throughout sleep cycle do not arouse patient; may be associated with restless legs syndrome.
Movement disorders	Tics: various types of movements or twitches can be behaviorally reproduced and can be at least temporarily suppressed.
	Paroxysmal kinesiogenic choreoathetosis: usually unilateral movement precipitated by onset of voluntary movement, such as getting up from chair or beginning to walk.
	"Stiff-man" syndrome, syndromes of continuous muscle fiber activity: rare, usually autoimmune, episodes of tonic posturing without change in consciousness.
	Dystonias (paroxysmal torticollis, activity-related dystonias, dystonia musculorum deformans, and drug related): dystonic posturing without alteration of awareness. Some are consistently reproducible by specific activity.
	Pseudohypoparathyroidism: hypocalcemia precipitates dystonic posturing. Although lifelong, often not detected until teens.

(continued)

TABLE 21.2

(Continued)

Paroxysmal Event	Typical Features Distinct from Seizures
	Restless legs syndrome: feelings of discomfort and need to move, relieved by walking, worse in evening and when tired. No alteration in consciousness.
Pseudoseizures (psychogenic or nonepileptic events)	More often involving agitated kicking, flailing, bilateral but non-synchronous movements, eyes closed (nearly all seizures have eyes open), pelvic thrusting common.
ADHD: episodic "staring" and inattention	Inattention is situation-specific, can be interrupted with strong stimuli and generally does not occur during activity, in contrast to absence seizures, which interrupt activity.

ADHD, attention deficit hyperactivity disorder; REM, rapid eye movement.

DIAGNOSIS

Epilepsy is primarily a clinical diagnosis based on the history.

1. Review the following with the observers and patient: (a) Activity and state at onset. Time of day of onset. (b) Relation to sleep state. At sleep onset? In deep sleep? Upon awakening? (c) What was the first abnormality noted: By patient? By observers? (d) Describe the episode: Body movements? Response to commands? At what point did unresponsiveness start? How long did unconsciousness last? (e) Incontinence? (f) Postictal state: Return of consciousness, paralysis, memory impairment; (g) Precipitating events: Sensory stimulation, activity, drugs, meals, medications, sleep pattern, stress, and menses. (h) Prior seizures or similar events.
2. Family history of epilepsy, neurocutaneous syndromes, and other neurologic conditions
3. Perinatal history
4. History of CNS infections or trauma
5. Drug history, including prescribed, over-the-counter, and "street" drugs and alcohol
6. Any other recent changes in health or function: any changes in cognition, motor function, or others to suggest onset of neurologic disease other than the seizure
7. Travel history and/or household exposure to recent immigrants

Physical Examination. Looking for systemic disease including

1. cardiac exam
2. skin: neurocutaneous syndromes (café-au-lait spots, depigmented macules, adenoma sebaceum, shagreen patch, and subungual fibromas)
3. eyes: funduscopic examination for papilledema

4. neurologic examination: look for focal abnormalities, observe gait and movements at rest and with activity for evidence of movement disorder as alternative explanation of symptoms
5. vital signs: blood pressure and pulse, rest and orthostatic
6. hyperventilation: hyperventilate for 2 to 3 minutes (petit mal suspected)

Laboratory Tests

1. Baseline CBC and liver function tests prior to starting an anticonvulsant medication
2. Tests of low yield in well teen with seizures: electrolytes, phosphorus, and magnesium. Rarely, seizure-like episodes are due to hypocalcemia in teens with pseudohypoparathyroidism. Test blood sugar if hypoglycemia is suspected, draw blood while patient is symptomatic
3. EEG: preferably both awake and asleep, with hyperventilation and photic stimulation. Sleep-deprived EEG increases the yield.
4. Neuroimaging: CT scan or MRI is indicated for newly diagnosed partial seizures or any seizure associated with neurologic abnormalities, papilledema, neurocutaneous stigmata, or suspected degenerative conditions
5. Lumbar puncture: acutely if infection or hemorrhage is suspected

TREATMENT

Anticonvulsant Therapy

General Guidelines

1. Start with a single anticonvulsant medication at lowest reasonable dose, considering both the seizure type and the potential side-effect profile
2. Increase medication slowly until seizures are controlled or toxicity occurs
3. Serum levels are useful only as guidelines. Clinical response and toxicity are more important
4. Divide daily dosing based on half-life. Consider using slow-release formulations
5. Follow-up for monitoring of seizure frequency, drug toxicity, and psychosocial issues
6. Change medications only when the first is pushed to tolerance without controlling the seizure unless allergic or serious idiosyncratic effects are evident. Polytherapy is reserved for refractory epilepsy unresponsive to trials of monotherapy
7. Discontinuation criteria: Assess the risks and benefits of continued therapy with anticonvulsants and consider tapering medication when patient is seizure-free for 2 to 4 years. Risk for recurrence on tapering is 30% to 40%. Risk factors for recurrence include mental retardation, large number of seizures before control, partial seizures with or without secondary generalization, and abnormal EEG. Medication should be tapered one drug at a time over 6 weeks to 3 months.

See Tables 21.3 and 21.4 for drugs used to treat specific types of seizures.

Side Effects of Anticonvulsant Drugs

Adverse effects of anticonvulsants can be divided into two major groups: dose-related reactions and idiosyncratic reactions unrelated to drug level. Mild sedation, which wanes over a few weeks, is common with initiation of any anticonvulsant. Potential reproductive effects are important in teenage girls.

TABLE 21.3

Metabolism, Uses, and Dosing Guidelines for Older Antiepileptic Drugs Used as Monotherapy[a]

Generic Name (Brand Name)	Primary Indications	Secondary Indications	Serum Half-Life (hr)	Time to Steady State	Therapeutic Levels	Toxic Levels	Daily Dosage	Preparations
Phenytoin (Dilantin)	Partial seizures with or without generalization	Generalized convulsions (avoid in JME)	24 ± 12	5–10 d	10–20 µg	>20 µg/mL	Pediatric: 3–8 mg/kg/d Adult: 250–400 mg/d	Dilantin capsules: 100 mg, 30 mg (slow release) Dilantin Infatabs: 50 mg Liquid: 125 mg/5 mL Generic capsules: 100 mg, rapid release; 300 mg slow release
Phenobarbital (Luminal)	Partial or generalized convulsive epilepsy[b]		72 ± 16	14–21 d	15–40 µg/mL	>40 µg/mL (much higher may be tolerated if used chronically)	Pediatric: 1–5 mg/kg/d Adult: 90–200 mg/d	Tablets: 15 mg, 30 mg, 60 mg 100 mg (essentially all generic) Liquid: 20 mg/5 mL
Primidone (Mysoline)	Partial or generalized convulsive epilepsy		12 ± 6 for primidone[c] 72 ± 16 for phenobarbital metabolite	14–21 d for metabolites	8–12 µg/mL primidone 15–40 g/mL phenobarbital metabolite	>15 µg/mL primidone	Pediatric: 10–15 mg/kg/d Adult: 500–1,000 mg/d	Tablets: 50 mg, 250 mg Liquid: 250 mg/5 mL

Drug	Indication 1	Indication 2	Half-life (h)	Time to steady state	Therapeutic level	Toxic level	Dose	Preparations
Carbamazepine (Tegretol, Epitol, Carbatrol, Tegretol XR)	Partial seizures with or without generalization	Generalized convulsions (avoid in JME)	12 ± 3 chronic; 36 ± 12 naive[d]	3–5 d	5–13 µg/mL	>15 µg/mL	Pediatric: 20 mg/kg/d (start lower) Adult: 400–1,800 mg/d	Tablets: 100 mg, 200 mg carbamazepine (fast release) Liquid: 100 mg/5 mL Sprinkle capsules, slow release (Carbatrol) 100 mg, 200 mg, 300 mg Tablets, slow release, Tegretol XR, 100 mg, 200 mg, 400 mg
Ethosuximide (Zarontin)	Typical absence (petit mal)	none	30 ± 6	7–14 d	40–100 µg/mL	>150 µg/mL	Pediatric: 10–40 mg/kg/d Adult: 500–1,500 mg/d	Capsules: 250 mg Liquid: 250 mg/5mL
Valproic acid (Depakene, Depakote, Depakote ER)	Primary generalized seizures, absence (typical or atypical), myoclonic seizures; first line for JME	Partial onset seizures	12 ± 6[e]	2–5 d	50–120 µg/mL	>120 µg/mL	Pediatric: 15–60 mg/kg/d Adult: 750–3,000 mg/d	Depakote capsules: 125 mg, 250 mg, 500 mg Depakote ER 250 mg, 500 mg Depakote sprinkle capsules: 125 mg (may be opened and mixed with food)

(continued)

TABLE 21.3

(Continued)

Generic Name (Brand Name)	Primary Indications	Secondary Indications	Serum Half-Life (hr)	Time to Steady State	Therapeutic Levels	Toxic Levels	Daily Dosage	Preparations
								Depakene or generic capsules 250 mg; Depakene or generic liquid valproic acid, 250 mg/5 mL.
Clonazepam (Klonopin)		Absence, myoclonic seizures	24 ± 12	5–10 d	Not helpful[f]	Not helpful	Pediatric: 0.02–0.05 mg/kg/d; Adult: 1–20 mg/d	Tablets: 0.5 mg, 1 mg, 2 mg

JME, juvenile myoclonic epilepsy.

[a]Monotherapy pharmacokinetics differs for chronic-use vs. antiepileptic drug–naive patient. Patients switched to monotherapy with phenytoin, barbiturates, or carbamazepine from another enzyme-inducing antiepileptic drug generally need higher doses.

[b]Phenobarbital is not considered a first-line medication for most indications despite wide-spectrum coverage, because of the potential for sedation and depression. However, it is first line in most of the developing world due to very low cost and ability to dose once daily.

[c]Primidone has several active metabolites including phenobarbital and PEMA. While primidone has a relatively short half-life, other metabolites have long half-lifes and a steady state may take 14–21 d to achieve.

[d]Carbamazepine metabolism autoinduces in many patients (much more rapid elimination after first few wk of treatment). Repeated dosage adjustments are often necessary in the first few mo of use.

[e]Depakote is of slow release with variable absorption and later peaks but is metabolized to valproic acid with the same elimination kinetics as Depakene and generics.

[f]Serum levels of benzodiazepines are not helpful in predicting therapeutic response. Alterations in receptors produce marked tolerance. Serum levels are occasionally useful in suspected ingestions or overdose, or to check compliance.

TABLE 21.4

Metabolism, Uses and Doses of Newer Anticonvulsant Medications

Generic Name (Brand Name)	Primary Indications	Secondary Indications	Serum Half-Life	Time to Steady State	Daily Dose	Usual Dosing Schedule	Preparations Available in the United States
Gabapentin (Neurontin)	Partial onset seizures, adjunctive	Partial onset seizures, monotherapy	5–7 hr[a]	2–3 d	Pediatric: 15–60 mg/kg/d Adult: 900–4,800 mg/d	t.i.d.–q.i.d.	100 mg, 300 mg, 400 mg, 600 mg, and 800 mg tabs; 250 mg/5 mL solution
Lamotrigine (Lamictal)	Generalized convulsive epilepsy; JME	Partial onset seizures, absence (typical or atypical) monotherapy or adjunctive	30 hr (markedly prolonged by coadministration of VPA; shortened by use of EIAED[b])	5–6 d	Pediatric: 5–15 mg/kg/d (2–5 mg/kg/d in combination with VPA) Adult monotherapy: 100–400 mg/d; up to 700 mg/d with EIAED	b.i.d.	5 mg, 25 mg chewable tabs; 25 mg, 100 mg, 150 mg, and 200 mg tablets
Topiramate (Topamax)	Generalized convulsive epilepsy; partial onset epilepsy (monotherapy or adjunctive)		21 hr	4 d	Pediatric: 5–20 mg/kg/d Adults: 200–400 mg/d	b.i.d.	25 mg, 100 mg, 200 mg tabs; 15 mg and 25 mg sprinkle capsules may be opened onto a spoon of food
Tiagabine (Gabitril)	Partial onset seizures	Partial onset seizures (adjunctive)	5–8 hr	2 d	Pediatric: 0.5–1 mg/kg/d Adults: 32–56 mg/d	b.i.d.	2 mg, 4 mg, 12 mg, 16 mg, and 20 mg tabs
Zonisamide (Zonegran)	Generalized or partial onset epilepsy (convulsive or nonconvulsive), adjunctive	Generalized or partial onset epilepsy (convulsive or non-convulsive), monotherapy	60 hr	10–12 d	Pediatric 5–12mg/kg/d Adults: 100–400 mg/d	q.d. or b.i.d.	25 mg, 50 mg and 100 mg capsules (brand or generic)

(continued)

225

TABLE 21.4

(Continued)

Generic Name (Brand Name)	Primary Indications	Secondary Indications	Serum Half-Life	Time to Steady State	Daily Dose	Usual Dosing Schedule	Preparations Available in the United States
Levetiracetam (Keppra)	Partial onset seizures (adjunctive)	Partial or generalized onset seizures, (adjunctive or monotherapy)	6–8 hr	1–2 d	Pediatric: 40–60 mg/kg/d Adults: 500–2,500 mg/d	b.i.d.	250 mg, 500 mg, 750 mg tabs; 500 mg/5 mL solution
Felbamate (Felbatol)		Refractory mixed generalized or multifocal seizures; Lennox Gastaut Syndrome (adjunctive or monotherapy)	20–23 hr	5–7 d	Pediatric: 40–60 mg/kg/d Adults: 2,000–4,000 mg/d	b.i.d.	400 mg and 600 mg tabs; 600 mg/5 mL solution
Oxcarbazepine (Trileptal)	Partial onset seizures (adjunctive or monotherapy)		2 hr for parent compound; 9 hr (for active metabolite MHD[c])	2–3 d	Pediatric: 10–40 mg/kg/d Adults: 300–1,800 mg/d	b.i.d.	150 mg, 300 mg, and 600 mg tabs; 300 mg/ 5 mL solution

JME, juvenile myoclonic epilepsy.

[a]Prolonged with renal dysfunction.

[b]EIAED, enzyme-inducing antiepileptic drugs, typically carbamazepine, phenytoin, phenobarbital or primidone; VPA, valproic acid

[c]MHD, monohydroxy derivative of oxcarbazepine; 10-hydroxycarbazepine is the primary compound.

Dose-Related Side Effects

1. Toxic CNS effects are shared among most anticonvulsants: (a) Excessive levels (or deliberate overdoses): ataxia, nystagmus, sedation progressing to coma, respiratory and cardiac depression at extremely high doses. (b) Movement disorders (chorea) and tremor at toxic levels.
2. Non-CNS dose-related effects: (a) Alterations in vitamin D metabolism with osteopenia. (b) Folate metabolism is altered. (c) Thyroid function tests (but not thyroid function) are commonly altered. (d) Gastrointestinal (GI): Gastric distress may be minimized by dividing dose and giving with food.
3. Drug interactions are common: (a) Most anticonvulsants induce P450 enzymes, increasing clearance of themselves (autoinduction), each other, and various other medications including steroids, estrogens, anticoagulants. (b) Exceptions are gabapentin (Neurontin), and levetiracetam (Keppra). (c) P450 inhibitors reduce clearance of carbamazepine (Tegretol), lamotrigine (Lamictal), and phenytoin. (d) Addition of erythromycin, other macrolide antibiotics, propoxyphene, or grapefruit juice may cause significant carbamazepine toxicity. (e) Isoniazid (INH) inhibits both carbamazepine and phenytoin metabolism.

Idiosyncratic (Non–Dose-Related) Side Effects

The following side effects may occur with any anticonvulsant:

1. Allergic reactions: skin rash, Stevens-Johnson syndrome, lupus-like syndromes
2. Bone marrow toxicity: usually reversible. Fatal aplastic anemia has been reported with carbamazepine and felbamate, primarily in older adults. Valproic acid: reversible bone marrow suppression, thrombocytopenia
3. Hepatotoxicity and metabolic abnormalities: most common in infants on valproic acid, but may rarely occur with any anticonvulsant at any age
4. Adenopathy: "mononucleosis syndrome" and pseudolymphoma are associated with hydantoins
5. Hair loss: moderate hair thinning with valproic acid
6. Weight changes: weight gain is most frequent with valproic acid but has been reported with many anticonvulsants, as has weight loss with felbamate, topiramate, zonisamide
7. Pancreatitis: valproic acid

Reproductive Effects

Increased risk of abnormal pregnancy outcome in women with epilepsy regardless of treatment:

1. Facial malformations: particularly cleft palate, microcephaly, congenital heart disease, and minor malformations such as hypoplastic nails
2. Open neural tube defects: valproic acid. Folic acid may reduce risk
3. No medication is "completely safe": risk of fetal damage must be balanced against the risk of recurrent convulsions
4. When prescribing oral contraceptives, higher estrogen doses may be needed

Other Problems with Anticonvulsant Therapy

1. Adherence problems are common
2. Antiepilepsy drugs may increase preexisting behavioral problems and occasionally cause depression.

Alternative Treatments of Refractory Epilepsy. Refer to epilepsy center for consideration of vagal nerve stimulation, ketogenic diet, and epilepsy surgery.

Other Treatment Issues

Dispelling Myths and Educating. (1) Epilepsy is not contagious. (2) The seizures may disappear with age. (3) Most seizures can be prevented with medication. (4) Epilepsy does not lower the teenager's intelligence. (5) He or she can participate in most activities. (6) Epilepsy is not a "mental illness."

The Teen and Family Should Be Educated about the Following. (1) Diagnosis. (2) Careful observation and record keeping. (3) Avoidance of precipitating factors. (4) Side effects of medication. (5) Prognosis and follow-up. (6) Precautions and restrictions, particularly regarding driving, swimming, and bicycle and motorcycle riding until seizure control is attained. Reports to Department of Motor Vehicles should be explained. Restrictions may need to be imposed regarding use of hazardous equipment, such as power tools. (7) For women and adolescent girls of childbearing age, the need for adequate birth control while receiving most anticonvulsants. Supplement with folic for female epilepsy patients with childbearing potential.

Family Members Should Be Aware of First Aid for Seizure Episodes. (1) Help the person into a lying position if there is adequate warning. (2) Do not try to restrain the person. (3) Clear the area of dangerous objects. (4) Remove glasses and loosen tight clothing. (5) Turn the head to one side (or roll the person onto his or her side) to allow saliva to drain. (6) Do not put anything into the person's mouth. (7) Report what you observe; try to time the episode with a watch. (8) Family members should be given specific individualized criteria to call for paramedic help. If the seizure lasts longer than 5 to 10 minutes or if seizures cluster without recovery, call for emergency medical help. (9) In teens who have clusters of seizures or prolonged breakthrough seizures, family can be taught to use rescue medication. In the United States, Diastat rectal diazepam gel is available (for teens the dosage is 0.2 mg/kg, maximum of 20 mg/dose). (9) For partial seizures (simple and complex), do not restrain the teen. (10) Protect from harm. (11) For absence (petit mal), myoclonic seizures, generally no first aid is needed.

Community Resources. Teenagers and parents should be provided with references and community resources. Local chapters of the Epilepsy Foundation have videotapes, pamphlets, and other educational materials for patients and families.

Miscellaneous Concerns. (1) Sports and activity: No need for restriction of activities once seizures are controlled, except for swimming alone, surfing, scuba diving, mountain climbing, or bicycling in areas with traffic. Contact sports are generally restricted until seizures are controlled. (2) Medical identification: Medical identification bracelet or necklace may avoid unnecessary trips to emergency facilities. (3) Driving: The wish to be seizure free to receive a license may enhance compliance. Laws regarding mandatory reporting to the state's Department of Motor Vehicles vary among the states. (4) School: Should be informed if seizures are a recurring problem. (5) Alcohol: Excessive use may increase the risk of seizures. (6) Anticipate other concerns: seizures, because of their unpredictable and abrupt onset, threat of injury, and embarrassment, can have profound effects on the developing adolescent. (7) Adherence suggestions: (a) Clear explanations of medications and their expected side effects. (b) Give adolescent responsibility for taking medications. (c) Discuss possible consequences of noncompliance. (d) Referral to a teen support group. (e) "Day of the week" pill boxes, filled and checked weekly with parental supervision, may enable the teen to manage his or her own medications. (f) Simplify dosing schedules (slow-release or once-a-day formulations).

WEB SITES AND REFERENCES

http://www.epilepsyfoundation.org. From the Epilepsy Foundation.

http://www.nlm.nih.gov/medlineplus/epilepsy.html. National Institutes of Health site.

http://www.cdc.gov/Epilepsy/index.htm. Information from the Centers for Disease Control and Prevention on epilepsy, including an excellent "Toolkit" entitled "You Are Not Alone."

http://www.aesnet.org. The American Epilepsy Society's official Web site.

French JA, et al. Efficacy and tolerability of the new antiepileptic drugs: I. Treatment of new onset epilepsy. *Neurology* 2004;62:1252.

French JA, et al. Efficacy and tolerability of the new antiepileptic drugs: II. Treatment of refractory epilepsy. *Neurology* 2004;62:1261.

Nadkarni S, LaJoie J, Devinsky O. Current treatments of epilepsy. *Neurology* 2005; 64(Suppl 3):S2.

CHAPTER **22**

Headaches

Wendy G. Mitchell, Kiarash Sadrieh, and Lawrence S. Neinstein

Recurrent headaches are a frequent problem. By the teens, most people have had at least one headache. Most recurrent headaches are not associated with severe organic pathology while the single severe acute headache may be due to significant CNS or systemic disease.

PAIN-SENSITIVE AREAS: WHAT HURTS IN THE HEAD

In general, the brain parenchyma is insensitive to pain. Pain-sensitive areas include the following:

1. Intracranial including cranial nerves, dura, dural vessels and intracavernous and proximal intracranial portions of the carotid arteries.
2. Extracranial soft tissues including skin, fascia, muscles and blood vessels of the scalp and neck, upper cervical nerve roots, sinuses and teeth; eyes and eye muscles; and ears

MECHANISMS OF PAIN

These include vascular dilation, muscular contraction, traction and inflammation

EPIDEMIOLOGY

1. *Prevalence:* By age 7 years, 40% of children have headaches, 66% by age 12 years, and 75% by age 15 years. For migraine headaches, 4% to 11% prevalence in ages 7 to 11 years; 8% to 23% in ages 11 to 16 years.
2. *Gender:* Equal prior to puberty; more common in females after puberty
3. *Types:* Acute headaches: Associated with a systemic disease, viral illness or sinusitis. Most recurrent headaches are either migraines, muscular contraction headaches, or a combination. Brain tumors rarely present as intermittent headache. Cluster headaches usually start late adolescence or later and are far more common in males. Depressive headaches may present without other depressive symptoms.

TABLE 22.1

International Headache Society Criteria for Migraine with Aura

A. At least two attacks that fulfill criteria B
B. Migraine aura fulfilling the following:
   1. Aura consisting of at least one of the following, but no motor weakness:
      a. Fully reversible visual symptoms including positive features (e.g., flickering lights, spots, or lines) and/or negative features (i.e., loss of vision)
      b. Fully reversible sensory symptoms including positive features (i.e., pins and needles) and/or negative features (i.e., numbness)
      c. Fully reversible dysphasic speech disturbance
   2. At least two of the following:
      a. Homonymous visual symptoms and/or unilateral sensory symptoms
      b. At least one aura symptom develops gradually over 5 min and/or different aura symptoms occur in succession over 5 min
      c. Each symptom lasts 5 to 60 min
C. Not attributed to another disorder

From Headache Classification Subcommittee of the International Headache Society. The international classification of headache disorders (2nd edition). *Cephalagia* 2004;8(Suppl 1):9.

DIFFERENTIAL DIAGNOSIS AND CHARACTERISTICS

(See Table 22.1)

Acute, Nonrecurrent (First or Worst) Headaches

1. *Febrile:* CNS infection: meningitis (bacterial, viral, TB and aseptic), brain abscess, epidural empyema or other intracranial infection, encephalitis. Non-CNS infection: sinusitis, nonspecific headache due to fever; and headaches associated with other infections (e.g. strep throat, mononucleosis, influenza, HIV).
2. *Afebrile:* Intracranial hemorrhages: subarachnoid hemorrhage, intraparenchymal, subdural or epidural hemorrhage; postictal headache; cerebral ischemia; severe hypertension; acute dental disease; eye or orbit problems (e.g. acute glaucoma or inflammation); and other (cysticercosis or acute obstructive hydrocephalus).

Recurrent Headaches (Episodic, Complete Recovery between Episodes)

Muscle Tension Headaches
1. Band-like, bilateral, steady pain
2. Lacking features of migraine
3. Often gradual in onset and related to stress or fatigue
4. Sometimes precipitated by minor trauma, whiplash, muscle strain, or temporomandibular joint dysfunction

TABLE 22.2

International Headache Society Criteria for Migraine without Aura

A. At least five attacks that fulfill criteria in B to D
B. Headache attacks that last 4–72 hr (untreated or unsuccessfully treated)
C. Headache has at least two of the following characteristics:
  1. Unilateral site
  2. Pulsating quality
  3. Moderate to severe intensity
  4. Aggravation by or causing avoidance of routine physical activity
    (e.g., climbing stairs)
D. During headache, at least one of the following symptoms:
  1. Nausea or vomiting (or both)
  2. Photophobia and phonophobia
E. Not attributed to another disorder

From Headache Classification Subcommittee of the International Headache Society. The international classification of headache disorders (2nd edition). *Cephalagia* 2004;8(Suppl 1):9.

Migraine (Also Known as Vascular Headache)

1. *Migraine with aura:* 10% to 15% (see Table 23.1)
   a. "Aura" of sensory disturbances: visual changes, numbness, tingling, dizziness, vertigo, and syncope are common.
   b. Throbbing, unilateral, and usually frontal or temporal pain occurs.
   c. Anorexia, nausea, and vomiting
   d. Phonophobia and photophobia are common.
   e. Relieved by sleep
   f. Positive family history
   g. Many have motion sickness or cyclic vomiting.
   h. Pattern varies over time. May be precipitated by puberty, life stresses or minor head injury. Food sensitivities (uncommon): chocolate, tyramine-containing cheeses, red wines, monosodium glutamate (MSG), nitrates, or nitrites.
2. *Migraine without aura ("common migraine"):* 80% to 90% characterized by the items above, but lacking aura; may be bilateral and variable in pain distribution (see Table 22.2).
3. *Variant migraine:* 5% to 10% including hemiplegic migraine, confusional migraine, abdominal migraine, basilar migraine, and ophthalmoplegic migraine.

Cluster Headaches (<5% in Children and Adolescents)

1. Male predominance
2. Steady burning or pain, usually localized behind one eye, sudden onset, extremely severe but brief
3. Rhinorrhea, lacrimation, and conjunctival injection on the same side is common.
4. Horner syndrome ipsilaterally during attack

5. During clusters, multiple daily episodes, often in early morning hours, awakening patient from sleep.
6. Differential diagnosis includes occult dental disease, acute glaucoma, and tic douloureux.

Chronic Headaches (Variable but Essentially Continuous or Increasing Since Onset)

Intracranial Mass Lesions
1. Patients with brain tumors may have headaches but very few patients with headaches have brain tumors.
2. Headaches are usually accompanied by other neurologic signs and symptoms.

Hydrocephalus (with or without Mass)
1. May be relatively constant, often worse in the morning
2. Aqueductal stenosis may present in adolescents, even if congenital.
3. Head may be large.
4. Pain is usually dull, vertex, and not very severe.
5. Pain may be increased by straining, bowel movements, coughing, or bending.

Post–Lumbar Puncture Headaches or Spontaneous "Low Pressure" Headache Due to CSF Leak
1. Positional, relieved by recumbency
2. Headache, nausea, and vomiting severe when upright.
3. Spontaneous or posttraumatic CSF leaks may occur in Marfan syndrome.
4. Opening pressure on a spinal tap is extremely low.

Pseudotumor Cerebri
Also called benign intracranial hypertension: Increased intracranial pressure without mass.

1. Papilledema is common. Visual fields may be abnormal, including enlarged blind spot or constricted fields.
2. Visual obscuration (transient dimming or loss of vision with straining or position change) may be present. Cranial nerve palsies (VI and VII) may be associated.
3. Pain is usually dull and vertex.
4. More common in females, obese patients.
5. Precipitants: vitamin A or vitamin D intoxication, rapid steroid taper, tetracycline, minocycline, isotretinoin (Accutane).
6. Risk of permanent visual loss if untreated.
7. Treatment: lumbar puncture (postimaging) may be both diagnostic and therapeutic. Carefully measure opening pressure with the patient in a relaxed position.

"Transformed Migraine". Migraine changes from episodic essentially continuous pain.

Analgesic Overuse Headache. Chronic daily headache due to analgesic overuse.

Depressive Headaches. Characterized by: "All day, all the time, every day, no relief"; other overt depressive symptoms may be absent. Excessive disability and family history of affective disorders common; may respond to antidepressants or psychotherapy.

Posttraumatic (Head Trauma). Mixed migrainous and "tension" quality; onset within a few days of head trauma, continuing for weeks to months.

Local Extracranial Disease
1. Chronic sinusitis
2. Dental disease, including temporomandibular joint dysfunction
3. Glaucoma or orbital inflammatory lesions
4. Vasculitis involving extracranial vessels

HIV or AIDS. Chronic or recurrent headaches may be due to HIV, coexisting infections (intracranial, sinus, or ear), or treatment, including antiretroviral agents.

Pregnancy. Early pregnancy may be associated with headache, nausea, and vomiting. Pregnancy may exacerbate migraines.

Chronic Meningitis. Also other inflammatory conditions (TB, fungal, or recurrent or chronic "aseptic" meningitis or sarcoidosis).

Headaches Due to Substance or Drug Abuse. Both excessive use and withdrawal may cause headaches.

Headaches Due to Obstructive Sleep Apnea. Headaches are often worst upon awakening.

Intermittent or Continuous Headaches Due to Other Medical Conditions. Hypoxia, hypercarbia, significant hypertension, severe anemia, uremia, and dialysis. Chemotherapy, antiretroviral therapy, and immunosuppressants.

DIAGNOSIS

In the evaluation of the patient with headaches, the history is (nearly) everything. The rest is the examination. (See Tables 22.1 and 22.2 for International Headache Society (IHS) criteria for migraines.)

1. *Onset:* Age at first episode; events or illnesses surrounding onset; temporal pattern of headaches (time of day, day of week, and season); frequency
2. *Pattern and chronology of symptoms:* Have the patient describe a typical episode in detail including: location (quality: pounding, dull, sharp, or sticking), associated symptoms (sweating, pallor, flushing, and palpitations), nausea, vomiting, and anorexia; duration and diurnal variation; severity, limitation of activities, response to medications and sleep
3. *Preceding and accompanying symptoms:* Particularly visual changes, numbness, weakness, etc.; prodrome if any.

4. *Precipitants of specific episodes:* Including stressors, illnesses, foods/diet/ eating pattern (food additives, chocolate, nuts, cheeses, specific suspect foods; skipping meals); medications including OTCs, exertion and orgasm, caffeine intake or withdrawal, alcohol intake, toxic exposures and physical exposures (bright or flashing lights, temperature changes, and strong odors).

5. *Other associated illnesses or symptoms:* Including HIV risks, changes in menstrual pattern, or galactorrhea.

6. *Medications* (prescribed and OTC) including analgesics, birth control pills, other medications used for headaches (acute or prophylactic) and medications for acne (tetracycline, minocycline, Accutane).

7. *Vitamin consumption*, unusual diets, supplements

8. *Substance abuse*

9. *Depression* or mood disorders

10. *School phobia* or avoidance, other secondary gains

11. *Behavior:* recent personality or cognitive change.

12. *Family history for migraines*, other headaches, epilepsy, affective disorders or other neurologic conditions.

Physical Examination. Patient needs a good general physical exam and careful neurological examination, including funduscopic exam.

Laboratory Tests

1. For recurrent headaches, with asymptomatic periods in between and with normal physical and neurologic exam: no lab test are needed. For acute episodes, lab evaluation is guided by history and physical.

2. Neuroimaging (CT or MRI) is indicated for an acute severe or increasing headache, abnormal neurologic examination, papilledema, or unexplained macrocephaly.

THERAPY

Rule 1A: Not having a headache is better than getting rid of it once it occurs. Rule 1B: Not taking pills every day is better than taking pills. Look for precipitants, particularly avoidable ones.

Rule 2: Take the preferred abortive medication at the onset of the headache, the earlier the better.

Rule 3: Do not underestimate the role of reassurance. Adolescents and parents are often concerned that the headache is caused by a brain tumor. General strategies for headache management are as follows:

1. *Headache diary:* The patient should be encouraged to understand causes and precipitants for headaches. The diary should be for at least three to five headache cycles, including *detailed* diary of headaches, medication intake, and results, as well as activities, foods, stresses, sleep pattern, and physical environment.

2. *Treatment:* tension headaches
   a. A brief period of relaxation or a nap often brings relief.
   b. Simple physical measures: Massage or stretching neck muscles or warm or cold compresses

    c. Analgesics (e.g., acetaminophen, nonsteroidal antiinflammatory drugs, aspirin)

    d. Avoid combined analgesic-sedative drugs [butalbital (Fiorinal)].

    e. Mixed tension–vascular headaches, if very frequent and disabling: consider prophylactic low-dose tricyclic antidepressants.

3. Things to try for migraines:

    a. Sun and glare avoidance: sunglasses, brimmed hat, or visor outdoors in sun. Avoid strobe lights or strobe-like conditions.

    b. Eliminate MSG, nitrates, and nitrites from diet.

    c. Stabilize caffeine intake or wean off completely.

    d. Eliminate alcohol.

    e. Stabilize sleep pattern to approximately the same amount of sleep daily.

4. Acute abortive treatment of episodic migraine

    a. Analgesics, (e.g., acetaminophen, ibuprofen, or other NSAIDs). Avoid overuse (rebound) by restricting to 3 to 4 days/week. Caffeine may potentiate the effect of the analgesic.

    b. Antiemetic should be combined with or precede an analgesic if nausea or vomiting is prominent.

    c. Avoid sedative-analgesic combinations.

    d. Triptans: Several triptans for parenteral, oral or intranasal use are available, all selective serotonin receptor agonists. Avoid overuse.

    e. Ergot derivatives: Ergotamine must be used at the onset of symptoms. (Sublingual, oral, rectal, or inhaled).

    f. Dihydroergotamine (DHE) IV, IM or nasal spray. *Do not use for hemiplegic migraines.*

    g. Inhaled high-flow oxygen: specific for cluster headaches

    h. Intravenous valproic acid (Depacon): Abortive medication in adolescent migraines. Dose = 1,000 to 1,500 mg. There are no randomized, controlled studies to date.

Warning: If headaches are frequent (i.e., more than twice a week), beware of analgesic or ergot overuse syndromes. This may convert intermittent migraines to chronic "transformed" migraines.

5. Prophylactic treatment: For severe recurrent attacks causing significant school absenteeism or functional limitations, or migraines accompanied by significant neurological deficits (e.g., hemiplegic migraines). Continue treatment until the headache pattern has markedly improved for approximately 6 months, then consider tapering.

    a. Beta-blockers: Propranolol

    b. Tricyclic antidepressants (amitriptyline, imipramine, desipramine, nortriptyline)

    c. Low-dose daily aspirin or NSAIDs (e.g., ibuprofen and naproxen)

    d. Cyproheptadine (Periactin)

    e. Anticonvulsants: Low doses of valproic acid (Depakote), low-dose phenobarbital, topiramate (Topamax), levetiracetam (Keppra)

    f. Calcium channel blockers (e.g., verapamil and nimodipine). Only flunarizine (not available in the United States) has been proven effective in a double-blind placebo controlled trial.

    g. Methysergide (Sansert): Significant risks make this a last choice in most circumstances.

    h. Lithium carbonate prophylactic for cluster headaches

i. Combinations of high dose riboflavin (vitamin B2) and magnesium. A commercial preparation of magnesium oxide, riboflavin and the herb feverfew is available as a food supplement.
6. "Transformed migraines," chronic migraines, rebound headache if severe and disabling. Use (a) intravenous dihydroergotamine plus antiemetic given over 2 to 4 days on an adjusted q8h schedule. (b) Short courses of high-dose corticosteroids. (c) Withdrawal of chronic overused analgesics, triptans, and ergots is essential. (d) Psychological supportive therapy, relaxation therapies, and physical exercise programs

PROGNOSIS

Up to 40% to 50% of childhood-onset migraines may remit during adolescence or young adulthood. Adolescent-onset migraines often continue into adulthood. However, adolescents should be reassured that even people with a strong tendency to have migraines do not have frequent attacks throughout life. Patterns of occurrence are highly variable. The goal is to avoid offending agents, use effective medication in appropriate doses, and lead a functional lifestyle.

WEB SITES AND REFERENCES

http://www.headaches.org/. Web site of the National Headache Foundation.
http://www.familydoctor.org/flowcharts/502.html. Flowcharts on headaches from the American Academy of Family Physicians.
Gladstein J, Holden EW, Winner P, et al. Chronic daily headache in children and adolescents: current status and recommendations for the future. Pediatric Committee of the American Association for the Study of Headache. *Headache* 1997;37:626.
Guidetti V, Galli F. Evolution of headache in childhood and adolescence: an 8-year follow-up. *Cephalalgia* 1998;18(7):449–454.
Headache Classification Subcommittee of the International Headache Society. The International Classification of Headache Disorders, 2nd ed. *Cephalalgia* 2004; 8(Suppl 1):9.
Lewis DW, Ashwal S, Dahl G, et al. Practice parameter: evaluation of children and adolescents with recurrent headache. *Neurology*. 2002;59:490.
Lewis, S., Ashwal, A., Hershey, et al. Practice Parameter: Pharmacological treatment of migraine headache in children and adolescents: Report of the American Academy of Neurology Quality Standards Subcommittee and the Practice Committee of the Child Neurology Society. *Neurology* 2004;63:2215.
Rothner AD. Headaches in children and adolescents: update 2001. *Semin Pediatr Neurol* 2001;8(1):2.

CHAPTER 23

Syncope and Sudden Cardiac Death

Amy D. DiVasta, Wendy G. Mitchell, and Mark E. Alexander

Cardiac symptoms in the adolescent are common; true cardiac disease is not. Syncope is a frequent complaint, often raising concerns of future sudden cardiac death (SCD). The clinician's critical task is to distinguish between benign and significant syncope.

SYNCOPE

Etiology. Syncope is a sudden, transient loss of consciousness and postural tone, lasting several seconds to a minute, followed by spontaneous recovery. Syncope is common, with a female predominance and peak incidence between 15 to 19 years. Any condition that leads to decreased cerebral perfusion may cause syncope.

Classification. There are three major causes of syncope: (1) neurocardiogenic, including vasovagal/reflex and postural orthostatic tachycardia; (2) cardiovascular, including structural and arrhythmogenic; and (3) noncardiovascular, including epileptic and psychogenic.

Syncope of unknown origin or simple syncope and neurocardiogenic syncope account for 85% to 90% of events. Ineffective cerebral blood flow, resulting from inadequate cardiac output, leads to loss of consciousness. Only 1% to 5% of patients have significant cardiac disease. Seizures and psychiatric diagnoses account for a small number as well.

History and Physical Examination. Key elements of the history include (1) onset and frequency of episodes; (2) circumstances such as exercise, posture, or other precipitating factors; (3) prodromal symptoms such as dizziness, diaphoresis, nausea, color changes, palpitations, chest pain, dyspnea; (4) complete or incomplete loss of consciousness, duration, time to recovery; (5) abnormal movements, incontinence, or injury (see Table 23.1 for common faint versus seizure); (6) past medical history and medications; and (7) family history of sudden death (particularly under age 40 years), similar episodes, or early onset heart disease. "Warning signs" that suggest a more serious etiology: syncope during exercise, syncope in supine position, family history of sudden death, personal history of cardiac disease, or an event precipitated by a loud noise, intense emotion, or fright.

TABLE 23.1

Neurocardiogenic Syncope versus Seizure

Characteristics	Neurocardiogenic Syncope	Seizure
Warning	Usually prodromal symptoms	Aura common
Duration	Brief	Prolonged
Position at onset	Usually erect	Any position
Color change	Pallor frequent	Flushing or cyanosis
Convulsions	Rare, opisthotonic/myoclonic	Common, may be focal
Urinary incontinence	Rare	Common
Postictal state	Residual symptoms common	Disorientation, headaches

Physical examination should include orthostatic vital signs, neurologic assessment, and a dynamic cardiac examination.

NEUROCARDIOGENIC SYNCOPE

Most common form of syncope, also known as vasovagal syncope, common faint, or reflex syncope.

1. *Duration:* Few seconds to minutes
2. *Onset:* Gradual, typically with a prodrome
3. *Precipitating factors:* Fear, anxiety, pain, hunger, overcrowding, fatigue, injections, the sight of blood, and prolonged upright posture
4. *Prodromal symptoms:* Nausea, dizziness, visual spots or dimming, feelings of apprehension, pallor, yawning, diaphoresis, and feelings of warmth
5. *Syncopal event:* Brief loss of consciousness, gradual loss of muscle tone
6. *Seizure:* Rarely, a brief tonic or clonic seizure will be precipitated by syncope after the preceding syncopal symptoms.
7. *Recovery:* Rapid, often with residual fatigue, malaise, weakness, nausea, and headache
8. *Pathophysiology:* Not understood; presumed to be a temporary derangement of cardiac and/or vascular regulation

Diagnostic Evaluation of Neurocardiogenic Syncope. Adolescents with a true syncopal event should have an electrocardiogram (ECG). A normal diagnostic screen (reassuring history, benign physical examination, and normal ECG) is generally sufficient to exclude cardiac disease. More tests needed only if continuing concerns of cardiac disease.

1. No labs, electroencephalogram (EEG), or intracranial imaging needed
2. *Echocardiogram:* Low yield; not for routine evaluation
3. *In some patients:* 24-hour Holter monitor for frequent, daily symptoms
4. *Exercise testing:* If syncopal episodes occur during exercise

5. *Tilt-table testing:* Variable sensitivity and poor specificity (40% of normal adolescents have a positive tilt test)
6. *Implantable loop recorder:* Invasive; reserved for severe, recurrent episodes

Management of Neurocardiogenic Syncope. Management includes: (1) reassurance; (2) hydration and caffeine/alcohol avoidance; (3) recognition of prodromal symptoms and assumption of supine position or use of postural techniques (isometric contractions of the extremities, folding the arms, or crossing the legs); (4) upright weight-bearing exercise, and (5) drug therapy, reserved for refractory cases that do not respond to supportive therapy (Table 23.2).

POSTURAL ORTHOSTATIC TACHYCARDIA SYNDROME

Postural orthostatic tachycardia syndrome (POTS) is a heterogeneous disorder of autonomic regulation. Patients complain of fatigue, dizziness, and exercise intolerance with upright position.

1. Marked pulse change (>30 bpm) or excessive tachycardia (>120 bpm) with upright position
2. Little or no blood pressure change
3. Abnormal autonomic regulation may be acquired, genetic, or both
4. Significant overlap between chronic fatigue syndrome and POTS
5. Treatment: Fluids, vasoconstrictors, beta blockers

ORTHOSTATIC HYPOTENSION

Uncommon in adolescents without comorbidities (e.g., malnutrition, medications, or neurologic disorders). Defined as drop in systolic blood pressure >20 mm Hg and drop in diastolic pressure >10 mm Hg with assumption of upright posture.

CARDIOVASCULAR SYNCOPE

Cardiovascular syncope is an acute collapse with few premonitory symptoms, often in association with exercise or exertion, suggesting cardiac syncope. Usually secondary to arrhythmia, obstructed left ventricular (LV) filling, obstructed LV outflow, or ineffective myocardial contraction (Table 23.3). If cardiac disease is suspected, refer to a cardiologist. Restrict patients with high-risk presentations from strenuous physical activity or competitive athletics until evaluated by the cardiologist. Adolescents should also avoid driving a motor vehicle until evaluation is complete. A few key conditions:

Hypertrophic Cardiomyopathy (HCM)
1. *Definition:* An inherited cardiac muscle disorder
2. *Natural history and prognosis:* Genetically and phenotypically heterogeneous. Generally asymptomatic. If symptoms develop, they are usually exertional chest pain, exercise intolerance, shortness of breath, and syncope.
3. *Diagnostic findings in HCM:*
   a. Systolic ejection murmur at the left lower sternal border (increasing with standing and decreasing with squatting), prominent LV lift

TABLE 23.2

Pharmacological Treatment Options for Neurocardiogenic Syncope

Drug	Dose	Proposed Mechanism of Action	Side Effects	Quality of Data
Fludrocortisone	0.1–0.2 mg/d	↑ Renal Na$^+$ absorption ↑ Circulating blood volume	Bloating or edema Hypokalemia Hypertension	+
Midodrine	5–10 mg q4h Maximum four doses/d	α-Agonist ↑ Peripheral vascular resistance	Piloerection Scalp pruritus Hypertension Urinary retention Difficult adherence to treatment	++
β-Blockers Atenolol Metoprolol	25–50 mg daily 25–50 mg b.i.d.	Blocks excess sympathetic response (paradoxical effect)	Fatigue Depression	±
SSRIs Fluoxetine Sertraline	20 mg daily 50 mg daily	↑ Extracellular serotonin leads to down-regulation of receptor density	Headache Insomnia GI effects	±

SSRIs, serotonin reuptake inhibitors; GI, gastrointestinal.
+, moderate data to support efficacy; ++: strong data to support efficacy; ± mixed data to support efficacy.

TABLE 23.3

Differential Diagnosis of Cardiac Syncope

Electrical	*Structural*
Heart block	Inadequate LV filling
Congenital	Pulmonary hypertension
Acquired	Pulmonic stenosis
Wolff-Parkinson-White syndrome	Inadequate LV output
Dysrhythmias	Aortic stenosis
Long QT syndrome	Hypertrophic cardiomyopathy
Inherited	Dilated cardiomyopathy
Secondary	Coronary artery anomalies
Brugada syndrome	Myocarditis
Postoperative congenital heart disease	Tumors
Arrhythmogenic right ventricular dysplasia	Marfan syndrome

LV, left ventricle.

  b. ECG: LV hypertrophy, ST-T wave changes, or atrial enlargement (25%)

  c. Echocardiogram: Nearly the "gold standard." Key findings include thickened interventricular septum and LV free wall, asymmetric septal hypertrophy, dynamic left ventricular outflow tract obstruction.

4. *Sudden death:* Rare in HCM, but HCM is the most common cause of SCD in ages 15 to 35. Mechanism of cardiac arrest is ventricular fibrillation. Risk factors for sudden death include previous cardiac arrest, positive family history of sudden death, and exertion-related syncope.

5. *Treatment:* All family members should be screened. Patient should avoid athletic participation even if asymptomatic. For patients at high risk of SCD, an implantable defibrillator is recommended.

Long-QT Syndrome

1. *Definition:* Long-QT syndrome (LQTS) is a disorder of delayed ventricular repolarization which leads to risk of arrhythmias, syncope, seizure, and sudden cardiac death. Patients may be asymptomatic.

2. *Hereditary LQTS:* Both autosomal recessive and autosomal dominant.

3. *Acquired LQTS:* Related to underlying disease state (such as myocarditis, eating disorders, and traumatic brain injury) or secondary to drug effect

4. *Diagnosis:* ECG is diagnostic tool of choice. Long QT interval ≥ 0.46 sec is most accurate in identifying gene carriers.

5. *Treatment of LQTS:* All patients should be referred to a cardiologist and treated, even if asymptomatic, to decrease mortality rate.

  a. Restriction from competitive athletics

  b. Avoidance of drugs/medications known to prolong the QT interval (for frequently updated information, see www.torsades.org)

  c. ECG evaluation of all family members

  d. Beta blockers: Initial treatment of choice

e. Implantable cardioverter-defibrillator (ICD)
f. Left cervicothoracic sympathetic ganglionectomy

Noncardiovascular Syncope

1. *Hyperventilation:* A frequent cause of dizziness in the adolescent, true syncope is rare.
2. *Metabolic disturbances:* Hypokalemia, hypomagnesemia, hypoglycemia
3. *Psychogenic syncope:* Graceful slump to the floor, without anxiety, injury, or vital sign instability
4. *Subclavian steal syndrome*
5. *Micturition syncope*
6. *Cough syncope:* Rare in adolescence except with chronic lung disease.
7. *Cerebrooclusive disease*
8. *Migraine:* Syncope, vertigo, or dizziness may precede or accompany the headache.

SUDDEN DEATH IN ADOLESCENTS AND YOUNG ADULTS

SCD represents only approximately 10% of the overall sudden death rate in the pediatric and young adult population, with an incidence of approximately 1/100,000 patient-years. Hypertrophic cardiomyopathy is the most common cause for ages 15 to 35 years. Etiologies include:

1. Structural or functional abnormalities, often familial, including hypertrophic cardiomyopathy, arrhythmogenic right ventricular dysplasia, coronary artery abnormalities, primary pulmonary hypertension, myocarditis/dilated cardiomyopathy, restrictive cardiomyopathy, Marfan syndrome with aortic dissection and aortic valve stenosis
2. Primary electrical abnormalities including long-QT syndromes, Brugada syndrome, Wolff-Parkinson-White syndrome, arrhythmogenic right ventricular dysplasia, primary or idiopathic ventricular tachycardia/fibrillation, catecholamine–exercise ventricular tachycardia, and heart block
3. Acquired conditions including commotio cordis, drug abuse, secondary pulmonary artery hypertension (Eisenmenger syndrome) and atherosclerotic coronary artery disease
4. Postoperative congenital heart disease
5. Postoperative cardiac transplantation

Any patient with a suspected cardiac condition should be referred to a cardiologist for a full evaluation, and determination of appropriate athletic and recreational activities.

History. Important historical details include a history of syncopal episodes, significant exercise intolerance, exertional chest discomfort, and a family history of premature coronary artery disease, sudden death in a person <40 years old, syncope, or hypertension.

Physical Examination. Clues to cardiac disease include hypertension, abnormal cardiac rhythm, heart murmur, or a body habitus suggestive of Marfan syndrome. However, the majority of patients at risk of sudden death will have a completely normal physical exam.

Laboratory Tests. The ECG is a useful screening tool but is often normal. Exercise electrocardiography is useful in an adolescent with symptoms of exertional chest discomfort, syncope, exercise intolerance, or worrisome palpitations. Routine screening with echocardiography or chest x-ray study is not accepted in U.S. practice. For further recommendations on limitations of these conditions for athletics, see Chapter 19.

Prevention. The accuracy of presymptomatic diagnostic testing and cost-effectiveness of a widespread preparticipation screening program are controversial issues. Current opinion in the United States is that existing data do not demonstrate that screening with ECGs, echocardiograms, or exercise testing prevents sudden death. In 1996, the American Heart Association concluded that the best screening for cardiovascular disease in athletes is a complete personal history, with thorough evaluation of cardiac or exercise-associated symptoms, a thorough family history, and a careful physical examination. Pilot studies continue with the use of screening echocardiography. Additional prevention strategies include chest protectors, maintenance of adequate hydration, the use of automatic electrical defibrillators, emergency response plans for schools, and training of personnel in basic cardiopulmonary resuscitation.

WEB SITES AND REFERENCES

http://cpmcnet.columbia.edu/dept/syncope/. A comprehensive clinical center for patients who have fainted, who are recurrently lightheaded, or who have related cardiovascular disease. Much information on syncope.

http://www.acponline.org/journals/annals/15jun97/ppsyncop.htm. *Annals of Internal Medicine* position paper on clinical guidelines for diagnosing syncope.

Boehm KE, Morris EJ, Kip KT, et al. Diagnosis and management of neurally mediated syncope and related conditions in adolescents. *J Adolesc Health* 2001;28:2.

DiVasta AD, Alexander ME. Fainting freshmen and sinking sophomores: cardiovascular issues of the adolescent. *Curr Opin Pediatr*, 2004;16:350.

Nishimura RA, Holmes DR Jr. Clinical practice. Hypertrophic obstructive cardiomyopathy. *N Engl J Med* 2004;350:1320.

Stewart JM. Transient orthostatic hypotension is common in adolescents. *J Pediatr* 2002;140:418.

CHAPTER 24

Sleep Disorders

Shelly K. Weiss

Sleep disturbances are common in adolescents. Many young people, when asked, acknowledge difficulties with sleep even though this is not the chief complaint. Sleep disorders are classified into four categories: (1) dyssomnias (range of disorders including difficulty initiating or maintaining sleep), early morning waking (insomnias), and excessive sleepiness; (2) parasomnias (associated with physical phenomena—motor or autonomic—that occur exclusively or predominantly during sleep); (3) sleep disorders associated with medical/psychiatric disorders; (4) proposed sleep disorders.

SLEEP PHYSIOLOGY

Sleep is divided into rapid-eye-movement (REM) sleep and non–rapid-eye-movement (NREM) sleep. REM sleep occupies 20% to 30% of sleep time in adolescents. Most dreams occur during REM sleep. NREM sleep occupies 70% to 80% of sleep time and is divided into four stages. Stages 1 and 2 are very light and medium-deep sleep, respectively. Stages 3 and 4 are progressively deeper "slow wave" sleep.

SLEEP PATTERN AND CHANGES DURING ADOLESCENCE

One of the important changes in sleep during adolescence is a delay in the circadian timing system. With progressive adolescent sexual development, there is a tendency for lengthening the internal day. This—coupled with the increasing time devoted to academic, employment, social, and extracurricular activities—can cause progressive delay in bedtime.

SLEEP HISTORY

1. Sleep complaint: (a) description by both teen and parent; (b) age at onset, timing during sleep, duration, frequency, and intermittent or continuous nature; (c) prior treatment and result.

2. General sleep history including prior sleep problems, bedroom environment and bedtime routines (e.g., TV/computer in room), description of sleep (e.g., time to fall asleep and amount of sleep), nocturnal arousals, snoring/restlessness, daytime symptoms (e.g., daytime naps or sleepiness, intake of caffeine, nicotine, and other drugs).
3. Medical (including over-the-counter medications, herbal products, dietary supplements, weight-loss products, performance-enhancing substances, other stimulants), psychiatric and surgical history (including history of tonsillectomy and adenoidectomy).
4. Psychosocial and academic history.
5. Family history, including history of sleep problems.

PHYSICAL EXAMINATION

Targeted exam depending on the complaint.

SLEEP DIARY

Keep a 1- to 2-week sleep diary listing bedtimes, nighttime symptoms, time on awakening, daytime fatigue or sleepiness, and naps.

SLEEP DISORDERS IN ADOLESCENTS

Dyssomnias

Dyssomnia Due to Inadequate Sleep
- Inadequate sleep is the most common cause of excessive daytime sleepiness.
- Poor sleeping habits or late bedtimes
- Chronic sleep deprivation
- Difficulty falling asleep or early morning waking may be due to stress, anxiety, or depression
- Physical illness associated with pain or discomfort
- Medication use (selective serotonin reuptake inhibitors, stimulants, sympathomimetics, and corticosteroids)
- Substance abuse or withdrawal (particularly stimulants, alcohol, or sedatives)

Dyssomnia Due to Delayed Sleep Phase Syndrome
- Daytime sleepiness can result from delayed bedtime with ensuing difficulties arising in the morning.
- Adolescents are prone to this delay due to busy schedules and an intrinsic biological preference for a later bedtime.
- Can be associated with sleep-onset insomnia, which occurs when the adolescent is asked to go to sleep at a normal bedtime

Dyssomnia Due to Obstructive Sleep Apnea Syndrome
The main cause of sleep-disordered breathing (SDB) is obstructive sleep apnea syndrome (OSAS), which is the presence of complete or partial obstruction of the upper airway during sleep and associated with habitual snoring with

labored breathing, observed apnea, restless sleep, and daytime neurobehavioral abnormalities or sleepiness. Physical examination may reveal evidence of growth abnormalities, signs of nasal obstruction, adenoidal facies, enlarged tonsils, and increased pulmonic component of second heart sound.

Narcolepsy

Narcolepsy is a genetically complex chronic neurologic disorder characterized by excessive and overwhelming daytime sleepiness and intrusion of REM sleep phenomenon into wakefulness. Onset is between 10 and 25 years. The first and primary manifestation is excessive daytime sleepiness. The disorder is characterized by four classic symptoms: sleep attacks, cataplexy, sleep paralysis, and hypnagogic and/or hypnopompic hallucinations. In addition, people with narcolepsy may have automatic activity during periods of altered consciousness.

Narcolepsy is diagnosed by history, overnight polysomnography (excludes other sleep disorders, such as sleep apnea), and daytime multiple sleep latency test (most specific test for narcolepsy, which shows a shortened time to sleep onset and early onset of REM sleep).

Parasomnias

Sleepwalking (Somnambulism) and Night Terrors (Sleep Terrors, Pavor Nocturnus)

Both are disorders of impaired and partial arousal from deep slow-wave sleep.

- Occur in the first third of the night, during the rapid transition from deep NREM sleep to light NREM sleep
- No recall of the experience in the morning
- Usually begins in childhood or early adolescence and disappears by older adolescence
- Positive family history in one or both parents in >60% of cases
- More likely associated with psychopathology if onset during adolescence or adulthood

Sleepwalking. Episode lasts from 1 to 30 minutes; person usually has a low level of awareness manifest by clumsiness and a blank expression, with indifference to the environment.

Night Terrors. Appearance of intense anxiety, fear, and sensation of doom that start suddenly, autonomic discharge (tachycardia, tachypnea, and sweating), vocalizations in the form of screams, moans, or gasps.

- Psychological disturbances are more likely a cause of the night terrors or sleepwalking if the onset is after age 12 years, the condition has persisted for several years, there is a negative family history, and/or there is maladaptive daytime behavior.
- A more alert state, more purposeful movements, and longer duration suggest hysterical phenomena such as fugue states.

REM-Related Parasomnia

Nightmares (Dream Anxiety Attacks)
- The most common type of REM related parasomnia

- Frequent nightmares affect about 5% of the population and are more common in children than adults.
- Onset is usually before 10 years of age
- Often associated with fears of attack, falling, or death
- Nightmares occur in the last third to half of the sleep period.
- Drug withdrawal—particularly from benzodiazepines, barbiturates, or alcohol—can lead to nightmares.

Sleep Paralysis, Hypnagogic and Hypnopompic Hallucinations
- Although frequently seen in narcolepsy, they can occur in nonnarcoleptics.

Nocturnal Enuresis (See Chapter 26)
- 2% to 3% of 12-year-old children and 1% to 3% of older adolescents are enuretic, independent of stage of sleep; this may be primary or secondary.

TREATMENT OF SLEEP DISORDERS

Preventive counseling can preclude the development of certain sleep disorders that are secondary to poor sleep habits. See "Sleep-Smart Tips for Teens" from the National Sleep Foundation (http:www.sleepfoundation.org).

Dyssomnias
Insomnia/Excessive Daytime Sleepiness Due to Inadequate Sleep
1. Counseling regarding any existing situational stresses
2. Regularize bedtime and awakening hours
3. Encourage regular mealtimes, especially breakfast in the morning, and avoid heavy late night meals. A light carbohydrate snack may help induce sleep at bedtime.
4. Teach relaxation techniques.
5. Daily exercise, but not close to bedtime
6. Curtail nicotine, alcohol, food or beverages that contain caffeine, and other stimulants.
7. Bedroom environment should be for sleep (e.g., no TV, or computer in the bedroom).
8. Keep bedroom dark and quiet. Morning exposure to bright light is also helpful.
9. Avoid daytime naps.
10. Medications. Behavioral techniques should be used to treat insomnia in adolescence unless there are specific medical, psychiatric or other sleep disorders (e.g., restless leg syndrome) that require medications. There has been a paucity of research on the use of medications for sleep disorders in adolescents.

Insomnia Due to Delayed Sleep Phase Syndrome
Review all of the above suggestions for the treatment of insomnia. An expert in sleep disorders may carry out chronotherapy (advancing bedtime and wake time by 15-minute intervals or by delaying bedtime by 2- to 4-hour adjustments every few days, forcing the adolescent to sleep around the clock until reaching an appropriate bedtime with 8.5 to 9.5 hours of sleep). There has been

limited research on the efficacy of this treatment. A referral to psychologist or psychiatrist may be required for evaluation of underlying psychological issues.

Insomnia Due to OSAS
Treatment requires a team effort. Weight loss, tonsillectomy and adenoidectomy, constant positive airway pressure, and bi-level pressure ventilation are all modalities used to treat OSAS. Consultation is suggested with pulmonology, otolaryngology or a sleep laboratory. An echocardiogram (to rule out pulmonary artery hypertension or right ventricular hypertrophy), and a lateral x-ray of the soft tissues of the neck are useful.

Parasomnias
Arousal Disorders (Sleepwalking and Night Terrors)
1. Take precautions to prevent injury.
2. Reassure, educate, and explain the phenomena.
3. Evaluate precipitating factors.
4. Scheduled awakenings (fully waking adolescent 15 to 30 minutes before expected arousal time may be tried). There is limited research on the efficacy of this treatment.
5. Encourage stress reduction/relaxation.
6. Refer for psychological evaluation and treatment when there is evidence of psychopathology.
7. Pharmacotherapy is rarely needed. Some medications (e.g. benzodiazepine, tricyclic antidepressant) have been reported to have efficacy when used short-term to "break the cycle" or to decrease the chance of arousal.

Nightmares (Sleep Anxiety Attacks)
Evaluation and treatment of underlying psychological stresses or fears and associated alcohol or other drug abuse problems.

Nocturnal Enuresis (See Chapter 26)

Sleep Disorder Clinics
For severe sleep disorders or diagnostic dilemmas, referral to a sleep disorder clinic can help. Updated lists are available from the National Sleep Foundation (www.sleepfoundation.org), the American Sleep Disorders Association (www.asda.org) or the Canadian Sleep Society www.css.to/sleep/centers.htm.

WEB SITES AND REFERENCES

http://www.aasmnet.org/. American Academy of Sleep Medicine.
http://www.nhlbi.nih.gov/health/dci/Browse/sleep.html. National Center on Sleep Disorders Research.
http://www.css.to. Canadian Sleep Society.
http://www.nhlbi.nih.gov/about/ncsdr/. NIH site about sleep disorders.
http://www.sleepnet.com/disorder.htm. Information about various sleep disorders.
American Academy of Sleep Medicine. *International classification of sleep disorders, revised: diagnostic and coding manual.* Chicago, Illinois: American Academy of Sleep Medicine, 2001.

National Institutes of Health, National Institute of Neurological Disorders and Stroke. *Understanding sleep.* NIH publication no 98-3440-c. Washington, DC: NIH, 1998.

National Sleep Foundation. Adolescent sleep needs and patterns. Research report and resource guide. Washington, DC: The National Sleep Foundation, 2000. Available at www.sleepfoundation.org.

Owens J, Babcock D, Blumer J, et al. The use of pharmacotherapy in the treatment of pediatric insomnia in primary care: rational approaches. A consensus meeting summary. *J Clin Sleep Med* 2005;1;49.

Genitourinary Tract Infections

Lawrence J. D'Angelo and Lawrence S. Neinstein

CYSTITIS

Epidemiology

1. Occurs three to five times more commonly in women and more so in adolescent females.
2. 10% to 20% of adolescent girls have at least one episode of acute cystitis.

Risk Factors

1. *Females:* greater risk due to a short urethra. Other potential risk factors include (a) poor perineal hygiene; (b) coital behaviors including diaphragm use, coital frequency, use of spermicide-coated condoms, and not voiding after intercourse; (c) pregnancy; (d) nonsecretion of ABO blood group antigens; (e) instrumentation of the urethra; (f) anatomic abnormalities.
2. *Males:* In non–sexually active male adolescents, infections are more likely a result of structural abnormality. Other factors include blood group B or AB nonsecretion, P_1 blood group phenotype, insertive anal intercourse, sexual partner with vaginal colonization by uropathogens, and lack of circumcision.

Microbiology

1. *Females: Escherichia coli* (75% to 90%); *Staphylococcus saprophyticus* (5% to 15%); other gram-negative organisms (0% to 5%).
2. *Males:* Gram-negative bacilli (75%); gram-positive organisms (15% to 25%, particularly enterococci and coagulase-negative staphylococci); *Trichomonas vaginalis, Gardnerella vaginalis* (rare).

Symptoms and Signs

1. *Females:* (a) Dysuria; (b) frequency, hesitancy, and urgency; (c) suprapubic pain; (d) pyuria; (e) hematuria.
2. *Males:* Male patients may also have symptoms associated with infections in the prostate, epididymis, or testicles.

Differential Diagnosis of Acute Dysuria

1. *Females* (Table 25.1): (a) Acute vulvovaginitis, (b) local dermatitis (from chemicals and other agents such as soap, contraceptive agents and foams, feminine hygiene products); (c) subclinical pyelonephritis; (d) acute urethral syndrome ("low-count," 10^2 to 10^4 bacteriuria/pyuria syndrome). However, many women with symptomatic cystitis have $<10^5$ CFU/mL, and 10^2 CFU/mL may be the appropriate microbiologic criterion for determining the presence of a UTI. The small group of symptomatic women with no growth on urine culture deserve evaluation for urinary or genital tract infections with *Chlamydia trachomatis, Mycobacterium tuberculosis,* herpes simplex virus, *Candida,* or *T. vaginalis.*)
2. *Males:* (a) Urethritis (secondary to STD organisms); (b) prostatitis; (c) irritation from agents such as spermicidal foam; (d) trauma (usually associated with masturbation).

Diagnosis

1. *History:* (a) In females, vaginal discharge or itching; in males: past urinary tract problems, or trauma; (b) medication, local soaps, or hygiene products that could cause a local dermatitis; (c) history of sexual activity; (d) fever and flank pain suggesting acute pyelonephritis.
2. *Physical examination:* In females, includes assessment of abdominal and flank tenderness; genital exam for local dermatitis or pelvic exam if clinically indicated. In males, inspection and palpation of the genitals for urethral discharge, meatal erythema, inflammation of the glans penis, penile lesions, an enlarged or tender epididymis or testis, or inguinal lymphadenopathy. A rectal examination is necessary if a diagnosis of prostatitis is under consideration.

Laboratory Studies

1. Microscopic examination of urine:
   a. The presence of one or more bacteria/oil immersion field of *uncentrifuged* urine.
   b. More than 10 organisms/oil immersion field on a *centrifuged* unstained sediment.
   c. Pyuria with five or more leukocytes/high-power field of urine sediment on spun urine is less correlated with bacteriuria.
   d. Leukocyte esterase dipstick has a sensitivity of about 75% to 96% and specificity of 94% to 98% in detecting pyuria associated with an infection.
2. *Urine culture:* Bladder or renal infection usually characterized by a urine culture with >100,000 CFU/mL of a typical urinary pathogen, but well established that >100 CFU/mL of a pure culture of an organism indicates an infection in the presence of symptoms and pyuria. A urine culture is not mandatory for the diagnosis and treatment of a female adolescent with signs and symptoms of a UTI. If therapy fails, if the infection represents a

TABLE 25.1

Differential Diagnosis of Acute Dysuria in Women

Condition	Pathogen	Pyuria	Hematuria	Urine Culture	Signs, Symptoms
Cystitis	*Escherichia coli, Staphylococcus saprophyticus, Proteus, Klebsiella* sp	Usually	Sometimes	10^2 to $>10^5$	Acute onset, severe symptoms, dysuria, frequency, urgency, suprapubic or low back pain, suprapubic tenderness
Urethritis	*Chlamydia trachomatis, Neisseria gonorrhoeae,* herpes simplex virus	Usually	Rarely	$<10^2$	Gradual onset, mild symptoms, vaginal discharge or bleeding, lower abdominal pain, new sexual partner, cervical or vaginal lesions on examination
Vaginitis	*Candida* sp, *Trichomonas vaginalis*	Rarely	Rarely	$<10^2$	Vaginal discharge or odor, pruritus, dyspareunia, external dysuria, no frequency or urgency, vulvovaginitis on examination

From Stamm WE, Hooton TM. Management of urinary tract infections in adults. *N Engl J Med* 1993;329:1329, with permission.

recurrence within the 3 months after an initial infection, or if the patient is a male, a culture is recommended. Cultures are also indicated for female patients with pyuria without bacteriuria. In patients who become asymptomatic with therapy, posttreatment cultures are unnecessary. Follow-up cultures are indicated for patients with acute pyelonephritis, a complicated infection, or during pregnancy.

3. *Other tests:* In females, <12 years of age, three infections within 1 to 2 years may be an indication for a more complete evaluation; however, in postpubertal females with uncomplicated cystitis, evaluation after recurrent episodes is unlikely to reveal significant abnormalities that would change either therapy or prognosis (Fig. 25.1). In males, an investigation with more invasive tests is probably not indicated after the first infection unless there is evidence in the history or physical examination of a possible renal abnormality or there is no response to therapy.

Recurrent Infections in Female Adolescents

About 20% of young women will have recurrent infections. Recurrent cystitis within 3 months of the original infection should result in a urine culture. Those female patients with a relapse (recurrent infection with original pathogen within 2 weeks after completion of therapy) should also have their urine cultured and in either case should have careful follow-up.

PYELONEPHRITIS

The clinical and laboratory manifestations usually include the following: symptoms of acute cystitis, fever, costovertebral tenderness, elevated leukocyte count and erythrocyte sedimentation rate, urinalysis showing leukocytes and bacterial casts and positive urine culture result.

If fever and flank pain persist after 72 hours of treatment, cultures should be repeated and ultrasonography or CT should be considered to evaluate for an abscess. Blood cultures should be obtained from those with uncertain diagnosis, a suspected hematogenous source, or an immunosuppressed or hospitalized patient. Additional indications for imaging include recurrent pyelonephritis, persistent hematuria, or poor response to treatment. Indications for hospitalization include persistent vomiting, suspected sepsis, uncertain diagnosis, urinary tract obstruction.

TREATMENT OF GENITOURINARY INFECTIONS

Acute, Uncomplicated Infection in Female Patients

A growing number of urinary tract pathogens have developed resistance to commonly used antibiotics, particularly trimethoprim/sulfamethoxazole and amoxicillin. Local resistance patterns should be consulted before prescribing any antibiotic as first-line treatment of UTI.

1. *No complicating factors:* Use a 3-day oral regimen of one of the following: (a) trimethoprim-sulfamethoxazole (160/800 mg every 12 hours) or trimethoprim (100 mg every 12 hours), (b) cefpodoxime (200 mg every 12 hours), (c) nitrofurantoin (100 mg every 6 hours). In older adolescents (>16 years),

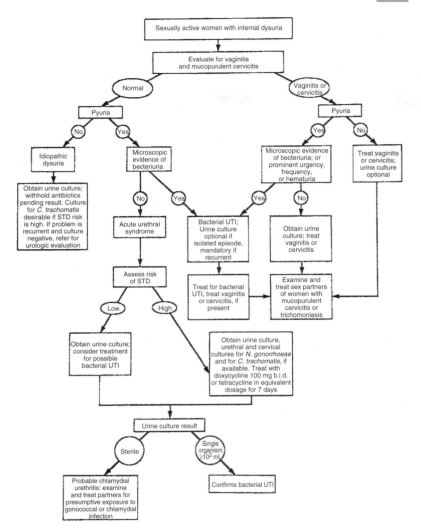

FIGURE 25.1   Flow diagram for the evaluation of women with internal dysuria. (From Holmes KK. Lower genital tract infection in women: cystitis, urethritis, vulvovaginitis, and cervicitis. In: Holmes KK, Mardh PA, Sparling PF, et al., eds. *Sexually Transmitted Diseases.* New York: McGraw-Hill, 1990, with permission.)

a 3-day regimen of a quinolone would also be appropriate, including either norfloxacin (400 mg every 12 hours), ciprofloxacin (250 mg every 12 hours), or ofloxacin (200 mg every 12 hours).

2. *For patients with potentially complicating problems* (diabetes, sickle cell disease, a history of a previous UTI, or symptoms for >1 week, etc.), 7-day regimen of a previously mentioned medication.

3. *Pregnancy:* Use a 7-day regimen of either nitrofurantoin (100 mg four times a day), cefpodoxime (200 mg every 12 hours) or trimethoprim/sulfamethoxazole (160/800 mg every 12 hours).
4. *Three-day course versus single-dose antibiotics:* A 3-day course of antibiotics appears to ensure greater success than the single-dose antibiotic regimens.
5. *Three-day course versus longer course of antibiotics:* No significant differences in the short- or longer-term frequency of positive urine cultures between a short (2- to 4-day) and standard duration oral antibiotic therapy (7 to 14 days). In adult patients, there is no difference in symptomatic cure but a slightly higher efficacy in bacteriological cure with prolonged treatment.

Acute, Uncomplicated Pyelonephritis in Female Patients

Due to *Escherichia coli, Proteus mirabilis, Klebsiella pneumoniae, Staphylococcus. saprophyticus*: Avoid amoxicillin and first-generation cephalosporins because 25% to 35% of these organisms are resistant to such antibiotics.

1. *Mild to moderate illness with no nausea or vomiting:* Oral therapy for 10 to 14 days with either Trimethoprim-sulfamethoxazole (160/800 mg every 12 hours), cefpodoxime (200 mg every 12 hours) or quinolones can be utilized in older adolescents and young adults including: norfloxacin (400 mg every 12 hours for 10 to 14 days), ciprofloxacin (500 mg every 12 hours for 10 to 14 days), ofloxacin (200 to 300 mg every 12 hours for 10–14 days) or levofloxacin (500 mg daily for 10 to 14 days).
2. *Severe pyelonephritis or other complicated UTI requiring hospitalization* (e.g., patients with diabetes, sickle cell disease, or immunodeficiency): Parenterally administered antibiotics including either: trimethoprim/sulfamethoxazole (160/800 mg every 12 hours), ceftriaxone (1 to 2 g/day), ciprofloxacin (250 to 500 mg every 12 hours), gentamicin (1 mg/kg every 12 hours with or without ampicillin), ticarcillin/clavulanate (3.1 g every 8 hours) or imipenem (500 mg every 8 hours). Use these until fever has resolved for 24 to 48 hours and then switch to either oral trimethoprim/sulfamethoxazole (160/800 mg every 12 hours), cefpodoxime (200 mg every 12 hours), norfloxacin (400 mg every 12 hours). For patients 16 years of age or older, ciprofloxacin (500 mg every 12 hours), or ofloxacin (200 to 300 mg every 12 hours).
3. *Pregnancy:* Hospitalization is highly recommended, with parentally administered antibiotics including one of the following: ceftriaxone (1 to 2 g/day), aztreonam (1 g every 8 to 12 hours), or gentamicin (1 mg/kg every 12 hours). Use these until fever has resolved for 24 to 48 hours and then treat with oral antibiotics for 14 days of therapy using one of the following: cefpodoxime proxetil (200 mg every 12 hours) or trimethoprim/sulfamethoxazole (160/800 mg every 12 hours).

Recurrent Infections

Recurrent cystitis in female patients should be managed by either *continuous prophylaxis, postcoital prophylaxis, or therapy initiated by the patient.*

1. *Continuous prophylaxis:* Use one of the following: trimethoprim (100 mg daily), trimethoprim/sulfamethoxazole (40/200 mg daily) or nitrofurantoin (50 to 100 mg daily).
2. *Postcoital prophylaxis*: Use either trimethoprim/sulfamethoxazole (40/200 mg) or nitrofurantoin (50 to 100 mg).

3. *Nonantibiotic measures:* voiding after intercourse, discontinuing use of a diaphragm, emptying the bladder frequently, and acidifying the urine.

Treatment of UTIs in Male Patients

Male patients should probably receive a 7- to 10-day course of antibiotics, although a 3-day regimen of trimethoprim/sulfamethoxazole or a quinolone such as norfloxacin in age-appropriate patients could be used.

Cautions and Contraindications

1. Fluoroquinolone antibiotics are not approved for use in adolescents <16 years and *should not be used in pregnancy.*
2. Trimethoprim/sulfamethoxazole is not approved in pregnancy but has been widely used.
3. Gentamicin should be used in pregnancy with great caution because of the possibility of toxicity to the eighth nerve of the developing fetus.
4. Local resistance patterns will influence the ultimate choice of antibiotics.

ASYMPTOMATIC BACTERIURIA

The prevalence of asymptomatic bacteriuria (reproducible growth of $>10^5$ CFU/mL) is 1% to 7%. Treatment is mainly indicated for pregnant patients, male patients, and female patients with either an underlying renal tract abnormality or an immunocompromising disease. Treatment should be with appropriate antibiotics selected on the basis of culture sensitivities.

NONGONOCOCCAL URETHRITIS

Nongonococcal urethritis (NGU) is an infectious inflammation of the urethra characterized by dysuria and by a mucopurulent penile discharge. The etiology is typically *C. trachomatis, Ureaplasma urealyticum, Mycoplasma genitalium, G. vaginalis, herpes simplex* virus, *S. saprophyticus, E. coli, or T. vaginalis.*

1. *Epidemiology:* Extremely common among sexually active men, with an estimated 3 to 4 million cases yearly in the United States.
2. *Clinical manifestations:* These include discharge, dysuria, rarely, hematuria and epididymitis, prostatitis (rare), and Reiter syndrome (very rare).
3. *Diagnosis:* Made by (a) clinical history; (b) Gram stain of urethral discharge (lack of intracellular gram-negative diplococci suggests NGU); (c) >10 white blood cells per high-power dry field of the urine sediment or positive leukocyte esterase dipstick suggest urethritis; (d) urethral culture if the Gram stain result of the discharge is negative.
4. *Therapy (see Chapter 60):* This includes either doxycycline (100 mg orally twice daily for 7 days) or azithromycin (1 g orally in a single dose) or ofloxacin (400 mg orally twice daily for 7 days).

PROSTATITIS

An inflammatory reaction confined to the prostate gland, unusual in adolescents. Although it is often assumed that STDs, and particularly infection with

N. gonorrhoeae and *C. trachomatis,* cause a large percentage of the cases of acute prostatitis in adolescents and young adults, evidence to support this is inadequate. Coliform bacteria, *S. saprophyticus, Mycoplasma hominis, U. urealyticum,* and *T. vaginalis,* have also been implicated as causative agents.

1. Symptoms:
    a. *Pain:* Penile/scrotal, suprapubic, perineal, groin, or back pain or pain that occurs during ejaculation
    b. *Bladder symptoms:* Frequency, dysuria, and hesitation
    c. *Systemic symptoms:* Chills, fever, and malaise
    d. *Other symptoms:* Hematospermia and hematuria
2. *Diagnosis:* "Segmental culture" technique (four separate specimens with prostatic massage after third specimen; *not* routinely done).
3. *Treatment:* includes either trimethoprim/sulfamethoxazole (160/800 mg every 12 hours for 7 days) or ofloxacin (400 mg every 12 hours for 7 days) or doxycycline (100 mg every 12 hours for 7 days) or erythromycin (500 mg every 6 hours for 7 days). If symptoms persist, more aggressive attempts to obtain specific diagnostic samples need to be undertaken, including the segmental culture technique described above.

HEMATOSPERMIA

Bloody ejaculate with a reddish discoloration of semen either after masturbation or on removing a condom. Usually either idiopathic and self-limited or related to an infection such as a gonococcal or chlamydial urethritis. No treatment is necessary.

WEB SITES AND REFERENCES

http://www.niddk.nih.gov/health/urolog/pubs/cpwork/cpwork.htm. National Institutes of Health information on prostatitis.

Hooton TM, Scholes D, Stapleton AE, et al. A prospective study of asymptomatic bacteriuria in sexually active young women. *N Engl J Med* 2000;343:992.

Sheffield JS, Cunningham FG. Urinary tract infection in women. *Obstet Gynecol* 2005; 106:1085.

CHAPTER 26

Enuresis

Diane Tanaka

Enuresis is defined as the involuntary passage of urine, usually during sleep, occurring more than once a month. Current urology literature uses the following terminology:

- *Primary nocturnal enuresis:* nighttime wetting without prior periods of dryness
- *Secondary nocturnal enuresis:* nighttime wetting with at least 6 months of prior dryness
- *Monosymptomatic nocturnal enuresis (MNE):* isolated nocturnal enuresis
- *Polysymptomatic nocturnal enuresis (PNE):* nighttime wetting associated with other bladder symptoms such as urgency, frequency, instability, or voiding dysfunction
- *Diurnal enuresis:* involuntary or intentional urination into clothing while awake

ETIOLOGY OF MONOSYMPTOMATIC ENURESIS

Organic Causes. Only 2% to 3% of patients have a true organic cause. Myelomeningocele is the most common neurologic cause. Urologic abnormalities include recurrent UTIs, urethral obstruction or posterior urethral valves, detrusor instability, or incomplete bladder emptying. Other organic causes include renal concentrating defects (e.g., sickle cell anemia), diabetes mellitus, and diabetes insipidus.

Genetic Causes. Genetic studies have shown that the most common mode of inheritance is autosomal dominant with high penetrance. One third of cases appear to be due to sporadic occurrence.

Sleep Disorder. Enuretic episodes can occur at random throughout the night and can occur in all stages of sleep, but they occur primarily during non–rapid-eye-movement (non-REM) sleep.

Maturational Delay. It has been postulated that a developmental delay in adequate neuromuscular maturation of the bladder as well as an immaturity of the CNS inhibition of the micturition reflex is responsible for enuresis.

Small Functional Bladder Capacity. The current thinking among enuresis experts is that affected teens either produce large nighttime volumes of urine with a normal bladder capacity or produce large nighttime volumes with a small bladder capacity.

Psychological Factors. Most enuretic patients are psychologically normal, and psychological stressors do not cause enuresis.

Vasopressin Levels. It has been postulated that as children approach adolescence, a faulty circadian rhythm of arginine vasopressin (AVP) secretion may be the paramount pathogenetic factor.

Detrusor Instability. If a patient has refractory primary MNE, bladder dysfunction should be considered.

ETIOLOGY OF DIURNAL ENURESIS

Primary Diurnal Enuresis. Possible etiologies include neurogenic bladder, congenital urethral obstruction (characterized by a weak or interrupted urinary stream), ectopic ureter (affected patients complain of constant wetness and dampness), and congenital diabetes insipidus.

Secondary Diurnal Enuresis. Possible etiologies include constipation, urinary tract infections, giggle incontinence, stress incontinence, emotional stress, Hinman syndrome (the bladder behaves like a neuropathic bladder even though there are no neurologic deficits), traumatic or infectious urethral obstruction, diabetes mellitus, acquired diabetes insipidus, and myogenic detrusor failure (seen commonly in neurogenic bladders and in patients with posterior urethral valves).

EPIDEMIOLOGY

By adolescence, the prevalence of enuresis is 1% to 2%. The male-to-female ratio is 3:2. More African-American teens are affected than whites. Some 80% to 85% of teens have nocturnal enuresis only, whereas 15% to 20% have nocturnal and daytime enuresis.

DIAGNOSIS

A thorough history, a focused physical examination, and simple laboratory tests will usually suffice to evaluate enuresis.

History. The history should include the following: severity of enuresis (how many dry nights per month, most consecutive dry nights, frequency of urination, urgency of urination), type of enuresis, symptoms of organic disease, history of UTIs, family history of enuresis or small bladders, nighttime awakening to use the toilet, prior therapeutic modalities and results, history of sleep disorders, timing of wetting (if the teen wets after voiding, think of vaginal reflux of urine, labial fusion, or postvoid dribble syndrome), type of urinary stream, and whether there is dribbling or hesitancy (seen with posterior urethral valves).

Physical Examination

This should include:

1. blood pressure.
2. abdomen (check for masses).
3. genitourinary tract (check the urethral meatus for evidence of stenosis); observe urinary stream to see whether it is full and forceful or narrow and dribbling.
4. look for midline defects in the lumbosacral area, abnormalities of the gluteal fold, or abnormal tufts of hair.
5. perform a neurologic examination (check gait, deep tendon reflexes, perineal sensation, rectal sphincter tone, and bulbocavernosus reflex).

Laboratory Tests

1. *Urinalysis:* Every patient evaluated for enuresis should have a urinalysis.
2. *Urine culture:* Obtain a urine culture if the urinalysis suggests a UTI.
3. *Uroflowmetry:* Patients void into a special toilet with a pressure-sensitive rotating disk at the base. A normal uroflow study shows a single bell-shaped curve with a normal peak and average flow velocity for age and size.
4. *Bladder capacity:* The patient drinks 12 ounces of water and then the volume of urine is measured when the patient needs to void.
5. *Imaging studies:* Radiologic studies are not needed routinely. If a urethral obstruction or a neurogenic bladder is suspected, a voiding cystourethrogram is indicated (the neurogenic bladder will appear as a trabeculated "Christmas tree" or "pine cone" configuration). If a neurogenic bladder is suspected and there is no obvious cause, obtain a spinal MRI to look for spinal cord abnormalities. Ultrasonography is indicated for patients with persistent daytime wetness or for those with failure to empty the bladder. A prevoiding and postvoiding bladder ultrasound can be obtained to rule out partial emptying (normal residual bladder volume is <10 mL).

THERAPY

1. *Motivational counseling:* Studies indicate that motivational counseling alone leads to a 25% to 70% remission rate. The relapse rate is 5%. If there is a lack of improvement after 3 to 6 months, other methods should be tried. In this program, the practitioner reassures the adolescent and family members that this problem is common to many teens, gives the adolescent an active role by putting him or her in charge of changing the sheets and placing them in the laundry machines, gives positive reinforcement for dryness, and provides close initial follow-up with the teen and family.
2. *Self-awakening programs:* The teen lies in bed and imagines that it is the middle of the night and a full bladder is trying to wake him or her, at which point the teen goes to the bathroom and urinates. Or the teen goes to bed when the urge to urinate arises, pretends to sleep, "awakens," and then walks to the bathroom to urinate.
3. *Parent-awakening programs:* If self-awakening is not effective, then parent awakening can be used. The parent awakens the teen, but the teen must locate the bathroom alone. Parents need to awaken their child at the parents' bedtime each night until the teen awakens quickly to sound for 7 consecutive nights. At that point, the teen is either cured or ready for an enuresis alarm.

4. *Alarm systems:* Enuresis alarms have the highest cure rate of any available treatment for enuresis (long-term cure rates average 70%). Alarm failure rates range from 20% to 30%. Alarms need to be used for 2 to 3 months and continued until 3 weeks after dryness has been achieved. If the teen's family cannot afford to buy an enuresis alarm, then a clock radio or alarm clock set for 3 hours after going to sleep can be used. The alarm works by causing contraction of the external sphincter when the teen awakens. In order for enuresis alarms to be effective, the teen must be able to awaken to touch or sound.
5. *Medications:* There is no drug that is safe and effective enough to cure enuresis. The major drugs available include the following:
    a. *DDAVP:* A synthetic analog of vasopressin. Its mechanism of action is to reduce urine production by increasing water retention and urine concentration in the distal tubules. DDAVP is tasteless and odorless and can be administered either intranasally or orally. It is given in the late evening to reduce urine production during sleep. The medication comes as a nasal spray that delivers 10 μg per spray or as a graduated intranasal tube (Rhinal Tube) that delivers doses of 5, 10, 15, and 20 μg per spray. The usual initial dose is 20 μg, or one spray in each nostril, at bedtime. The dose can be increased by 10 μg weekly to a maximum dose of 40 μg. The duration of action is 10 to 12 hours.
    b. *Oral desmopressin:* The initial dose of oral desmopressin is 0.2 mg, given 1 hour before bedtime. If there is no response within a week, increase the dose by 0.2 mg to a maximum of 0.6 mg nightly. Seventy percent of patients with nocturnal enuresis who receive desmopressin stop their bed-wetting completely or reduce it significantly. A positive effect of the medication is seen within a few days and is maintained as long as the drug is administered. Most patients relapse after drug withdrawal, particularly if the drug is stopped abruptly (relapse rate can be as high as 50% to 95%). Therefore, the drug should be tapered slowly. During long-term therapy, treatment-free windows of approximately 3 months are essential to avoid treating a child who has become dry.
    c. *Imipramine (Tofranil):* This drug combines an anticholinergic effect that increases bladder capacity with a noradrenergic effect that decreases bladder detrusor excitability. Imipramine is also thought to increase excretion of antidiuretic hormone from the posterior portion of the pituitary gland. Imipramine is taken 1 hour before bedtime. The duration of action is 8 to 12 hours. Start the patient at 25 mg/day and increase the dose weekly, as needed, to a maximum dose of 75 mg/day. A sustained-release form of imipramine, Tofranil-PM, is also available. Response rate is 25% to 40%; relapse rate can be as high as 75%. The relapse rate is higher when the drug is stopped abruptly or prematurely. The maximal effect of imipramine usually occurs in the first week of therapy. However, one should continue therapy for 1 to 2 weeks before deciding on efficacy and whether to adjust the dose. The current recommendation is to treat for 9 months and then taper the drug by 25 mg decrements over 3 to 4 weeks. If the patient has a relapse, an additional course of therapy can be prescribed. The drug is most beneficial for occasional use when dryness is necessary (e.g., trips, vacations, sleepover parties).
    d. *Oxybutynin (Ditropan):* Oxybutynin provides an anticholinergic, antispasmodic effect that reduces uninhibited detrusor muscle contractions and

increases bladder capacity. Therefore, it may be most beneficial for patients with small-capacity bladders who also have daytime frequency or enuresis associated with uninhibited bladder contractions. A sustained-release formulation of oxybutynin is available (10 mg/day), as well as a conventional formulation (5 mg twice daily). A success rate of 90% was reported in one study of individuals with daytime enuresis, bladder instability, or both. This drug is to be used in teens with PNE, urge syndrome, or neurogenic bladder.

e. *Combined drug therapy with enuresis alarms:* Combining drugs with an alarm is very effective in the treatment of enuresis. Teens who have frequent enuresis are candidates for this therapy. After the adolescent is dry for 3 weeks, the drug is tapered gradually (if using desmopressin, decrease by one spray every 2 weeks; if using imipramine, decrease by 25 mg every 2 weeks).

TREATMENT RELAPSES AND FAILURES

Treatment relapse is defined as the recurrence of enuresis after having been dry for at least 1 month. The remedy is to reinstitute the treatment that was effective previously.

PROGNOSIS

Adolescent enuretics have a spontaneous cure rate of 15% per year.

CHAPTER 27

Asymptomatic Proteinuria and Hematuria

Lawrence J. D'Angelo and Lawrence S. Neinstein

ASYMPTOMATIC PROTEINURIA

Asymptomatic proteinuria—defined as proteinuria not associated with hematuria, hypertension, other symptoms or renal insufficiency—is a common finding on a screening urinalysis in adolescent patients. For the majority of these teens, no significant renal disease is present and the long-term prognosis is excellent. The objective in evaluating these adolescents is to establish the significance of the proteinuria, search noninvasively for treatable underlying conditions, and select those few patients who need referral for more extensive evaluation, including renal biopsy.

Etiology

1. Increased glomerular permeability, as in primary or secondary glomerulopathies [e.g., minimal change disease, systemic lupus erythematosus (SLE), membranous nephropathy]
2. Increased production of abnormal proteins (e.g., monoclonal gammopathies)
3. Decreased tubular reabsorption of proteins, as in tubular disease (e.g., Fanconi syndrome, aminoglycoside nephrotoxicity) or chronic interstitial nephritis
4. Miscellaneous—functional proteinuria (e.g., fever, exercise, congestive heart failure) and orthostatic proteinuria

Epidemiology. Up to 10% to 19% of healthy adolescents have protein in their urine on a dipstick test of a random urine sample.

Clinical Manifestations. Small amounts of protein in the urine are normal, and most individuals excrete 30 to 130 mg of protein per day. *Isolated asymptomatic proteinuria* refers to excretion of >150 mg/day by a person without clinical signs or symptoms. The leading causes of this condition are "benign persistent proteinuria" and orthostatic proteinuria. Orthostatic (postural) proteinuria, which is proteinuria while upright but not while recumbent, is common in adolescents. The etiology is unclear, although exaggerated hemodynamic response to the upright position and functional compromise of the left renal vein have been postulated as two possible causes. This is an asymptomatic condition characterized by an onset at 10 to 20 years, a positive dipstick or other measures of protein excretion while upright which disappear after the subject is recumbent for at least 4 hours, and normal renal function.

Differential Diagnosis

1. Mild asymptomatic proteinuria (expected excretion of protein: <500 mg/m^2 in 24 hours) including: benign persistent proteinuria, orthostatic or postural proteinuria (proved with split 24-hour urine collection), pyelonephritis (usually with fever and pyuria), renal tubular disorders, chronic interstitial nephritis, congenital dysplastic lesions, and other (exercise, trauma with hematuria, fever, congestive heart failure).

2. Moderate proteinuria (expected excretion of protein: 500 to 2,000 mg/m^2 in 24 hours), including acute poststreptococcal glomerulonephritis (PSGN), primary glomerulonephritis, hereditary chronic nephritis (Allport syndrome), and systemic diseases (e.g., SLE).

3. Severe proteinuria (expected excretion of protein: $>2,000$ mg/m^2 in 24 hours; usually >3.5 g), typically associated with edema, hypoalbuminemia, and hypercholesterolemia (nephrotic syndrome).

    a. Idiopathic glomerulonephritis: Minimal change disease, focal sclerosis, membranous or membranoproliferative glomerulonephritis

    b. Systemic disease: SLE, amyloidosis (in setting of chronic inflammatory disease or familial Mediterranean fever)

    c. Less commonly: infection (bacterial endocarditis, hepatitis, malaria, human immunodeficiency virus) and toxins (mercury, heroin, gold, penicillamine)

    d. Uncommon conditions, including allergens: Bee stings, mechanical (pericarditis, renal vein thrombosis), cancer (Hodgkin disease, lymphoma), pregnancy and congenital (Fabry disease and Alport syndrome)

Diagnosis. Confirm an initial positive test result twice. If proteinuria is confirmed, then a thorough history, physical examination, and lab evaluation are indicated. In addition, false-positive test results should be considered (Table 27.1).

1. *Urinalysis:* A repeat UA should be analyzed for glucose, casts, and cells.

2. *Protein:creatinine ratio:* A random urine sample is analyzed for protein and creatinine. When both are expressed in milligram amounts, a ratio of <0.2 is normal and a ratio >1.0 signifies nephrotic-range proteinuria. If the urine protein/creatinine ratio is >0.5 with no definitive postural change, then further evaluation is indicated including a timed urine collection (ideally 24 hours), BUN and creatinine concentrations; complete blood cell count; concentrations of albumin, antinuclear antibody, and cholesterol; hepatitis B screening tests; complement levels (CH_{50}, C3, C4); and an antistreptolysin O titer.

3. *Orthostatic proteinuria:* To screen for orthostatic proteinuria, a first-void specimen obtained immediately on arising is compared with a second specimen obtained at least 4 hours after arising. If the latter is at least five times the first specimen, this supports a diagnosis of orthostatic proteinuria. Follow-up should be done every 6 to 12 months.

4. *Renal ultrasound:* Indicated for abnormal renal function or nonpostural proteinuria.

TABLE 27.1

Causes of False-Positive Test Results for Proteinuria

Cause	Dipstick Method	Protein Precipitation Methods
Highly concentrated urine*	+	+
Gross hematuria	+	+
Contamination with antiseptic (chlorhexidine or benzalkonium)	+	−
Highly alkaline urine	−	−
Radiographic contrast medium (affects specific gravity more than proteinuria)	−	+
High levels of cephalosporin or penicillin analogs	−	+
Sulfonamide metabolites	−	+

*Because the dipstick provides only a qualitative reading, proteinuria (2+) in a highly concentrated urine with a specific gravity of 1.030 may have different (less) significance than proteinuria (2+) in a dilute urine of specific gravity 1.010.

Adapted from Abuelo JF. Proteinuria: diagnostic principles and procedures. *Ann Intern Med* 1983;98:186.

5. *Renal biopsy:* Refer the patient to a nephrologist for further evaluation and consideration for renal biopsy in the following situations: (a) a spot urine/creatinine ratio of >1.0 (suggesting a 24-hour protein concentration is >1,000 mg); (b) the diagnosis is unclear and significant disease is suspected; (c) the nephrotic syndrome is present and has not responded to a therapeutic trial of corticosteroids; (d) renal function is deteriorating; (e) the patient, family, or both express a need for prognostic information.

Prognosis and Follow-Up

Isolated Proteinuria. In general, the prognosis for asymptomatic orthostatic or persistent proteinuria (excretion of <500 mg protein in 24 hours) is good. Table 27.2 addresses the risk of chronic renal disease based on the pattern of proteinuria and suggests recommendations for follow-up.

Nonisolated Proteinuria. The prognosis depends on the underlying cause of the proteinuria and is rarely dictated by the level of the proteinuria. The exception is proteinuria related to diabetic nephropathy, in which the prognosis worsens as the level of protein excretion rises.

HEMATURIA

Hematuria is defined as the excretion of abnormal quantities of RBCs in the urine. Usually 2 to 4 erythrocytes per high-power field (HPF) on a

TABLE 27.2

Risk of Chronic Renal Disease and Recommended Follow-Up

Pattern of Protein Excretion	Risk of Chronic Renal Failure	Recommended Evaluation	Interval (yr)
Transient	None		
Intermittent			
<150 mg/day	None	None	
150 mg/day	Very slight if any	Blood pressure, urinalysis	1
Constant	20% after 10 yr (depending on exact lesion)	Blood pressure, urinalysis, blood urea nitrogen, serum creatinine	0.5–1
Orthostatic	Very slight if any	Blood pressure, urinalysis, monitor change in pattern or amount of proteinuria	1–2

Adapted from Abuelo JF. Proteinuria: diagnostic principles and procedures. *Ann Intern Med* 1983;98:186.

resuspended centrifuged urine sediment specimen is considered normal. The orthotoluidine-impregnated paper strips give a positive result with a specimen that contains as few as 2 to 5 RBCs/HPF. Hematuria must be differentiated from pigmenturia (i.e., myoglobinuria, hemoglobinuria or porphyrinuria).

Epidemiology. <3% of healthy individuals excrete >3 RBCs/HPF.

Clinical Manifestations and Differential Diagnosis. Usually asymptomatic in adolescents but if present, symptoms often suggest a cause. Possibilities include lower or upper UTI; trauma, and renal stones. Rarer causes: SLE, Henoch-Schönlein disease and IgA nephritis, and intrinsic renal disease (Alport syndrome, polycystic kidney disease, medullary sponge kidney), malignant hypertension, and arteriovenous malformations. Hematuria can also be seen with sickle cell disease and certain coagulopathies (acquired or iatrogenic).

False Hematuria. False hematuria can be caused by vaginal bleeding, factitious hematuria, or pigmenturia, including endogenous (porphyrinuria, hemoglobinuria, myoglobinuria) and exogenous (foods and drugs) forms of pigmenturia. In true hematuria, there is positive dipstick and RBCs on spun urine and clear spun serum. In false hematuria related to hemoglobinuria, myoglobinuria, and porphyrins, no RBCs are seen on microscopic urine although the spun urine appears red or orange. With hemoglobinuria, there is pink spun serum.

Diagnosis

History. Includes the pattern of hematuria, family history of renal disease or hematuria, associated symptoms (dysuria, renal colic, fever, joint pain, hearing loss), and drug history.

Physical Examination. Includes (1) blood pressure—elevated blood pressure associated with hematuria suggests renal abnormality; (2) skin: rashes may indicate connective tissue disease. Ecchymosis is suggestive of Henoch-Schönlein purpura, while petechiae are suggestive of thrombocytopenia; (3) corneal and lens abnormalities and hearing loss suggest hereditary nephritis; (4) abdomen—masses and renal enlargement may suggest polycystic disease.

Laboratory Tests. Significant hematuria should be confirmed on repeated urinalyses before an extensive evaluation is undertaken. Urine should be examined to determine the presence or absence of RBC casts and proteinuria. RBC casts and >10% dysmorphic RBCs suggest a renal parenchymal origin, usually either glomerulonephritis or interstitial nephritis, and the need for further evaluation. Significant associated proteinuria would also suggest a glomerular cause and the need for further evaluation. If there are no RBC casts or a qualitative proteinuria (>1+), the evaluation will depend on the findings from the history and physical examination. In the presence of RBC casts and significant proteinuria, a renal biopsy is indicated, as it is if hypertension accompanies either of these two symptoms. Without such a history, almost all individuals will have either normal biopsy findings or changes not indicative of significant pathology. If gross hematuria persists without an obvious cause, renal angiography can be considered in looking for vascular causes of the hematuria.

Specific Conditions

Marathon Runner's (Athlete's) Hematuria. Gross or microscopic hematuria is associated with many forms of exercise, including baseball, track, football, hockey, boxing, cross-country skiing, swimming, crew, lacrosse, rugby, and basic military training. The typical history is one of a normal urine before exercise, with hematuria on the first specimen voided after exercise, lasting up to 24 to 48 hours, possibly in association with dysuria and suprapubic discomfort. The cause is unclear. The prognosis is excellent unless another renal problem is the underlying cause.

Loin-Pain Hematuria Syndrome. This is a cause of hematuria found mainly in young females receiving oral contraceptives. The condition occurs with recurrent bouts of gross or microscopic hematuria with or without dysuria but almost always with unilateral or bilateral loin pain. Treatment has not been satisfactory, although nonsteroidal anti-inflammatory agents and calcium-hannel blockers may be of some use. The use of birth control pills should be discontinued.

Immunoglobulin A Nephropathy (Berger Disease). IgA nephropathy is a relatively common cause of gross hematuria in young adults. It is associated with IgA and IgG deposits in the mesangium. Renal function is usually normal, but a moderate percentage of individuals (40%) may progress to renal insufficiency. Poor prognostic signs include hypertension, renal insufficiency, and persistent proteinuria (protein excretion >1 g/day). Serum IgA levels are elevated in 50% of patients. The diagnosis is made by characteristic history or renal biopsy. No treatment is available. Henoch-Schönlein purpura can cause similar renal lesions, but it is associated with nonthrombocytopenic vasculitic purpura, arthralgias, and abdominal pain.

Hereditary Nephritis (Alport Syndrome) and Polycystic Kidney Disease. The adult form of polycystic kidney disease usually manifests in the second or third decade of life with hematuria and hypertension. It is an autosomal dominant disease. Familial nephritis in males often causes an early onset of renal insufficiency. The renal disease is often accompanied by abnormalities of the lens and retina and high-frequency hearing loss.

Benign Familial Hematuria. This is a condition characterized by glomerular hematuria (RBC casts), nonprogressive renal disease, and normal renal function in many affected family members. It is often associated with thinning of the glomerular basement membrane. The inheritance is autosomal dominant. The diagnosis is suggested by (a) the presence of hemoglobin or RBC casts in the urine of the adolescent and in that of a parent or sibling, (b) absence of renal insufficiency in the patient, and (c) no history of renal failure or auditory abnormalities in the affected family members. The disease is more common in females.

WEB SITES AND REFERENCES

http://www.niddk.nih.gov/kudiseases/pubs/proteinuria. National Institutes of Health (NIH) site on proteinuria.

http://www.niddk.nih.gov/kudiseases/pubs/hematuria. NIH education site on hematuria.

http://www.kidney.org/atoz/index.cfm. National Kidney Foundation Web site on kidney diseases.

http://www.keepkidshealthy.com/welcome/commonproblems/hematuria.html. Information site for parents on hematuria in children.

Ahmed Z, Lee J. Asymptomatic urinary abnormalities: hematuria and proteinuria. *Med Clin North Am* 1997;81:641.

Bergstein JM. A practical approach to proteinuria. *Pediatr Nephrol* 1999;13:697.

Hogg RJ. Adolescents with proteinuria and/or the nephrotic syndrome. *Adolesc Med* 2005;16:163.

CHAPTER 28

Scrotal Disorders

William P. Adelman and Alain Joffe

MALE GENITAL EXAMINATION

The male genitalia are readily accessible for palpation and the anatomy is straightforward; if unclear, ultrasonography can be used to clarify anatomy.

SCROTAL SWELLING AND MASSES (FIG. 28.1)

History
1. Pain: abrupt onset is suggestive of torsion; gradual onset suggests epididymitis or orchitis, lack of pain suggests a tumor or cystic mass.
2. Trauma.
3. Recent change in testicular size or scrotum. Reactive hydroceles are common secondary to trauma, orchitis, testicular cancer, and epididymitis.
4. Sexual activity: epididymitis in adolescence is usually sexually transmitted.
5. Prior history of pain: torsion is often preceded by episodes of mild pain.

Physical Examination
1. Inspect testes: in torsion, the affected testis is often higher and displaced more anteriorly than that on the contralateral side. Also, the affected testis and often the contralateral testis lie horizontally instead of in the usual vertical position owing the congenital defect involved. With infections, the affected testis is often lower.
2. Palpate the testicular surfaces, the epididymis, and the cord and head of the epididymis.
   a. Isolated swelling and tenderness of the epididymis suggests epididymitis.
   b. A tender, pea-sized swelling at the upper pole suggests torsion of the appendix testis.
   c. Generalized swelling and tenderness of both the testis and the epididymis can be found in either testicular torsion or epididymitis with orchitis.
   d. Presence of a cremasteric reflex makes torsion unlikely.
   e. Prehn sign: relief of pain with elevation of the testis suggests epididymitis.
   f. Nausea or vomiting with testicular pain is usually caused by torsion.
3. If a painless mass is present (Fig. 28.1):
   a. Palpate to assess location: (i) a mass within the testis is a tumor until proven otherwise; (ii) a mass palpable separate from the testis is

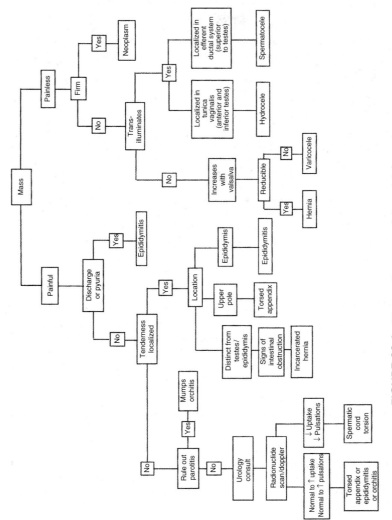

FIGURE 28.1 Diagnostic approach to scrotal masses.

unlikely to be a tumor; (iii) a "bag of worms" or "squishy tube" on the left spermatic cord is a varicocele; (iv) a mass located near the head of the epididymis, above and behind the testis, is probably a spermatocele; (v) a mass anterior to the testis or surrounding the testis is probably a hydrocele; (vi) a mass that is separate from the testis/epididymis, intensifies with straining (Valsalva), and is reducible is probably a hernia;

b. Transilluminate the mass: clear transillumination suggests a hydrocele or a spermatocele. Absence of transillumination suggests a testicular tumor or, if the mass is separate from the testis/epididymis, a hernia or large spermatocele.

Laboratory Evaluation

1. *Urinalysis:* Positive leukocyte esterase or presence of leukocytes is suggestive of epididymitis.
2. *Gram stain:* Gram-negative diplococci suggest a gonococcal epididymitis. A Gram stain with white blood cells without gram-negative bacteria suggests a chlamydial epididymitis; a negative Gram stain suggests an orchitis or torsion.
3. *Color-flow Doppler ultrasound and nuclear scans:* These should be obtained only after consultation with a urologist. If a reasonable suspicion of torsion exists, the primary therapy should be surgical exploration. In cases of torsion, the scan and Doppler study will show a decreased flow to the affected side.

TORSION

Etiology. Testicular torsion is a twisting of the testis and spermatic cord resulting in venous obstruction, progressive edema, arterial compromise, and, testicular infarction. Aside from torsion at the spermatic cord, appendages of the testes or of the epididymis can occasionally undergo torsion (Fig. 28.2A). Torsion can be difficult to differentiate from epididymitis (Table 28.1).

Epidemiology. Two thirds of cases occur between 12 and 18 years, with peak at 15 to 16 years.

Clinical Manifestations. (1) onset is usually abrupt; (2) 50% of teenagers have had brief prior episodes of scrotal pain; (3) pain may be isolated to the scrotum or radiate to the abdomen; (4) nausea and/or vomiting may occur; (5) physical examination shows the following:

a. The testis is tender and swollen.
b. The affected side is often higher than the contralateral side because of the elevation from the twisted spermatic cord.
c. The epididymis, if palpable, is often out of the usual posterolateral location.
d. The affected testis and often the contralateral testis lie in a horizontal plane.
e. The cremasteric reflex is absent.
f. Fever and scrotal redness are usually absent.

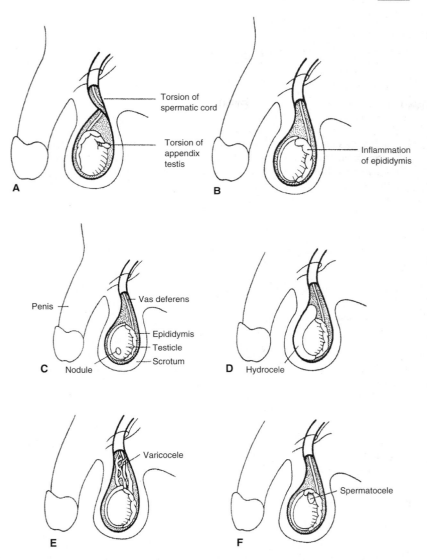

FIGURE 28.2 **A:** Torsion. **B:** Epididymitis. **C:** Testis tumor. **D:** Hydrocele. **E:** Varicocele. **F:** Spermatocele.

Diagnosis. Testicular torsion is a surgical emergency. The diagnosis of torsion should be suspected in any adolescent with a painful swelling of the scrotum. If the history and physical examination are consistent with torsion, a urology consultation should be immediately obtained and decisions made for further testing or direct surgical exploration (Table 28.1).

TABLE 28.1

Differentiating Torsion from Epididymitis

Symptoms and Other Findings	Torsion	Epididymitis
Pain	Severe	Severe
Onset	Sudden/abrupt	Hours to days
Prior episodes	50% of cases	Usually not
Nausea or vomiting	Frequent	Less frequent
Time to presentation	Short (<24 hr)	Longer (>24 hr)
Cremasteric reflex	Usually absent	Usually present
Epididymal abnormality	Obscured or anterior	Palpable and tender
Prehn sign	Absent: No relief of or increase in pain with elevation of the scrotum	Present: Pain relief with elevation of the scrotum
Urethral symptoms	Absent	May have dysuria, discharge
Urethral Gram stain	Negative	May be positive for gram-negative intracellular diplococci or white blood cells
Urinalysis	Usually negative	First-catch urine positive for white blood cells and/or leukocyte esterase

Therapy. Immediate surgery to save testicular function depends on early surgical intervention. If surgery is performed within 6 hours after symptoms begin, recovery is the rule.

EPIDIDYMITIS

Etiology. An inflammation of the epididymis caused by infection or trauma; it is primarily a problem of sexually active adolescents and is usually caused by *Chlamydia trachomatis* or *Neisseria gonorrhoeae*. Epididymitis due to *Escherichia coli* or other bowel flora can be secondary to unprotected insertive anal intercourse and be difficult to differentiate from torsion (Table 28.1).

Epidemiology. Epididymitis is uncommon in prepubertal males and also in non–sexually active males without a history of genitourinary tract abnormalities

Diagnosis. Suggested by the presentation of a sexually active teenager with subacute onset of pain in the hemiscrotum, inguinal area, or abdomen with epididymal swelling and tenderness, a reactive hydrocele, urethral discharge, dysuria, possibly fever, and pyuria (Fig. 28.2B). The laboratory evaluation should include:

1. Gram staining of an endourethral swab specimen for diagnosis of urethritis and for presumptive diagnosis of gonococcal infection.
2. A culture of intraurethral exudates or a nucleic acid amplification test on an intraurethral swab or urine for *N. gonorrhoeae* and *C. trachomatis*. Because of their higher sensitivity, amplification tests are preferred for the detection of *C. trachomatis*.
3. Examination of first void urine for leukocytes. If the urethral Gram stain is negative, send for Gram stain and culture.
4. Syphilis serology and HIV counseling and testing.

Therapy. Information on STD guidelines is available from the CDC at http://www.cdc.gov/std/treatment.

1. Scrotal support, bed rest, and analgesics are adjuncts to antimicrobial therapy.
2. Ceftriaxone 250 mg is given intramuscularly once and doxycycline 100 mg is given orally twice a day for 10 days.
3. Failure to improve within 3 days requires reevaluation.
4. Sexual partners should be treated.

TESTICULAR TUMORS

Etiology. Most testicular neoplasias are malignant and of germ-cell origin (95%). (Fig. 28.2C).

Epidemiology
1. Most common solid tumor in males age 15 to 35 years; incidence of 2.3 to 10 per 100,000 males.
2. Testicular cancer is 4.5 times more common in Caucasian men than in African-American men.
3. The risk of testicular tumor is increased 10- to 40-fold in teens with a history of cryptorchidism.

Diagnosis. The diagnosis of tumor should be suspected in any male with a firm, circumscribed, painless area of induration within the testis that does not transilluminate. Swelling is noted in up to 73% of cases at presentation but is usually considered asymptomatic by the patient. Testicular pain is the presenting symptom in 18% to 46% of patients who have germ cell tumors.

Therapy. Therapy involves a direct biopsy for confirmative diagnosis and cell type and a coordinated effort involving the urologist, the primary care specialist, and the oncologist.

HYDROCELE

Etiology. A hydrocele is a collection of fluid between the parietal and visceral layers of the tunica vaginalis, which lies along the anterior surface of the testicle and is a remnant of the processus vaginalis—the embryonic sleeve through which the testes descend (Fig. 28.2D).

Diagnosis. A hydrocele is usually a soft, painless, fluctuant scrotal mass that is anterior to the testis, transilluminates, and appears cystic on ultrasonography. Long-standing hydroceles are usually benign. The presence of a new hydrocele should alert the examiner to check for a possible underlying cause such as a hernia, testicular tumor, trauma, or infection.

Therapy. Usually no therapy is required for an asymptomatic long-standing hydrocele. A painful or tense hydrocele that might reduce circulation to the testis, a bulky mass that is uncomfortable and uncosmetic for the teenager, or a hydrocele associated with a hernia (a communicating hydrocele) is corrected with surgical resection of the parietal tunica vaginalis.

VARICOCELE

Etiology. A varicocele, or dilated scrotal veins, results from increased pressure and incompetent venous valves in the internal spermatic veins (Fig. 28.2E).

Epidemiology. Common in the 10- to 20-year age group, with a prevalence of 15%. Some 85% of varicoceles are clinically evident on the left side and 15% are bilateral.

Diagnosis. Varicoceles are detected in adolescents on routine examination or secondary to a patient's discovery. Occasionally a patient complains of pain from the varicocele. On exam, a visible varicocele (grade 3 or large) has a "bag of worms" appearance and feel. A palpable varicocele that is not visible is classified as grade 2 (moderate). More subtle varicoceles may feel like a thickened or asymmetric spermatic cord. The distention usually decreases when the patient lies down.

Therapy. No therapy is indicated for an adolescent with a normal semen analysis, but this may not be practical in teens. Loss of testicular volume or failure of the testis to grow during puberty has been the traditional indication for surgical correction of a varicocele during adolescence.

SPERMATOCELE

A spermatocele is a retention cyst of the epididymis that contains spermatozoa. Most are small (<1 cm in diameter), painless, cystic, freely movable, and will transilluminate (Fig. 29.2F). If it is large, the teen may complain of a "third testicle." It is usually felt as a smooth, cystic sac above and posterior to the testis, at the head of the epididymis. No therapy is indicated unless it is large enough to annoy the patient, in which case a urologist may excise it.

TESTICULAR SELF-EXAMINATION

The recommendations for self-examination by the American Cancer Society are as follows:

1. Examine the testes during or after a hot bath or shower.
2. Examine each testicle with the fingers of both hands, using the index and middle fingers on the underside of the testicle and the thumbs on the top of the testicle.
3. Gently roll the testicle between the thumbs and fingers.
4. Be on the lookout for lumps, irregularities, change in size, or pain in the testicles.
5. The epididymis should not be mistaken for an abnormality.
6. If any abnormality such as a lump is found, it should be reported immediately.
7. Testicular self-examination should be performed once a month.

WEB SITES AND REFERENCES

http://tcrc.acor.org/tcexam.html. Testicular Cancer Self Exam.

Adelman WP, Joffe A. The adolescent male genital examination: what's normal and what's not. *Contemp Pediatr* 1999;16:76–92.

Adelman WP, Joffe A. The adolescent with a painful scrotum. *Contemp Pediatr* 2000;17:111–128.

Infectious Respiratory Illnesses

Terrill Bravender and Emmanuel Walter

INFECTIOUS MONONUCLEOSIS (IM)

IM is usually an acute, self-limited, benign disease that commonly occurs in adolescence or young adulthood. Although Epstein-Barr virus (EBV) is responsible for IM in approximately 90% of cases, the syndrome may also be caused by other infectious agents, such as cytomegalovirus (CMV), *Toxoplasma*, human herpesvirus 6, and adenovirus.

Etiology. Transmission of EBV occurs primarily through exposure to oropharyngeal secretions; the incubation time is 30 to 50 days. The virus initially infects oral epithelial cells and then spreads to B lymphocytes, which disseminate the infection throughout the lymphoreticular system. EBV remains in the body for life. Virus is shed by 70% to 90% of individuals for 8 to 24 weeks after resolution of the clinical syndrome. After this, 60% to 100% of normal, asymptomatic EBV-seropositive individuals shed virus intermittently.

Clinical Manifestations. The majority of EBV infections are either asymptomatic or associated with mild, nonspecific symptoms such as malaise, fever and chills, and anorexia.

The traditional triad of IM includes:

1. Fever, lymphadenopathy, and pharyngitis
2. Lymphocytosis with atypical lymphocytes
3. Antibody response indicated by heterophil antibodies or EBV-specific antibodies.

279

In those who develop clinical symptoms, there is often a prodromal period of 3 to 5 days of malaise, headache, anorexia, myalgia, and fatigue, followed by more severe symptoms and signs as the immune response mounts.

Symptoms. (In order of prevalence): sore throat (70% to 80%), malaise (50% to 90%), anorexia (50% to 80%), nausea (50% to 70%), headache (40% to 70%), myalgias (12% to 30%), cough (5% to 15%), abdominal pain (2% to 14%), arthralgias (5% to 10%), and photophobia (5% to 10%)

Clinical Signs. Lymphadenopathy (93% to 100%), fever (80% to 100%), tonsillopharyngitis (69% to 91%), palpable splenomegaly (11% to 60%), hepatomegaly (10% to 25%), palatal petechiae (25% to 35%), periorbital edema (25% to 35%), liver or splenic tenderness (15% to 30%), jaundice (5% to 10%), rash (usually maculopapular, 3% to 15%; risk of rash is higher if ampicillin or amoxicillin has been given), and pneumonitis (<3%)

Complications. Overall, the complication rate is about 1% to 2% and may include neurologic problems, significant hematologic abnormalities, carditis, airway obstruction, parotitis, or orchitis.

1. *Splenic rupture* is seen in about 0.1% to 0.2% of cases between days 4 and 21 of the illness, and at least 50% of cases are spontaneous, without any history of trauma or unusual physical exertion. Clinical severity, laboratory results, and physical examination are not reliable predictors of risk. Patients should refrain from vigorous physical activity for at least 1 month after the onset of symptoms or until palpable splenomegaly resolves, whichever is later.
2. *Airway obstruction.* An uncommon but life-threatening complication of IM related to massive lymphoid hyperplasia and mucosal edema.
3. *Streptococcal pharyngitis.* Reported rates of coinfection vary from 4% to 33%.

Laboratory Evaluation
The total white blood cell count is elevated, in the range of 10,000 to 20,000/mm^3. About 95% of patients will demonstrate a lymphocytosis, with 10% or more being atypical lymphocytes. Anemia is uncommon. Mild hepatitis is very common and is seen in about 90% of individuals. Transaminase levels may be as high as two to three times normal; alkaline phosphatase and lactate dehydrogenase levels may also be elevated. Liver function test abnormalities peak at about week 2 or 3 of symptoms and usually resolve by the end of the fourth week. Entirely normal findings from liver chemistries may suggest a diagnosis other than EBV infection.

Heterophil Antibodies. These tests detect immunoglobulin M (IgM) antibodies induced by EBV infections. The MonoSpot test has a sensitivity of 86% and a specificity of 88% to 99%, but the sensitivity is lower during the first week of illness, and it is also lower (about 80%) in adolescents <16 years of age. EBV serology is best reserved for measurement in adolescents when (1) clinical IM is present and a heterophil test result is negative or (2) the clinician is investigating clinical situations such as thrombocytopenia, pneumonia, or a neurologic condition to exclude the diagnosis of acute EBV disease.

Specific Epstein-Barr Virus Antibodies. Table 29.1 and Figure 29.1 show the pattern of serologic results in various EBV stages.

TABLE 29.1

Patterns of Serology

Type of Infection	Heterophil Antibody	VCA-IgG	VCA-IgM	Early Antigen		EBNA
				D-EA	R-EA	
Susceptible (nonimmune)	–	–	–	–	–	–
Acute primary infection	+	++	+	+	–	–
Remote past infection	–	+++	–	–	–	+
Reactivated infection	+/–	+++	–	+	++	+/–

D-EA, diffuse early antigen; EBNA, Epstein-Barr nuclear antigen; Ig, immunoglobulin; R-EA, restricted early antigen; VCA, viral capsid antigen.

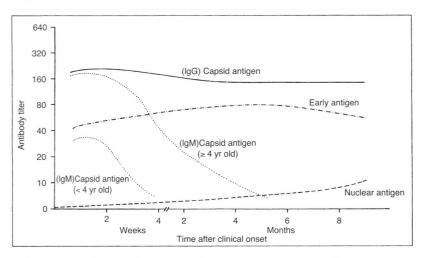

FIGURE 29.1 The evolution of antibodies to various EBV antigens in patients with IM is shown above. The titers are geometric mean values expressed as reciprocals of the serum dilution. IgM and IgG antibody responses to EBV capsid antigen develop during the acute phase, as does an IgG response to EBV early antigen in most cases. The IgG response lasts for life, but the IgM response is transient and is shortest in very young children. Antibody response to nuclear antigen lasts for life and is typically quite late in onset. (From Sumaya CV. Epstein-Barr serologic testing: diagnostic indications and interpretations. *Pediatr Infect Dis* 1986;5:337–342 with permission.)

Differential Diagnosis. Causes of EBV-negative mononucleosis-like syndrome include CMV, *Toxoplasma gondii,* rubella, adenovirus, herpes simplex virus 6, drug side effects, and acute HIV infection. Other considerations include group A beta-hemolytic streptococcal pharyngitis, viral tonsillitis, *Mycoplasma pneumoniae,* Vincent angina (necrotizing ulcerative gingivitis), diphtheria, viral hepatitis, and lymphoproliferative disorders or leukemia.

Diagnosis
1. Clinical symptoms: IM should be suspected in an adolescent with fatigue, fever, splenomegaly, adenopathy, and pharyngitis.
2. Abnormal white blood cell count: Patients will usually have the following:
   a. Relative lymphocytosis >50%.
   b. Absolute lymphocytosis >4,000/mm^3.
   c. Atypical lymphocyte counts >10% of the white blood cell count differential.
3. Positive serology: If a patient continues to be symptomatic and heterophil antibodies are negative, titers for EBV (including Viral Capsid Antigen (VCA) and Epstein-Barr Nuclear Antigen (EBNA)) should be evaluated.

Management. Only supportive care is required for most patients with IM.

1. Symptomatic care

a. *Rest* as needed during the acute phase. Acute symptoms usually resolve over 1 to 2 weeks, although the associated fatigue may persist for up to 2 months. Between 9% and 22% have persistent fatigue 6 months after the onset of symptoms.

b. *Nonsteroidal anti-inflammatory agents* or acetaminophen may be used as needed for fever and pain.

2. *Corticosteroids:* In general, steroids are not indicated for management of IM. Prednisone, initially 40 mg to 60 mg daily, then tapered over 1 to 2 weeks may be used in patients with significant pharyngeal edema that threatens or causes respiratory compromise.

3. *Return to activity*

a. Light, nonimpact activities may be resumed after 3 weeks of illness, and full participation in non-impact activities may be resumed after 4 weeks of illness.

b. Contact sports should be delayed for 4 to 6 weeks, even in the absence of splenomegaly. Ultrasound evaluation of the spleen is not of proven benefit.

MYCOPLASMA PNEUMONIA

Mycoplasma pneumoniae is a common cause of upper respiratory infections and pneumonia in adolescents; it is often referred to as "walking pneumonia."

Etiology. Transmission to the respiratory tract is via aerosolized inhalation. There is a high rate of transmission to family members and close contacts, with an incubation period of 3 to 4 weeks.

Epidemiology. *M. pneumoniae* infects patients of all ages, but lower respiratory disease is more common in adolescents and young adults. The illness is responsible for up to 20% of all pneumonias in middle and high school and up to 50% of pneumonias among college students and military recruits.

Clinical Manifestations

1. *Symptoms:* The onset of symptoms can be insidious.

a. *General:* Malaise, fever, chills, and headache occur early.

b. *Respiratory:*

- A cough develops 3 to 5 days after the onset of general symptoms. It usually starts as nonproductive but may lead to frothy white sputum. Sputum production is not as copious as in typical bacterial pneumonias. The cough may become paroxysmal, and occasionally chest pain and hemoptysis occur.
- Dyspnea is common.
- In those who are predisposed, infection may lead to reactive airway disease.
- Nasal congestion and rhinorrhea are uncommon.
- Bilateral bullous myringitis is highly suggestive but rare.

2. *Signs:* Patients do not generally appear very ill. Chest finding are often minimal. Other signs include: pharyngitis (75%), conjunctivitis (50%), and lymphadenopathy (25% to 50%).

3. *Complications:* Nonrespiratory infections and complications usually occur 1 to 21 days after initial symptoms and may involve the musculoskeletal, gastrointestinal, cardiovascular, or central nervous systems. Patients may develop an erythematous maculopapular rash or other exanthems.

Laboratory Evaluation. Serologic testing, although not routine, is the most specific of the laboratory tests. Enzyme-linked immunoassay (EIA) detects IgM and IgG antibodies against *Mycoplasma pneumoniae.* The IgM test does not become positive until 7 to 10 days after the onset of symptoms, so it may not be useful in guiding initial therapy.

1. Direct antigen testing is increasingly available, including polymerase chain reaction (PCR) assays.
2. White blood cell count is usually normal, although a mild leukocytosis may be present.
3. Chest x-ray examination: Variable; appearance is usually a nonlobar, patchy, or interstitial pattern; occasionally a pleural effusion is present. Major consolidation is rare.
4. Bacterial cultures are of little use for diagnostic purposes.

Differential Diagnosis. Differential diagnosis includes infection by *Streptococcus pneumoniae* viral infections, including adenovirus, parainfluenza and influenza, *Chlamydia pneumoniae,* and *Legionella;* less common causes include tuberculosis infection, Q fever *(Coxiella),* rickettsial infections, and fungal infections.

Diagnosis. The diagnosis is most often based on the patient's clinical presentation. In some instances, a more precise diagnosis may be required, and cold agglutinin tests may be performed quickly, even at the bedside. PCR assays will likely become the diagnostic test of choice as they become more available.

Management. Although most infections with *M. pneumoniae* are self-limited and resolve without treatment, antibiotic therapy has been shown to decrease the length and severity of illness.

a. Azithromycin: 500 mg on day 1, then 250 mg daily on days 2 through 5.
b. Clarithromycin: 500 mg twice per day for 7 days.
c. Erythromycin: 500 mg four times per day for 7 days.
d. Tetracycline: 500 mg four times per day for 7 days.
e. Doxycycline: 100 mg twice per day for 7 days

PERTUSSIS

Pertussis infection continues to cause fatal illness in neonates and incompletely immunized infants, and adolescents and young adults are likely a major source of infection for these vulnerable populations.

Etiology. *Bordetella pertussis* is the sole cause of epidemic pertussis, and the usual cause of sporadic pertussis. Transmission is via close contact with respiratory secretions, and intrafamilial spread is quite common in both immunized and unimmunized individuals. Pertussis is most contagious from about 1 to 2 weeks before the onset of cough and for 2 to 3 weeks after coughing begins.

Thus infected persons often transmit the disease to others before they are diagnosed and treated. The incubation period is commonly 5 to 10 days but may be as long as 21 days.

Epidemiology. From 1990 to 2004, there has been an 18.8-fold increase in the diagnosis of Pertussis among 10- to 19-year-olds. This increase is largely due to improved recognition and diagnosis of the illness, but it may also be due to a true increase in the number of pertussis infections. In adolescents with prolonged cough illness, between 13% and 20% are due to *B. pertussis* infection.

Clinical Manifestations. The clinical severity of pertussis varies widely. Classic pertussis is divided into three stages: Catarrhal, paroxysmal, and convalescent. Adolescents, particularly those who have been immunized, are unlikely to show distinct stages of illness. The adolescent may complain only of coughing episodes, with no history of fever or upper respiratory congestion, but the illness often leads to days or weeks of interrupted sleep and time away from school. The physical examination in between coughing episodes may be completely normal. Adolescents rarely develop serious complications.

Laboratory Evaluation
1. *Blood cell counts:* Profound leukocytosis with white blood cell counts from 15,000 to as high as 100,000/mm^3 due to an absolute lymphocytosis may be seen.
2. *Culture:* The incubation period is 10 to 14 days; therefore, culture rarely guides treatment decisions.
3. *Direct immunofluorescence assay (DFA):* DFA of nasopharyngeal secretions may help guide early treatment decisions, but the test is unreliable owing to variable sensitivity and low specificity; culture confirmation of the test should be attempted.
4. *Serology:* No single test is diagnostic, and in order to achieve acceptable sensitivity and specificity, acute and convalescent titers must be obtained.
5. *DNA amplification:* If available, the polymerase chain reaction (PCR) for the diagnosis of pertussis has shown great promise, being rapid, and having a sensitivity of 97% and specificity of 93%.

Differential Diagnosis. Adenovirus, *Mycoplasma pneumoniae*, *Chlamydia pneumoniae*, and influenza.

Diagnosis. Pertussis should be suspected in any adolescent with a complaint of a cough lasting >1 to 2 weeks, regardless of immunization status. A history of posttussive vomiting and a lymphocytosis on laboratory evaluation support the diagnosis, as do the absence of other symptoms such as fever as well as a lack of findings on physical examination. The diagnosis is often made based on clinical evaluation. Increasing use of PCR as a diagnostic tool may improve the ability to make a more timely diagnosis.

Management. All cases of suspected or confirmed pertussis should receive appropriate antibiotic therapy. Treatment may provide some clinical benefit and clearly decreases the spread of infection.

1. Erythromycin 500 mg four times daily for 14 days has been the traditional treatment.
2. Azithromycin has been shown to be as effective as erythromycin and is better tolerated. Dose is 500 mg on the first day and 250 mg daily for 4 additional days.
3. Clarithromycin 500 mg twice daily for 7 days is another alternative.
4. Trimethoprim/sulfamethoxazole is an alternative for those who are unable to tolerate treatment with macrolides. Dose is 1 double-strength tablet twice daily for 14 days.

Control Measures
1. Treatment with a full course of antibiotics is indicated for all household contacts regardless of immunization status, and can limit secondary transmission.
2. Students with pertussis should be excluded from school. Patients are considered no longer infectious after 5 days of antibiotic therapy, and may return to school at that time. If they are unable to take antibiotics, they are considered infectious for 21 days after the onset of cough.

Immunization
Natural and vaccine-induced immunity to pertussis wane over time, leaving adolescents and adults susceptible to infection. Two acellular pertussis vaccines have recently been licensed for use in adolescents (Tdap). Tdap is indicated for routine use in adolescents at 11 to 12 years of age replacing the standard Td booster previously administered at this age. Tdap is also indicated for older adolescents who have not received a prior vaccination, provided that it has been at least 2 years since a previous dose of Td vaccine. Further information on the Tdap vaccine is found in Chapter 4.

INFLUENZA

Although most influenza infections in adolescents are self-limited, those patients with chronic illness such as asthma or cardiac disease may develop a serious life-threatening infection.

Etiology. Influenza viruses are classified as A, B, or C. Influenza A and B are responsible for seasonal epidemics, whereas C is responsible for mild common cold like illnesses. Influenza A and B are indistinguishable clinically. Transmission is via person to person via respiratory droplets or by direct contact with articles recently contaminated by nasopharyngeal secretions. The incubation period is only 1 to 4 days. Patients are most infectious during the 24 hours prior to symptoms, and during the peak of symptoms. Viral shedding continues for about 7 days after the onset of symptoms.

Epidemiology. Although influenza may be sporadically identified through the year, epidemics typically occur annually during the winter months.

Clinical Manifestations
1. *Clinical symptoms* include: Sudden onset of fever and chills, non-productive cough, myalgias, sore throat, malaise, and headache. Nausea, vomiting, diarrhea are more common in younger patients

2. *Clinical signs* include: patient appears unwell, hyperemic mucous membranes, injected conjunctiva, clear rhinorrhea. Fever is often as high as 40 C, peaks within 24 hours of the onset of symptoms, and may last up to 5 days. The dry, hacking cough may persist for up to one week after the other symptoms have resolved.
3. *Complications* include primary viral pneumonia, encephalitis, encephalopathy, Guillain-Barre syndrome, Reye syndrome, and myositis.

Laboratory Evaluation
1. Viral culture is impractical for use in clinical care.
2. Direct fluorescent antibody (DFA) and indirect fluorescent antibody (IFA) staining have low sensitivity (62% to 74%), but high specificity (97% to 98%).
3. Two rapid diagnostic tests are available:
   a. Immunoassay: Sensitivity varies widely, from 40% to 100%, as does specificity, ranging from 63% to 100%.
   b. Viral neuraminidase detection: Sensitivity varies from 48% to 96%, and specificity ranges from 63% to 93%.

Differential Diagnosis
This includes bacterial infections (*Streptococcus pneumoniae, Chlamydia pneumoniae, and Mycoplasma pneumoniae*) and other viral infections (e.g., adenovirus, parainfluenza, respiratory syncytial virus, and rhinovirus)

Diagnosis
The clinical diagnosis of influenza can be difficult, even during peak influenza activity, because many other circulating respiratory viruses exhibit similar symptoms and it is impractical to test every patient with signs and symptoms of influenza. During a seasonal outbreak, the diagnosis should be considered in any adolescent who presents with the sudden onset of fever and a dry, nonproductive cough.

Management
The majority of adolescents require supportive care only. Patient should be cautioned against the use of aspirin because of the potential for the development of Reye syndrome. Patients who have underlying illness or otherwise healthy patients who present for treatment within 48 hours of the onset of symptoms may benefit from treatment with antiviral medications. These medications have been shown to decrease the time to symptom resolution by 1 to 2 days.

1. Amantadine
   a. May cause CNS disturbance
   b. Adolescent treatment dose: 100 mg by mouth twice per day for 5 days.
2. Rimantadine
   a. Causes less CNS disturbance than amantadine
   b. Adolescent treatment dose: 100 mg by mouth twice per day for 5 days.
3. Oseltamivir
   a. Adolescent treatment dose: 75 mg by mouth twice per day for 5 days.
4. Zanamivir
   a. Orally inhaled powder

b. Should not be used in patients with underlying respiratory diseases such as asthma because bronchospasm may occur.

c. Adolescent dose: Two inhalations (5 mg each inhalation) twice per day for 5 days.

Immunization

The primary means for the prevention of influenza is through immunization. In years when there is an ample vaccine supply, influenza vaccine should be encouraged for all adolescents without contraindications to vaccination. Vaccine should be prioritized for adolescents who are at increased risk of developing severe complications due to influenza.

There are two options for immunization: trivalent inactivated influenza vaccine (TIV) and live attenuated influenza vaccine (LAIV). Both vaccines are trivalent, containing two A antigens (representing both the H1N1 and H3N2 subtypes) and a B antigen, and both vaccine viruses are grown in chicken eggs. TIV is a killed virus product administered by intramuscular injection, whereas LAIV is a live attenuated virus product administered intranasally. Neither vaccine should be given to those with a history of an anaphylactic hypersensitivity to eggs or to other specific vaccine components. TIV can be used for both healthy adolescents as well as those with high-risk medical conditions. Use of LAIV should be restricted to healthy adolescents only and should not be administered to those with high-risk medical conditions. In addition, LAIV should not be administered to those with a history of Guillain-Barré syndrome (GBS). The decision to use TIV in patients with a history of GBS should be made on an individual basis. For those at low risk of complications due to influenza and for those who experienced GBS within 6 weeks after receipt of a prior influenza vaccine, TIV should be avoided. Immunization information is updated annually and is available at www.cdc.gov.

REFERENCE

Centers for Disease Control and Prevention. Prevention and control of influenza: recommendations of the Advisory Committee on Immunization Practices (ACIP). *MMWR* 2005;54(No. RR-8):1–40.

CHAPTER 30

Hepatitis

Praveen S. Goday

EPIDEMIOLOGY (TABLE 30.1)

Overall, the U.S. prevalence of hepatitis B is 0.3%; the number of chronically infected persons is estimated at 1.25 million. A decline of 67% from 1990 to 2002 has been noted, reflecting the success of the vaccination program. The prevalence of antibodies to hepatitis C in the United States is about 2%. Injection drug use is responsible for the majority of hepatitis C transmission with a prevalence of antibodies to hepatitis C in users of about 80% to 90%. Aside from drug use, 18% of hepatitis C is associated with sexual exposure, 4% with occupational exposure, and 9% unknown. Screening of organ, tissue, and blood donors for hepatitis C has essentially eliminated the risk of transmission from transplantation and transfusion.

CLINICAL MANIFESTATIONS

It is not possible to distinguish among the types of hepatitis based on clinical presentation. If the date of exposure is known, incubation periods may be helpful in diagnosis: hepatitis A virus (HAV), 2 to 6 weeks; hepatitis B virus (HBV), 2 to 6 months; and hepatitis C virus (HCV), 2 weeks to 6 months.

Symptoms. Common early symptoms of viral hepatitis include fatigue, lassitude, anorexia, nausea, dark urine, drowsiness, low-grade fever, right upper abdominal discomfort, myalgia, and arthralgias. In viral hepatitis B, immune complexes can lead to arthralgias, arthritis, and a rash.

Signs. Icteric sclera, tender hepatomegaly, splenomegaly (10% of cases), arthritis, and rash.

Laboratory Findings. Relative lymphocytosis; elevated serum transaminases; elevation in total and conjugated bilirubin and serum alkaline phosphatase. In severe disease, decreased serum albumin and prothrombin time.

Viral Antigens and Antibodies
1. *Hepatitis A (HAV):* Antibody patterns are shown in Figure 30.1 and Table 30.2.
2. *Hepatitis B* (Fig. 30.2 and Table 30.2)

TABLE 30.1

Clinical and Epidemiological Comparison of Hepatitis Viruses

Characteristics	Hepatitis A	Hepatitis B	Hepatitis C	Hepatitis D	Hepatitis E
Transmission					
Usual	Fecal-oral	Parenteral	Parenteral	Parenteral	Fecal-oral
Alternative	Parenteral (rare)	Frequently nonparenteral (venereal, perinatal)	Venereal, perinatal	Venereal	Possibly parenteral
Distribution	Point-source outbreaks, random cases	Prevalent in young adults and urban populations	Injection drug use, venereal, perinatal	Worldwide; not highly endemic in the United States	Primarily Asia, Africa, Mexico; rare in the United States
Incubation period (d)	15–50	45–160	49–63	Coinfection, 45–60 Superinfection, 14–136	15–60
Onset	Acute	Often insidious	Insidious	Acute or insidious	Acute
Severity	Usually mild, often anicteric	More severe than hepatitis A; less often anicteric	Mild to moderate	Often severe or fulminant	Variable; severe in pregnancy

Chronic disease	None	90% of perinatal cases; 10% of adult cases	50%–60% of cases	Yes	None
Carrier state	None	Yes	Yes	Unknown	Unknown
Case-fatality rate	0%–0.2%	0.3%–15%	Unknown	Unknown	Unknown
Estimated incidence trend in the United States	Decreasing	Decreasing	Decreasing	Unknown	Not endemic in the United States
Estimated proportion of acute hepatitis cases in the United States	~25%	~50%	~20%	Unknown	None

From Koff RS. Hepatitis B today: clinical and diagnostic overview. *Pediatr Infect Dis J* 1993;12:428. Adapted from Hoofnagle JH. Type B hepatitis: virology, serology, and clinical course. *Semin Liver Dis* 1981;1:1.

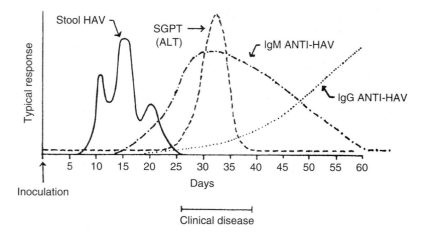

FIGURE 30.1 Course of hepatitis A infection. Anti-HAV, anti-hepatitis A viral antibody; IgG, immunoglobulin G; IgM, immunoglobulin M; SGPT (ALT), alanine transaminase. (Adapted from Centers for Disease Control. Hepatitis Surveillance Report No. 42. Washington, DC: CDC, June 1978.)

a. Hepatitis B surface antigen (HBsAg) positivity indicates either acute or chronic infection and signifies that the patient is capable of transmitting HBV.

b. Anti–hepatitis B surface antigen (anti-HBs) indicates past infection or immunity from immunization.

c. Anti–hepatitis B core antigen (anti-HBc) is extremely helpful in differentiating between acute and past infections. The detection of anti-HBc (IgM) indicates an acute infection, whereas if only anti-HBc (IgG) is present, the illness must be of at least 6 months' standing. Anti-HBc may be the only test that is positive in some individuals during the window period when HBsAg has become negative and before anti-HBs has become positive.

d. Hepatitis e antigen (HBeAg) is usually seen during the incubation phase and correlates with increased viral replication. Persistence of HBeAg beyond 12 weeks is probably indicative of progression to a chronic carrier state or development of chronic HBV infection and high infectivity.

e. Anti–hepatitis B e antigen (anti-HBe) appears with the disappearance of HBeAg and suggests reduced viral replication and a lower infectivity.

3. *Hepatitis C (HCV):* The enzyme immunoassay (EIA) for antibodies against HCV (anti-HCV) serves as a screening test. False-positive tests (e.g., in autoimmune diseases) and false-negative tests (e.g., in immunodeficiency and early hepatitis C) can occur. Qualitative HCV RNA testing is used to confirm the diagnosis of hepatitis C infection.

4. *Delta hepatitis:* Laboratory diagnosis of hepatitis delta virus (HDV) infection is based on tests for anti-HDV or HDV RNA or delta antigen in serum.

TABLE 30.2

Interpretation of Hepatitis Antibody Test Results

IgM Anti-HAV	IgG Anti-HAV	HBsAg	Anti-HBc (IgM)	Anti-HBc (IgG)	Interpretation
+	–	–	–	–	Acute hepatitis A
–	+	–	–	–	Prior hepatitis A infection
–	–	+	–	–	• Person is immune to hepatitis A Acute hepatitis B; early state or chronic carrier with hepatitis of another origin
–	–	+	+	+	Acute hepatitis B
–	–	+	–	+	Chronic carrier state
–	–	–	+	+	Recent hepatitis B
–	–	–	–	–	Non-A, non-B hepatitis, other viruses, or other causes

Anti-HAV, antibody to hepatitis A virus; anti-HBc, antibody to hepatitis B core antigen; HBsAg, hepatitis B surface antigen; Ig, immunoglobulin.

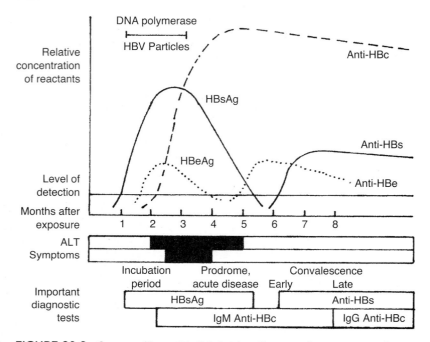

FIGURE 30.2 Course of hepatitis B infection. Pattern of symptoms and serologic tests. ALT, alanine aminotransferase; Anti-HBc, hepatitis B core antibody; Anti-HBe, hepatitis B e antibody; Anti-HBs, hepatitis B surface antibody; HBeAg, hepatitis B e antigen; HBsAg, hepatitis B surface antigen; HBV, hepatitis B virus; Ig, immunoglobulin. (From Hollinger FB. Hepatitis markers: guide to test selection. *Diagnosis* 1986; Aug:58.)

CLINICAL COURSE

1. *Viral hepatitis A:* The clinical course is summarized in Figure 30.1.
    a. More than 75% of adolescents and adults are symptomatic (compared with children <3 years of age, who are usually asymptomatic).
    b. Some 95% of patients have a 4- to 6-week course.
    c. Clinical symptoms appear as IgM antibodies, and liver enzymes rise.
    d. As clinical symptoms disappear and IgM antibodies fall, IgG antibodies rise.
    e. The virus is maximally excreted 2 weeks prior to the onset of symptoms. Patients are usually considered noninfectious 1 week after the onset of jaundice.
2. *Viral hepatitis B:* The typical clinical course is summarized in Figure 30.2.
    a. HBsAg and HBeAg titers rise 4 to 8 weeks after exposure and 4 to 8 weeks before clinical symptoms appear.
    b. Liver transaminases rise and clinical symptoms appear.
    c. HBsAg may peak and fall in uncomplicated cases or remain positive in chronic carriers.

    d. Anti-HBc titers rise as HBsAg titers fall.

    e. Anti-HBs appears weeks to months after HBsAg disappears.

    f. A "window phase" may exist in which HBsAg is negative before anti-HBs appears. During this phase, anti-HBc IgM will be positive.

    g. Chronic HBV infection is defined as either the presence of HBsAg in serum for at least 6 months or the presence of HBsAg in the absence of anti-HBc IgM. Age is a factor in the likelihood of developing chronic HBV infection; <5% of acutely infected adolescents and adults develop chronic infection. However, chronic HBV infection can lead to cirrhosis or hepatocellular carcinoma.

3. *Hepatitis C*

    a. The clinical course varies from asymptomatic infection (up to 70%) to icteric hepatitis (25%) to fulminant liver failure (rare).

    b. Chronic disease develops in about 60% of patients.

    c. Some 10% to 25% of patients with chronic disease develop cirrhosis.

    d. HCV is strongly associated with the development of hepatocellular carcinoma.

4. *Delta hepatitis:* HDV in association with HBV can cause a more severe form of acute hepatitis than HBV alone and can lead to accelerated progression of HBV-related chronic liver disease.

DIFFERENTIAL DIAGNOSIS

This includes drug-induced hepatitis, alcoholic hepatitis, toxic hepatitis, any of the "alphabet" viruses (hepatitis A, B, C, E; HDV may occur along with or complicate HBV infection), and other viruses (e.g., herpes simplex, cytomegalovirus, Epstein-Barr virus, varicella, enteroviruses such as coxsackie B or echovirus, rubella, and adenovirus).

DIAGNOSIS

1. Clinical history may suggest a toxin, drug, or exposure to a source of hepatitis A, B, or C.

2. Order IgM anti-HAV, HBsAg, anti-HBc IgM, anti-HCV EIA, and a mononucleosis spot test (Table 30.2). If hepatitis C is suspected, a qualitative RNA test will be needed, as there is high likelihood of a false-negative EIA in this scenario.

PREGNANCY CONSIDERATIONS WITH HEPATITIS B AND C

1. *Hepatitis B:* Transmission of HBV infection from mother to infant during the perinatal period is extremely high. Presence of HbeAg in HbsAg-positive mothers substantially increases the risk of perinatal transmission. Recommendations to prevent perinatal transmission include the following:

    a. All pregnant women should be routinely tested for HBsAg at the first prenatal visit of each pregnancy. If at high risk, HBsAg testing can be repeated later in the pregnancy.

b. Infants born to HbsAg-positive mothers are treated with both hepatitis B immune globulin (HBIG) and hepatitis B vaccine. Dose recommendations are given in Table 30.3.

c. Testing of infants for HBsAg and anti-HBs is recommended at 9 to 15 months of age to evaluate the success of therapy. If HBsAg is not detectable and anti-HBs is present, the child can be considered protected.

d. Breast feeding can be allowed even prior to the first dose of HBIG and can continue following immunizations.

2. *Hepatitis C:* Transmission to the infant occurs in 5% of pregnant women with HCV. Coinfection with human immunodeficiency virus (HIV) increases transmission.

a. An anti-HCV EIA should be performed at the first prenatal visit for pregnant women at high risk for exposure. HCV RNA testing should be performed if anti-HCV is positive. Women at high risk include those with a history of injection drug use, repeated exposure to blood products, prior blood transfusion, or organ transplants.

b. Breast feeding poses no important risk of HCV transmission if nipples are not traumatized and maternal hepatitis C is quiescent.

c. Infants of women with hepatitis C should be tested for HCV RNA on two occasions, between the ages of 2 and 6 months and again at 18 to 24 months.

PREVENTION

Hepatitis A

1. Good hand hygiene is central to the prevention of hepatitis A for those working in environments with possible exposure (e.g., day care centers). Food hygiene is also important.

2. *Hepatitis A prophylaxis:* Human immune serum globulin (HISG) and hepatitis A vaccine are available for prophylaxis against hepatitis A. The indications for both HISG and the vaccine are given in Table 30.4. Whenever postexposure prophylaxis is attempted, HISG should be used, as data are limited on the effectiveness of the vaccine alone.

a. HISG is at least 85% effective in preventing hepatitis A when given intramuscularly within 2 weeks after exposure and also affords short-term protection against hepatitis A. HISG should be given along with hepatitis A vaccine (at a separate anatomic site) for those with risk for further exposures to hepatitis A. The usual dose of HISG is 0.02 mL/kg of body weight, which provides effective protection for up to 3 months.

b. Two inactivated hepatitis A vaccines are available: Havrix (SmithKline Beecham Biologicals) and Vaqta (Merck, Inc.). Havrix is approved for children over 2 years of age and Vaqta is approved for children over 12 months of age. Both are available in adult and pediatric formulations. Two doses are recommended. Persons are considered to be protected by 4 weeks after the initial dose of hepatitis A vaccine. For long-term protection, a second dose is needed 6 to 12 months later. Also available is Twinrix, which includes both hepatitis A and B vaccines. Using three doses of Twinrix produces similar seroprotection for hepatitis A and B as using vaccines for A and B separately. Recommended dosing is at 0, 1, and 6 months.

TABLE 30.3

Recommended Doses of Currently Licensed Hepatitis B Vaccines[a]

Group	Recombivax-HB		Engerix-B	
	μg	mL	μg	mL
Infants of HBsAg-negative mothers, children, and adolescents (<20 yr)	5	0.5	10	0.5
Infants of HBsAg-positive mothers; (HBIG [0.5 mL] also recommended)	5	0.5	10	0.5
Adults (>20 yr)	10	1.0	20	1.0
Dialysis patients and other immunocompromised persons	40	1.0[b]	40	2.0[c]

HBsAg, hepatitis B surface antigen; HBIG, hepatitis B immune globulin.

[a]Both vaccines are routinely administered in a three-dose series. Engerix-B has also been licensed for a four-dose series administered at 0, 1, 2, and 12 mo.

[b]Special formulation.

[c]Two 1-mL doses administered at one site, in a four-dose schedule at 0, 1, 2, and 6 mo.

Adapted from American Academy of Pediatrics. Committee on Infectious Diseases. *Red Book 2003*. AAP, 2003:318.

TABLE 30.4

Persons Needing Hepatitis A Vaccine or Immune Globulin

Hepatitis A vaccine

Children at least 2 years of age living in a state (Alaska, Arizona, California, Idaho, Nevada, New Mexico, Oklahoma, Oregon, South Dakota, Utah, or Washington) or a county with a high rate of infection (≥20 cases per 100,000 population from 1987 through 1997)

Travelers at least 1 year of age to countries with high or intermediate rates of disease

Men who have sex with men

Users of illicit drugs, both injecting and noninjecting

Persons who have chronic liver disease

Persons who use clotting factor concentrates

Laboratory personnel who work with the hepatitis A virus

Military personnel

Day care attendees older than 1 yr

Immune globulin

Persons who will be traveling to countries with high or intermediate rates of disease within the next 2 wk

Children younger than 1 yr who will be traveling to countries with high rates of disease

People who need the vaccine but are allergic to it or do not wish to take it

For postexposure prophylaxis, within 14 d of exposure:

a. Persons who have been exposed to food that was handled by someone with acute hepatitis A, who had either poor hygiene or diarrhea

b. Persons exposed to a family member with acute hepatitis A

Adapted from Craig AS, Schaffner W. Prevention of hepatitis A with the hepatitis A vaccine. *N Engl J Med* 2004;350:476.

Hepatitis B

1. *Preexposure prophylaxis:* Hepatitis B vaccine is recommended for all babies at birth and for all children and adolescents not previously vaccinated. The vaccine is usually given in three separate doses at 0, 1, and 6 months. These three doses induce protective antibodies (anti-HBs) in >90% of healthy adults and >95% of infants, children, and adolescents. The deltoid muscle is the recommended site for the vaccination in adults and adolescents. Pregnancy or lactation is not a contraindication to vaccination.

2. *Hepatitis B postexposure prophylaxis:* Prophylactic treatment to prevent hepatitis B in unimmunized persons should be considered in the following situations:

   a. Perinatal exposure of an infant born to an HBsAg-positive mother (see above).

   b. Persons with acute exposure to blood: For greatest effectiveness, passive prophylaxis with HBIG (0.06 mL/kg) should be given as soon as possible after exposure. The first dose of the vaccine should be given

simultaneously but at a different site (see http://www.cdc.gov/mmwr/
PDF/rr/rr5011.pdf).

   c. Sexual contacts with HBsAg-positive persons: Screening of sexual partners for hepatitis antibodies (anti-HBc or anti-HBs) before treatment is
recommended but should not delay treatment beyond 14 days after last
exposure. Treatment consists of HBIG (0.06 mL/kg) along with the hepatitis vaccine series.

   d. Household contacts of persons with acute infection: Prophylaxis is not
indicated unless there is exposure to blood of the index case (e.g., sharing
of toothbrushes or razors). If indicated, treatment is with both HBIG and
vaccine. If the index patient becomes a carrier, all household contacts
should receive hepatitis B vaccine.

Delta Hepatitis

Because HDV is dependent on HBV for replication, prevention of HBV infection
suffices to prevent delta hepatitis.

GENERAL APPROACH TO MANAGEMENT

1. Restriction of physical activity is not needed; activity as tolerated.
2. *Diet:* There is no evidence that any special diet affects the course of the
disease.
3. Adolescents should avoid alcoholic beverages, oral contraceptives,
steroids, and all hepatotoxic drugs until transaminases return to normal.
4. Severe disease is indicated by (a) elevated prothrombin time (this is the only
truly prognostic liver function test); (b) albumin <2.5 g/dL; or (c) evidence
of ascites, edema, or encephalopathy.
5. Most cases of hepatitis in adolescents can be managed at home. If severe
disease is present or if hydration cannot be maintained in the outpatient
setting because of nausea and vomiting, hospitalization is indicated.
6. When the prothrombin time is elevated, it must be followed closely and
the patient may have to be hospitalized. If the prothrombin time is normal
(or once it returns to normal), the concentrations of serum bilirubin and
transaminases should be monitored weekly during the acute illness, then
every 2 to 3 weeks as the teen improves and enzymes fall. Monitoring can
be stopped when liver enzymes return to normal.
7. Treatment of chronic hepatitis is beyond the scope of this book. Therapy
should be managed by a specialist in the treatment of chronic hepatitis.

COMPLICATIONS

1. Systemic complications such as pancreatitis, myocarditis, atypical pneumonia, aplastic anemia, transverse myelitis, and glomerulonephritis
2. Hepatic complications such as
   a. Fulminant hepatitis
   b. Chronic carrier state (HbsAg-positive for >6 months)
   c. Chronic hepatitis
   d. Cirrhosis and its complications, including chronic liver failure and hepatocellular carcinoma

WEB SITES AND REFERENCES

http://www.cdc.gov/ncidod/diseases/hepatitis/. CDC hepatitis resource page.

Centers for Disease Control and Prevention. Hepatitis B virus: a comprehensive strategy for eliminating transmission in the United States through universal childhood vaccination. Recommendations of the Immunization Practices Advisory Committee (ACIP). *MMWR Morb Mortal Wkly Rep* 1991;40[No. RR-13]:1.

CHAPTER 31

Human Immunodeficiency Virus Infections and Acquired Immunodeficiency Syndrome

Marvin E. Belzer, Miguel Martinez, and Lawrence S. Neinstein

Acquired immunodeficiency syndrome (AIDS) is one of the largest pandemics to hit modern society. The last decade has seen a dramatic reduction in the mortality from AIDS in developed countries. When taken correctly, combinations of antiretroviral medications called highly active antiretroviral therapy (HAART) enable most infected patients to have long, healthy lives. The greatest challenges for care providers of adolescents infected with human immunodeficiency virus (HIV) involve identifying infected persons, engaging them in care, and helping them with long-term adherence to these medications. Unfortunately, only a fraction of the estimated 20,000 annual new cases of HIV infection in 13- to 25-year-olds in United States receive care while these patients are still adolescents or young adults. Internationally, the impact on youth is even higher, with an estimated 50% of new HIV infections occurring in youth. Developing countries have limited access to the lifesaving medications. Special issues are important to consider in relation to the adolescent population and infection with HIV, including a host of legal and ethical dilemmas regarding testing, disclosure of information, and consent for treatment in research protocols. For HIV-infected adolescents, there is also the problem of availability of age-appropriate services. Adolescents are in danger of contracting HIV because of their risky sexual behaviors, drug use, or both. The treatment of HIV has become so complex that recommendations have been made that all HIV-infected persons should be treated by physicians with expertise in HIV medications, their side effects, and interactions as well the psychosocial interventions required to maintain adherence.

EPIDEMIOLOGY

1. *Cases:* Through the end of 2005, a total of 956,019 persons in the United States had been reported as having AIDS. About 13.8% of HIV/AIDS cases were reported in 13- to 24-year-olds at their age of diagnosis. In addition,

about 12.3% of HIV/AIDS cases involve 25- to 29-year-olds at their age of diagnosis. The number of AIDS cases reported annually among teens aged 13 to 19 increased between 1998 to 2003 but dropped in 2004, and rose again in 2005. For those between the ages of 20 and 24, there has been an increase every year from 2000 to 2005.

2. *Gender and ethnicity:* In 2005, males made up over 64% of HIV/AIDS in 13- to 19-year-olds and 72% in 20- to 24-year-olds. This difference increases with age and for all adults 25 years and older; in 2005, over 75% were males with HIV/AIDS. African Americans are overrepresented, making up 69% of all cases of HIV/AIDS in youth aged 13 to 19 years in 2005.

3. *Transmission:* Most new cases in male adolescents and adults (85%) are in men who have sex with men and injection drug users, with about 13% representing the latter group only. Heterosexual contact (80%) is the main reported mode of transmission among female adolescents and adults, with about 19% representing injection drug use.

Blood, semen, vaginal secretions, and breast milk are the only fluids documented to be associated with HIV infection. Although HIV is found in saliva, tears, urine, and sweat, no case has been documented that implicates these fluids as agents of infection. The CDC has provided guidelines for reducing the spread of HIV and hepatitis through the sharing of needles (http://www.cdc.gov/hiv/topics/research/prs/index.htm). Within the hierarchy of risk for HIV transmission, receptive anal intercourse without condoms is riskiest, followed by insertive anal intercourse and vaginal intercourse. Oral sex is categorized as less risky in this model but has been shown to transmit HIV. Studies have shown that the proper and consistent use of latex condoms or dental dams can markedly reduce the risk for HIV transmission during sex.

The risk to health professionals of infection caused by needle sticks from HIV-infected patients is estimated to be 1 in 200 to 1 in 500. Injuries involving injection of blood are much riskier than simple pricks. Current CDC recommendations include consideration of rapid treatment within hours, with multiple medications, after the occurrence of a needle stick from a known HIV-infected patient (postexposure prophylaxis), with consultation with an HIV expert (http://www.ucsf.edu/hivcntr/PEPline/index.html) and hotline (888-448-4911). These resources can also be used for nonoccupational exposure to HIV though exposure to blood, genital secretions, or infectious body fluids.

DEVELOPMENTAL ISSUES RELATED TO HIV INFECTIONS IN ADOLESCENTS

Although most youth do not undergo extreme turmoil and distress in their teenage years, adolescence provides many opportunities for risk for youth with regard to HIV infection owing to (1) cognitive and emotional development; (2) social, behavioral, and physiologic development; and (3) family relationships.

Cognitive and Emotional Development. Factors that put teens at increased risk for AIDS include: (1) Greater experimentation and a greater degree of influence by peer behaviors; (2) naïveté and lack of good judgment; (3) feelings of immortality and invulnerability; (4) ignorance of modes of AIDS transmission and prevention; (5) denial of personal risk; (6) identification with moral codes (i.e., those of peers) other than those of parents.

Social, Behavioral, and Physiologic Development. Adolescent behaviors that increase teens' risk for HIV infection include the following:

1. *Sexual activity:* A high percentage of adolescents engage in sexual intercourse, often without a barrier contraceptive or any contraceptive. In 2005, 46.8% of high school students (http://www.cdc.gov/HealthyYouth/yrbs/index.htm) reported that they had had sexual intercourse. Many adolescent males (17% to 37%) report having had at least one same-sex experience. Although reported condom use at last sex has increased from 46.2% in 1991 to 63% in 2005, there is still risk for HIV infection through unprotected intercourse.
2. *Sexually transmitted diseases (STDs):* The high prevalence of STDs (one in four) among adolescents is an indicator of high-risk behavior and the lack of condom use.
3. *Illicit drug use:* Estimates are that 1 in 50 high school juniors and seniors have injected drugs, while 23.3% of high school students have reported use of alcohol or drugs before last sex.
4. *Runaway behavior:* About 1 million teenagers run away each year; many of these are involved in high-risk behaviors, including injection drug use and survival sex (sex for money, food, or a place to stay).
5. *Physiologic factors:* Adolescent girls may be at increased risk of HIV infection because of (a) differences in the cervix of the adolescent female (more columnar epithelium); (b) alterations of the vaginal pH as compared with that in the adult; (c) differences in menstrual patterns.

Family Relationships. Unresolved issues can lead to powerful conflicts between parents and adolescents. Sometimes the dysfunctional nature of the teen's family significantly increases the chances of the teen's involvement in high-risk behavior.

HIV TESTING

Most laboratories offer enzyme immunosorbent assay (EIA) screening with a confirmatory Western blot analysis for any blood specimen with two consecutive positive EIA test results. A positive EIA test result should never be reported to a patient as a positive test result for HIV. A positive Western blot has almost 100% specificity. Western blot tests can be indeterminate. This is common for patients in the "window" phase between acute infection and seroconversion. However, many patients with indeterminate tests will later test HIV negative by EIA or Western blot. It is recommended that testing be repeated until a definitive positive or negative test occurs. This can be performed after 1, 3, and 6 months for an indeterminate Western blot. The time delay from HIV infection to positive Western blot averages 21 days with newer test reagents. False-positive serology results may occur in 1 of 200,000 cases. Factitious reporting of HIV infection occurs as well. In confusing cases—including indeterminate results, false reporting, and patients who are potentially in the window period—HIV DNA or RNA determination by polymerase chain reaction (PCR) may be helpful in clarifying serostatus.

The technology for HIV testing has expanded greatly. In addition to blood tests, tests of oral secretions and urine are approved by the U.S. Food and Drug

Administration (FDA). Oral secretion tests have sensitivity and specificity similar to those of blood, while urine tests are slightly less sensitive. Positive tests must be confirmed, and this must be incorporated into pretest counseling. The CDC website (http://www.cdc.gov/hiv/topics/testing/rapid/) has extensive information on the use of rapid HIV testing, including specific recommendation for providers regarding the Clinical Laboratory Improvement Amendments (CLIA) program, counseling, and quality assurance guidelines. As of 2006, the current tests include (1) OraQuick Advance Rapid HIV-1/2 Antibody test (Oral fluid, whole blood or plasma); (2) Reveal G-2 Rapid HIV-1 Antibody test (serum or plasma); (3) Uni-Gold Recombingen HIV test (Whole blood, serum or plasma; and (4) Multispot HIV-1/HIV-2 Rapid test (serum or plasma). All of these tests have sensitivities in the 99% to 100% range and specificities in the 98.6% to 99.9% range. One benefit to rapid testing is that it nearly eliminates the problem of youth not returning for their results. Most rapid tests have CLIA waivers, although some states may have additional regulations.

Consent and Confidentiality. Health care practitioners must balance the protection of adolescents' rights against the amount of information needed to deliver proper care.

1. *Individuals >18 years of age who are competent:* These individuals must give an informed consent for HIV testing, which involves a dialogue concerning the risks and benefits of the test, the implications of the test, and alternatives to the test. However, in 2006, the CDC recommended that adults, adolescent, and pregnant women in all health care settings receive HIV testing after being informed and given a chance to opt out (http://www.cdc.gov/mmwR/preview/mmwrhtml/rr5514a1.htm). The CDC also recommended that separate written consent (from the general medical consent) not be required and that prevention counseling should not be required for HIV diagnostic testing or as part of HIV screening programs.
2. *Individuals between 12 and 17 years of age:* The laws vary widely from state to state. In most states, the adolescent can and must give his or her own consent; however, as with any informed consent, the individual must be considered by the practitioner as competent to give an informed consent.
3. *Individuals <12 years of age and incompetent adolescents:* For these individuals, a third party (parent or guardian) authorizes the testing. However, this authorization may be restricted by state laws.

To Whom Should HIV Testing Be Offered? In 2006, as indicated above, the CDC modified its recommendations to advise that HIV testing be routinized for all sexually active adolescents and adults under age 64 when they access health care. Youth should be advised that they will be tested and given the option to decline. Separate written consent is no longer recommended by the CDC but many states have laws requiring written informed consent. The following groups are high risk and should have repeat testing at least annually: (1) men who have sex with men (as many youth in this group may not self-identify as gay or bisexual); (2) youth who share needles (including tattooing, ear piercing, steroid injection, and recreational drugs); (3) youth with partners from the above two groups; (4) youth who have had intercourse or shared needles with HIV-infected persons; (5) youth with STDs; (6) sexually active youth from economically disadvantaged areas or areas of high seroprevalence; (7) youth with multiple sexual partners.

Who Should Have HIV Testing Deferred? (1) Suicidal teens and those who seriously state they would be suicidal if HIV positive; (2) intoxicated and drug-withdrawing youth; (3) severely mentally ill youth who cannot provide consent for testing.

Methods for HIV Testing
1. *Anonymous testing:* Patients are not identified by name but are given a number.
2. *Confidential testing:* Pretest and posttest counseling is done, and the results are part of the medical record. Normal laws regarding patient confidentiality still protect clients.
3. *Youth-specific testing:* Many testing sites now have counselors (including peers) who are specifically trained to work with adolescents and are located where other services are available for teens (e.g., homeless shelters, free clinics, schools, recreation centers, mobile testing vans).

HIV COUNSELING AND TESTING

The primary goals of HIV testing include identifying patients who are infected with HIV and providing linkage to appropriate health care and supportive services. The CDC is moving in a direction of increasing the ability and frequency of detecting HIV and avoiding prevention counseling as a possible impediment to HIV testing. Although HIV prevention counseling is no longer required for HIV testing, Donna Futterman, MD, has developed the ACTS (Assess, Consent, Test, Support) system to assist practitioners with brief HIV counseling and testing for adolescents (Table 31.1).

Posttest Counseling for Positive Tests. HIV-positive youth need counseling on the treatment of HIV, prevention of transmission, and disclosure to family, friends, and sexual partners.

MANAGEMENT OF HIV INFECTION IN ADOLESCENTS

Management of youth infected with HIV is best conducted by an HIV specialist. Primary care providers need to understand issues around primary care and evaluation of acute medical concerns that may be associated with having HIV. The specialty clinic should have a multidisciplinary team including a physician, social worker, nurse, and other caregivers.

Vaccinations
1. *Hepatitis A*: Recommended for all at-risk individuals.
2. *Hepatitis B*: Recommended for all patients without evidence of hepatitis B immunity or chronic infection. Retrospective studies demonstrate that many youth with HIV do not develop antibodies to hepatitis B after three immunizations. Physicians can consider a fourth immunization or repeating the series after the patient begins HAART.

TABLE 31.1

ACTS: A Rapid System for HIV Counseling and Testing

Assess need for HIV testing, care, or prevention counseling
- Explain benefits of testing for patient's health and prevention.
- Discuss modes of HIV transmission (e.g., sex, needles, perinatal).
- Review risk assessment form or explain to patient that HIV testing is advisable if the patient has: (a) ever had sex, (b) has had inter-course without a condom, (c) has ever used recreational drugs intra-venously, or (d) shared intravenous syringes and works.
- Recommend testing, discuss HIV prevention, and provide referrals as appropriate.

Counsel and obtain consent
- Clarify the meaning of positive and negative results and explore patient's potential reactions.
- Assess readiness for immediate testing, including patient's social support network.
- Review health department requirements, such as the difference between confidential and anonymous testing and names reporting, partner notification, and domestic violence screening.
- Obtain consent.

Test
- Describe/provide HIV test (e.g., blood, oral, urine, rapid).
- Make appointment to deliver results in person, by phone, or have patient wait for rapid results.

Support during testing and afterward

HIV-negative patients
- Clarify need to retest in 3 months (e.g., window period, based on risk assessment).
- Provide prevention strategies and referrals; HIV testing alone is not prevention.

HIV-positive patients
- Provide support and link to care and prevention.
- Review HIV reporting, partner notification, and domestic/partner violence issues.

Complete ACTS training materials are available at www.adolescentaids.org.

HIV, human immunodeficiency virus.
From Futterman DC. HIV and AIDS in adolescents. *Adolesc Med Clin* 2004;15:369 with permission.

3. *HPV:* HIV infection is not a contraindication (it is not a live vaccine), and in the HIV-infected population, it could be a real positive. However, it is not clear if the efficacy in the immune-suppressed population will be as high as the non–immune-suppressed population. Although HPV vaccine is currently FDA-approved only for females between the ages of 9 and 26,

the significant morbidity and even mortality associated with HPV-related disease in men who have sex with men argues for the early adoption of vaccination for men into clinical practice.

4. *Influenza:* Should be offered annually in October or November to all HIV-infected individuals. In patients not receiving HAART, the viral load may increase transiently after vaccination, but it returns to baseline in approximately 1 month. Intranasal vaccination is contraindicated.

5. *Measles-mumps-rubella (MMR):* All patients should have received two MMR vaccinations in their lifetimes. MMR is considered safe in patients with HIV but should not be used if severe immunosuppression is present (severe immunosuppression is not defined, but one might use a CD4 under 200 in this setting).

6. *Meningococcal vaccination:* Persons with HIV are likely at increased risk for meningococcal disease. They may elect to receive the conjugate quadrivalent vaccine, although its efficacy in this population is unknown.

7. *Pertussis (acellular pertussis):* Adolescents and young adults are being recommended to be revaccinated with Tdap. HIV is not a contraindication (it is not a live virus), but the response in those who are immunosuppressed might be suboptimal.

8. *Pneumococcal*: Should be given once to previously unimmunized individuals.

9. *Polio:* Patients requiring primary or booster immunizations should receive the inactive form, inactivated poliovirus (IPV), not the oral poliovirus vaccine (OPV).

10. *Tetanus-diphtheria*: Same as if uninfected.

11. *Varicella (chickenpox):* The vaccine for prevention of varicella (Varavax, which is live attenuated varicella virus vaccine) is *not* advised for use in those with acquired or primary immunodeficiencies. Research using this vaccine in persons previously infected with varicella is in progress. Zostavax (live attenuated varicella vaccine for those over age 60) is used for the prevention of shingles and is contraindicated in those with immunosuppressive diseases including AIDS.

Early manifestations of HIV infection include the following:

Chronic lymphadenopathy	Pruritic papular eruptions
Unexplained weight loss	Oral hairy leukoplakia
Xerosis	Frequent tinea
Severe molluscum contagiosum	Leukopenia
Seborrheic dermatitis	Exacerbations of psoriasis
Isolated thrombocytopenia	Fatigue and malaise

Opportunistic diseases, including infections and neoplasms, typically occur after immune suppression reaches a certain level (Table 31.2).

Management of Sexually Transmitted Infections. See Chapter 60 and (http://www.cdc.gov/STD/treatment/). Cervical dysplasia has been shown to be very prevalent in women with HIV; spontaneous regression appears to be less common. Annual screening after initiating sexual activity (rather than delaying for 3 years, as is now recommended for HIV-negative patients), and referral for colposcopy for both low- and high-grade squamous intraepithelial lesions or recurrent atypical results on Pap smears are recommended.

TABLE 31.2

Opportunistic Diseases

CD4+ T-cell Count (per mm³)	Condition
200–500	Thrush Kaposi sarcoma Tuberculosis reactivation Herpes zoster Bacterial sinusitis/pneumonia Herpes simplex
100–200	*Pneumocystis carinii* pneumonia All of the above
50–100	Systemic fungal infections Primary tuberculosis Cryptosporidiosis Cerebral toxoplasmosis Progressive multifocal leukoencephalopathy Peripheral neuropathy Cervical carcinoma
0–50	Cytomegalovirus disease Disseminated *Mycobacterium avium* complex Non-Hodgkin lymphoma Central nervous system lymphoma AIDS dementia complex

AIDS, acquired immunodeficiency syndrome.
From Phari JP, Murphy RL. *Contemporary diagnosis and management of HIV/AIDS infections*. Newton, PA: Handbooks in Health Care, 1999 with permission.

Management of Family Planning. With the marked improvements in prevention of maternal-child transmission of HIV, family planning has changed. Many youth now acknowledge their interest in having children despite having HIV. The risk of maternal-child transmission of HIV is about 23% without antiretroviral treatment. The current standard of care is to treat infected women who desire pregnancy with HAART (minimum of three antiretrovirals). The risk of transmission has been shown to be <4% for women taking HAART, and it is probably <1% when a patient conceives while following an effective HAART regimen (i.e., viral load is undetectable) (http://www.cdc.gov/mmwr/PDF/rr/rr5118.pdf) and maintains the program during pregnancy. Data from a cohort of HIV-infected adolescents indicated that the majority of adolescents reported condoms as their main method of contraception, but they were frequently used irregularly. Contraceptives utilizing estrogen may be less effective in patients using protease inhibitors (which increase estrogen metabolism).

Travel. Visiting regions outside one's normal community can expose an individual to many pathogens. In developing countries, opportunities for exposure to enteric pathogens exist, including *Cryptosporidium* and *Isospora*. Risk for certain respiratory infections such as coccidioidomycosis, histoplasmosis, and TB also increases in many developing countries and in certain geographic regions of the United States (CDC international travelers' hotline at telephone 877-FYI-TRIP and http://www.cdc.gov/travel/). Patients should discuss preventive strategies to: (1) avoid contaminated food and drink (i.e., tap water); (2) receive appropriate immunizations; (3) take appropriate medications and telephone numbers for emergency care; (4) seek medical attention promptly if fever, diarrhea, or other illness occurs during or after travel.

Sports Participation. There have been no documented cases of HIV transmission during athletic participation. We would not withhold a youth from competitive sports (even full-contact sports like wrestling or football) solely on the basis of HIV-positive status. However, no participant with an open wound should compete, and universal precautions should be followed.

Evaluation of Specific Syndromes
Pulmonary (Cough or Shortness of Breath)
1. If the CD4+ T-cell count is ≤200/mL or the percentage of CD4+ T cells percent is ≤14%, the patient requires the following: (a) Chest radiographic examination for interstitial or other infiltrates; (b) pulse oxymetry or arterial blood gas determination for hypoxemia; (c) consideration of induced sputum or bronchoscopy for *Pneumocystis jiroveci* pneumonia.
2. In patients with a CD4+ count ≥200/mL and a percentage ≥14%, it is unlikely to be PCP: Consider (a) evaluation for bronchitis, sinusitis, TB, and bacterial pneumonia; (b) chest radiographic examination or sinus films; (c) subsequent PPD; (d) sputum for culture and sensitivity, acid–fast bacillus.

Fever. Evaluation in patients who have severe immunosuppression (CD4+ T-cell count <200/mL) but lack of specific organ system signs or symptoms includes (1) chest radiographic examination for interstitial infiltrates consistent with *Pneumocystis jiroveci* pneumonia, *Mycobacterium avium* complex (MAC), or CMV, focal infiltrates consistent with TB, or bacterial pneumonia; (2) complete blood count: anemia is common in MAC; (3) chemistry panel: elevated lactate dehydrogenase is common in *Pneumocystis*; elevated alkaline phosphatase is common in MAC; (4) blood cultures for bacteria, virus (CMV), fungus, and acid-fast bacillus; (5) serum cryptococcal antigen.

If fever persists and the above tests are inconclusive, consider the following: (1) lumbar puncture for cryptococcal infection; (2) bone marrow biopsy for disseminated MAC, CMV, or fungus; (3) ophthalmology consultation for CMV; (4) body CT for lymphoma; (5) sinus films. In patients with mild immunosuppression (CD4+ T-cell count 200 to 500/mL), look for common illnesses (viral or bacterial) and TB, sinusitis, and pneumonia. In patients with minimal immune suppression (CD4+ T-cell count > 500/mL), avoid costly workups unless conservative evaluation fails.

Diarrhea. (Always assess whether this could be medication-related.) In patients with severe immunodeficiency (CD4+ T-cell count <200/mL): (1) If mild, consider empiric treatment with diphenoxylate (Lomotil) or loperamide (Imodium). (2) If severe, check stool for ova and parasites, culture and sensitivity, *Cryptosporidium, Cyclospora* or *Isospora* infection. (3) If tests are inconclusive, consider colonoscopy looking for CMV, MAC, *Microsporidium*, and *Isospora.*

In patients without severe immunodeficiency: (1) Diarrhea is usually self-limited and costly evaluations should be avoided. (2) Consider stool ova and parasites, stool for *Clostridium difficile* toxin, bacterial culture, and sensitivity if the patient is sexually active, is homeless, or has had recent foreign travel.

Neurologic (New Headaches, Seizures, Focal Neurological Signs). In patients with severe immunodeficiency (CD4+ T-cell count <200/mL): (1) emergency CT or MRI of head for toxoplasmosis and primary central nervous system lymphoma; (2) lumbar puncture for cell count, protein, cryptococcal antigen, Gram stain, routine acid-fast bacillus and fungal cultures, and VDRL.

Dysphagia. In patients with severe immunodeficiency (CD4+ T-cell count <200/mL): (1) If oral thrush is present, consider empiric treatment for *Candida* organisms with fluconazole or ketoconazole. (2) If there is no oral thrush or empiric treatment fails, try endoscopy with evaluations for fungus, CMV, and herpes simplex virus.

Prophylaxis

Prophylaxis is one of the most important ways that patients with severe immunosuppression can maintain their health. Patients who have severe immune suppression but are not ready for HAART should still be encouraged to use prophylaxis.

Primary Prophylaxis. The CDC frequently publishes updated guidelines for primary prophylaxis (http://aidsinfo.nih.gov/ContentFiles/OIpreventionGL. pdf).

Antiretroviral Therapy. The CDC regularly updates guidelines on the use of antiretrovirals for adolescents and adults and should be consulted (http://aidsinfo.nih.gov/ContentFiles/AdultandAdolescentGL.pdf) with the assistance of an HIV specialist. The National AIDS Clearing has a report titled, *Helping Adolescents with HIV Adhere to HAART* (http://www.cdc.gov/mmwr/preview/mmwrhtml/00001789.htm).

Initiating Highly Active Antiretroviral Therapy (HAART). Although the U.S. Department of Health and Human Services publishes guidelines for the initiation of HAART with adolescents and adults that are based primarily on a patient's immune status (CD4+ T-cell count) and risk for disease progression (viral load, HIV RNA), there has been considerable attention to the issue of a patient's ability to adhere strictly to a regimen over the long term. Decisions to initiate therapy must be made jointly by a well-informed patient and his or her health care providers.

HIV Prevention

Primary. Until a vaccine is found, behavioral interventions, comprehensive school-based health education, blood supply screening, postexposure prophylaxis, and access to sterile needles are the main tools to reduce the risk of infection.

Appropriate educational interventional goals for HIV-negative adolescents include the following: (1) Reducing misinformation and prejudice against HIV-infected persons. (2) Helping to reduce high-risk behavior, including recommendations to decrease sexual activity, numbers of sexual partners, and experimentation with drugs. (3) Supporting those who choose abstinence. (4) Increasing the use of condoms in those who are having intercourse. (5) Encouraging those in sexual relationships to get tested for HIV with their partners and to maintain monogamy.

HIV/AIDS prevention education must be conducted at schools, religious organizations, youth organizations, medical facilities, and meetings with parents. Media (television, radio, magazines) are powerful methods to impart information that may change adolescents' attitudes. Meetings of youth, where they congregate, with outreach workers can be an especially effective method of reaching high-risk populations such as homeless youth, gang youth, or out-of-school youth. Topics include the following: (1) Epidemiology of HIV/AIDS; (2) sexual transmission and prevention, including abstinence, safer sex, and condom use; (3) transmission through needles, drug use prevention; (4) HIV and pregnancy; (5) testing and counseling; (6) medical aspects of HIV/AIDS; (7) peer pressure and dating skills; (8) community resources.

The information must be simple, accurate, and direct. In recent years, the federal government has put a lot of resources into *abstinence-only* prevention education. Unfortunately, there has never been any research documenting the long-term benefit from such programs. In fact, one study of abstinence-only education showed that it increased the level of sexual activity in youth. *Abstinence-based* education, which also provides information on how to reduce risk if one is sexually active, has been shown to delay the onset of sexual activity in some studies.

Effective school-based sex education programs were those that reflected the following: (1) use of social learning theory as a foundation for program development; (2) focus on reducing sexual risk-taking behaviors that may lead to HIV, STDs, or pregnancy; (3) provision of basic, accurate information about the risks of unprotected intercourse and methods of avoiding unprotected intercourse through experiential activities designed to personalize this information; (4) activities addressing social or media influences on sexual behavior; (5) strengthening of individual values and group norms against unprotected sex; 6) modeling and practice in communication and negotiation skills.

Many youths are not in school. Street youth service workers who have regular contact with these teens may be effective AIDS educators, and involving peers can be helpful. Principles of youth development have shown promise in the prevention of a variety of adolescent high-risk behaviors. They can help to (1) build competencies and self-efficacy; (2) teach families and communities to send consistent messages for positive behavior; (3) expand opportunities for youth who engage in positive behavior and activities; (4) provide structure in program activities; (5) offer opportunities for engagement of youth in the development of services. Programs are more effective if they last a minimum of 9 months.

Secondary. Providers working with HIV positive youth should monitor and attempt to influence potential risk behaviors while building a trusting provider/patient relationship in order to influence behavior change, following these guidelines: (1) Be persistent in efforts to engage and retain youth in services. (2) Conduct a comprehensive interview at intake and update as needed. (3) Ask HIV-positive adolescents about their social lives at every visit. (4) Talk to youth about your concerns regarding their health. (5) Explore the reasons for risky behavior and those that prevent youth from changing their behavior and disclosing their status.

Recommendations for Primary Care Physicians. (1) Obtain a sexual history and perform counseling on safer sexual behaviors. (2) Perform pretest and posttest HIV antibody counseling. (3) Comanage individuals with HIV infections with HIV specialists. (4) Initiate the evaluation of common AIDS-related symptoms. (5) Be familiar with community resources.

WEB SITES AND REFERENCES

http://AIDSinfo.nih.gov. DHHS HIV treatment guideline for Adolescents and Adults (Oct 2004), Use of antiretrovirals in pregnancy (June 2004).

http://www.cdcnpin.org. National Prevention Information Network.

http://www.cdc.gov/hiv. Guidelines for counseling and testing.

http://www.cdc.gov/mmwr/preview/mmwrhtml/rr5402a1.htm. Postexposure prophylaxis.

http://www.unaids.org. United Nations Programme on HIV/AIDS (UNAIDS).

http://www.cdc.gov/hiv/resources/guidelines/index.htm#occupational. Information on universal precautions.

Cote J, Godin G. Efficacy and interventions in improving adherence to antiretroviral therapy. *Int J STD AIDS* 2005;16:335–343.

Hammer SM. Management of newly diagnosed HIV infection. *N Engl J Med* 2005; 353:1702.

Lyon ME, D'Angelo LJ, eds. *Teenagers, HIV and AIDS*. Westport, CT: Praeger, 2006.

CHAPTER 32

Obesity

Marcie Schneider

Obesity is a serious medical problem increasing in prevalence in the adolescent and adult populations. In children and adolescents, the term obesity has been replaced by overweight. The prevalence of overweight in American teenagers ranges from 12.7% to 24.7%, depending primarily on gender and race. With overweight teens, the psychobiological cues for eating are discordant with energy requirements. It is recommended that overweight adolescents and those at risk for overweight be screened using the body mass index (BMI): BMI = weight in kilograms/height in meters squared.

For children and adolescents, "at risk for overweight" is defined as a BMI between the 85th and 95th percentiles for age and gender, while overweight is defined as BMI exceeding the 95th percentile for age and gender. BMI-for-age charts are available on the Centers for Disease Control (CDC) Web site: www.cdc.gov/growthcharts/.

A triceps skinfold thickness for age and gender above the 95th percentile suggests excessive weight (Table 32.1). Skinfold measurement can be inaccurate due to interobserver error and does not take into account regional distribution of body fat, which has been correlated with obesity-related health risk in adults.

PUBERTAL CHANGES

Effects of Puberty on Body Composition. During adolescence, lean body mass increases in both sexes. The maximum increase occurs at about the time of peak height velocity (PHV) in both sexes, whereas the maximum fat deposition occurs 2 years before PHV. In females, fat deposition continues throughout puberty, and females ultimately have more body fat than males.

TABLE 32.1

Triceps Skinfold Measurements in Children and Adolescents

Age in Years	95% Skinfold Thickness in Males (mm)	95% Skinfold Thickness in Females (mm)
6–6.9	14.6	16
7–7.9	16.7	18
8–8.9	17	20
9–9.9	19.9	22
10–10.9	21	24
11–11.9	22	26
12–12.9	23	28
13–13.9	24	30
14–14.9	23	31
15–15.9	22	32
16–16.9	22	33
17–17.9	22	34
18–18.9	22	34
19–19.9	22	35

Adapted from Barlow SE, Dietz WH. Obesity evaluation and treatment: expert committee recommendations. *Pediatrics* 1998;102:e29.

Effects of Obesity on Puberty. Overweight adolescents tend to be taller, larger in skeletal mass, and more advanced in skeletal development. Shortness in an overweight preadolescent or early adolescent should raise a "red flag" for possible endocrine disease. Overweight female adolescents tend to experience earlier sexual maturation. Menstrual irregularities are often seen in overweight adolescents. Many have anovulatory cycles characteristic of polycystic ovary syndrome.

ETIOLOGY

Obesity is a chronic condition with multiple factors contributing to its etiology. Only 5% of overweight children and adolescents have an underlying cause identified: 3% with endocrine problems (e.g., hypothyroidism, Cushing syndrome, hypogonadism) and 2% with rare syndromes (e.g., Prader-Willi, Laurence-Moon-Biedl, Fröhlich, Alström, and Kallmann syndromes).

Familial or Genetic. There is an increased incidence of obesity among people with obese parents and among twins, even when reared apart. Identified genes linked to obesity include mutations in leptin, leptin receptor, neuropeptide Y, pro-opiomelanocortin, prohormone convertase 1, and melanocortin receptor MC4R. Obesity loci have been found on chromosomes 2, 5, 10, 11, and 20.

Activity, Energy Expenditure, and Calorie Intake. One study reported that the most powerful predictor of the development of overweight in adolescence was the time that a child (6 to 11 years old) spends viewing television. For every extra hour of television watched by 12- to 17-year-olds, there is a 2% increase in prevalence of overweight. Another study found that decreasing sedentary behavior led to a decrease in intake. Caloric intake is variably elevated in overweight adolescents and is dependent on where they eat.

Behavior. Overweight adolescents often eat fast, skip meals, eat when not hungry, eat when depressed or anxious, eat while watching television, underestimate their calorie consumption, overindulge in "fast foods," participate in unhealthy weight-control practices, and are often sedentary.

EPIDEMIOLOGY

1. Data from the NHANES 1999 to 2002 showed that approximately 16.1% of adolescents aged 12 to 19 years were overweight (BMI >95%) and 14.8% were at risk for overweight (BMI 85% to 95%). More Mexican Americans were overweight (22.5%) than non-Hispanic blacks (21.1%) or non-Hispanic whites (13.7%). Overweight was more common in Mexican-American males, non-Hispanic white males, and non-Hispanic black females than their corresponding gender counterparts.
2. *Trends (Table 32.2):* Data from the NHANES done in 1976 to 1980, 1988 to 1994, and 1999 to 2002, have shown that the prevalence of overweight in 12 to 19 year olds increased from 5% to 10.5% to 16.1%, respectively.
3. Fifty percent to 85% of overweight adolescents will be obese adults.
4. BMI ≥30 and age 18 in a woman carries three times the risk of premature death compared to a BMI of 18.5 to 21.9.

TABLE 32.2

Overweight in Children Aged 6 to 11 and Adolescents Aged 12 to 19 Years (United States National Health and Nutrition Examination Surveys)

	NHANES II *1976–1980*	*NHANES III* *1988–1994*	*NHANES* *1999–2002*
Females 6–11	6.4	11.0	14.7
Females 12–19	5.3	9.7	15.4
Males 6–11	6.6	11.6	16.9
Males 12–19	4.8	11.3	16.7
Males/females 6–11	6.5	11.3	15.8
Males/females 12–19	5.0	10.5	16.1

Adapted from Ogden CL, Flegal KM, Carroll MD, et al. Prevalence and trends in overweight among US children and adolescents, 1999–2000. *JAMA* 2002;288:1728, and Hedley AA, Ogden CL, Johnson CL, et al. Prevalence of overweight and obesity among US children, adolescents, and adults, 1999–2002. *JAMA* 2004;291:2847.

5. In a study of weight-loss practices among American adolescents, 30,000 adolescents in Minnesota, 12% of females and 2% males reported chronic dieting, 30% females and 13% males reported binging, 12% females and 6% males reported self-induced vomiting, and 2% females and 0.5% males reported diuretic or laxative use. In a study of 4,746 Minnesota adolescents, 3.1% of females and 0.9% males stated that they met criteria for binge eating disorder. Of this self-identified group, 41.2% males and 15% females had BMIs >95%; 85% to 90% had dieted in the preceding year, and 70% to 80% were currently trying to lose weight.

INFLUENCE OF OBESITY ON HEALTH

Complications due to obesity in adolescents include the following: (1) cardiovascular—dyslipidemias and hypertension; (2) endocrinologic—hyperinsulinism, insulin resistance, impaired glucose tolerance, type 2 diabetes mellitus, menstrual irregularities, polycystic ovary syndrome. Metabolic syndrome is a combination of dyslipidemias (HDL <40 mg/dL, triglycerides >110 mg/dL), elevated blood pressure, fasting glucose >110 mg/dL, and overweight; (3) orthopedic—slipped capital femoral epiphysis, Blount disease; (4) respiratory—sleep apnea, snoring, Pickwickian syndrome, asthma, obesity, hypoventilation syndrome; (5) gastroenterologic—gallbladder disease, steatohepatitis; (6) psychological—depression, eating disorders, social isolation, poor self-esteem.

MEDICAL EVALUATION

The medical evaluation includes an assessment of factors that contribute to weight gain, inhibit weight loss, and comorbid factors that exist and can benefit from weight loss or maintenance.

1. *History:* (a) family history of obesity, cardiovascular disease, hyperlipidemia, hypertension, type 2 diabetes, thyroid disease, colorectal or breast cancer; (b) past weight loss efforts; (c) onset of obesity; (d) triggers for weight gain (e.g., illness or injury, depression, medication use); (e) diet history including diet recall, family eating patterns; (f) unhealthy eating attitudes and weight-related behaviors including dieting, binge eating, purging; (g) exercise history; (h) sedentary activity time including evaluation of screen time (computer, video games, handheld electronic games); (i) medication use or abuse; (j) history of potential secondary causes (e.g., thyroid disease, Cushing disease); (k) full review of systems including headaches (R/O pseudotumor cerebri), orthopedic complaints, snoring, daytime sleeping, abdominal pain, hip pain, urinary frequency, polydipsia, polyuria, irregular menses or amenorrhea.
2. *Physical examination:* (a) Weight, height, and BMI calculation should be plotted on the appropriate CDC growth curves (short stature suggests hypothyroidism or Cushing syndrome); (b) blood pressure should be checked with the appropriately sized cuff; (c) waist circumference may be helpful in those >20 years; (d) triceps skinfolds can be done if the examiner has expertise

with this measurement (Table 32.1); (e) sexual maturity rating should be determined (undescended testicles are seen in Prader Willi males; delayed puberty in females suggests Turner syndrome); (f) skin, hair, and ligaments (acanthosis nigricans suggests insulin resistance and polycystic ovary syndrome; striae that are violet in color and located on the abdomen, buttocks, and thighs are suggestive of Cushing syndrome; hirsutism is suggestive of polycystic ovarian syndrome; polydactyly suggests Bardet-Biedl syndrome, as does mental retardation); (g) papilledema suggests pseudotumor cerebri; (h) thyromegaly suggests hypothyroidism; (i) developmental delay suggests Prader-Willi syndrome or other genetic syndromes.

3. *Laboratory tests:* (a) Thyroid-stimulating hormone, thyroxine, fasting blood glucose, fasting lipid profile, liver function tests; (b) for further evaluation for insulin resistance, particularly if there is acanthosis nigricans or a strong family history of diabetes, a 2-hour glucose tolerance test is recommended. After the ingestion of a 75-g glucose load, a blood glucose >140 mg/dL at 2 hours reflects impaired glucose tolerance, and a blood glucose >200 mg/dL is most likely representative of diabetes. Fasting insulin levels and glucose/insulin ratios have also been used to predict insulin resistance; (c) Patients with polycystic ovarian syndrome may have amenorrhea or irregular menstrual periods, hirsutism, and acne. An elevated free testosterone, DHEAS or androstenedione can be helpful in the diagnosis of polycystic ovary syndrome. An LH:FSH ratio of >3.0 is present in only half of patients and lacks sensitivity and specificity; (d) If a teen is cushingoid, a 24-hour urine free cortisol and overnight dexamethasone suppression test are in order; (e) If obstructive sleep apnea is present, overnight oximetry or sleep study is warranted.

TREATMENT

Adolescents with morbid obesity—those with twice normal weight, BMI >40, or >100 lb (45.5 kg) overweight—are at significant risk for medical problems and need to be encouraged to lose weight. Goal weight should be <85% BMI for age and gender. This can often be accomplished by weight maintenance over a period of time, while for others a slow weight loss of 1 lb per month should be encouraged. Severe calorie restriction during adolescence, particularly during a growth spurt, can halt growth and the progression of puberty. Therefore understanding where an adolescent is with respect to his or her pubertal development and growth spurt is critical in developing appropriate weight goals.

Critical areas to assess treatment readiness in the adolescent include motivation, support, compliance, and realistic goals.

Diet and Physical Activity. An energy deficit is needed for weight loss. The type of calorie restriction should take into account current food types, eating habits, situation-dependent eating, and family and cultural preferences. To support growth and development, there must be good nutritional balance among the food groups.

Approximate daily energy needs in the postpubertal adolescent can be calculated from the weight in kilograms (W), as follows:

$$\text{Males} = [900 + (10 \times W)] \times \text{activity factor}$$
$$\text{Females} = [800 + (7 \times W)] \times \text{activity factor}$$

where the activity factor is 1.2, 1.4, or 1.6 for low, moderate, and high activity levels, respectively. The energy requirement to maintain each extra kilogram of body weight is approximately 22 kcal. A balanced weight-reduction or maintenance diet should be recommended and should include foods from all five food groups (milk, meat, bread, fruits, and vegetables), at least three meals per day, and less total calories than previously consumed. Every weight-reduction program should include regular physical activity.

Cognitive Behavioral Therapy or Behavior Modification Techniques. These are most effective when used in combination with diet and medical therapies. They usually consist of a contract and reward system for weight loss, a food diary, an increase in eating awareness, and appropriate behavioral changes.

Groups. When part of the weight-loss program, membership in a group can provide encouragement, support, and an opportunity to release feelings as well as peer contact and acceptance. There is no evidence of the effectiveness of structured commercially based weight-loss programs in adolescents.

Medications for the Treatment of Obesity. Sibutramine and orlistat are the two drugs approved for the treatment of obesity. Sibutramine—a serotonin, norepinephrine, and dopamine reuptake inhibitor—has been studied in overweight adolescents 16 years of age and older. The starting dose is 10 mg once daily, which is increased after 4 weeks to 15 mg once daily. This approach is more successful if weight loss is demonstrated in the first 4 weeks. Improvement has also been documented in levels of triglycerides, high-density lipoprotein, cholesterol, insulin, and insulin sensitivity. Adverse effects include headache, dry mouth, constipation, insomnia, and increases in blood pressure. Contraindications include anorexia nervosa, hypersensitivity to drug, therapy with monoamine oxidase inhibitors or other serotonergic drugs, coronary heart disease, congestive heart failure, stroke, arrhythmia, uncontrolled hypertension, severe hepatic or renal disease, pregnancy, and lactation. Caution is advised in people with a history of seizures. The medication is not indicated for mildly or moderately overweight individuals in the absence of medical complications.

Orlistat is a lipase inhibitor that blocks the absorption of dietary fat by inhibiting gastrointestinal lipases. The medication has no effect on the absorption of carbohydrates, proteins, or phospholipids. It increases fecal fat from 5% to 30%. The use of orlistat has been studied in overweight adolescents 12 years and older; if tolerated, it can lead to increases short-term weight loss. Dosage is 120 mg orally three times a day. Contraindications include malabsorption syndromes, cholestasis, known hypersensitivity, pregnancy, and lactation.

Many selective serotonin reuptake inhibitors including fluoxetine, fluvoxamine, sertraline, and citalopram have been used to decrease binging in patients with binge eating disorder. Sibutramine and topiramate have been found to decrease binging in this population as well.

Gastrointestinal Procedures: Bariatric Surgery

Pediatric and surgical specialists have published guidelines for bariatric surgery in adolescents (Inge, 2004). Potential candidates include skeletally mature adolescents who have failed >6 months of dietary weight management and have a BMI >40, with serious comorbid conditions that would resolve with sustained weight loss, and who have both a supportive family and personal maturity. Those with BMI >50 with less serious comorbid conditions could be considered. A multidisciplinary team including the bariatric surgeon as well as specialists in adolescent obesity, psychology, and nutrition are essential to the process. Potential procedures include Roux-en-Y gastric bypass and laparoscopic adjustable gastric banding. The Roux-en-Y gastric bypass is performed laparoscopically, separating the stomach into a small-volume upper pouch, and connects the stomach to a limb of jejunum. Approximately 85% of people lose at least 50% of their excess weight at 4 years. Micronutrient supplementation is needed. The laparoscopic adjustable band uses a small Silastic band around the upper stomach, which is inflated with saline via a subcutaneous port. Although it is reversible and removable, there have been technical issues as well as patient management problems.

PREVENTION

(1) Encourage healthy nutritional practices in early puberty including adequate calcium, increased fruits and vegetables, and decreased amounts of saturated fat. Reduce the intake of soft drinks and caloric-dense food. (2) Identify unhealthy eating behaviors. (3) Encourage a lifestyle of activity and participation, including an increase in the frequency and intensity of activity during physical education classes in schools. Increase access to recreational facilities within communities. (4) Discourage screen time (TV, computer, video games), and other sedentary pastimes. (5) Support better food choices in schools, including school lunches and vending machines. (6) Encourage family meals and activities.

WEB SITES AND REFERENCES

http://www.nhlbi.nih.gov/guidelines/obesity/ob_home.htm. Clinical Guidelines on the Identification, Evaluation, and Treatment of Overweight and Obesity in Adults, from NIH.

http://www.niddk.nih.gov/health/nutrit/nutrit.htm. National Institute for Diabetes and Digestive and Kidney Diseases, publications on weight control.

http://www.aafp.org/afp/990215ap/861.html. From *American Family Physician*, evaluation and treatment of childhood obesity.

http://www.obesity.org/Obesity_Youth.htm. American Obesity Association.

http://www.aap.org/obesity Resources for physicians on obesity.

http://www.nasso.org The obesity society, a scientific society for research, education, advocacy and organizational development whose journal is *Obesity Research*.

http://www.obesityonline.org. Online collection of evidence-based obesity education resources.

Barlow S, Dietz W. Obesity evaluation and treatment: expert committee recommendations. *Pediatrics* 1998;102:e29.

Dietz WH, Robinson TN. Overweight children and adolescents. *N Engl J Med* 2005; 352(20):2100.

Inge TH, Krebs NF, Garcia VF, Skelton JA, et al. Bariatric surgery for severely overweight adolescents: concerns and recommendations. *Pediatrics* 2004;114:217.

CHAPTER 33

Anorexia Nervosa and Bulimia Nervosa

Debra K. Katzman and Neville H. Golden

ANOREXIA NERVOSA

Anorexia nervosa (AN) is an eating disorder that primarily affects adolescent girls. The core features are self-induced weight loss accompanied by distorted body image, intense fear of weight gain, denial of the seriousness of weight loss, and amenorrhea (absence of at least three consecutive menstrual periods in the postmenarcheal female). Anorexia nervosa is subdivided into a restrictive subtype and a binge eating and purging subtype (Table 33.1).

Etiology

The multifactorial etiology of AN includes biological, psychological, and sociocultural contributing factors (Fig. 33.1).

Epidemiology

1. *Prevalence:* The estimated prevalence in young women is 0.3% to 0.5%.
2. *Age:* Most eating disorders begin during adolescence and over 90% of individuals with eating disorders are diagnosed before the age of 25 years old. Peak age of onset is midadolescence (13 to 15 years).
3. *Gender:* Approximately 85% to 90% of adolescents with eating disorders are female.
4. *Comorbidity:* AN may coexist with other psychiatric and medical conditions such as anxiety disorders, depression, obsessive-compulsive disorder, substance abuse, diabetes mellitus, and cystic fibrosis.

Clinical Manifestations
Typical Presentation
The common behaviors, signs, and symptoms associated with adolescents with AN are outlined below:

Behaviors. Dieting, relentless pursuit of thinness, distorted body image, unusual eating attitudes and behaviors, increased physical activity, purging behaviors (vomiting, excessively exercising, fasting for a day or days after a binge, taking laxatives, diuretics, ipecac, diet pills, herbal remedies or complementary and alternative medicines), frequent weighing, wearing baggy clothes, poor self-esteem, isolation, inflexibility, irritability, and mood changes.

321

TABLE 33.1

DSM-IV Diagnostic Criteria for Anorexia Nervosa

1. Refusal to maintain body weight at or above a minimally normal weight for age and height (e.g., weight loss leading to maintenance of body weight <85% of that expected), or failure to make expected weight gain during period of growth, leading to body weight <85% of that expected.
2. Intense fear of gaining weight or becoming fat, although underweight.
3. Disturbance in the way in which one's body weight or shape is experienced, undue influence of body shape and weight on self-evaluation, or denial of the seriousness of current low body weight.
4. In postmenarcheal females, amenorrhea, that is, the absence of at least three consecutive menstrual cycles. (A woman is considered to have amenorrhea if her periods occur only following hormone, e.g., estrogen administration.)

Specify type

Restricting type: During the current episode of anorexia nervosa, the person has not regularly engaged in binge eating or purging (i.e., self-induced vomiting or the misuse of laxatives, diuretics, or enemas).

Binge eating/purging type: During the current episode of anorexia nervosa, the person has regularly engaged in binge eating or purging (i.e., self-induced vomiting or the misuse of laxatives, diuretics, or enemas).

Reprinted with permission from the American Psychiatric Association. *Diagnostic and statistical manual of mental disorders*, 4th ed. Text Revision, Copyright, 2000.

Signs and Symptoms

1. *Signs:* Weight loss (any significant or unexpected weight loss in an adolescent is cause for concern), amenorrhea (loss of menses for >3 months in a postmenarcheal female), pubertal delay, lack of growth or poor growth, changes in body hair (lanugo hair, hair loss or thinning), skin changes (dry skin, hyperkeratotic areas, yellow or orange discoloration, pitting or ridging of the nails), recurrent fractures, hypothermia (temperature as low as 35°C), bradycardia, hypotension, acrocyanosis, peripheral edema, systolic murmur sometimes associated with mitral valve prolapse.
2. *Symptoms:* Cold intolerance, postural dizziness, fainting; early satiety, abdominal bloating, discomfort and pain; fatigue, muscle weakness, muscle cramps; poor concentration.

Laboratory Features

1. *Hematologic:* Leukopenia, anemia, thrombocytopenia, decreased serum complement C3 levels, decreased erythrocyte sedimentation rate (ESR <4 mm/hr).
2. *Chemistry:* Increased blood urea nitrogen (BUN) concentration, mildly increased serum glutamic-oxaloacetic transaminase and serum glutamic-pyruvic transaminase levels, hypophosphatemia, depressed serum

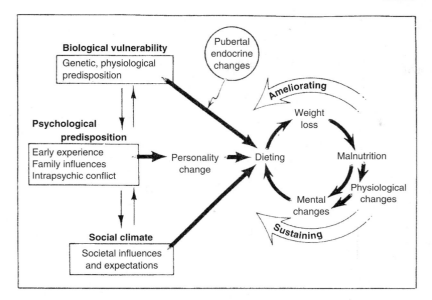

FIGURE 33.1 Biopsychosocial model for anorexia nervosa. (From Lucas AR. Toward the understanding of anorexia nervosa as a disease entity. *Mayo Clin Proc* 1981;56:254, with permission.)

magnesium and calcium concentrations, increased cholesterol, increased serum carotene level, decreased vitamin A level, decreased serum zinc and copper levels.

3. *Endocrine:* The hormonal changes in AN reflect an adaptive response to malnutrition.
   a. Thyroid: Normal thyrotropin (TSH), normal or slightly low thyroxine (T4), often low 3,5,3'-triiodothyronine (T3).
   b. Growth hormone (GH): Decreased IGF-1 levels, normal or elevated GH levels.
   c. Prolactin: Normal.
   d. Gonadotropins: Low basal levels of luteinizing hormone (LH) and follicle-stimulating hormone (FSH); prepubertal 24-hour LH secretory pattern, blunted response to gonadotropin-releasing hormone.
   e. Sex steroids: Low estradiol in females (<30 pg/mL), low testosterone in males.
   f. Cortisol: Normal secretion on stimulation. Basal levels are within the reference range or occasionally slightly high.
4. *Cardiac:* Electrocardiographic (ECG) changes including bradycardia, low-voltage changes, prolonged QTc interval, T-wave inversions, and occasional ST-segment depression; echocardiographic changes including decreased cardiac size, left ventricular wall thickness; increased prevalence of mitral valve prolapse, and pericardial effusion.
5. *Gastrointestinal (GI):* Usually normal findings on upper GI tract series, with occasional decreased gastric motility; normal findings on barium enema.

6. *Renal and metabolic:* Decreased glomerular filtration rate, elevated BUN concentration, decreased maximum concentration ability (nephrogenic diabetes insipidus), metabolic alkalosis, and alkaline urine.
7. Low bone mineral density (BMD).

Differential Diagnosis

Includes medical and psychiatric conditions.

1. *Medical conditions:* Inflammatory bowel disease, malabsorption, endocrine conditions (hyperthyroidism, Addison disease, diabetes mellitus), collagen vascular disease, CNS lesions (hypothalamic or pituitary tumors), malignancies, chronic infections (tuberculosis, HIV), immunodeficiency.
2. *Psychiatric conditions:* Mood disorders, anxiety disorders, somatization disorder, substance abuse disorder, psychosis.

Evaluation

History. Helpful questions include:

1. Why has the teen and/or family come for an assessment?
2. How does the teen feel about the way she or he looks?
3. Is the teen trying to change the way she or he looks?
4. Has there been any change in the teen's weight? If yes, what methods has the teen used to control his or her weight?
5. How much does the teen want to weigh?
6. Does the teen binge? Describe a "binge"? How often does the teen binge?
7. Is there any purging behavior (vomiting, laxative abuse, diuretic use, ipecac use, diet pills, herbal medications or other complementary and alternative medicines)?
8. What was the most and least the teen has weighed and when was that?
9. Do the teen's feelings about her or his body affect her or his mood?
10. Is the teen uncomfortable with any particular part of his or her body (e.g., buttocks or thighs)?
11. How much does the disordered eating interfere with the teen's life? How much time does he or she spend preparing food, exercising, and weighing himself or herself?
12. How much does the teen worry about weight or food?
13. Exercise history? Type, amount, and frequency?
14. What has the teen eaten in the past 24 hours?
15. Has the teen ever had a menstrual period? If yes, when was her last normal menstrual period? How often does she get her period? Has there been any change in her periods? Is she on oral contraceptive pills?
16. Is there a family medical and psychiatric history including a history of an eating disorder, mental illness or substance abuse?
17. Any history of sexual, physical, or emotional abuse?
18. How does the family understand the teen's eating problem? What have the parent(s)/caregiver/family members done to support the teen?
19. Where does the teen get help? With whom does she or he share information?

Physical Examination. Height and weight should be carefully measured and plotted on growth charts. Previous growth curves are very helpful. Body mass index should be calculated (BMI = weight in kilograms/height in meters squared) and plotted on the CDC growth curves. The percentage of ideal or standard body weight should be determined from the National Center for

Health Statistics tables. Sexual maturity rating should be completed on each adolescent.

Laboratory Assessment. Suggested laboratory tests include complete blood count (CBC) and platelet count, ESR, BUN and serum creatinine, urinalysis, serum electrolytes and liver function tests, serum calcium, phosphate, magnesium and phosphorus concentrations, serum albumin level, carotene level; T3, T4 and TSH level; LH, FSH, estradiol, and prolactin level if amenorrheic; ECG; BMD in females with AN who have been amenorrheic for >6 months.

Optional. Upper GI tract series and small bowel series; barium enema; celiac screen; CT or MRI of the head.

Nutritional Assessment. The nutritional assessment should include a 24-hour dietary recall, an assessment of both foods and beverages consumed, and anthropometric measurements such as height, weight, BMI, and skinfold measures.

Complications

1. *Fluid and electrolytes:* Dehydration, hypokalemia, hyponatremia, hypophosphatemia, hypomagnesemia, hypoglycemia
2. *Cardiovascular:* Sinus bradycardia (sinus arrhythmia), orthostatic hypotension, ventricular dysrhythmias, reduced myocardial contractility, sudden death secondary to arrhythmias, cardiomyopathy secondary to ipecac use, mitral valve prolapse, ECG abnormalities (including low voltage, prolonged QT interval, and prominent U waves), pericardial effusion, congestive heart failure
3. *Renal:* Increased BUN, decreased glomerular filtration rate, renal calculi, edema, renal concentrating defect
4. *GI:* Delayed gastric emptying, constipation, elevated liver enzymes, superior mesenteric artery syndrome, rectal prolapse, gallstones
5. *Hematologic:* Anemia, leukopenia, thrombocytopenia
6. *Endocrine or metabolic:* Primary or secondary amenorrhea, pubertal delay, thrombocytopenia euthyroid sick syndrome (low-T3 syndrome), hypercortisolism, decreased serum testosterone level, partial diabetes insipidus, elevated cholesterol level
7. *Low bone mass:* Females with anorexia nervosa have reduced bone mass and increased fracture risk
8. *Neuromuscular:* Generalized muscle weakness, seizures secondary to metabolic abnormalities, peripheral neuropathies, syncope in absence of orthostatic hypotension, movement disorders, structural brain changes (MRI studies have demonstrated enlargement of the lateral ventricles and sulci and significant deficits in both gray- and white-matter volumes in the low-weight stages. Increases in sulcal volume and decreases in gray-matter volume may not be fully reversible with weight recovery.)

Treatment

1. *Team approach:* An interdisciplinary team skilled and knowledgeable in working with adolescents with eating disorders and their families. The timeline for resolution of the medical complications is shown in figure 33.1.
2. *Diagnosis:* Recognize and address the eating disorder as soon as possible.

3. *Medical and nutritional intervention:* Nutritional rehabilitation, weight restoration and reversal of the acute medical complications.
4. *Psychological intervention:* Includes family psychoeducation, interpersonal therapy, and family therapy. Family-based treatment has been found to be effective in adolescents.
5. *Pharmacologic treatment:* Fluoxetine does not appear to be effective in treating the primary symptoms of AN. Studies using fluoxetine have shown inconsistent results with respect to preventing relapse in older adolescents. The most common medications used have included the selective serotonin reuptake inhibitors (SSRIs), such as fluoxetine, sertraline, paroxetine, fluvoxamine, and citalopram. These medications are also useful in treating comorbid depression or obsessive-compulsive disorder (OCD).
6. *Treatment setting:* Includes inpatient treatment, outpatient treatment, partial hospitalization, and residential treatment. Indications for hospitalization are outlined in Table 33.2.

TABLE 33.2

Indications for Hospitalization in an Adolescent with an Eating Disorder

One or more of the following justify hospitalization:
1. Severe malnutrition (weight ≤75% average body weight for age, sex, and height)
2. Dehydration
3. Electrolyte disturbances (hypokalemia, hyponatremia, hypophosphatemia)
4. Cardiac dysrhythmia
5. Physiological instability
   Severe bradycardia (heart rate <50 beats/min daytime; <45 beats/min at night)
   Hypotension (<80/50 mm Hg)
   Hypothermia (body temperature <96°F)
   Orthostatic changes in pulse (>20 beats/min) or blood pressure (>10 mm Hg)
6. Arrested growth and development
7. Failure of outpatient treatment
8. Acute food refusal
9. Uncontrollable binging and purging
10. Acute medical complications of malnutrition (e.g., syncope, seizures, cardiac failure, pancreatitis)
11. Acute psychiatric emergencies (e.g., suicidal ideation, acute psychosis)
12. Comorbid diagnosis that interferes with the treatment of the eating disorder (e.g., severe depression, obsessive-compulsive disorder, severe family dysfunction)

Reprinted with permission from Golden NH, Katzman DK, Kreipe RE, et al. Eating disorders in adolescents. Position paper of the Society for Adolescent Medicine. *J Adolesc Health* 2003;33:496.

7. *Treatment of amenorrhea and low BMD:* Weight restoration results in resumption of menses, usually within 3 to 6 months of achieving treatment goal weight. Hormone replacement therapy has not been proven to be effective in increasing BMD. Recommendations include weight restoration, resumption of spontaneous menses, calcium and vitamin D supplementation, and moderate weight-bearing exercise.
8. *Advice for parents/caretakers:* (a) Be patient, recovery often takes 5 to 6 years. (b) Avoid blaming. (c) Avoid comments (regarding adolescent's weight and appearance). (d) Promote a positive body image and healthy attitude toward eating and activity. (e) Encourage family meals as often as reasonably possible. (f) Avoid making food the struggle. (g) Work with your health care team.

Outcome

The prognosis for adolescents with AN is better than that for adults, owing in part to the shorter duration of symptoms in adolescents. Approximately 50% of adolescents have a "good" outcome; 30% have a "fair" outcome and 20% a "poor" outcome. The time to full recovery is prolonged and can range from 57 to 79 months. The mortality rate ranges from 2% to 8%, with longer-term studies revealing a mortality as high as 15%. The most common causes of death are suicide and the medical complications of starvation. Factors associated with prognosis include:

1. *Good prognosis:* (a) short duration of illness; (b) early identification and intervention; (c) early onset (<14 years old); (d) no associated comorbid psychological diagnoses; (e) no bingeing and purging; (f) supportive family.
2. *Poor prognosis:* (a) longer duration of illness; (b) bingeing and purging; (c) comorbid mental illness (affective disorder, substance abuse); (d) lower body weight at diagnosis.

BULIMIA NERVOSA

Bulimia nervosa (BN) is an eating disorder characterized by binge eating coupled with compensatory behaviors intended to promote weight loss such as self-induced vomiting, laxative abuse, excessive exercise, or prolonged fasting (Table 33.3). Approximately one third of patients with AN "cross over" to BN at some other time in their illness.

Epidemiology

1. *Prevalence:* Lifetime prevalence in females is 1% to 4%.
2. *Age:* Onset is usually during late adolescence or early adulthood, with a modal age of onset of 18 to 19 years. BN is rare under the age of 14 years.
3. *Gender:* 90% to 95% are female.
4. *Comorbidity:* Approximately 80% of individuals with BN report a lifetime prevalence of another psychiatric condition including affective disorders (50% to 80%), anxiety disorders (13% to 65%), personality disorders (20% to 80%) and substance abuse (25%). Patients with BN tend to be more impulsive than those with AN.

TABLE 33.3

DSM-IV Diagnostic Criteria for Bulimia Nervosa

1. Recurrent episodes of binge eating. An episode of binge eating is characterized by both of the following:
    a. Eating, in a discreet period of time (e.g., within any 2 hour period), an amount of food that is definitely larger than most people would eat during a similar period of time and under similar circumstances.
    b. A sense of lack of control over eating during the episode (e.g., a feeling that one cannot stop eating or control what or how much one is eating).
2. Recurrent inappropriate compensatory behavior to prevent weight gain, such as self-induced vomiting; misuse of laxatives, diuretics, enemas, or other medications; fasting; or excessive exercise.
3. The binge eating and inappropriate compensatory behaviors both occur, on average, at least twice a wk for 3 mo.
4. Self-evaluation is unduly influenced by body shape and weight.
5. The disturbance does not occur exclusively during episodes of anorexia nervosa.

Two types have been identified:
1. Purging type: During the current episode of bulimia nervosa, the person has regularly engaged in self-induced vomiting or the misuse of laxatives, diuretics, or enemas.
2. Nonpurging type: During the current episode of bulimia nervosa, the person has used other inappropriate compensatory behaviors, such as fasting or excessive exercise, but has not regularly engaged in self-induced vomiting or the misuse of laxatives, diuretics, or enemas.

Reprinted with permission from the American Psychiatric Association. *Diagnostic and statistical manual of mental disorders*, 4th ed. Text Revision, Copyright, 2000.

Clinical Manifestations

Typical Presentation

Behaviors

1. Binging and purging: A binge is the rapid consumption of a large amount of high-calorie food in a short period of time and associated with self-perceived loss of control over eating. The individual often experiences feeling of being "out of control" during the binge episode.
2. Evidence of purging: Frequent trips to the bathroom after eating, signs and/or smells of vomit and the presence of laxatives or diuretics.
3. Evidence of binge-eating: Often family members report the disappearance of food or the presence of empty wrappers and containers indicating the consumption of large amounts of food. In addition, adolescents with BN may steal, hoard, or hide food and eat in secret.
4. Frequently weighing self.
5. Preoccupation with food.
6. Overly concerned with food, body weight, shape, and size.

Signs and Symptoms
These may be minimal but can include:

1. *Signs:* (a) body weight is usually normal or above normal; (b) calluses on the dorsum of the hand secondary to abrasions from the central incisors when the fingers are used to induce vomiting (Russell sign); (c) painless enlargement of the salivary glands, particularly the parotids; (d) dental enamel erosion (perimolysis); (e) weight fluctuations; (f) edema (fluid retention).
2. *Symptoms:* (a) weakness and fatigue; (b) headaches; (c) abdominal fullness and bloating; (d) nausea; (e) irregular menses; (f) muscle cramps; (g) chest pain and heartburn; (h) easy bruising (from hypokalemia/platelet dysfunction); (i) bloody diarrhea (laxative abusers)

Table 33.4 contrasts AN with BN.

TABLE 33.4

Anorexia Nervosa versus Bulimia Nervosa: Similar and Contrasting Features

Area	Anorexia Nervosa	Bulimia Nervosa
Epidemiology	90% Female patients	Same
	Increased prevalence of eating disorders and depression in families	Same
	Onset early to midadolescence	Slightly older onset
	Prevalence <1%	Prevalence 1%–4%
Psychopathology	Intense fear of gaining weight or becoming fat	Same
	Introverted, obsessional, perfectionistic, rigid	More outgoing, impulsive, prone to acting-out behaviors (shoplifting, sexual promiscuity, self-destructive acts)
	Poor self-esteem	Same
	Secretive about behaviors	Same
	Binge eating not necessary	Binge eating must be present
	Level of denial high	Aware of problem; wants help
Physical signs		
Weight	Underweight; must be <85% expected weight	Usually of normal weight Weight can be normal, high, or low
Menses	Must be amenorrheic	May have normal, irregular, or absent menses

Differential Diagnosis

Includes medical and psychiatric conditions:

1. *Medical conditions:* (a) chronic cholecystitis; (b) cholelithiasis; (c) peptic ulcer disease; (d) gastroesophageal reflux disease; (e) superior mesenteric artery syndrome; (f) malignancies (including CNS tumors); (g) infections—acute bacterial and viral gastrointestinal infections, parasitic infections, hepatitis; (h) pregnancy; (i) oral contraceptives—nausea can be a side effect of oral contraceptives and hormone replacement therapy; (j) some medications have side effects that may include nausea and vomiting, or food cravings.
2. *Psychiatric conditions:* (a) anorexia nervosa binge/purge subtype; (b) binge eating disorder; (c) major depressive disorder with atypical features; (d) borderline personality disorder; (e) Kleine-Levin syndrome.

Evaluation

Evaluation includes a complete history, physical examination, and laboratory screening including CBC, BUN and creatinine, electrolytes, glucose, calcium, phosphorus, serum amylase, ECG with rhythm strip, urinalysis (specific gravity).

Complications

1. *Fluid and electrolytes:* dehydration, hypokalemia (the most frequently seen electrolyte abnormality), hyponatremia, hypophosphatemia.
2. *Cardiovascular:* cardiac arrhythmias, ipecac cardiomyopathy.
3. *Gastrointestinal:* parotid gland enlargement and increased serum amylase, esophagitis, Mallory-Weiss tears, rupture of the esophagus or stomach, acute pancreatitis, paralytic ileus secondary to laxative abuse, cathartic colon, Barrett esophagus.
4. *Pulmonary:* aspiration pneumonia secondary to vomiting, pneumomediastinum secondary to vomiting.
5. *Dental:* erosion of dental enamel, dental caries.

Treatment

1. *Interdisciplinary team approach.*
2. *Medical and nutritional intervention:* Includes careful medical monitoring, the correction of any medical complications (electrolyte abnormalities), and a structured meal plan to include eating three normal meals a day.
3. *Psychological intervention:* In adults, cognitive-behavioral therapy (CBT) reduces binge eating and purging activity in approximately 30% to 50% of patients.
4. *Pharmacologic treatment:* Fluoxetine is the only medication approved by the FDA for the treatment of BN and is most effective at a dose of 60 mg daily. A combination of antidepressant medication and CBT appears to be superior to either modality alone.
5. *Treatment settings:* The majority of adolescents with bulimia nervosa can be treated in an outpatient setting (outpatient clinic or partial hospitalization).

Outcome

Most adolescents with BN recover over time with recovery rates ranging from 35% to 75% at 5-year follow-up. BN tends to be a chronic relapsing condition and approximately one third of affected individuals relapse within 1 to 2 years. Comorbidity is frequent but mortality is low. Compared with AN, BN has higher rates of both partial and full recovery.

EATING DISORDERS NOT OTHERWISE SPECIFIED (EDNOS)

EDNOS refers to the diagnostic category of those patients who have problems with eating or body image but who do not meet full DSM-IV criteria for AN or BN. This category accounts for the majority of adolescents presenting for treatment.

Binge Eating Disorder

Binge eating disorder (BED) is a newly recognized disorder and only recently appeared in the DSM (1994). The DSM-IV–proposed criteria include the following:

1. Recurrent episodes of binge eating. An episode of binge eating is characterized by both of the following:
   a. Eating, in a discrete period of time (e.g., within any 2-hour period), an amount of food that is definitely larger than what most people would eat during a similar period and under similar circumstances.
   b. A sense of lack of control over eating during the episode (e.g., a feeling that one cannot stop eating or control what or how much one is eating).
2. The binge eating episodes are associated with three or more of the following:
   a. Eating more rapidly than normal
   b. Eating until feeling uncomfortably full
   c. Eating large amounts of food when not physically hungry
   d. Eating alone because of embarrassment
   e. Feeling disgusted with self and depressed
3. Marked distress regarding binge eating is present.
4. The binge eating occurs, on average, at least 2 days a week for 6 months.
5. The binge eating is not associated with the regular use of inappropriate compensatory behaviors (e.g., purging, fasting, and excessive exercise) and does not occur exclusively during the course of AN or BN.

Community-based surveys suggest that BED occurs in 1% to 2% of adolescents between the ages of 10 and 19. Most people with BED are obese, but normal-weight people also can be affected. Up to 20% of individuals who present for treatment of obesity meet criteria for binge eating disorder. The causes of BED are still unknown.

Males and Eating Disorders

Approximately 10% of older adolescents suffering from eating disorders are male. The percentage of males with eating disorders is higher among young adolescent males than in adult males. Eating disorders in adolescent males are clinically similar to eating disorders in females. Body image concerns appear to be one of the strongest variables in predicting eating disorders in males.

At-risk males include those (1) involved in athletic activities where there is a focus on body weight and body image—body builders, wrestlers, dancers, swimmers, runners, rowers, gymnasts and jockeys; (2) struggling with sexual identity conflict; (3) diagnosed with comorbid mental disorders, and (4) with a family history of an eating disorder.

Although males of all types of sexual orientation develop eating disorders, several studies report that there is an increased incidence of homosexuality among males with eating disorders.

Female Athlete Triad

The female athlete triad is a syndrome consisting of disordered eating, amenorrhea, and osteoporosis in female athletes. The key feature is insufficient caloric intake for the amount of energy expenditure, resulting in hypothalamic amenorrhea (primary or secondary) and a low estrogen state. The low estrogen state is associated with osteoporosis and increased fracture risk.

Females at greatest risk are those participating in sports that emphasize a lean physique (e.g., figure skating, gymnastics, ballet, long-distance running, and swimming). Treatment includes increasing caloric intake, calcium and vitamin D supplementation, restricting the intensity of training (if necessary), and monitoring for resumption of menses.

WEB SITES

http://www.aedweb.org. The Academy for Eating Disorders.

http://www.edap.org/. The National Eating Disorders Association (NEDA).

http://www.adolescenthealth.org/Eating_Disorders_in_Adolescents.pdf.

http://www.nationaleatingdisorders.org The National Eating Disorders Association (NEDA).

http://www.anred.com Anorexia Nervosa and Related Eating Disorders Inc. (ANRED).

http://www.iaedp.com. International Association of Eating Disorder Professionals.

http://www.mentalhealth.com/book/p45-eat1.html. Information from the National Institute of Mental Health.

Psychosomatic Illness in Adolescents

David M. Siegel

It is important to have an organized and consistent approach to somatizing adolescents, with goals of carrying out a judicious yet complete diagnostic evaluation as well as formulating a management plan that ameliorates symptoms and maintains (or restores) function and quality of life. Some teens will experience periods of significant struggle as they try to adapt to the changes of adolescence. These challenges, if sufficiently disruptive, can be characterized as an adjustment disorder and can sometimes be expressed in somatic terms.

CLASSIFICATION

As stipulated in the *Diagnostic and Statistical Manual of Mental Disorders, Text Revision* (DSM-IV-TR, 2000) (APA, 2000) there are three broad categories of psychosomatic disorders:

1. *Psychophysiologic:* Psychological conflict affects the development or recurrence of an existing physical condition.
2. *Somatoform:* Somatic complaints and/or dysfunctions are not under conscious control and physical findings are absent or insufficient to explain all symptoms and complaints.
3. *Factitious:* Somatic and/or psychological symptoms are consciously controlled.

Psychophysiologic Disorders. In psychophysiologic disorders, physical symptoms are observable and often fall into biologic processes that are understood by the clinician. For example, the patient with asthma experiences

333

increased bronchospasm when under stress. The connection between the psychological and the physical, once shared with and understood by the patient and family, is not typically rejected or denied. The clinician must try to help (including mental health consultation as appropriate) the adolescent and parent(s) to identify those sources of stress and anxiety that are contributing to inadequate control of the primary disease and its symptoms.

Somatoform Disorder. Symptoms in somatoform disorders are seen as associated with, or reflective of, *unconscious* conflict. Somatoform disorders include somatomization disorder, undifferentiated somatoform disorder, conversion disorder (hysteria), hypochondriasis, body dysmorphic disorder, and somatoform pain disorder. Among adolescents, patients with undifferentiated somatoform disorder are more common than patients who meet the restrictive criteria for somatization disorder.

Factitious Disorders. These result from the conscious falsification of symptoms and signs and involve a different behavior from the unconscious process of somatoform disorders. The intentional creation of the sick role is thought to be motivated by the unconscious need to be cared for.

EVALUATION

With adolescents complaining of single or multiple somatic symptoms, both biomedical and psychosocial factors should be part of the initial evaluation— i.e., a biopsychosocial assessment. The eventual diagnosis of a psychosomatic disorder is more acceptable to families if this conclusion does not arise late in the evaluation process only as a diagnosis of exclusion. Focusing on the symptoms does not reinforce the illness but rather can give the teen the message that the provider is taking his or her symptoms seriously. Laboratory and imaging studies should be chosen based on the history and physical examination and should be limited to the fewest minimally invasive tests required to clarify the diagnosis.

When this biopsychosocial assessment leads the clinician away from a definable biologic, pathophysiologic abnormality to explain the patient's symptom(s), and somatizing is suspected, an initial consideration should be whether this represents psychiatric disease. Mood disorders and anxiety disorders can manifest with somatization and, when significant, warrant formal intervention, which may include mental health consultation.

Somatization can also be associated with certain personality (axis II) disorders. Those patients with obsessive-compulsive personality disorder or histrionic personality disorder are at higher risk for developing somatization. Adolescents with personality traits of dependency or neurotic preoccupation with self also have a greater tendency to experience and describe unexplained physical symptoms. Somatizing in parents, family members, or peer contacts should be examined as possible models for, and contributors to, the teen's own symptoms and behaviors.

Approach to the Patient

The clinician's initial history gathering takes into account a differential diagnosis of physiologic causes but also includes sensitivity for psychosomatic etiology. As the physical examination proceeds, a lack of positive physical findings may elevate the likelihood of emotional distress as a major contributor to the symptoms and also helps guide the clinician's diagnostic testing. However, even if the initial history suggests emotional upset, the clinician should avoid statements suggesting that this is the exclusive cause of the physical symptoms. When an adolescent presents with a specific symptom, it is important that the problem be addressed in the terms expressed by the patient and that any diagnostic or therapeutic recommendations be offered in that context. When a psychological element is suspected to be contributory, this can be constructively introduced to the patient and family without discrediting or trivializing the identified symptoms. In our adolescent practice setting, we have clinical psychologists available on-site for consultation, and I will often let patients and families know about this if I think mental health referral is likely at a subsequent visit. The aim is to acknowledge the teen's emotional distress and to foster acceptance by the adolescent and parent(s) of a psychological dimension that will be integrated into the treatment. The patient/family may or may not come to endorse the psychological process as primary and the physical symptoms as secondary. Identifying sources of stress, depression, and emotional distress and how to cope with them may be seen by the adolescent and parent(s) as a parallel (rather then integrated) process leading to improvement in the symptom, but the emotional–psychological–physical connection has been framed in terms that fit with the parent's and/or patient's insight, defensive structure, and level of sophistication, allowing treatment to proceed.

The vast majority of somatizing adolescents can be successfully managed as outpatients, making use of appropriate consultation. Inpatient admission should be reserved for the small minority of patients who fail a multidisciplinary outpatient program and/or for those whose deterioration places them at significant risk for chronicity. Hospitalizing a somatizing patient with the goal of expediting the diagnostic evaluation and convincing the patient and family that the problem is psychological rather than physical risks setting up an eventual confrontation with the clinician that is unlikely to facilitate either short-term improvement or a successful long-term outcome. Although the admitting physician may be reassured by the many negative tests and consultations garnered in hospital, patients and families paradoxically may view the decision to admit the adolescent as "proof" of physiologic severity and may therefore be even more resistant to any subsequent psychological explanation and intervention.

CONCLUSION

Those caring for adolescents should take a methodical and pragmatic approach to the identification of psychosomatic illness. Although patience and persistence are often called for from clinicians, patients, and families, eventual improvement is a realistic expectation in most instances.

REFERENCES AND ADDITIONAL READINGS

American Psychiatric Association. Somatoform disorders. In: *Diagnostic and Statistical Manual of Mental Disorders, Text Revision* (DSM-IV-TR, 2000). 4th ed. Washington, DC: American Psychiatric Association, 2000.

Kreipe RE. The biopsychosocial approach to adolescents with somatoform disorders. *Adolesc Med Clin* 2006;17:1

Von Hahn L, Harper G, McDaniel SH, et al. A case of factitious disorder by proxy: the role of the health-care system, diagnostic dilemmas and family dynamics. *Harvard Rev Psychiatry* 2001;9:124.

CHAPTER 35

Fatigue and the Chronic Fatigue Syndrome

Martin Fisher

Fatigue is common among adolescents. Up to 70% indicate that they are sleepy during the day. In most instances, fatigue in adolescence is due to a deficit in hours of sleep. The key to the evaluation of the adolescent with fatigue is to distinguish those patients who need merely reassurance and perhaps a change in schedule from those who require further management for organic or psychiatric disorders or who have signs and symptoms of chronic fatigue syndrome (CFS).

CAUSES OF FATIGUE

Adolescent Sleep Patterns. The most common cause for fatigue is insufficient sleep.

1. Total sleep duration decreases from a mean of 10.1 hours at 9 years of age to a mean of 8.1 hours at 16 years of age.
2. Most adolescents sleep more on weekends than they do during the week. Adolescents sleep as much as 2 hours less per night on weekdays during the school year than during the summer.
3. Fifteen percent of adolescents report falling asleep in the car or bus on the way to school; 25% report falling asleep on the way home.

Psychological Causes. In adolescents, psychological causes are responsible for most cases of fatigue that are unrelated to too little sleep and/or too much activity. Psychological causes of fatigue include (a) depression, (b) anxiety, (c) stressful situations, and in some cases (d) other psychiatric disorders.

Organic Causes. These are infrequent during adolescence, but fatigue may result from (a) medications (especially antihistamines, sedatives, antidepressants, and other psychotropic medications), alcohol, or illicit drugs; (b) infectious diseases (especially mononucleosis, hepatitis, chronic infectious diseases such as HIV, tuberculosis or Lyme disease, or bacterial endocarditis); (c) endocrine disorders, including thyroid disease, adrenal disease, or diabetes mellitus; and (d) other systemic illnesses (e.g., connective tissues diseases, anemia, neoplasms, congenital heart disease, asthma, inflammatory bowel disease, or kidney or liver failure).

Sleep Disorders. These are increasingly being recognized as a cause of fatigue and/or daytime sleepiness in adolescents. The following are included in this category:

1. *Insomnia* is defined as decreased sleep quality and/or quantity due to trouble falling asleep and/or maintaining sleep. Insomnia may be a symptom of an underlying medical or psychological disorder, part of a delayed sleep phase syndrome (DSPS), or unexplained. DSPS is a common disorder "in which an individual's internal circadian pacemaker is not in synchrony with internal or environmental time" (Millman et al., 2005).
2. *Obstructive sleep apnea* occurs in up to 1% to 3% of adolescents and may be caused by enlarged tonsils and adenoids, obesity, retrognathia, or nasal obstruction.
3. *Other sleep disorders* are uncommon; they include narcolepsy, idiopathic hypersomnia, "periodic leg movements during sleep," and "restless leg syndrome."

Chronic Fatigue Syndrome. CFS is a poorly understood and sometimes controversial diagnosis that has increasingly been reported in adolescents. The Centers for Disease Control and Prevention has developed a working definition of chronic fatigue syndrome (Fukuda et al., 1994):

1. Fatigue of at least 6 months' duration
2. Limits the individual to 50% of premorbid activity levels
3. May be persistent or recurrent
4. No other cause found to account for the fatigue
5. Four of the following symptoms: recurrent pharyngitis, tender lymph nodes, new-onset headaches, impaired memory or concentration, joint pains, muscle pains, nonrefreshing sleep, postexertion fatigue

Epidemiology. Mean age of onset in adolescents is 14 to 15 years. Sixty percent to 70% of patients are female. Patients will often have had symptoms for years prior to presentation, and some will have had premorbid problems with school attendance.

Symptoms. Patients often have multiple symptoms, including fatigue, headache, sore throat, abdominal pain, fever, impaired cognition, myalgia, diarrhea, adenopathy, anorexia, nausea/vomiting, dizziness, arthralgia, sweats, chills, and depression.

Etiology. No specific etiology has been identified as the cause of CFS. It is likely that the underlying cause may be multifactorial, including an acute infectious illness that acts as a precipitant, a background of psychological distress, and an underlying physiologic vulnerability (in the cardiovascular, neurologic, endocrine, and/or immune systems). Etiologies that have been considered include the following:

1. *Infection:* Infection, most notably that due to Epstein-Barr virus or influenza, can serve as the precipitant for the onset of CFS. In other parts of the world, other viral infections have been implicated as triggers for CFS. Any acute illness can cause an exacerbation of symptoms during the course of the syndrome.

2. *Cardiovascular system:* Underlying cardiovascular instability may be a factor in the cause of CFS. Orthostatic symptoms are common and tilt-table testing is often positive.

3. *Endocrine system:* Decreased hypothalamic-pituitary-adrenal axis function has been proposed as an etiology in CFS but has never been clearly demonstrated.

4. *Immune function:* Studies have shown in vitro abnormalities in lymphocyte function and cytokine production in CFS; however, reproducible abnormalities and opportunistic infections have not been found and treatment with immunoglobulins and other immune modulators have not shown clear benefits in CFS.

5. *Depression:* A history of depression is found in many adults with CFS and depression may create a psychological vulnerability necessary for the onset of CFS. There is substantial overlap in the symptoms of CFS and depression, leading to the possibility that some patients with depression will be misdiagnosed with CFS and vice versa. Some believe that CFS is merely a manifestation of primary depression.

6. *Other psychological risk factors:* Premorbid psychosomatic symptoms are found in some children and adolescents with CFS. Separation anxiety and/or school phobia may be a factor in some children and adolescents.

EVALUATION OF FATIGUE

Evaluation of the adolescent with a complaint of fatigue is aimed at distinguishing those who are merely not getting enough sleep from those who may have specific disorders of sleep or other psychological or medical causes.

History. This should evaluate sleep patterns and activity levels (hours of sleep at night, naps during the day, time going to sleep, time arising, difficulty falling asleep, waking up during the night, patterns on weekdays, patterns on weekends, school schedule, out-of-school schedule), alcohol and illicit drug use, caffeine intake, medical history, medications, snoring, systemic symptoms, and unexplained leg movements. A comprehensive psychological history should be obtained, looking for evidence of depression and/or anxiety or recent stressors. Finally, determine if the patient meets criteria for the diagnosis of chronic fatigue syndrome (see above).

Physical Examination. Fatigue associated with nonorganic causes is usually accompanied by a normal physical examination.

Laboratory Testing and Other Studies

1. *Screening tests:* complete blood count, erythrocyte sedimentation rate, urinalysis, comprehensive metabolic panel, T4 and TSH, screening for mononucleosis.

2. Additional tests are done based on the history and physical examination and may include studies such as tuberculosis testing (PPD), ECG, chest x-ray, sinus x-rays, HIV testing, antinuclear antibody and rheumatoid factor (RH), cortisol level, and Lyme titers.

3. Specialized studies that may be indicated include sleep studies (polysomnography), tilt-table testing in those with orthostatic symptoms (especially

in CFS), or MRI or CT of the brain in those with headaches or accompanying neurologic symptoms.

TREATMENT

General Causes of Fatigue. Managing the adolescent with fatigue is based on the diagnosis.

1. *Adolescent sleep patterns:* Reassure families and advise healthy sleep patterns and daytime schedules.
2. Specific interventions are provided to those whose fatigue has treatable medical or psychological causes.
3. Guidance on changing sleeping patterns is provided to those with DSPS (See Table 35.1). Use of melatonin and/or bright lights has been studied for the treatment of DSPS, but results are variable. Use of continuous positive airway pressure (CPAP) and/or orthodontic appliances at night may help some adolescents with obstructive sleep apnea syndrome.

Chronic Fatigue Syndrome. No specific treatment has been found to shorten the course of CFS in adolescents. Emphasize that the prognosis for adolescent CFS has generally been shown to be substantially better than that

TABLE 35.1

Techniques to Reverse Sleep-Wake Cycle in Adolescents with Delayed Sleep Phase Syndrome

1-Day Plan[*]	*1-Week Plan*[†]
1. Fall asleep at usual time (e.g., 4 A.M.).	1. Day 1: Stay awake until 3 hours after usual sleep time (e.g., go to sleep at 7 A.M.).
2. Set alarm and wake up 6 hours later (e.g., 10 A.M.).	2. Day 2: Stay awake until 3 hours after previous bedtime (e.g., go to sleep at 10 A.M.).
3. Remain awake all day.	3. Day 3: Go to sleep three hours later than previous day (e.g., 1 P.M.).
4. Go to sleep at midnight (will have slept only 6 hours in past 36 hours so should be tired).	4. Day 4: Again go to sleep three hours later (e.g., 4 P.M.)
5. Set alarm and wake up at 8 A.M. (will again need to be active to stay awake 2 days in a row).	5. Day 5: Go to sleep 3 hours later (e.g., 7 P.M.)
	6. Day 6: Go to sleep 3 hours later (e.g., 10 P.M.)
	7. Day 7: Go to sleep at Midnight and wake up at 8 A.M.

[*]Personal communication, R. Fisher.
[†]Czeisler et al., 1981.

in adults. (a) Reassure patients and families that symptoms are real and generally improve over time. (b) Help families to minimize "doctor shopping," unnecessary testing, and unproven therapies. (c) Antidepressant medication may be used to decrease symptoms of depression in CFS, but studies do not show that they change the course or outcome of the illness. (d) Anti-inflammatory medications can be used for treatment of symptoms; medications for sleep should be used sparingly. (e) Patients with orthostatic changes and/or a positive tilt-table test may benefit from medication or an increase in salt and water intake. (f) Many adolescents with CFS require home tutoring or partial school programs in order to function educationally. (g) Graded exercise programs are beneficial to some adolescents with CFS; (h) Cognitive-behavioral therapy, family therapy, or individual therapy is sometimes helpful.

WEB SITES AND REFERENCES

http://www.cdc.gov/ncidod/diseases/cfs/index.htm. The CDC Website for CFS.

http://www.niaid.nih.gov/publications/cfs.htm. NIH state-of-the-art consultation.

Czeisler CA, Richardson GS, Coleman RM, et al. Chronotherapy; resetting the circadian clocks of patients with delayed sleep phase insomnia. *Sleep* 1981;4:1.

Fukuda K, Straus SE, Hickie I, et al. The chronic fatigue syndrome: a comprehensive approach to its definition and study. *Ann Intern Med* 1994;121:953.

Krilov LR, Fisher M. Chronic fatigue syndrome in youth: maybe not so chronic after all. *Contemp Pediatr* 2002;19:61.

Millman RP, Working Group on Sleepiness in Adolescents/Young Adults, American Academy of Pediatrics Committee on Adolescence. Excessive sleepiness in adolescents and young adults: causes, consequences, and treatment strategies. *Pediatrics* 2005;115:1774.

CHAPTER 36

Chronic Abdominal Pain

Paula K. Braverman

Chronic abdominal pain is a common complaint among teenagers and young adults. The approach is challenging in the adolescent population as often (90–95% of cases) no specific organic abnormality is found.

DEFINITION

The differential diagnosis of chronic abdominal pain includes functional gastrointestinal disorders (FGIDs) and organic disorders related to anatomic abnormalities, inflammation, or tissue damage.

DIFFERENTIAL DIAGNOSIS AND CLINICAL MANIFESTATIONS OF CHRONIC ABDOMINAL PAIN

Functional Gastrointestinal Disorders (FGIDs)

Epidemiology

Older studies commonly used the term *recurrent abdominal pain* (RAP) to refer to entities that are now being described as FGIDs. The exact prevalence of FGIDs in adolescents is unknown. In one study, the prevalence of RAP in patients between 6 and 19 years old was 12.1% in males, 16.7% in females, and 5% in 16- to 17-year-olds. More recently, a community-based study of 7th and 10th graders who self-reported gastrointestinal symptoms found similar results; 13% to 17% reported at least weekly pain, and 17% to 24% reported pain severe enough to affect activities.

Proposed Etiologies of Functional Gastrointestinal Disorders

(1) Visceral hypersensitivity or hyperalgesia; (2) altered gastrointestinal motility; (3) autonomic dysfunction with disordered brain-gut communication

Diagnostic Criteria

The Rome II criteria define FGID in children and adolescents as abdominal pain lasting for at least 12 weeks (not necessarily consecutive weeks) during the previous 12 months. The following disorders are listed in Rome II criteria in the category "Abdominal Pain."

Functional Abdominal Pain

1. *Epidemiology:* Functional abdominal pain is the most common FGID.
2. *Diagnostic criteria:* (a) at least 12 weeks of continuous or nearly continuous pain either not related or only occasionally related to physiologic events such as eating, menses, and defecation; (b) the pain is not malingering; (c) loss of some daily functioning may occur; (d) criteria for other FGIDs are not met.

Irritable Bowel Syndrome (IBS)

1. *Epidemiology:* IBS occurs in 10% to 20% of adolescents and adults.
2. *Diagnostic criteria:* Abdominal pain/discomfort without metabolic or structural abnormalities associated with disordered defecation and meets two of the following three criteria: (a) pain relief with defecation; (b) pain onset with associated changes in stool frequency; (c) pain onset with associated changes in form or appearance of stool

Functional Dyspepsia

1. *Epidemiology:* The exact prevalence in adolescents is unknown.
2. *Diagnostic criteria:* (a) pain in upper abdomen above the umbilicus; (b) no evidence of organic disease (e.g., normal upper endoscopy); (c) pain not relieved by defecation and not associated with change in stool frequency or form
3. *Types of dyspepsia:* (a) ulcer-like dyspepsia–predominant symptom is upper abdominal pain; (b) dysmotility-like dyspepsia—nonpainful discomfort in upper abdomen with upper abdominal fullness, early satiety, bloating, or nausea; (c) nonspecific dyspepsia—symptomatic patients not fitting criteria for ulcer-like or dysmotility type

Abdominal Migraine

1. *Epidemiology:* The exact prevalence in adolescents is unknown.
2. *Diagnostic criteria:* (a) Must have at least three episodes in 12 months and be asymptomatic for weeks to months between episodes; (b) must have two of the following: (i) headache during episode; (ii) photophobia during episode; (iii) family history of migraine; (iv) unilateral headache; (v) an aura with either visual, sensory, or motor disturbance; (c) no evidence of metabolic, gastrointestinal, or central nervous system structural or biochemical diseases

Aerophagia

1. *Epidemiology:* The exact prevalence in adolescents is unknown.
2. *Diagnostic criteria:* At least 12 weeks in the preceding 12 months of at least two of the following: (a) air swallowing; (b) abdominal distension from intraluminal air; (c) belching and/or flatus

Organic Causes of Chronic Abdominal Pain

Causes of Chronic Pain Commonly Associated with Dyspepsia

(1) Gastroesophageal reflux; (2) peptic ulcer disease; (3) biliary tract obstruction; (4) gallbladder dyskinesia; (5) chronic pancreatitis; (6) gastroparesis; (7) chronic hepatitis

Causes of Chronic Pain Commonly Associated with Altered Bowel Pattern

(1) Lactose intolerance; (2) inflammatory bowel disease (IBD); (3) celiac disease; (4) colitis; (5) complications of constipation—encoporesis, megacolon; (6) infection—parasites and bacteria

Causes of Chronic Pain Commonly Associated with Paroxysmal Abdominal Pain

(1) Musculoskeletal pain; (2) bowel obstruction; (3) ureteral obstruction

The differential diagnosis includes gynecological conditions, referred pain from the lungs or spine and systemic conditions such as diabetic ketoacidosis or sickle cell crisis.

DIAGNOSIS

The Subcommittee on Chronic Abdominal Pain in Children reviewed the existing literature and was unable to produce an evidence-based procedural algorithm for the diagnostic evaluation of chronic abdominal pain. The following conclusions were drawn by the subcommittee regarding the diagnostic value of history, physical examination, and screening laboratory tests:

History

1. Some patients have features of more than one FGID.
2. The pain frequency, severity, location or impact on lifestyle cannot distinguish functional and organic disorders. Timing of the symptoms, including postprandial pain and nighttime awakening, were not found to be helpful.
3. "Alarm symptoms or signs" suggestive of organic disease requiring further diagnostic testing include but are not limited to (a) involuntary weight loss; (b) family history of IBD; (c) deceleration in linear growth; (d) unexplained fever; (e) gastrointestinal blood loss; (f) significant vomiting—cyclical vomiting, bilious emesis; (g) chronic severe diarrhea; (h) persistent right-upper or right-lower-quadrant pain
4. Family history: (a) Parental history of anxiety, depression, and somatization is not helpful in distinguishing between functional and organic disorders. (b) Overall family functioning (e.g., cohesion, conflict, marital satisfaction) does not differ between those with FGIDs and healthy families or those with acute illness.
5. Issues regarding the relationship of pain to current stress and emotional and behavioral concerns include (a) History of anxiety, depression and more negative life event stress do not distinguish functional from organic abdominal pain. (b) There is a relationship between daily stress and pain episodes as well as increased negative life events and persistent symptoms. (c) There is no evidence to support the concept of emotional/behavioral symptoms predicting the severity of pain, course of the pain episode, or response to treatment. (d) There is evidence to support that adolescents with FGIDs are at risk for emotional problems and psychiatric disorders (e.g., anxiety and depression) later in life.
6. Pain diary: It can be helpful to have the teen document the pattern, timing, severity, association with food or beverage and precipitating factors of the pain for 1 to 3 weeks.

Physical Examination

FGIDs are usually associated with normal findings on physical examination or mild pressure tenderness without rebound commonly located in the upper abdomen.

Laboratory Tests/Radiologic Studies/Diagnostic Tests

1. No studies have been done to specifically evaluate the use of laboratory tests to distinguish between functional and organic abdominal pain even with alarm signals.
2. There is no evidence that ultrasound of the abdomen or pelvis, endoscopy and biopsy, or pH monitoring in the absence of alarm signals significantly detects organic disease.
3. FGID can be diagnosed by a primary care clinician when there are no alarm symptoms, the physical exam is normal, and there is a negative stool sample for occult blood.

Approach to the Evaluation of Functional Gastrointestinal Disorders

If, after a careful history and physical examination, there is no obvious organic source for the chronic abdominal pain, the practitioner should explain to the teen that the evaluation seems to indicate a FGID. Although a serious underlying disease is not suspected, the teen should appreciate that the symptoms being experienced are real. It is also useful to explain the concepts of visceral hypersensitivity, altered motility, and autonomic dysfunction with disordered brain–gut communication in terms that the adolescent and family can understand. If further clarification of the history is needed, the teen should be asked to keep a pain diary. If there are alarm signals or further diagnostic tests are necessary for reassurance, selected screening utilizing laboratory tests and/or radiologic studies can be performed.

TREATMENT/THERAPEUTIC APPROACHES

FGIDs are best treated in the context of a biopsychosocial model, which may include psychological interventions, dietary changes, and some specific pharmacologic therapy to reduce the frequency and severity of the symptoms. Pharmacologic therapy should be used judiciously for specific symptomatology and specific functional gastrointestinal conditions. The goal of treatment is to resume normal functioning and return to daily activities rather than focusing on the pain itself.

Conclusions on Treatment from the Subcommittee on Chronic Abdominal Pain

The Subcommittee on Chronic Abdominal Pain in Children found a paucity of studies evaluating pharmacologic and dietary treatments in children and adolescents. They concluded the following:

(1) Two weeks of treatment with peppermint oil capsules may be beneficial for children with IBS. (2) Evidence for benefit of H_2-receptor antagonists is inconclusive, but such treatment may be beneficial for patients with severe dyspepsia. (3) Evidence for benefit of fiber supplementation in decreasing frequency of pain attacks is inconclusive. (4) Lactose intolerance and recurrent pain appear to be two different entities. The evidence that a lactose-free diet decreases symptoms for patients with recurrent abdominal pain is inconclusive.

Other Pharmacologic Treatment Options for Functional Gastrointestinal Disorders

Medications with some evidence of effectiveness from pediatric and adult studies include the following:

(1) Pizotifen, propanolol and cyproheptadine may be used prophylactically for abdominal migraine. (2) The 5-HT$_4$ antagonist (tegaserod) has been helpful in adult women with constipation predominant IBS. (3) 5-HT$_3$ antagonist (alosetron) has been helpful in adult women with severe diarrhea predominant IBS. (4) Tricyclic antidepressants (imipramine, amitriptyline) have been used in low doses in adults with IBS with refractory diarrhea.

Psychological Interventions

The practitioner should stress that the pain is not "in the adolescent's head" but is a real manifestation that can be exacerbated by stress. It is important to reassure the adolescent that he or she is physically healthy and can continue with all activities. If the teen is missing a lot of school, the family, teachers and school nurse should work together with the teen to keep him or her in school. If significant depression, anxiety, or family problems are uncovered, the teen and family can be referred for further psychological or family assessment. However, psychological intervention may be helpful even in less severe cases. Cognitive behavioral therapy has been demonstrated to be successful for treating functional disorders in children and adolescents. Other techniques that have been used include teaching relaxation, self-management, and behavior management techniques. Ultimately the goal is to reduce illness behavior and to help the parents reinforce good coping behavior. Long-term follow-up studies have shown that >25% to 50% of teens with functional chronic abdominal pain continue to have symptoms as adults.

WEB SITES AND REFERENCES

http://www.acg.gi.org/. Home page for American College of Gastroenterology.

http://www.iffgd.org/. Home page for the International Foundation for Functional Gastrointestinal Diseases.

http://www.merck.com/. *Merck Manual* on line. Enter topic of interest.

http://www.naspgn.org/. Home page of North American Society for Pediatric Gastroenterology and Nutrition. Position papers on various topics online, including functional abdominal pain.

Boyle JT. Abdominal pain. In Walker WA, et al., eds. *Pediatric gastrointestinal disease.* Ontario: BC Decker, 2004:225–243.

Campo JV, Di Lorenzo C, Chiappetta L, et al. Adult outcomes of pediatric recurrent abdominal pain: do they just grow out of it? *Pediatrics* 2001;108:E1.

Di Lorenzo C, Colleti RB, Lehman HP, et al. Chronic abdominal pain in children, subcommittee on chronic abdominal pain. *Pediatrics* 2005;115:370 (Technical Report) and 812.

Lesbros-Pantoflickova D, Michetti P, Fried M, et al. Meta-analysis: the treatment of irritable bowel syndrome. *Aliment Pharmacol Ther* 2004;20:1253.

Rasquin-Weber A. Hymen PE, Cucchiara S, et al. Childhood functional gastrointestinal disorders, *Gut* 1999;45(Suppl II):1160.

Weydert JA, Bail TM, Davis MF, et al. Systematic review of treatments for recurrent abdominal pain. *Pediatrics* 2003;111:1.

CHAPTER 37

Chest Pain

John Kulig and Lawrence S. Neinstein

Chest pain is reported by about 5% of adolescents. Cardiac chest pain is uncommon among adolescents but many teens have fears of heart disease or cancer.

DIFFERENTIAL DIAGNOSIS

Musculoskeletal (31%)

Well-localized, sharp pain with insidious onset. Movement and breathing may increase the pain.

1. *Precordial catch/"stitch":* Common, with sudden onset; at rest, a sharp stabbing pain lasting seconds to minutes, localized to left sternal border.
2. *Muscle strain/overuse:* Strain of chest wall or upper back after exercise. Localized tenderness increased by arm movements.
3. *Costochondritis (8%):* Focal tenderness from the second through sixth anterior ribs. Usually unilateral; may radiate to the back or abdomen. Tenderness over the involved articulations at the costochondral junction. May be preceded by an upper respiratory infection.
4. *Tietze syndrome:* Rare. Associated with tender solitary swelling at second or third costal cartilage. Unilateral, increasing with breathing and movement. May persist for days to months.
5. *Slipping-rib syndrome:* Uncommon syndrome caused by slipping of the eighth to tenth ribs on the immediately superior rib. Pain is sharp and stabbing, in the upper quadrant of the abdomen.
6. *Fibromyalgia syndrome:* See Chapter 38. Chronic pain associated with aching, fatigue, and morning stiffness.
7. *Thoracic outlet obstruction*
8. *Malignant disease of bone*

Idiopathic/Psychogenic (25%)

(1) Stress or anxiety: often described as a tightness or heaviness in the chest or intermittent sharp, knifelike pains. (2) Hyperventilation: may cause chest pain associated with light-headedness, shortness of breath, paresthesias, and syncope. (3) depression; (4) bulimia nervosa: esophagitis or Mallory-Weiss tear from frequent self-induced emesis.

Pulmonary (21%)

Usually associated with other symptoms, including cough, fever, and dyspnea. Pulmonary causes include cough (10%), asthma (4%), pneumonia/bronchitis (7%), pleural effusion, pleurodynia, spontaneous pneumothorax/pneumomediastinum, acute chest syndrome in sickle cell disease, pulmonary embolism/infarction, and Lemierre syndrome (pharyngeal abscess complicated by thrombophlebitis of the internal jugular vein).

Gastrointestinal (7%)

Gastrointestinal causes include reflux esophagitis, esophageal foreign body, esophageal spasm, caustic ingestion, gastritis, peptic ulcer disease, nonulcer dyspepsia, cholecystitis, and pancreatitis.

Trauma (5%)

Including rib contusion or fracture, sternal contusion, clavicular contusion or fracture, and hepatic or splenic trauma.

Breast (5%)

Including pubertal gynecomastia, premenstrual or pregnancy-associated breast tenderness, fibrocystic breast changes, breast mass, especially fibroadenoma and mastitis.

Cardiac (4%)

Uncommon in teens. The pain may be associated with exertion and accompanied with, syncope, palpitations, and dizziness. Causes include (1) mitral valve prolapse; (2) dysrhythmias; (3) pericarditis: sharp pain aggravated by respiratory motion: sitting up and leaning forward often lessens the pain; (4) myocarditis or cardiomyopathy; (5) left ventricular outflow obstruction; (6) ischemic heart disease: very rare in teens without predisposing factors; (7) Kawasaki disease; (8) dissecting aortic aneurysm: extremely rare in teens except with a predisposing connective tissue disorder (e.g., Marfan syndrome); (9) anomalous origin of the coronary arteries.

Miscellaneous (2%)

Including mediastinitis, mediastinal mass, herpes zoster (shingles), cigarette smoking, carbon monoxide poisoning, and illicit drug use (e.g., cocaine, "ecstasy," amphetamine, anabolic steroids).

DIAGNOSIS

History

Careful history is critical:

1. *Characterization of the pain*
   a. *Pain quality:* Localized sharp, aching pain suggests chest wall etiology. Deep, gnawing pain suggests visceral cause.
   b. *Onset:* Sudden onset more likely indicates an organic etiology.
   c. *Severity:* Restriciton of teen's usual activities?

d. *Location:* T1 to T4 dermatome distribution often referred from myocardium, pericardium, aorta, or esophagus. Pain in T5-to-T8 distribution may arise from diaphragm, gallbladder, liver, pancreas, duodenum, or stomach.

e. *Timing and duration*

f. *Precipitating and alleviating factors:* Substernal pain when lying down suggests reflux esophagitis. Pain increasing with breathing or cough suggests pleural or chest wall pain. Pain increasing with stress suggests anxiety, while pain awakening teen suggests organic cause.

2. *Recent activity:* e.g., activity causing chest wall strain, such as lifting weights or exercising.

3. *Recent trauma*

4. *Recent infections or systemic illness*

5. *Medications or drugs*

6. *Associated symptoms:* Light-headedness, paresthesias, or tingling in extremities suggesting hyperventilation syndrome?

7. *Previous treatment*

8. *Family history:* Known cardiovascular disease? Hypertension? Lipid disorder? Coagulopathy? Sudden deaths?

9. *Recent stress*

10. *Fears and concerns:* Is the teen worried about heart disease or cancer?

Physical Examination

Detailed examination with attention to the chest wall.

1. *General state:* Evidence of anxiety, hyperventilation, cyanosis, or pallor?

2. *Vital signs*

3. *Chest wall palpation:* Examine for localized tenderness or swelling along the ribs and intercostal spaces. Check for trauma. Perform the hooking maneuver to check for "slipping" rib. (Pain is reproduced when the examiner hooks his or her fingers under the affected ribs and pulls anteriorly.) In males, examine for palpable breast tissue.

4. *Cardiopulmonary examination:* Including (a) Heaves or thrills/peripheral pulses; (b) asymmetric breath sounds: pneumothorax, pleural effusion, and empyema; (c) rales: pneumonia and pulmonary embolism; (d) pleural friction rub: pleurisy and pulmonary embolism; (e) cardiac friction rub/distant heart sounds: pericarditis and effusion; (f) midsystolic click, late-systolic murmur: mitral valve prolapse; (g) other cardiac murmurs: aortic stenosis, for example; (h) cardiac dysrhythmia.

5. *Breast examination:* Symmetry, masses, tenderness, discharge.

6. *Abdominal examination*

Laboratory Testing

Usually no evaluation other than a detailed history and physical examination is required. If a specific organic cause is suggested, consider appropriate testing, including chest radiograph, electrocardiogram, echocardiography, 24-hour Holter monitoring, exercise stress testing, cardiac enzymes (troponin 1, CPK-MB), lipid profile, urine drug screening, pulse oximetry, D-dimer, abdominal ultrasonography, or upper GI tract endoscopy.

THERAPY

Chest pain is rarely life-threatening in teens and rarely necessitates emergent intervention. Referrals are rarely needed. Reassurance is the most important intervention. Otherwise therapy depends on the specific diagnosis.

REFERENCES AND ADDITIONAL READINGS

Cava JR, Sayger PL. Chest pain in children and adolescents. *Pediatr Clin North Am* 2004;51:1553.

Gumbiner CH. Precordial catch syndrome. *South Med J* 2003;96:38.

Owens TR. Chest pain in the adolescent. *Adolesc Med State of the Art Rev* 2001;12:95.

CHAPTER 38

Fibromyalgia Syndrome and Reflex Sympathetic Dystrophy

David M. Siegel

FIBROMYALGIA SYNDROME

Fibromyalgia syndrome (FS) is predominately a disorder of females character-ized by widespread pain, fatigue, poor sleep, and some or all of a variety of other somatic complaints. Prevalence of FS in a general population of adults has been estimated at 3.4% in women and 0.5% in men. Wolfe et al. identified two major diagnostic criteria for FS; widespread (defined as above and below the waist and on both sides of the body) pain for at least 3 months and a min-imum of 11 out of 18 tender points on physical examination. In adolescents, we and others have maintained that in the presence of other consistent data, detecting <11 tender points does not eliminate FS as a credible diagnosis.

Presentation and Diagnosis

The typical adolescent with FS is a young woman who describes the gradual onset of diffuse achiness in the periarticular soft tissue or in the joints them-selves. There is no redness or warmth, but patients frequently describe a de-gree of muscle or joint swelling that is not perceived by the health professional. Associated with pain and fatigue are numerous somatic complaints including recurrent headache, abdominal pain with cramping and alternating diarrhea and constipation (irritable bowel syndrome), dysmenorrhea, joint stiffness, in-termittent subjective swelling of hands and feet, Raynaud phenomenon, mood disturbance, and difficulty with concentration.

Although the above symptoms are frequently volunteered by the patient and parent(s), a key abnormality is the quality of sleep and whether the ado-lescent feels fatigued much of the time. The adolescent with FS reports being tired in the morning. If asked "How many hours of sleep do you need in or-der to feel rested and refreshed?" the FS patient will typically reply that "No matter how many hours of sleep I seem to get, I am always tired. Even if I nap during the day [and many of these individuals are engaged in quite a bit of purposeful daytime sleeping], I am never able to regain any energy." This phenomenon is known as *nonrestorative sleep* and in our study was found in

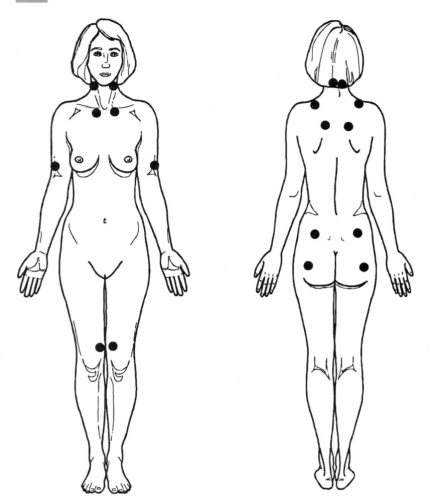

FIGURE 38.1 Locations of tender points in fibromyalgia.

98% of adolescents with FS (Siegel et al., 1998). Questioning will often uncover that the patient is restless during the night, with multiple awakenings and bed covers significantly disheveled or even entirely off the bed in the middle of the night or in the morning. This restless, nonrestorative sleep pattern represents inadequate delta-wave or stage IV sleep because of the intrusion of lighter alpha-wave sleep.

The review of systems is negative for fever, weight loss, oral lesions, or joints with swelling, warmth, erythema, or limitation of motion. A comprehensive physical examination in FS should incorporate a systematic palpation of each of the 18 tender points (Fig. 38.1) as well as some control points. Proper technique involves identifying the cutaneous location and then applying 4 kg of pressure using the examiner's thumb or another finger. *The force required results in a degree of discomfort even in patients without the diagnosis. However, in those with FS, the examination experience is much more unpleasant and characterized by marked grimacing and withdrawal.*

Laboratory and imaging studies in FS are consistently normal, and no diagnostic interventions are absolutely confirmatory of the illness. In a patient with presumptive FS, judicious laboratory testing consists of a complete blood count with differential, an erythrocyte sedimentation rate (and/or C-reactive protein), and perhaps thyroid function studies. If depression is a comorbid concern, a standardized metric such as the Beck Depression Inventory is a prudent step to better define the severity of affective disorder and the possible need for formal mental health intervention.

Treatment

1. *Sleep hygiene:* This is the first priority and includes a consistent bedtime and morning wake-up time on both weekdays and weekends. We strongly discourage napping as well as intake of caffeine, nicotine, alcohol, or stimulants.
2. *Medications:* The majority of patients will also require medication, the effect of which is to facilitate stage IV sleep. The most commonly used preparations are tricyclic antidepressants given in low doses 1 to $1\frac{1}{2}$ hours prior to bedtime. Cyclobenzaprine at a dose of 10 to 20 mg nightly is often very effective in these patients, although some adolescents may require higher doses. The initial benefit observed is a diminution in both nighttime awakening and disruption of bed covers. Usually, after 2 to 3 weeks of quieter, more restful sleep, an increase in energy begins to occur as well as a decrease in pain. If the quality of sleep is not changing within a couple of weeks, then upward titration of the dose in 5- to 10-mg increments is in order. Other classes of drugs that have been studied and found to be variably successful include selective serotonin reuptake inhibitors and serotonin/norepinephrine reuptake inhibitors. Although tramadol and sedative hypnotics (e.g., zolpidem tartrate) have been shown to be beneficial in FS, we discourage their use in adolescents because of the potential for dependency. Nonsteroidal anti-inflammatory drugs and acetaminophen are not reliably helpful in these patients, but for the individual teen, these analgesics may offer some interim relief until definitive therapy takes hold.
3. *Exercise:* In addition to correcting the sleep defect, regular moderate exercise has also been shown to improve the status of patients with FS, both in the physical and psychological realms. A low-intensity aerobic exercise routine, such as brisk walking for 20 to 30 minutes three times per week, is an example of appropriate physical activity to incorporate into the treatment plan for FS.
4. *Psychological support:* Many of those with FS will benefit from some degree of psychological support and intervention. The health care provider should assess the emotional dimension of the problem and undertake initial counseling for the patient and family. For some patients, formal mental health consultation will be necessary to fully address the psychological morbidity of the illness.

Prognosis

Over a period of weeks following initiation of treatment, the adolescent with FS will become increasingly less symptomatic with regard to pain and fatigue although restoring complete exercise tolerance may take longer. If new symptoms or signs appear that suggest alternative diagnoses, the clinician should readdress the correctness of the FS label. The majority of adolescents with FS should be able to return to their previous, premorbid status.

REFLEX SYMPATHETIC DYSTROPHY

RSD (also known as neurovascular dystrophy, or more recently, complex regional pain syndrome, type I) is a noninflammatory musculoskeletal syndrome of pain, hyperesthesia, vasomotor disturbances, and eventually dystrophic changes. It is most common in adolescent girls but can occur in younger children and in patients of either sex.

Predisposing Factors

1. *Personality factors:* Characteristically, adolescents with RSD are overachievers.
2. *Trauma:* When preceding trauma has occurred, it may be of any type (burn, contusion, fracture, laceration, and nerve injury) but is often minor, may antedate RSD symptoms by weeks (or longer) and often results in the patient and family not immediately identifying or remembering the inciting event.
3. *Neurologic factors:* These include multiple sclerosis, peripheral neuropathy, tumors, and cerebrovascular accidents, but they occur in only few adolescents with RSD.
4. *Other precipitating factors:* Local cold injury, revascularization of an ischemic injury or postoperative wound.

The precipitating factor in RSD is frequently trivial and the pain response is dramatically out of proportion to the injury.

Clinical Manifestations

Most characteristic of the syndrome is exquisite tenderness to the lightest touch (allodynia). Objective changes (caused by vasomotor instability) include swelling, blotchiness or bluish discoloration, reduced skin temperature, and decreased pulses. Perspiration may be either decreased or increased in the involved area. Pain is present in 98% of cases, decreased motion in 75%, and vasomotor changes in 67%. Early symptoms include burning or aching pain, swelling, and hyperthermia or hypothermia. Diffuse osteoporosis due to disuse is a common sequel.

Differential Diagnosis

This includes Raynaud disease, chronic arterial insufficiency, phlebothrombosis, rheumatic disorders such as systemic lupus erythematosus, and localized infections.

Treatment

Outcome is improved if treatment is initiated early. Pain generally is not amenable to direct therapeutic intervention; narcotic analgesics in particular should not be used. The basic therapeutic approach is to employ a combination of physical therapy and psychological counseling. It should be emphasized to adolescents that the more they use the involved extremity, the quicker the extremity is going to get better; conversely, disuse will worsen the condition.

Emphasize that the prognosis is good with treatment. Stress that without psychological intervention, the risk that RSD will recur or another pain amplification syndrome develop is increased. Helping the family deal with the emotional aspects of the disease is crucial to the achievement of an excellent outcome.

The literature on adults with RSD reports that some patients benefit from corticosteroids, ganglionic blocking agents, and chemical sympathetic blockers. However, except for the rare case in which emotional factors are not implicated, these forms of therapy should be avoided in adolescents. Nonsteroidal anti-inflammatory drugs usually have little effect on relieving the pain of RSD; their long-term use is especially discouraged.

In most cases, outpatient management will suffice. With severe and long-standing symptoms or failure of outpatient treatment, admission to an inpatient rehabilitation service for multidisciplinary treatment may be necessary. *Admission* is the time to be very clear about the emotional factors involved in most adolescents with RSD and to establish a "discharge goal." A typical example of a discharge goal for the adolescent with lower extremity involvement might be to walk for a reasonable distance, wearing shoes and socks, with no more than a minimal limp. Prosthetic devices and aids—such as wheelchairs, crutches, and braces—are quickly withdrawn. Patients are permitted to receive mild analgesics, such as acetaminophen if requested, but they are advised that drugs are not likely to provide major pain relief.

Role of the Therapeutic Team Members

Physician. The physician sets the overall direction of the patient's medical management, is a central participant in determining the discharge goal, regularly examines the patient, and consistently communicates with the patient and parents.

Nurse. The primary nurse plays a key role in the day-to-day coordination of the patient's in-hospital routine. These tasks include helping (often with social work) to schedule weekly team meetings, reinforcing and explaining or clarifying weekly objectives to the teen, and checking on the adolescent's progress in meeting these objectives. Most important, the nurse has a special role to fulfill in providing emotional support by encouraging the adolescent to talk about feelings and express anger in appropriate ways, listening to the teen's complaints of pain, and providing support to the family.

Physical Therapist. The physical therapist provides range-of-motion, strengthening, and weight-bearing exercises for the involved extremity and is often also someone with whom the adolescent can talk about the illness and treatment experiences. Desensitization techniques, such as vigorous toweling or immersion in contrast baths, are used. As frequently as is appropriate, the patient is given a choice of different treatment modalities (thereby fostering assertiveness and a shared responsibility in treatment and getting better); throughout the process, the therapist uses a firm but nonpunitive approach.

Occupational Therapist. The OT provides tasks requiring hand and arm use in much the same way as the physical therapist does for the lower extremities. Occupational therapy provides opportunities for the teen to make choices and exercise age-appropriate independence as well as to interact with other teens in a nonthreatening milieu.

Mental Health Professional. This person's role is crucial to the short-term but especially the long-term outlook; her or his first task is to evaluate the psychosocial dynamics of the patient and family. Studies have shown a high frequency of subtle family conflict, difficulty in expressing anger, and enmeshment with the mother. The father, on the other hand, is frequently viewed by teen and mother as powerful but remote. Although the patient may be the family member with symptoms ("the presenting patient" or "identified patient"), RSD should be seen as a family disorder, and family therapy is highly desirable.

The Parents. Without active parental participation, recovery tends to be slower or may not occur, and relapses are more common. The mental health professional on the team uses a family systems perspective and facilitates parental involvement appropriately in that framework.

The return to satisfactory functioning and a manageable (or absent) level of pain in these patients is usually fraught with patient and parent anxiety and resistance to treatment. Although there is a genuine desire to improve, aggressive physical therapy often strikes the family as counterintuitive ("My foot is exquisitely tender and painful and yet you tell me that the cure is for me to move, strengthen, and bear weight on that very part of my body that hurts the most!") By maintaining a supportive structure and a respectful but absolutely persistent adherence to the principles outlined above, a gradual and substantial recovery is a realistic treatment outcome.

WEB SITES AND REFERENCES

http://www.niams.nih.gov/Health-Info/Fibromyalgia/default.asp. NIH fact sheet on fibromyalgia.

http://www.afsafund.org/. American Fibromyalgia Syndrome Association.

http://www.fmnetnews.com. Fibromyalgia Network.

http://www.angelfire.com/on/teenfms/main.html. Teen guide to fibromyalgia.

http://www.rheumatology.org. American College of Rheumatology.

http://www.ninds.nih.gov/disorders/reflex_sympathetic_dystrophy/reflex_sympathetic_dystrophy.htm. NIH facts sheet on RDS.

http://www.rsds.org. Reflex Sympathetic Dystrophy Syndrome Association of America.

http://www.arthritis.org/conditions/diseasecenter/rsds.asp. Question and answers on RSD from the Arthritis Foundation.

http://www.angelfire.com/wi/rsdhopeteens/. Teen site on RSD.

http://www.rsds.org/gallery_page_1.htm. Photo gallery of RSD patients.

Bennett RM. The rational management of fibromyalgia patients. *Rheum Dis Clin North Am* 2002;28:181.

Siegel DM, Janeway D, Baum J. Fibromyalgia syndrome in children and adolescents: clinical features at presentation and status at follow-up. *Pediatrics* 1998;101:377.

Williams DA. Psychological and behavioral therapies in fibromyalgia and related syndromes. *Best Pract Res Clin Rheumatol* 2003;17:649.

Wolfe F, Smythe HA, Yunus MB, et al. The American College of Rheumatology 1990 criteria for the classification of fibromyalgia. *Arthritis Rheum* 1990;33:160.

CHAPTER **39**

Adolescent Sexuality

Martin M. Anderson and Lawrence S. Neinstein

Adolescents are sexual beings. Sexual behavior does not start during adolescence or adulthood but with childhood sexual curiosity. Understanding the sexual nature of adolescence is essential to developing the skills needed to answer teenagers' questions and address their sexual feelings and problems.

ADOLESCENT SEXUAL DEVELOPMENT

Preadolescence. Characteristics include (1) a low physical and mental investment in sexuality; (2) information gathering on the topic of sexuality; (3) prepubertal appearance; (4) masturbation, which occurs as a normal behavior.

Early Adolescence. Characteristics include (1) initiation of puberty; (2) extreme body concern and curiosity; (3) sexual fantasies, which are common and may elicit guilt; (4) masturbation in response to sexual feelings; (5) sexual activities, most often nonphysical.

Middle Adolescence. Characteristics include (1) full pubertal maturation; (2) sexual energy at a high level; (3) sexual behavior of an exploratory, experimental nature; (4) dating and noncoital sexual activities; (5) little attention to the adverse consequences of sexual behavior.

Late Adolescence. Characteristics include (1) completion of puberty; (2) more expressive sexual behavior; (3) possible development of intimate sharing relationships.

NONCOITAL SEXUAL BEHAVIORS

Data on rates of vaginal intercourse, pregnancy, and sexually transmitted diseases (STDs) are readily available, which is not the case with noncoital sexual activities.

Oral Sex

Surveillance data show that 46% of 15- to 17-year-old males were not sexually experienced while 36% had vaginal intercourse and 44% had oral sex (Table 39.1). Twenty-one percent of 15- to 17-year-old male virgins (no vaginal intercourse) and 85% of nonvirgins had engaged in oral sex. The data for female 15- to 17-year-olds indicate that 48.6% were not sexually experienced while 39% had had vaginal sex, 47% had had oral sex with a male, and 8% had had oral sex with a female (Table 39.2). The percent of females engaging in oral sex differed between virgins and nonvirgins. Eighteen percent of virginal women between 15 and 17 years of age had had oral sex with a male and 4.8% had had oral sex with a female. Eighty percent of nonvirgin 15- to 17-year-old females reported oral sex with a male and 14% had had oral sex with a female.

Anal Sex

The 2002 National Survey of Family Growth (NSFG) reported that 8.1% of males had had anal sex with a female and 3.9% had had anal or oral sex with a male. Among virgin males, the rate of anal sex with a female was 1% and oral or anal sex with a male was 2.6%. For nonvirgin males, the rate of anal sex with a female was 20.7% and oral or anal sex with a male was 6.4%. In addition, 5.6% of females had had anal sex with a male. For virgin females, the figure did not reach statistical significance; for nonvirgins, it was 28.6%.

COITAL SEXUAL BEHAVIORS

The 2005 Youth Risk Behavior Survey (YRBS at http://www.cdc.gov/mmwr/preview/mmwrhtml/ss5505a1.htm) surveyed "in-school" youth (Fig. 39.1) and found that 47% of students in grades 9 through 12 had vaginal intercourse (48% male, 46% female). This increased from 34% (29% female, 39% male) in ninth grade to approximately 63% by the senior year (62% female, 64% male). Four percent of females and 9% of males in grades 9 through 12 started having sex before age 13 (Fig. 39.2). Over 20% of high school seniors had four or more partners (Fig. 39.3).

The 2002 NSFG (http://www.cdc.gov/nchs/datawh/statab/pubd.htm-Sexual Activity) (Tables 39.1 and 39.2) surveyed both "in- and out-of-school" youth and found that 39% of 15- to 17-year-old females and 36% of 15- to 17-year-old males had engaged in vaginal intercourse. By the time these adolescents reached 17 years of age, 46.9% of the males and 49% of the females had had vaginal intercourse; by 18 years of age, this figure had increased to 62% for males and 70% for females.

Sexual Pressures

The Kaiser National Survey of Adolescents and Young Adults demonstrated that 29% (33% males, 23% females) of 15- to 17-year-olds felt pressured to have sex. Sixty three percent (66% males, 60% females) felt that waiting to have sex is a nice idea but that nobody really does. Almost 60% (59% males, 58% females) felt that there was pressure to have sex by a certain age, and 39% (50% males,

TABLE 39.1

Types of Sexual Contact for Males 15 to 19 Years Old Including Anal and Oral Sex

Characteristic	Number (in Thousands)	Any Opposite-Sex Sexual Contact	Opposite-Sex Sexual Contact						Any Oral or Anal Sex with a Male	No Sexual Contact with Another Person
			Vaginal	Any Oral	Oral		Anal	Female Touched Penis		
					Gave	Received				
Age										
15–19 years	10,208	63.9	49.1	55.2	38.8	51.5	11.2	52.4	4.5	35.4
15–17 years	5,748	53.2	36.3	44.0	28.2	40.3	8.1	42.7	3.9	46.1
15 years	1,930	43.2	25.1	35.1	15.5	30.3	4.6	35.4	2.2	55.9
16 years	1,998	53.3	37.5	42.0	27.0	39.4	7.3	43.2	3.1	46.3
17 years	1,820	63.5	46.9	55.7	43.2	51.9	12.9	50.1	6.6	35.6
18–19 years	4,460	77.7	65.5	69.5	52.4	66.0	15.2	65.0	5.1	21.6
18 years	2,392	74.4	62.4	65.4	50.5	61.7	15.1	59.2	4.3	24.6
19 years	2,067	81.6	68.9	74.2	54.6	70.9	15.3	71.6	6.0	18.0
Ever had vaginal intercourse with a female and age										
Yes	13,624	100.0	100.0	88.8	75.1	85.9	31.3	81.3	5.3	—
15–17 years	2,069	100.0	100.0	84.8	60.5	79.3	20.7	80.0	6.4	—
18–19 years	2,912	100.0	100.0	90.2	69.9	86.9	21.9	82.1	6.0	—
No	6,393	30.0	—	25.2	13.5	22.2	1.3	24.8	4.4	67.9
15–17 years	3,629	27.1	—	20.7	10.0	18.1	1.0	21.7	2.6	71.8
18–19 years	1,537	35.7	—	30.6	19.6	26.8	a	33.0	3.3	62.4

[a]Figure does not meet standards of reliability or precision.

Adapted from Mosher WD, Chandra A, Jones J. Centers for Disease Control and Prevention. Sexual behavior and selected health measures: men and women 15–44 years of age, United States, 2002. Adv Data Vital Health Stat 2005;362:1.

TABLE 39.2

Types of Sexual Contact for Females 15 to 19 Years Old Including Anal and Oral Sex

Characteristic	Number (in Thousands)	Any Opposite-Sex Sexual Contact	Opposite-Sex Sexual Contact Vaginal	Any Oral	Oral Gave	Oral Received	Anal	Any Oral or Anal Sex with a Male	No Sexual Contact with Another Person
Age									
15–19 years	9,834	63.3	53.0	54.3	43.6	49.6	10.9	10.6	35.5
15–17 years	5,819	49.8	38.7	42.0	30.4	38.0	5.6	8.4	48.6
15 years	1,819	33.8	26.0	26.0	18.3	23.9	2.4	7.2	63.7
16 years	1,927	49.6	39.6	42.4	30.4	39.3	6.9	13.1	48.8
17 years	2,073	64.0	49.0	55.5	41.1	49.1	7.3	5.1	35.2
18–19 years	4,015	82.9	73.8	72.3	62.0	66.7	18.7	13.8	16.5
18 years	2,035	78.2	70.3	70.2	61.3	62.4	18.8	13.7	21.2
19 years	1,980	87.8	77.4	74.4	64.2	71.1	18.6	13.9	11.7
Ever had vaginal intercourse with a male and age									
Yes	13,782	100.0	100.0	87.4	77.6	83.4	28.6	15.6	—
15–17 years	2,251	100.0	100.0	80.1	60.6	74.5	13.9	14.1	—
18–19 years	2,953	100.0	100.0	85.6	75.8	78.7	25.2	17.4	—
No	5,858	24.1	—	24.3	17.9	21.1	0.8	4.8	73.0
15–17 years	3,563	18.1	—	18.0	11.4	14.9	a	4.8	79.2
18–19 years	1,049	35.3	—	35.3	26.2	33.0	a	3.7	62.5

aFigure does not meet standards of reliability or precision.

Adapted from Mosher WD, Chandra A, Jones J. Centers for Disease Control and Prevention. Sexual behavior and selected health measures: men and women 15–44 years of age, United States, 2002. Adv Data Vital Health Stat 2005;362:1.

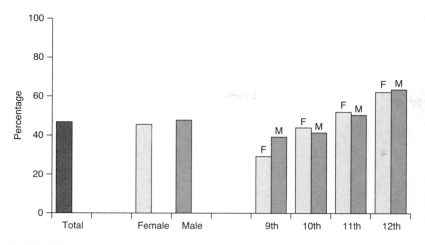

FIGURE 39.1 Percentage of high school students who had sexual intercourse, by sex and grade, 2005. (From the Centers for Disease Control and Prevention. Youth risk behavior surveillance–United States, 2005. *MMWR* 2006;55 #SS-5.)

27% females) agreed that "if you have been seeing someone for a while, it is expected that you will have sex."

Oral sex was viewed by 24% (18% males, 31% females) of 15- to 17-year-olds as a way to avoid vaginal intercourse. "Oral sex is not as big of a deal as sexual intercourse" was reported by 46% of all teens (54% of males, 38% of females). Almost 40% (47% males, 30% females) viewed oral sex as safer sex.

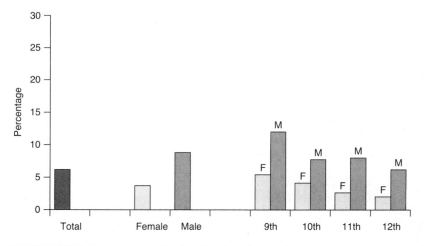

FIGURE 39.2 Percentage of high school students who engaged in their first sexual intercourse before age 13 years, by sex and grade, 2005. (From the Centers for Disease Control and Prevention. Youth risk behavior surveillance–United States, 2005. *MMWR* 2006;55 #SS-5.)

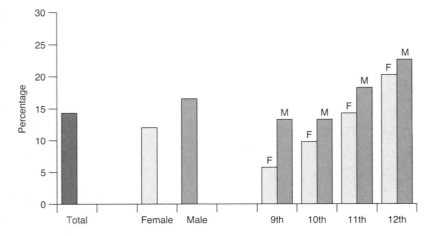

FIGURE 39.3 Percentage of high school students who have had four or more sex partners during their lifetime, by sex and grade, 2005. (From the Centers for Disease Control and Prevention. Youth risk behavior surveillance– United States, 2005. *MMWR* 2006;55 #SS-5.)

Forty seven percent (40% males, 54% females) of 13- to 14-year-olds felt pressure to have sex. Almost a quarter (27% males, 18% females) agreed with the statement, "If you have been seeing someone for a while, it is expected that you will have sex."

Another Kaiser report (http://www.kff.org/youthhivstds/3257-index.cfm) found that both casual and dating relationships were common among 15- to 17-year-olds. Twenty-six percent of the teens reported that oral sex was part of a dating relationship "almost always" or "most of the time"; 23% of teens surveyed reported that oral sex was part of a casual relationship.

Social and Demographic Factors Associated with Sexual Activity

Race/ethnicity, income, and family structure explained only 9.7% of the difference between younger teens who have or have not had sexual intercourse and 2.9% of the difference for older teens. A more comprehensive picture of the social and demographic factors that affect a teen's choice of whether to be sexually active is given in Table 39.3. Considered jointly, these factors explain 25% to 34% of the difference between males who have and have not had sexual intercourse and 35% to 49% of the difference between females.

Age Difference between Sexual Partners

The 2002 NSFG reported that 13% of females and 5% of males had a first sexual experience at 15 years or younger with an individual who was 3 or more years older (Fig. 39.4). The younger the teen at first sexual intercourse, the more likely that the partner was at least 3 years older (Fig. 39.5).

Even though many teens have their first sexual intercourse with an older partner, 77% of these older male and female partners were still in their teens. The minority of relationships occur when the adult partner is significantly older than the teen (Fig. 39.6).

TABLE 39.3

Factors Associated with Whether Youth had Sexual Intercourse[a]

	Males			Females		
	White[b]	Black	Hispanic	White[b]	Black	Hispanic
Individual sexual experience						
Opportunity						
Ever dated[c]	▲	▲			▲	▲
Ever kissed or necked[c]	▲	▲	▲[e,f]		▲	▲
Romantic relationship in 18 months before survey[c]	▲	▲		▲		▲
Motivation						
Made public or written virginity pledge	▲[g]	○[h]				
Perceived personal and social benefits to sex	○	▲[h]	▲[i]	○ ▲	○	▲
Perceived personal and social costs to sex		○[j]	○[j]	○		○[k]
Perceived costs of getting/making someone pregnant	○[l]	○[l]		○[l]	○[l]	○[l]
Perceived (not actual) knowledge of birth control[d]	▲	▲		▲	▲	▲
Individual						
Ever repeated a grade[c]			▲[i]			▲
Frequent problems with school work			○			○
Wants and expects to attend college						○[m]
Religious beliefs						▲
Physical maturity						
Peer context						
Number of best friends who drink	▲			▲	▲	▲
Prejudice among teens at school						

(continued)

TABLE 39.3

(Continued)

	Males			Females		
	White[b]	Black	Hispanic	White[b]	Black	Hispanic
Family context						
Parents disapprove of youth having sex at this time in their life						o
Positive parent/family relationships					o	
Number of siblings					o	

[a]The following risk and protective factors were not associated with ever having had intercourse in any gender/ethnic subgroup: whether would keep child if became pregnant; frequency of religious activities or physical recreation; believes successes were earned; self-esteem; parent presence after school; parent presence at dinner; sets own curfew; frequency of parent drinking; family member suicide or attempt; joint decision making; whether Spanish was the primary language at home (Hispanic).

[b]The following were not consistently related to ever having had intercourse among white youths when their sample size was matched to the Hispanic and black sample sizes: ever dated; virginity pledge; ever repeated a grade; hobbies; college plans; parent-family relationship; extended family in the home (adults); friend's suicide or attempt; number of best friends who drink; worked 20+ hr/wk.

[c]Dichotomous (yes/no) variable. History of rape was asked only of girls.

[d]Extent of perceived knowledge of birth control was only weakly related to extent of actual knowledge regardless of grade or sexual experience.

[e]Risk is enhanced if the youth sees a benefit to sex.

[f]Risk is enhanced if the youth repeated a year.

[g]Risk is enhanced if the youth feels knowledgeable about birth control.

[h]Risk is enhanced if the youth sees few social costs.

[i]Risk is enhanced if the youth had a romantic relationship.

[j]Protection is enhanced if the youth sees risk of pregnancy.

[k]Protection is enhanced if the youth has strong religious belief.

[l]Protection is enhanced if the youth has good school attendance.

[m]Protection is enhanced if the youth sees many social costs.

▲ = Risk; o = Protection.

From Blum RW, Beuhring T, Rinehart PM. Protecting teens: beyond race, income, and family structure, Center for Adolescent Health, University of Minnesota, 200 Oaks Street SE, Suite 260, Minneapolis, MN, University of Minnesota Printing Services, Minneapolis, MN 2000.

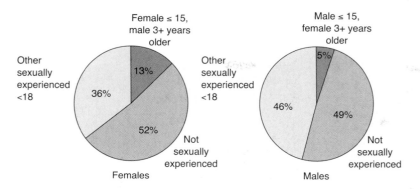

FIGURE 39.4 Prevalence of sex between young teens and older individuals.

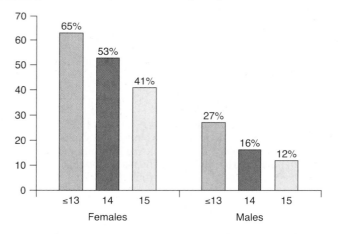

FIGURE 39.5 Percentage of young teens whose first sex was with an individual 3+ years older by age at first sex.

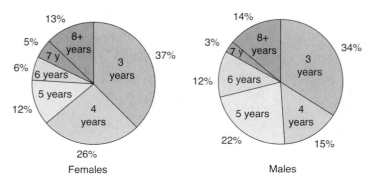

FIGURE 39.6 Distribution of age difference among young teens whose first sex was with an individual 3+ years older.

Wantedness of first sex

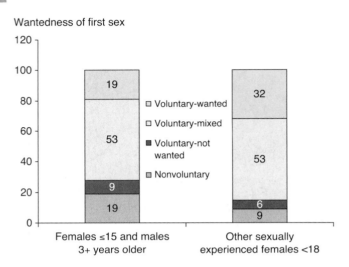

FIGURE 39.7 Wantedness of first sex among females who had sex before age 18.

Unwanted Sexual Experiences

The earlier a teen has sex, the more likely it is unwanted (Fig. 39.7 and Table 39.4). During adolescence, intercourse was involuntary in 61% of women who were 13 years old and younger at the time of first intercourse (Table 39.4). Sex with an older male partner increases the likelihood that it was forced (Fig. 39.7). In the NSFG, 15-year-olds who had their first sexual intercourse with a male at least 3 years older, were twice as likely to be forced to have intercourse

TABLE 39.4

Percentage of Sexually Experienced U.S. Females Aged 19 Years and Younger with History of Involuntary Intercourse

Age at First Intercourse	Involuntary Intercourse Only (%)	Both Voluntary and Involuntary Intercourse (%)	Voluntary Intercourse Only (%)
13 and younger	61	13	26
14 and younger	42	17	40
15 and younger	26	14	60
16 and younger	10	14	76
17 and younger	5	13	82
18 and younger	3	12	85
19 and younger	1	14	85

From Alan Guttmacher Institute. *Sex and America's teenagers*. New York: Alan Guttmacher Institute, 1994, using data from Moore KA, Nord CW, Peterson JL. 1987 National survey of children. *Fam Plann Perspect* 1989;21:110, with permission.

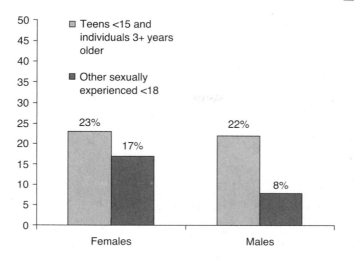

FIGURE 39.8 Percentage ever forced to have sexual intercourse among teens who had sex before age 18.

as compared to others who were <18 years old. One in five women who were 15 years old or younger and having sex with a male at least 3 years older reported this experience as "voluntary and wanted" compared to one in three of all sexually active women who were <18 years old. Of males <15 years old who had sex with an older female (>3 years older), 22% stated that it was unwanted as opposed to 8% of all sexually active males <18 years old (Fig. 39.8).

RECOMMENDATIONS

Suggestions to help children and adolescents better deal with their sexuality include the following:

Parent Education

1. *Infants and toddlers:* Use accurate anatomic terms to name the parts of the body. Children can be taught that their genitals are private and not to be touched in public, similar to covering their mouths when they cough or not pick their noses in public.
2. *Preschoolers:* Answer questions with simple and honest answers as they arise. Common examples of sex and procreation (i.e., family pet has a litter of puppies, a teacher is pregnant, or a sibling is born) may prompt discussion. Children should be taught the difference between "good" and "bad" touches. A "good" touch is one that feels comfortable and safe. A "bad" touch is one that makes the child feel "uncomfortable" or "confused." Children should also be encouraged to tell a trusted adult if they find themselves in an uncomfortable situation.
3. *Elementary school–aged children:* Television watching and computer use should be supervised and may prompt discussions about sex. School-aged children can begin to understand about germs, infections, and hygiene.

4. *Preteens:* Onset of puberty is a time when parents should begin frank and open discussions with their adolescents about STDs, HIV, pregnancy, and safe sex. They should know what intercourse is and that vaginal intercourse can result in pregnancy. There is no evidence that discussing sex makes children more likely to engage in it.

5. *Teenagers:* Parents should openly express their opinions concerning the appropriate time for their child to become sexually active, discuss rules about dating and curfews, and review contraception and disease prevention. Sexual values should be taught along with other values. Sexually responsible behavior is part of the overall assumption of adult responsibility.

6. *Timing:* Sexuality is a natural part of life from birth onward. Discuss sexuality as children grow up.

7. *Education:* Adolescents should be informed and knowledgeable—with the aid of parents, school, or community resources—in the following areas: (i) basic reproductive anatomy and physiology; (ii) basic sexual functioning and alternatives to intercourse; (iii) myths about sex and contraception—which should be replaced by medically accurate information; (iv) consequences of sexual activities, including pregnancy, STDs, HIV, parenthood; (v) contraception; (vi) the range of human relationships; (vii) components of decision making; (viii) the importance of self-esteem and respecting one's choices; and (ix) available resources to answer concerns, address questions, or tackle problems.

8. *Admit personal discomfort:* Adolescents respect honesty, and this will often allow for additional trust between the adolescent and the parent or counselor.

9. *Resources:* Be informed about available books, pamphlets, and other resources regarding adolescent sexuality. Some valuable references and organizations are listed at the end of this chapter and in Appendix II to this book.

10. *Privacy:* It is important to respect an adolescent's privacy and at the same time allow him or her the opportunity to discuss issues of sexuality comfortably without prying into details.

Community Resources

1. *Sex education:* Schools need to incorporate a curriculum on sex education that, in addition to including facts, stresses concepts of sexual responsibility and sexual decision making.

2. *Family planning clinics:* Increased availability of family planning clinics that serve and are sensitive to the needs of adolescents is essential.

3. *Professional education:* Health care providers continue to be educated regarding adolescent sexuality, resultant problems, and helpful resources.

4. *Contraceptive technology:* Development of continued safe, effective, easy-to-use contraception that would complement the adolescent's active lifestyle is needed (e.g., birth control patch and ring).

5. *Sexual history:* Should be taken of all patients (see Chapter 3 for the HEEADS approach). Confidentiality and its limits (e.g., sexual abuse and, in some states, statutory rape) must be clearly stated. Make no assumptions about sexuality or sexual practices. Teens should be asked if they are "now having" or "have ever had" sexual contact, both noncoital and coital. Adolescents should also be asked if they have ever been forced to have sex. A brief sexual history should be obtained even during episodic care. A teen's symptom of

abdominal pain or headaches could be the result of a prior history of sexual abuse or current relationship abuse (see Chapter 3).

6. *Sexual health of adolescents with chronic illness:* One study of the Add Health data set reported that teens with disabilities have rates of sexual activity similar to teens without physical disabilities. They also found that adolescent females with physical disabilities consistently have higher odds of experiencing forced sex. A review of studies on risk behaviors in teens with chronic illnesses found a substantial prevalence of sexual activity, but low level of knowledge and low prevalence of contraceptive use.

WEB SITES AND REFERENCES

www.goaskalice.columbia.edu. "Go Ask Alice" is a source of general health and sex information.

http://www.advocatesforyouth.org/. Advocates for Youth.

http://www.agi-usa.org/index.html. The Alan Guttmacher Institute home page.

http://www.kff.org/. The Henry J. Kaiser Family Foundation home page.

http://www.teenpregnancy.org. National Campaign to Prevent Teen Pregnancy.

http://www.cpc.unc.edu/. The National Longitudinal Study of Adolescent Health (1998).

http://www.plannedparenthood.org. Planned Parenthood Federation of America.

http://www.arhp.org/rap/. Resources for Adolescent Providers.

http://www.siecus.org/index.html. Sexuality Information and Education Council of the United States.

Centers for Disease Control and Prevention. Youth risk behavior surveillance—United States, 2005. *MMWR CDC Surveill Summ* 2006;55(SS05);1–108. www.cdc.gov/HealthyYouth/yrbs/

Kaiser Family Foundation, Holt T, Greene L, Davis J. *National survey of adolescents and young adults: sexual health knowledge, attitudes and experiences.* Menlo Park, CA: Henry J. Kaiser Family Foundation, 2003.

Mosher WD, Chandra A, Jones J. Sexual behavior and selected health measures: Men and women 15–44 years of age, United States, 2002. *Adv Data Vital Health Stat* 2005;362:1–56.

Society for Adolescent Medicine. Abstinence-only education policies and programs: a position paper of the Society for Adolescent Medicine. *J Adolesc Health* 2006; 38(1):83.

Valencia LS, Cromer BA. Sexual activity and other high-risk behaviors in adolescents with chronic illness: a review. *J Pediatr Adolesc Gynecol* 2000;13:53.

CHAPTER 40

Gay, Lesbian, Bisexual, and Transgender Adolescents

Eric Meininger and Gary Remafedi

HOMOSEXUALITY

Homosexuality is an emotionally charged issue and a difficult topic for the adolescent and his or her family and practitioner to discuss. Homosexuality usually reflects: "a persistent pattern of homosexual arousal accompanied by a persistent pattern of absent or weak heterosexual arousal." A bisexual person is attracted to both men and women. Sexual orientation should not be confused with gender identity, an individual's innate sense of maleness or femaleness.

Prevalence

Although sexual orientation is thought to be determined before adolescence, its expression may be postponed until early adulthood or indefinitely, making it difficult to determine the actual prevalence of homosexuality during adolescence. One study found that 2.5% of youths self-identified as gay, lesbian, or bisexual.

Four Stages of Acquisition of Homosexual Identity

1. *Stage I: Sensitization.* The child feels a sense of being different; by early adolescence, there may be awareness, including feelings and behaviors that would be considered homosexual.
2. *Stage II: Identity confusion.* The adolescent begins to identify behaviors and feelings that could be homosexual and may experience isolation or feel that no one else is like him or her.
3. *Stage III: Identity assumption.* The identity is adopted and possibly shared with others. This is known as "coming out."
4. *Stage IV: Commitment.* The individual experiences satisfaction, self-acceptance, and an unwillingness to alter his or her sexual identity.

Adolescents have reported first awareness of same-sex attractions by 10 or 11 years of age, self-identification at age 13 to 15, and first same-sex experiences near the time of self-identification.

Homophobia

Homophobia is an irrationally negative attitude toward homosexuals. One study found that 81% of GLB adolescents experienced verbal abuse; 38%, threats of physical harm; 15%, a physical assault (6% with a weapon); and 16%, a sexual assault.

Health Concerns

Breast Cancer. The risk of breast cancer among lesbians may be heightened by nulliparity, delayed pregnancy, alcohol use, obesity, and nonuse of screening services.

Eating Disorders. Gay males reported a significantly higher prevalence of poor body image, frequent dieting, binge eating, or purging than heterosexual males.

Pregnancy and Parenthood. In the 1987 Minnesota Adolescent Health Survey, lesbian or bisexual women were equally likely to have had intercourse with men, but more likely than their heterosexual peers to report a pregnancy (12% vs. 5%).

Runaway and Homelessness. Parental rejection, abandonment, and violence contribute to the disproportionately high numbers of GLBT teens in the homeless youth community.

School Problems. One report found that GLB middle and high school students were more likely to have been in a fight and were more likely to have witnessed violence.

Substance Abuse. GLBT adolescents are more likely to use tobacco and other illicit substances than their heterosexual peers. Substance use may result in unsafe sexual practices leading to sexually transmitted diseases (STDs) or HIV. There is a strong correlation between methamphetamine use and HIV transmission.

Suicide. Attempted suicides among homosexual youths are consistently higher than expected in the general population of adolescents, ranging from 20% to 42%. Identified risk factors are young age at first awareness of homosexuality, experience of orientation-based rejection, substance use, and perceived gender nonconformity.

HIV and Other STDs. Unprotected penile–anal intercourse has been shown to be the most efficient route of infection by hepatitis B, cytomegalovirus and HIV. Oral–anal or digital–anal contact can transmit enteric pathogens such as the hepatitis A virus. Unprotected oral sex also can lead to oropharyngeal disease and gonococcal and nongonococcal urethritis for the insertive partner. Certain STDs can facilitate the spread of HIV. Men who have sex with other men (MSM) continue to be at great risk for HIV infection. HIV prevalence was found to be higher in MSM of color than among Caucasian MSM.

Concordance between female sexual partners suggests that bacterial vaginosis is sexually transmitted among lesbians. Human papillomavirus and *Trichomonas* infections also may be transmitted between women.

Health Assessment

Begin by assuring the adolescent that all information will be kept in confidence (unless the adolescent poses a danger to himself or others). Inquiring about specific sexual practices will help determine the adolescent's risk and provides an opportunity to offer prevention education. Practitioners might routinely offer STD and HIV testing to high-risk populations such as incarcerated youth, youth in the sex industry, and institutionalized and homeless youth.

Specific STDs or Conditions

GLBT adolescents are at risk of contracting the same STDs as their heterosexual counterparts. Specific conditions related to sexual practices that are more common among gay adolescents include the following:

Enteric Illnesses. Teens engaging in unprotected oral or anal sex run a higher risk of contracting enteric pathogens. Evaluation may include stool cultures and microscopic evaluation for ova and parasites. Tests for gonococcal, chlamydial, and herpes infection should be obtained if proctitis is present. Also consider anoscopy, anal Pap smear, and testing for syphilis and HIV.

Chlamydia. Clinicians should be aware of lymphogranuloma venereum (LGV), a systemic disease caused by *Chlamydia trachomatis* (serovars L1, L2, and L3), which occurs only rarely in the United States. LGV should be considered in young MSM who have proctitis, proctocolitis, or painful inguinal lymphadenopathy as a presenting complaint.

Gonorrhea. Infections may be asymptomatic or associated with pharyngitis, urethritis, and proctitis. The Centers for Disease Control and Prevention (2007) no longer recommend fluoroquinolones in treating any gonococcal infections.

Syphilis. Regular syphilis screening is recommended for sexually active MSM. There is evidence that coinfection with HIV may alter the course of syphilis.

Hepatitis. Historically there has been a higher prevalence of hepatitis B in the gay male community than in the general population. Hepatitis A can be transmitted by the fecal–oral route during sex. The hepatitis A and B vaccine series is recommended for all MSM.

Cytomegalovirus. As many as 80% of homosexual males who engage in sex with multiple partners will acquire cytomegalovirus within a year. This infection is largely asymptomatic but may cause a mononucleosis-like illness in an HIV-seropositive teen.

Human Papillomavirus. HPV can cause dysplasia in the cervical, anal, or rectal mucosa, increasing the risk for carcinoma. Anal Pap smears can be used to screen for anal condyloma. The benefit of screening for anal carcinoma is under study. A vaccine for the prevention of HPV infections is now available for females between the ages of 9 and 26 years.

Herpes Simplex. HSV infections of the penis, vagina, mouth, or rectum can occur.

HIV. Discuss safer sexual practices including (1) abstinence from sex or risky sexual practices such as anal intercourse; (2) reducing the number of sexual partners (screen for Internet use as a means of meeting new partners); (3) avoidance of needle sharing—if needles must be used, they should be clean, fresh from a sealed pack, or flushed with household bleach and then water; (4) consistent use of latex condoms or barriers and water-based lubricants during sex; (5) avoidance of substance use during sex. Brainstorm harm-reduction techniques to increase the likelihood of condom use, and discuss the danger of sharing needles (see Chapter 31).

Counseling Issues

Given the opportunity to grow up in a supportive environment, gay and lesbian adolescents are no more likely to experience serious mental health problems than others. Homophobia engenders guilt, shame, and psychological problems. Practitioners must also be prepared to counsel parents as they attempt to understand their child.

Counseling the Teen

First, create an open environment in which the teen feels comfortable discussing issues of sexuality. Do not minimize the adolescent's concerns. Stating that "it's just a phase" may actually intensify the teen's confusion. Assuring him or her that questions about sexual orientation will resolve over time may take some of the urgency out of the issue "Am I or am I not?" The position of the American Psychiatric Association is that conversion therapy (i.e., attempts to repair or "cure" homosexuality) is not useful and may be damaging.

Regardless of the teens' uncertainty about their sexual orientation, helping to prevent the spread of HIV infection is critical. Not all homosexual teens experience difficulties with their orientation. As with other adolescents, well-adjusted homosexual individuals need sensitive and informed health care services.

Counseling Concerned Parents

- Help parents explore and address their feelings of anger, fear, shame, guilt, or grief.
- Offer correct information about homosexuality.
- Explain that not every problem manifested by a teen is a result of his or her sexual orientation.
- Challenge the dichotomous belief that homosexuality is bad and that heterosexuality is good.
- Explore religious beliefs and provide appropriate referrals. Affirming groups exist in most faiths and religious denominations.
- Discuss HIV/AIDS. Some make automatic connections between orientation and illness.
- Supplement counseling of parents by referring them to support groups such as Parents and Friends of Lesbians and Gays (PFLAG). Another useful resource is the National Youth Advocacy Coalition, which maintains a directory of local resources.

- Finally, the most important point to emphasize to concerned parents is that the adolescent who just "came out" is the same teen who sat before them before the disclosure.

TRANSGENDER ADOLESCENTS

General Considerations

The available literature on transgender adolescents is limited but growing. The American Academy of Pediatrics defines *gender identity* as a person's innate sense of maleness or femaleness. A person whose assigned sex at birth does not match gender identity is *transgender*. *Transitioning* is the process of changing one's appearance to better reflect one's gender identity. A *transsexual* is someone who has done something—either medically, surgically, or merely cosmetically—to express the gender with which he or she identifies. *Transgender* is a term that captures diverse individuals: those who have disclosed their gender identity to others, started mental health counseling, initiated medical hormone management, undergone sexual reassignment surgery (SRS), or some combination thereof. It is different from the paraphilia of cross-dressing or transvestitism, involving sexual pleasure from dressing or wearing clothes of the opposite gender. Although transgender individuals are typically identified by health professionals as male-to-female (conventionally, MTF) or female-to-male (FTM), affected youth may not even identify as transgender but only as male or female.

Unlike homosexuality, which was removed from the *Diagnostic and Statistical Manual* as a mental illness, the diagnosis of gender identity disorder (GID) has persisted, hopefully only to facilitate access to therapy and counseling specific to gender and transitioning issues and to enable individuals to receive medical and surgical management of their gender identity.

Prevalence

The most recent data from the Netherlands suggest that 1 in 11,900 males and 1 in 30,400 females meet the criteria for GID. However, little is known about the actual prevalence of transgender individuals in populations.

Etiology

Multiple studies have attempted to identify biological differences between transgender and nontransgender individuals. Except for intersexuality, variant gender identity is not necessarily associated with endocrinologic disorders, although some experts disagree.

Health Concerns

Transgender adolescents are at increased risk for multiple health problems.

Cancer. Little is known about the risks of malignancy in transgender people. Health educators may not perceive someone who is MTF as a woman and may neglect to offer education about breast self-examination. Likewise, an FTM individual who has not had chest reconstruction but who passes as a man also may not receive appropriate instruction.

Pregnancy. Transgender youth may be perceived as at low risk for pregnancy. However, it is important to ask about sexual practices and the biological gender of partners.

Smoking. Transgender youth appear to have a higher prevalence of smoking.

HIV. Risk factors include needle use to inject hormones or silicone, unprotected sex, and prostitution. Black transgender MTF young people have been identified as a subgroup with extraordinarily high rates of HIV, 63% in one study of Californians.

Runaway and Homelessness. For many of the same reasons as GLB youth, transgender youth have an increased likelihood of becoming homeless.

School Problems. A study in Philadelphia found that 96% of transgender youth reported verbal harassment and 83%, physical harassment; 75% had dropped out of school.

Substance Abuse. Substance abuse has been identified as a problem in the transgender adult community. No definitive studies of youth are available.

Suicide. Transgender youth may be at an even greater risk of attempted suicide than GLB youth. One study found that 62% of MTF and 55% of FTM adults met the criteria for depression. A third of each population had attempted suicide.

Hepatitis. Transgender youth may be at an increased risk for Hepatitis B and C if they are using injection hormones, silicone or other injection drugs and sharing needles.

Mental Health Concerns

The time delay between "coming out" as transgender and transitioning medically is a very unique stressor affecting the individual's mental health. Age-related emotional immaturity can adversely affect identity formation and decision-making skills.

Counseling the Teen. Create an open environment where adolescents feel comfortable discussing issues that trouble them. Do not make assumptions about names or pronouns or trivialize concerns about gender identity. Gender dysphoria can be very stigmatizing. Acknowledge adolescents' concerns and encourage them to take advantage of professional resources.

Puberty for transgender teens can be socially, emotionally, and physically stressful. It can feel as if the body were changing against one's will. Know the local resources for endocrinologic treatment and mental health counseling and support.

Because of discomfort with certain body parts, both transgender individuals and their health care providers may avoid examining the genitalia. Acknowledge the discomfort, and remind the adolescent that it is important to continue appropriate screening.

Counseling Concerned Parents. Help parents explore and address their feelings of anger, fear, shame, guilt or grief. Reassure them that they did not cause gender confusion. PFLAG chapters are often good places for parents to connect with other parents who have transgender children.

Medical and Surgical Management of the Transgender Teen

The Harry Benjamin Standards of Care, the most widely recognized approach to transgender management, encourages mental health evaluation and ongoing counseling as part of the process of medical and surgical transitioning. See the references below for additional information.

WEB SITES AND REFERENCES

www.pflag.org. Federation of Parents and Friends of Lesbians and Gays (PFLAG).

www.thetaskforce.org. National Gay and Lesbian Task Force (NGLTF).

www.biresource.org. Bisexual Resource Center (BRC).

www.glnh.org. Gay and Lesbian National Help Center (GLNH) 800-246-PRIDE.

www.youthresource.com. Advocates for Youth.

www.nyacyouth.org. National Youth Advocacy Coalition (NYAC).

www.wpath.org. World Professional Association for Transgender Health (WPATH).

American Academy of Pediatrics, Frankowski, BL, Committee on Adolescence. Sexual orientation and adolescents. *Pediatrics* 2004;113:1827.

Boehmer U. Twenty years of public health research: inclusion of lesbian, gay, bisexual, and transgender populations. *AJPH* 2002;92:1125.

Harry Benjamin International Gender Dysphoria Association (HBIGDA). Standards of care for gender identity disorders, sixth version. *J Psychol Hum Sexuality* 2001; 13:1. Available online at http://www.wpath.org/Documents2/socv6.pdf.

Ryan C, Futterman D. *Lesbian and gay youth: care and counseling.* New York: Columbia University Press, 1998.

Smith SD, Dermer SB, Astramovich, RL. Working with nonheterosexual youth to understand sexual identity development, at-risk behaviors, and implications for health care professionals. *Psychol Rep* 2005;96:651.

Tom Waddell Health Center protocols for hormonal reassignment of gender. Available online at http://www.dph.sf.ca.us/chn/HlthCtrs/HlthCtrDocs/TransGendprotocols122006.pdf.

CHAPTER 41

Teenage Pregnancy

Joanne E. Cox

Teen pregnancy, despite consistent declines over the last decade, remains an important medical, social, and public health issue in adolescent health.

EPIDEMIOLOGY OF ADOLESCENT PREGNANCY

1. *Teenage pregnancies:* There are approximately 800,000 pregnancies for females age 15 to 19 per year. Approximately 51% of these pregnancies result in a live birth, 35% end with an abortion, and 14% end with a miscarriage or stillbirth. For 10- to 14-year-old females, there are approximately 15,000 pregnancies per year.
2. *Pregnancy and birth rate trends:* The United States has set a national goal of decreasing the rate of teenage pregnancies to 43 pregnancies per 1,000 females between the ages of 15 and 17 years by 2010. In 2000, the teen pregnancy rate for 15- to 17-year-old females was 48.2. For 15- to 17-year-olds, the birth rate decreased from 38.6 in 1991 to 22.1 in 2004 (Fig. 41.1). In 2003, the birth rate per 1,000 females aged 10 to 14 years was 0.6 live births. The decline in teen pregnancy is due to both increasing use of effective contraception and decreased sexual activity. Analysis of 1991 to 2001 national data showed a 53% decline in adolescent sexual experience and a 46% increase in the use of contraceptives.
3. *Ethnicity:* Black and Hispanic females disproportionately experience pregnancy compared to whites. Hispanic females are most likely to experience birth before the age of 20.
4. *Geography:* Pregnancy rates vary considerably from state to state (Table 41.1) (www.teenpregnancy.org).
5. *Repeat pregnancy:* Of 561,330 births to teens between the ages of 15 and 19 years in 2003, 453,826 were first births and 107,512 were subsequent births.
6. *Prenatal care:* In 2003, 70% of teens aged 15 to 19 years and 49% of those below age 15 began prenatal care in the first trimester. Adequate prenatal care was lowest among non-Hispanic black teens and was directly proportional to age.
7. *Income levels:* Teens who give birth more often come from families that have low incomes (83%) as compared with teens who have abortions (61%) or teens overall (38%).

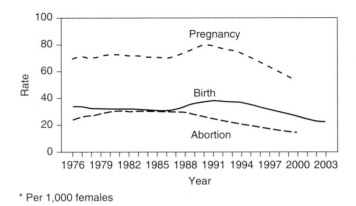

* Per 1,000 females

FIGURE 41.1 Pregnancy, birth, and abortion rates for teenagers 15 to 17 years old. (From National Campaign to Prevent Teen Pregnancy. *Fact sheet: recent trends in teen pregnancy, sexual activity, and contraceptive use.* Washington, DC: National Campaign to Prevent Teen Pregnancy, 2004. Available at: www.teenpregnancy.org/resources/reading/pdf/rectrend.pdf. Accessed June 19, 2005.)

FACTORS CONTRIBUTING TO ADOLESCENT PREGNANCY

1. *High rates of sexual activity:* According to the 2005 Youth Risk Behavior Survey (YRBS: www.cdc.gov/HealthyYouth/yrbs/), 47% of U.S. high school students had engaged in intercourse, representing a 13% decline since 1991. African-American teens have the highest rates of early sexual activity, followed by Latino and white teens. In 2005, about 91% of males and 83% of females used contraception at their most recent sex. Contraceptive use increases sharply with increasing age at first sex for females. However, condom use actually decreased with increasing age for males. In 2002, 36% of Latino girls used contraception at most recent intercourse, compared with 57% of African American girls and 72% of white teens.
2. *Physical and sexual abuse:* Nearly half of teen mothers have reported previous sexual abuse or coercive sexual experiences.
3. *Economic concerns:* A baby can represent success and hope for the future for teens facing economic and educational obstacles.
4. *Cultural values:* Early initiation of sexual activity is not unusual if other family members have a history of having become pregnant during adolescence. Other cultural factors include peer pressure, early dating, and lack of religious affiliation.
5. *Psychological factors:* Although psychological factors such as depression may have some influence on an adolescent's decision to become pregnant, the role of psychological and behavioral antecedents is unclear.
6. *Early puberty:* Earlier physical maturation has widened the gap between reproductive capacity and cognitive and emotional maturation and has increased the risk of unintended pregnancy in this age group.

TABLE 41.1

Teen Pregnancies, Births, Abortions, and Miscarriages and Stillbirths by Ethnicity and State and Abortion among Women Aged 15 to 19 by Race and Ethnicity

State	Pregnancies[a] Non-Hispanic White	Black	Hispanic	Births Non-Hispanic White	Black	Hispanic	Abortions[a] Non-Hispanic White	Black	Hispanic	Miscarriages and Stillbirths[a] Non-Hispanic White	Black	Hispanic
U.S. total	**346,980**	**235,650**	**204,980**	**204,056**	**118,954**	**129,469**	**92,830**	**84,460**	**45,110**	**50,090**	**32,240**	**30,400**
Alabama	7,310	6,600	390	4,976	4,380	305	1,210	1,220	20	1,120	1,000	60
Alaska	u	u	u	483	80	83	u	u	u	u	u	u
Arizona	6,670	930	9,480	3,732	559	6,585	1,990	240	1,440	950	140	1,460
Arkansas	5,470	2,890	460	3,942	1,992	358	670	460	30	860	440	70
California	u	u	u	10,279	5,406	36,919	u	u	u	u	u	u
Colorado	6,190	850	4,810	3,258	594	3,539	2,070	120	520	860	130	760
Connecticut	u	u	u	1,108	851	1,249	u	u	u	u	u	u
Delaware	1,160	1,120	240	589	577	158	420	390	40	160	150	40
District of Columbia	u	u	150	10	926	126	u	u	u	u	u	u
Florida	u	u	u	10,311	9,255	5,481	u	u	u	u	u	u
Georgia	11,510	12,890	2,580	7,593	8,213	2,004	2,180	2,760	160	1,740	1,920	420
Hawaii	470	130	u	164	57	414	250	50	100	60	20	b
Idaho	2,590	30	670	1,724	18	517	480	10	40	390	b	90
Illinois	u	u	u	7,063	7,647	5,832	u	u	u	u	u	110
Indiana	(11,600)	3,240	1,020	7,858	2,045	851	(1,970)	720	u	(1,770)	480	u
Iowa	(4,930)	410	410	3,061	272	344	(1,140)	70	u	(730)	60	u
Kansas	4,640	1,030	1,100	3,070	629	832	860	250	100	700	150	180
Kentucky	(8,740)	1,530	u	6,472	1,075	194	(890)	210	b	(1,380)	240	40
Louisiana	(6,350)	9,030	200	4,422	6,546	170	(950)	1,070	u	(980)	1,420	u
Maine	2,110	40	u	1,205	20	14	610	10	10	300	10	b
Maryland	u	8,840	640	2,645	3,934	533	u	3,740	u	u	1,160	u
Massachusetts	u	u	u	2,543	1,009	1,727	u	u	u	u	u	u

(continued)

379

TABLE 41.1

(Continued)

State	Pregnancies[a] Non-Hispanic White	Black	Hispanic	Births Non-Hispanic White	Black	Hispanic	Abortions[a] Non-Hispanic White	Black	Hispanic	Miscarriages and Stillbirths[a] Non-Hispanic White	Black	Hispanic
Michigan	u	u	u	7,204	4,545	1,152	u	u	u	u	u	u
Minnesota	5,580	1,400	920	3,280	779	660	1,500	420	120	810	200	140
Mississippi	4,280	7,140	110	3,075	4,796	80	540	1,260	10	670	1,090	20
Missouri	9,920	4,230	550	6,782	2,541	407	1,620	1,070	60	1,520	620	90
Montana	(1,530)	10	u	854	10	61	(460)	b	u	(220)	b	u
Nebraska	u	u	u	1,615	293	404	u	u	u	u	u	u
Nevada	u	u	u	1,518	445	1,658	u	u	u	u	u	u
New Hampshire	u	u	u	854	18	53	u	u	u	u	u	u
New Jersey	5,310	10,090	5,640	1,961	3,259	3,000	2,690	5,620	1,860	660	1,210	790
New Mexico	1,790	190	4,460	1,001	103	2,976	540	60	810	250	30	680
New York	18,300	22,890	14,660	6,010	7,325	7,251	10,080	12,820	5,410	2,210	2,750	1,990
North Carolina	u	9,400	u	7,229	5,621	1,996	u	2,420	u	u	1,370	u
North Dakota	770	10	10	472	9	20	180	b	10	110	b	b
Ohio	19,550	8,760	1,130	12,432	5,127	787	4,210	2,370	170	2,910	1,260	170
Oklahoma	u	1,560	u	4,619	1,076	813	u	240	u	u	240	u
Oregon	6,560	460	1,760	3,423	198	1,209	2,230	200	290	910	60	270
Pennsylvania	13,710	8,510	2,340	8,066	4,218	1,665	3,660	3,130	310	1,980	1,160	360
Rhode Island	u	340	u	540	170	385	u	120	u	u	50	u
South Carolina	5,970	6,200	470	3,738	4,217	361	1,350	1,040	30	880	950	80
South Dakota	1,030	20	60	698	14	41	180	94,056	10	160	b	10
Tennessee	10,540	5,680	690	7,224	3,631	536	1,700	1,210	50	1,620	850	110
Texas	23,910	12,660	42,430	14,811	8,065	30,924	5,580	2,710	4,840	3,520	1,880	6,670
Utah	4,010	90	1,270	2,924	55	962	460	20	100	630	10	200
Vermont	930	10	u	501	2	3	300	10	b	130	b	b

Virginia	u	6,880	u	4,656	3,987	864	u	1,900	u	u	990	u
Washington	u	u	u	4,806	536	1,968	u	u	u	u	u	u
West Virginia	(3,780)	250	u	2,663	161	5	(530)	50	u	(590)	40	u
Wisconsin	6,560	2,640	1,210	3,960	1,656	867	1,640	590	150	960	390	190
Wyoming	u	10	u	632	12	126	u	‡	u	u	u	u

From Guttmacher Institute. *U.S. teenage pregnancy statistics, National and state trends and trends by race and ethnicity.* New York: Guttmacher Institute, 2006.

<http://www.guttmacher.org/pubs/2006/09/12/USTPstats.pdf>. Accessed November 13, 2005.

u = unavailable.

Numbers of pregnancies include estimates of the numbers of miscarriages and stillbirths. Numbers of pregnancies and abortions in parentheses include abortions obtained by Hispanic women; in these states ≤10% of births to white women aged 15–19 years were to Hispanics. Even though abortions have been tabulated according to state of residence where possible, in states with parental notification or consent requirements for minors, the number of abortions and pregnancies may be too low because minors have traveled to other states for abortion services.

[a]Rounded to the nearest 10.

[b]<5 abortions.

7. *Developmental issues:* A limited ability to plan for the future or to foresee the consequences of their actions as well as a sense of personal invulnerability interfere with adolescent decision making regarding sexual activity and the successful use of contraceptives.
8. *Barriers to contraceptive use include* inaccurate information, poor accessibility or financial barriers, fears about side effects, partner concerns, and intended pregnancy or fear of infertility. Clinicians may fail to address sexuality and contraceptive use with their patients. Some providers are unwilling to prescribe contraceptives for their patients without parental knowledge or consent.

TEEN PREGNANCY PREVENTION INTERVENTIONS

Both primary (first pregnancy) and secondary (repeat pregnancy) interventions have been created and evaluated. Successful programs include elements of abstinence promotion, contraceptive information/availability, sexual education, education/school completion strategies, job training and other youth development strategies such as volunteerism, and involvement in the arts or sports. No research exists that links contraceptive education with increased sexual activity.

EVALUATION AND MANAGEMENT OF THE PREGNANT ADOLESCENT

Common Presentations of Pregnancy in Adolescents

The most frequent objective concern is a missed or an abnormal menstrual period. Others may report abdominal pain, fatigue, breast tenderness, vomiting, or appetite changes.

Pregnancy Tests

Pregnancy tests measure levels of human chorionic gonadotropin (hCG), a glycoprotein that is secreted by invasive cytotrophoblast cells. Most urine pregnancy tests detect hCG levels >25 mIU/mL, giving a positive test result around the first missed menstrual period.

1. *hCG levels during pregnancy:* Serum hCG is detectable by day 11 in >98% of women. Levels peak at 10 to 12 weeks' gestation and then decline rapidly until a slower rise begins at 22 weeks' gestation, which continues until term.
2. *hCG levels after pregnancy:* Levels gradually decrease after a delivery or abortion and the initial decrease is quite rapid. After 2 weeks, the serum hCG level should be <1% of the level when the pregnancy was terminated.
3. *Types of pregnancy kits*
   a. *Immunometric tests:* The urine test kits usually provide accurate qualitative response within 5 to 15 minutes and measure hCG levels as low as 5 to 50 mIU/mL. This can provide positive test results as soon as 10 days after fertilization.
   b. *Home pregnancy testing (HPT):* HPTs are popular, but their accuracy is not ideal. A percentage of urine hCG values during the fourth and fifth weeks is below the sensitivities of detection for common HPTs (range 25 to 100 mIU/mL).

c. *Quantitative beta-hCG RAI:* The most sensitive pregnancy test is a radioimmunoassay (RIA) that detects serum levels of the beta subunit of hCG as low as 7 mIU/mL. The major use is in identifying an abnormal pregnancy such as ectopic pregnancy, trophoblastic disease, or threatened miscarriage by checking either the doubling time or hCG disappearance over time.

4. *False-positive and false-negative results*
   a. False-negative tests occur with an hCG concentration below the sensitivity threshold of the specific test being used, a miscalculation of last menstrual period, delayed ovulation, or delayed menses from early pregnancy loss. Elevated lipids, immunoglobulin levels, and low serum protein levels can interfere with the serum test.
   b. False-positive test results with immunometric tests are very rare but can also occur with laboratory error. Very rarely, pregnancy test results are positive from hCG production from a nonpregnancy source such as tumors of the ovaries, breast, and pancreas.

5. The pelvic examination will help determine the gestational age of the fetus and will identify any problems that may require immediate attention.

6. *Uterine enlargement:* (a) 8 weeks of gestation, uterine enlargement detected; (b) 12 weeks of gestation, uterus palpated at symphysis pubis; (c) 20 weeks of gestation, fundal height at umbilicus. At this point, fetal movements should be detected and fetal heart sounds should be audible by Doppler study.

7. Other signs include softening of the cervix, discoloration of the cervix (purplish or hyperemic), and uterine softness.

Ascertaining the Gestational Age

The expected date of delivery (also called the expected date of confinement) can be obtained from the pregnancy wheel or is estimated using the Nägele rule. Add 7 days to the first day of the LMP, subtract 3 months from the month of the LMP, and add 1 year to the calculated date.

ALTERNATIVES FOR PREGNANT ADOLESCENTS AND PREGNANCY COUNSELING

Critical elements of counseling the pregnant adolescent include the following:

1. *A private assessment* of the adolescent's expectations and desires regarding the possible pregnancy. A preliminary assessment of any stressors or safety concerns is useful while counseling the adolescent about her test results.

2. *Support:* If the pregnancy test result is positive, adolescents should be encouraged to seek the support of parents, grandparents, or another trusted adult. The partner may also share in the decision-making process. It is vital, however, to screen the adolescent for safety in both their relationship and family domains.

3. *Confidentiality:* Adolescents should be reminded that any discussions about STDs or potential pregnancy (in a health facility) remain confidential unless the adolescent wishes to inform or include others. Occasionally, there are mental health concerns making it necessary to share information about the pregnancy with other health professionals and with the adolescent's adult caretakers (parents or guardians). Practitioners should familiarize

themselves with the medical confidentiality laws of their state, particularly in regard to statutory rape, parental consent for termination, and guidelines for judicial bypass.

4. *Nonjudgmental approach:* The provider should allow the adolescent to express her wishes for this pregnancy without imposing his or her personal values.

5. *Presenting options:* The adolescent needs to consider the following options:
   a. Carrying the pregnancy to term and assuming parental responsibility.
   b. Family-centered care for the adolescent and her new baby, thereby sharing child care responsibility with the baby's extended family.
   c. Placing the baby with adoptive parents after the baby is born.
   d. Terminating the pregnancy (e.g., induced abortion).

Adolescents Assuming Parental Responsibility

This is the most common outcome for pregnant adolescents, yet it is, in many respects, the most difficult commitment to fulfill, because it requires the adolescent to assume long-term responsibility for a baby. Essential elements for adolescent-focused prenatal programs include a complement of culturally sensitive medical, psychological, social, and educational services; staff knowledgeable in adolescent health; continuity of care through the postpartum period; and linkages to mother/infant programs.

Family-Centered Care for the Adolescent and the Newborn

Because adolescents are rarely able to assume independence after the birth of a baby, the adolescent's family (or community) will usually offer support to the young mother, her child, and if possible her partner. This supports the adolescent's personal development; however, it requires that she abdicate a significant amount of parental responsibility to other family members. Fathers should be included in services whenever possible. Providers who care for the adolescent parents will need to be linked to community-based services for extended families. Long-term continuous relationships with caring providers are essential to positive outcomes.

Adoption after Delivery

In most states and the District of Columbia, mothers who are minors may legally place their child for adoption without parental involvement. Less than 10% of the babies born to unmarried teens are placed in adoptive homes.

Terminating the Pregnancy

Unintended pregnancies account for >90% of pregnancies among 15- to 19-year-olds. Adolescents represent 19% of the approximately 1.3 million abortions that occur each year in the United States. Providers for patients who seek an abortion should be aware that careful follow-up and psychological support is needed while the adolescent explores this option.

Health care providers should be aware of their state's laws governing adolescents who seek abortion services. Many states require that parents of adolescents play an active role in securing an abortion for their daughter. Any financial barriers that may interfere with the adolescent's ability to obtain the abortion should also be reviewed. After a teen has decided to end her pregnancy, she may need help in selecting the best method. There are more options for those who have earlier terminations, but adolescents may delay abortion until later than 15 weeks.

Choice of Medical versus Surgical Early Abortion Methods

Medical Methods

Advantages of the medical method are that it avoids surgery and anesthesia, is less painful, may be easier emotionally, provides the girl with more control, is a more private process, and poses less risk of infection.

Disadvantages include bleeding, cramping, and nausea; more waiting and uncertainty; extra clinic visit; limited to pregnancies up to 7 to 9 weeks; and risk of methotrexate-induced birth defects if abortion is incomplete.

Types of medical methods (to be used during the first trimester) are as follows:

1. *Mifepristone-misoprostol:* Mifepristone is a progesterone antagonist that is an effective abortifacient. Efficacy increases with addition of a prostaglandin analog, such as misoprostol. The earlier in pregnancy these are used, the higher the efficacy. The technique involves at least three visits. Complications include infection, incomplete abortion, and heavy bleeding.
2. *Methotrexate and misoprostol:* methotrexate is a cytotoxic drug that is lethal to trophoblastic tissue. Combined with misoprostol, it is about 95% successful in terminating early pregnancies. This technique involves at least two clinic visits. Complications include incomplete abortion, infection, and heavy bleeding.

Surgical Methods

Advantages to using surgical methods are as follows: quicker (one visit); more certain; teen can be less involved; can be done under general anesthesia; and continuation of pregnancy is rare. Disadvantages include invasiveness (need for local or general anesthesia) and small risk of uterine or cervical injury or infection. These methods include the following:

1. Vacuum aspiration is the most widely used, standard first-trimester surgical method. It can be performed with local anesthesia in an office through 14 weeks gestation.
2. Dilation and evacuation is the most common second-trimester method. Laminaria or other osmotic dilators are inserted 1 day before the procedure to dilate the cervix. It is commonly used between 13 and 16 weeks.
3. Medical techniques for second-trimester abortions include hypertonic saline instillation, hypertonic urea instillation, and prostaglandin E2 suppository insertion. These techniques account for <1% of all abortions in the United States.

Abortion Risks and Complications

1. *Infection (up to 3%):* This can be minimized by prior diagnosis and treatment of gonorrhea and chlamydia, as well as by the use of prophylactic antibiotics.
2. Intrauterine blood clots (<1%)
3. *Cervical or uterine trauma:* Women younger than 17 years have an increased risk of cervical injury. Use of laminaria and skillful technique lowers the risk.
4. Bleeding (0.03% to 1%)
5. Failed abortion (0.5% to 1%). The mortality rate is <1 per 100,000 abortions.

MEDICAL MANAGEMENT OF THE PREGNANT ADOLESCENT

Prenatal care is a major factor predicting a positive outcome for a teen birth. In 2003, some 6.4% of all teens received late or no prenatal care. Factors associated with adequate teen prenatal care are increased age, a longer interpregnancy interval, partner/social support, and participation in a specialized adolescent pregnancy program.

1. *Initial evaluation:* Should include a personal medical history, family history of chronic illness, and a drug history for tobacco, alcohol, and substance use. A complete physical examination and pelvic examination should be performed. Laboratory evaluation should include the following: a complete blood count, urinalysis, blood type and group, syphilis serology, sickle cell test in black patients, test for Tay-Sachs disease for those of Mediterranean or Jewish heritage, rubella titer, Pap smear if a patient has been sexually active for 3 years, gonococcal and chlamydial test, hepatitis B serology, and HIV counseling and testing.

2. *Follow-up visits:* Topics to be covered on successive visits include physiology of pregnancy, maternal nutrition, substance abuse, sexually transmitted diseases (STDs) and HIV infection. Discussion should include referral to a prepared childbirth class, childbirth, breast-feeding and infant nutrition, infant care and development, contraception and sexuality, and postdelivery care needs.

3. *Nutrition*
   a. Ideal weight gain should be 25 to 40 lb.
   b. See Chapter 6 for specific changes in daily requirements for pregnancy.
   c. The teen should be advised against dieting during pregnancy.
   d. A prenatal vitamin supplement should be prescribed.
   e. Additional iron is required if iron deficiency is diagnosed.
   f. Adolescents consuming <1,000 mg of calcium per day should be given a calcium supplement.

4. *Prenatal visits:* Pregnant adolescents should have visits every 2 to 4 weeks, through the seventh month. Visits are every 2 weeks in the eighth month and weekly thereafter.

5. *Psychosocial aspects:* It is essential to consider that the pregnant teenager's acceptance of the pregnancy and her relationship with her parents or the father of the child may change during the course of the pregnancy.

6. *Substance abuse:* One large epidemiologic study found that adolescents were more likely than adult women to stop alcohol and drug use once pregnancy was confirmed.

7. *Medications during pregnancy:* Class A drugs have been tested and found to be safe during pregnancy; class B drugs have been frequently used in pregnancy and no adverse side effects have been documented; class C, drugs not yet tested and effects are largely unknown; class D, drugs have definite health risks, and class X, drugs should never be used in pregnancy.

8. *The chronically ill adolescent:* Pregnancy in chronically ill adolescents presents specific challenges and requires coordination with specialty care providers.

9. *HIV disease:* Pregnant women infected with HIV should be referred for appropriate treatment and supportive services. Owing to the risks of HIV

transmission through breast milk, breast feeding is not recommended for HIV-infected mothers.

10. *Battering:* Battering often starts or becomes worse during pregnancy. Prenatal risk assessment should include specific questions regarding family and partner violence.

MEDICAL COMPLICATIONS OF PREGNANCY IN ADOLESCENCE

Adolescents are not at a higher risk of developing complications during early pregnancy.

1. *Spontaneous abortion:* As with adults, a spontaneous abortion may occur in 20% of pregnancies. Abdominal cramping and vaginal bleeding characterize the early stages of a miscarriage or a spontaneous abortion. *Threatened abortion* refers to pregnancies complicated by bleeding and cramping, but the cervix remains long and closed. Should the condition progress, the pregnancy is nonviable and an abortion is "inevitable." A "complete abortion" occurs when all the products of conception have passed. A sonogram will confirm the absence of the fetus, and physical examination will show that cervical os is closed. If the miscarriage is considered an incomplete abortion, a dilation and evacuation procedure will be necessary to prevent blood loss and infection. Serum hCG levels should be followed until they are zero.

2. *Ectopic pregnancy (2% of all pregnancies):* Abdominal cramping and bleeding also suggest an ectopic, or extrauterine, pregnancy (see Chapter 56).

3. *Hydatidiform mole,* or gestational trophoblastic disease, may occur in 1 of 1,000 pregnancies each year.

OTHER CONSEQUENCES OF ADOLESCENT PREGNANCY

Child Outcomes. For teens over age 15, pregnancies do not have increased risk of adverse outcomes if adequate prenatal care is received. However, for teens under age 15 years, there are increased risks, independent of prenatal care, for prematurity, low birth weight, and mortality. Factors associated with pregnancy outcome are variations in prenatal care, nutritional status, prepregnancy weight, sexually transmitted disease exposure, smoking, and substance use. Owing to these factors, adolescents are at doubled risk for low infant birth weight and tripled risk for neonatal death.

The children of teen mothers face significant challenges with risks of developmental delay, behavioral problems, school failure, mental health problems, and high-risk behaviors during adolescence. Sons are at increased risk for incarceration and teen fatherhood and daughters are at increased risk for pregnancy.

Growth and Development. Although some recent studies have suggested small potential decreases in hip bone mineralization and ultimate height in the very young pregnant adolescents, no definitive data suggest that adolescent pregnancy adversely affects growth and development.

Education. Factors linked to higher educational attainment for adolescent mothers are race (blacks do better than whites), growing up in a smaller family, reading materials in the home, mother's employment, and higher parental educational level.

Socioeconomic Issues. Teen mothers are more likely to end up on welfare (80% receive assistance at some point in time). An estimated 50% of funds of the Temporary Assistance for Needy Families (TANF) budget is expended on families in which the mother was a teenager when her first child was born.

Subsequent Childbirth. Within 2 years, 10% to 40% of teen mothers become pregnant again. Protective factors against repeat adolescent pregnancy are older maternal age (>16 years), participation in a specialized adolescent parent program, use of effective contraception, school attendance, new sex partner, and avoidance of interpersonal violence.

WEB SITES AND REFERENCES

http://www.teenpregnancy.org/. National Campaign to Prevent Teenage Pregnancy.

http://www.plannedparenthood.org. Home page of Planned Parenthood, includes information in Spanish; also http://www.teenwire.com is for youth.

http://www.cdc.gov/reproductivehealth/unintendedpregnancy/. CDC site on teenage pregnancy.

http://www.urban.org/family/invmales.html. From the Urban Institute: Involving males in preventing teen pregnancy.

http://www.guttmacher.org/pubs/2006/09/12/USTPstats.pdf. Alan Guttmacher Institute, pregnancy trends.

http://www.childtrends.org. Research briefs and facts in at-a-glance sections.

http://www.nlm.nih.gov/medlineplus/teenagepregnancy.html. Bilingual site from the National Institutes of Health.

http://www.childtrends.org/Files/SexualActivityRB.pdf. Trends and recent estimates: sexual activity among U.S. teens.

http://childstats.gov. Forum on Child and Family Statistics.

Centers for Disease Control and Prevention, Department of Health and Human Services. Youth Risk Behavior Surveillance—United States, 2005. *MMWR Morbidity and Mortality Weekly Report* 2006;53(SS-5):1–108. (http://www.cdc.gov/HealthyYouth/yrbs/)

CHAPTER **42**

Contraception

Anita L. Nelson and Lawrence S. Neinstein

CURRENT TRENDS

Sexual Activity. The 2005 Centers for Disease Control and Prevention (CDC) Youth Risk Behavior Survey found that 46.8% of high school students had had sexual intercourse and 33.9% of students had sexual intercourse during the 3 months preceding the survey. Almost one third (29.3%) of ninth-grade girls had had intercourse; this rate rose to 62.4% for twelfth-grade girls. Many surveys do not ask about noncoital sexual practices, such as same sex practices, heterosexual anal intercourse, or oral–genital sexual pleasuring. While these practices do not result in pregnancy, they may expose the young person to sexually transmitted diseases (STDs). Oral sex among teens aged 15 to 19 is more common than vaginal intercourse. More than one in five teens age 15 to 19 who have not had vaginal intercourse report that they have had oral sex. Less than 10% of teens report using a condom the last time they had oral sex. Heterosexual anal intercourse was reported by about 11% of teens. Same-sex sexual contact was reported by 4.5% of male teens and 10.6% of female teens. Of significance is that >1 in 10 young women who first had sexual intercourse before age 15 described it as nonvoluntary and many more described it as unwanted.

Pregnancy Rates. There was a 28% reduction in U.S. adolescent pregnancy rates between 1991 and 2004, and these rates are currently the lowest in 30 years. The elective abortion rate peaked in 1983 at 30.7 per 1,000; it steadily declined by more than half to 14.5 per 1,000 by 2000. Of concern is that half of births to teen mothers involve men aged 20 to 24, and an additional one-sixth of those fathers are above age 25. Despite recent reductions in pregnancy rates, teen pregnancy rates in the United States are still much higher than they are in other developed countries. Estimates are that 78% of teen pregnancies are unintended and 28% are electively terminated.

Contraceptive Usage. The recent decline in adolescent pregnancies is due both to a decrease in sexual experience of adolescents (53% of decline) and to more effective contraception use (47% of decline). Condoms are the most popular method at first intercourse. About 67% of women and 71% of men reported using this method with first coitus. Even use of birth control pills increased from 52% to 61% between 1995 and 2002. Injectable contraception use increased among sexually experienced women from 10% to 21% between 1995 and 2002. Importantly, dual-method use (condom and hormonal method) more than doubled from 1995 to 2002 (8% to 20%). Contraception was less likely to be used (or used consistently) if the teenage girl had taken a virginity pledge, had an older partner, had a number of close friends who knew her partner, or reportedly had a relationship that was not romantic but had those trappings.

Contraceptive Education.   While parents, schools, and clinicians are all options for teens in obtaining contraceptive education, parents are often overlooked. Studies have shown ultimately better teen–partner communications and condom use when the parent was open, skilled, and comfortable with the discussion. Analysis of the abstinence-only school-based programs has demonstrated no long-term beneficial impact but has decreased access to contraceptive services.

CONTRACEPTIVE OPTIONS

The list of contraceptive options available in the United States has both expanded and retracted over the last decade (Table 42.1). Oral contraceptive pills and condoms are still the most frequently used methods, but new hormonal delivery systems such as transdermal patches, vaginal rings, and implants have been introduced to add convenience in use and hopefully increase efficacy.

Oral Contraceptive Pills

New oral contraceptive pill (OCP) formulations with lower doses of estrogen, different progestins, different pill utilization patterns and new noncontraceptive benefits have been introduced. The first nonandrogenic progestin (drospirenone) is now available in two different formulations. More pills with lower doses of ethinyl estradiol (20 and 25 μg) are available. New patterns of utilization are also available. Three low-dose pill formulations reduce the number of placebo pills in the 28-day packets to minimize estrogen withdrawal symptoms. Extended cycle use of pills with FDA-approved products and off-label use with other pill formulations and with rings reduces the number of episodes of withdrawal bleeding women have each year. Eliminating withdrawal bleeds offers significant health and quality-of-life benefits to adolescent women. However, careful counseling of teens is needed.

Implants and Injectable Contraceptives.   The implantable contraceptive system (Implanon) was approved by the FDA in July 2006. This is a single-rod system, which greatly simplifies insertion and removal procedures. The injectable progestin-only method [depot medroxyprogesterone acetate (DMPA), Depo-Provera] has been available off label for 30 years and since 1991 on label. A new formulation of DMPA with different buffers has been introduced with the name depo-subQ Provera 104. This formulation reduces the injection dose from 150 to 104 mg while maintaining intermediate-term (12 to 14 weeks) efficacy and replacing intramuscular injections with subcutaneous shots. Subcutaneous injections offer the potential for self-injection to streamline access and is also approved for the treatment of endometriosis. Concerns about the possible adverse effects that DMPA-induced hypoestrogenism may have on adolescent bone mineralization prompted a black-box warning on both formulations, as discussed in Chapter 47.

TABLE 42.1

Contraceptive Options

Category	Brand Name	Duration of Use
Intrauterine contraceptives		
Copper T-380A IUD	ParaGard	10 years
Levonorgestrel-releasing IUS	Mirena	5 years
Injections		
DMPA-IM	Depo-Provera	11–13 weeks
DMPA-SQ	depo-subQ provera 104	12–14 weeks
Implants	Implanon	3 years
Combined hormonal vaginal ring	NuvaRing	21 days
Combined hormonal transdermal patch	Ortho Evra	7 days
Combined hormonal pills	Multiple	1 day
Progestin-only pills	Multiple	1 day
Male condoms	Wide array	Single use
Female condoms	Reality	Single use
Cervical barriers	Diaphragms	24 hours
	Today sponge	Single episode
	Lea's Shield	48 hours
	FemCap	24 hours
Spermicides	Foams	Single episode
	Suppositories	Single episode
	Films	Single episode
	Today sponge	Single episode
Periodic abstinence and fertility awareness	Rhythm method	
	Billings method	
	Basal body temperature method	
	Standard Days Method	
	Symptomothermal method	
Withdrawal ("pulling out")	None	

IUD, intrauterine device; IUS, intrauterine system.

Intrauterine Contraceptive Devices. Changes in labeling for the copper IUD have made it a more attractive option for adolescent girls. There is no longer a recommendation that the IUD candidate be parous or in a stable monogamous relationship with no history of pelvic inflammatory disease (PID). The levonorgestrel intrauterine system (IUS) retains the more restrictive labeling but offers candidates significant reduction in menstrual blood loss.

Condoms. Male condoms have been greatly improved, with features such as ribs, scents, and different sizes/shapes to encourage more consistent and successful utilization. Simplified packaging helps to eliminate the chance that the condom will be incorrectly unrolled. Spermicide coating has been removed from many condoms because the spermicide added no benefit for contraception or STD risk reduction but increased cost. Adolescents should be told that condoms reduce the transmission of HIV and that correct and consistent use of condoms is a key component of safer sex practices. Two polyurethane condoms are available for couples with latex allergy.

Female Barrier Methods. Female barrier methods have also changed. Diaphragms may reemerge in the near future as a delivery system for microbicides. The female condom is available, but it is not as frequently utilized as the male condom because it is more expensive, more complicated to use, and less effective than the male condom. The latex cervical cap (Prentif Cervical Cap) is no longer available in the United States. However, the vaginal contraceptive sponge (Today), a cervical "shield" (Lea's Shield) and a silicone cervical cap (Fem Cap) have been introduced to be used with spermicide.

Fertility Awareness Methods. Fertility awareness methods such as periodic abstinence and periodic use of contraception are less reliable for adolescents because of their irregular cycling. However, for women with well-established cycles lasting 26 to 32 days, the "Standard Days" method with a ring of color-coded beads ("Cyclebeads") to help the couple identify at-risk days has greatly simplified the use of these methods. Other sexual practices, such as withdrawal, are quite prevalent with adolescents.

Emergency Contraception. One of the most important new products to be introduced in recent years is the emergency contraceptive (EC). The first FDA-approved EC, with estrogen and progestin (Preven), is no longer available. It has been replaced by the only other FDA-approved product (Plan B), a levonorgestrel-only EC. Plan B is safe and can be used by virtually every adolescent woman in need. EC provides a backup in case the couple's primary method did not function or was not correctly used. Since ECs works most effectively if taken as soon as possible after unprotected coitus, the optimal strategy is to provide an EC by advance prescription. Plan B has been approved for over-the-counter availability for people 18 years and over with government identification (proof of age).

SELECTING A CONTRACEPTIVE METHOD

Age alone should not limit contraceptive choices for young people. A brief description of how each method is used, how well it works to prevent pregnancy, what noncontraceptive benefits may accrue, and what side effects and health risks are possible are necessary for informed consent and for long-term contraceptive continuation. To help clinicians effectively counsel women and help them select optimal methods, the concept of "contraceptive fit" has been developed (i.e. the best method is the one with the greatest pregnancy protection that she will use consistently). The four dimensions include the following:

1. *Safety: What medical contraindications does she have?* A patient's medical conditions may exclude some options. For example, clinicians should not prescribe estrogen-containing methods to an adolescent with severe hypertension or breast cancer. Similarly, adolescents taking medications that have

significant drug-drug interactions with some contraceptives may not be offered those methods.

2. *The woman's reproductive stage: How soon does she want to become pregnant? How important is it to her to prevent pregnancy?* This question helps providers establish the concept that pregnancy should be planned and prepared for and also helps highlight or diminish the attractiveness of long-acting methods.

3. *Her lifestyle: What challenges does she have using contraceptives?* An adolescent mother may be overwhelmed by all the pressures and demands of child care. Convenience in the contraception may be important. An adolescent who has not disclosed her sexual activity to adult authority figures may need to use very discrete and private contraceptive methods. Episodic sexual activity patterns may discourage a woman from using methods that require daily administration, especially during weeks or months when she is not having coitus. A young adolescent may not be able to negotiate with her partner about sexual activities or use of condoms.

4. *The patient's own preferences: What has she heard from her friends and from the media?* While modifiable with education, this element may be the most critical in the equation to ensure an adolescent's commitment to using her contraceptive method.

IMPORTANT PROPERTIES OF CONTRACEPTIVES TO ADOLESCENT WOMEN

Convenience. Methods that require little forethought and/or preparation are most likely to be more successfully utilized by teens. Injections, implants, and intrauterine contraceptives all share this property. Once-monthly and once-weekly preparations are also attractive options. Among the combined hormonal methods, the once-a-month contraceptive vaginal ring is most convenient, followed by the once-a-week patch.

Effectiveness. Since pregnancy prevention is critical among teens, it is important to select methods with higher effective rates but that are still appealing. Emergency contraception should be provided by advance prescription to every sexually active teen and to each adolescent who may be contemplating sexual activity.

STD Risk Reduction. Adolescents are more likely to acquire STDs than other age groups due both to their intrinsic biological vulnerability and more risky sexual practices. For adolescents who are sexually active, pregnancy protection should not be sacrificed for the sake of STD risk reduction. Adolescents who are at risk for pregnancy *and* for STDs should be offered dual methods to minimize risk.

Maximize Noncontraceptive Benefits. Hormonal contraceptives provide important health benefits, improve a young woman's quality of life, and provide birth control. Some pills can be used to treat acne, reduce hirsutism, or regulate, eliminate, or minimize menses (for women with dysmenorrhea, catamenial seizures, menstrual migraine, premenstrual syndrome, or premenstrual dysphoric disorder). All women benefit from long-term health improvements, such as the reduction in the risk of ovarian and endometrial cancers. New designs of condoms may enhance sexual pleasure as well as reduce the risk of STDs.

Minimize Side Effects. Reduce the impact of contraceptive side effects by selecting a method with few side effects and also counsel women about potential side effects prior to initiation and to response quickly to complaints of "nuisance" side effects if they arise.

Flexibility in Contraceptive Initiation and Use. Health care providers can enhance contraceptive usage in teens using following principles and practices: (1) No pelvic exam is needed prior to the initiating a contraceptive method except intrauterine contraceptives, diaphragms and, perhaps, vaginal rings. (2) No cervical cytologic testing (Pap smear) is needed prior to the initiation of any method in an asymptomatic woman. Even a history of an abnormal Pap smear does not preclude use of any hormonal or barrier methods of contraception. Urine testing can be done to screen for STDs. (3) Immediate initiation of contraceptive methods should be offered, such as traditional barrier methods, Quick Start birth control pills, contraceptive vaginal rings, contraceptive transdermal patches, DMPA, and copper IUDs. Each of these methods can be started any day of a woman's cycle if it is relatively certain that she is not pregnant. Back-up methods for 7 to 9 days are needed after Quick Start of various methods. In addition, it is prudent to provide emergency contraception with Quick Start. (4) Extended cycling with combined hormonal contraceptives (pills and rings) can add health benefits and improve young women's quality of life. (5) Identify opportunities to provide contraception. (6) If possible, provide condoms generously. Give specific instructions for their use and storage.

CONTRACEPTIVE CONSIDERATIONS IN ADOLESCENTS WITH COMMON ILLNESSES OR DISABILITIES

The standard used to evaluate the safety of contraception in any individual situation is that the risks of using the method must be less than the risks presented by pregnancy. For women with serious medical problems, pregnancy may be hazardous. Therefore, it may be reasonable to accept higher risks with birth control with these women. Some methods are absolutely contraindicated. The appropriateness of use of any method must be evaluated considering how important pregnancy prevention is. The World Health Organization (WHO) Medical Eligibility Guidelines (Tables 42.2 and 42.3) represent a consensus of contraceptive experts based on current research. The guidelines are not intended to be a basis for individual risk recommendations but rather to provide national family planning organizations with recommendations on which to base their protocols.

Pulmonary Disease
Asthma. All methods of contraception may be used by women with asthma.

TABLE 42.2

WHO Categories for Temporary Methods

WHO Category 1   *Can use* the method. *No restriction on use.*

WHO Category 2   *Can use* the method. *Advantages generally outweigh theoretical or proven risks.* Category 2 conditions could be considered in choosing a method. If the client chooses the method, longer than usual follow-up may be needed.

WHO Category 3   *Should not use* the method unless a doctor or nurse makes a clinical judgment that the client can safely use it. *Theoretical or proven risks usually outweigh the advantages* of the method. Method of last choice, for which regular monitoring will be needed.

WHO Category 4   *Should not use* the method. Condition represents an *unacceptable health risk* if method is used.

Cystic Fibrosis. Concern exists in individuals with cystic fibrosis because progesterone can cause thick mucus and potentially thick bronchial mucus. A preliminary study suggested that OCPs containing <50 μg of ethinyl estradiol per dose may not exacerbate pulmonary disease. Another study examined the pharmacokinetics of sex steroids in women with cystic fibrosis using OCPs and found that these women receive contraceptive protection similar to that achieved by healthy women. However, hormonal contraceptives should be used with caution in these patients until further studies indicate that they are safe.

Inflammatory Bowel Disease. If disease is active and malabsorption of sex steroids is possible, OC use is not appropriate. Nonoral hormonal delivery systems bypass the enteric absorption problems and may, be used. In teens with stable, quiescent inflammatory bowel disease, OCs can be used with caution.

Diabetes. One study found that adolescents with diabetes mellitus were at higher risk to become pregnant at a time when their glucose control is suboptimal. Adolescents are also less likely to develop vascular complications than older diabetics and may be the best candidates to use low-dose hormonal methods. Implants may be attractive because of their limited impact on glucose and lipid profiles. Progestin injections have more notably deleterious effects on glucose control and lipid profiles. All women with diabetes using hormonal methods of birth control require ongoing glucose monitoring. They also need counseling to plan for pregnancy, because preconceptional glucose control has a profound impact on pregnancy outcome.

Hematologic Disorders

Iron Deficiency Anemia. Hormonal methods of birth control can be helpful for patients with iron deficiency anemia because they tend to limit menstrual loss. Long-term use of progestin injections and levonorgestrel-releasing intrauterine system (LNG-IUS) usually results in amenorrhea, which is extremely attractive to patients with anemia. Extended-cycle combined hormone methods reduce scheduled menstrual blood loss.

TABLE 42.3

Selected Conditions with Multiple Ratings for Contraceptive Methods

Condition	COC	P/R	POP	DMPA NET-EN	LNG/ETG Implants	Cu-IUD	LNG-IUD
Cardiovascular disease							
Multiple risk factors for arterial cardiovascular disease (such as older age, smoking, diabetes, and hypertension)	3/4	3/4	2	3	2	1	2
Hypertension							
1. Adequately controlled hypertension, where blood pressure CAN be evaluated	3	3	1	2	1	1	1
2. Elevated blood pressure levels (properly taken measurements)							
a. Systolic 140–159 or diastolic 90–99 mm Hg	3	3	1	2	1	1	1
b. Systolic >160 mm Hg or diastolic >100 mm Hg	4	4	2	3	2	1	2
3. Vascular disease	4	4	2	3	2	1	2
Deep venous thrombosis (DVT)/pulmonary embolism (PE)							
1. History of DVT/PE	4	4	2	2	2	1	2
2. Current DVT/PE	4	4	3	3	3	1	3
3. Family history (first-degree relatives)	2	2	1	1	1	1	1
4. Major surgery							
a. With prolonged immobilization	4	4	2	2	2	1	2
b. Without prolonged immobilization	2	2	1	1	1	1	1

Known thrombogenic mutations (e.g., factor V Leiden; prothrombin mutation; protein S, protein C, and antithrombin deficiencies)	4	4	2	2	2	1	2
Superficial thrombophlebitis	2	2	1	1	1	1	1
Current and history of ischemic heart disease	4	4	I 2 / C 3	3	I 2 / C 3	1	I 2 / C 3
Stroke (history of cerebrovascular accident)	4	4	I 2 / C 3	3	I 2 / C 3	1	2
Known hyperlipidemias (screening is NOT necessary for safe use of contraceptive methods)	2/3	2/3	2	2	2	1	2
Valvular heart disease							
1. Uncomplicated	2	2	1	1	1	1	1
2. Complicated (pulmonary hypertension, atrial fibrillation, history of subacute bacterial endocarditis)	4	4	1	1	1	1	2

(continued)

TABLE 42.3

(Continued)

Condition	COC		P/R		POP		DMPA NET-EN		LNG/ETG Implants		Cu-IUD		LNG-IUD	
	I	C	I	C	I	C	I	C	I	C	I	C	I	C
Neurological conditions														
Headaches														
1. Non-migrainous (mild or severe)	1	2	1	2	1	1	1	1	1	1	1		1	1
2. Migraine														
a. Without aura (age <35)	2	3	2	3	1	2	2	2	2	2	1		2	2
b. With aura (at any age)	4	4	4	4	2	3	2	3	2	3	1		2	3
Reproductive tract infections and disorders														
Unexplained vaginal bleeding (suspicious for serious condition)														
Before evaluation	2		2		2		3		3		4	2	4	2
Cervical cancer (awaiting treatment)	2		2		1		2		2		4	2	4	2
Breast cancer														
1. Current	4		4		4		4		4		1		4	
2. Past and no evidence of current disease for 5 years	3		3		3		3		3		1		3	
Endometrial cancer	1		1		1		1		1		4	2	4	2
Ovarian cancer	1		1		1		1		1		3	2	3	2

Condition					Cu-IUD		LNG-IUD	
					I	C	I	C
Current pelvic inflammatory disease (PID)	1	1	1	1	4	2	4	2
Sexually transmitted diseases (STDs)								
1. Current purulent cervicitis or chlamydial infection or gonorrhoea	1	1	1	1	4	2	4	2
2. Increased risk of STDs	1	1	1	1	2/3	2	2/3	2
AIDS	1	1	1	1	3	2	3	2
Endocrine conditions								
Diabetes								
1. Nephropathy/retinopathy/neuropathy	3/4	2	3	2	1	1	2	2
2. Other vascular disease or diabetes of > 20 years duration	3/4	2	3	2	1	1	2	2
Gastrointestinal conditions								
Current symptomatic gall-bladder disease	3	2	2	2	1	1	2	2
Past history of COC-related cholestasis	3	2	2	2	1	1	2	2
Active viral hepatitis	4	3	3	3	1	1	3	3
Cirrhosis								
1. Mild (compensated)	3	2	2	2	1	1	2	2
2. Severe (decompensated)	4	3	3	3	1	1	3	3

(continued)

TABLE 42.3

(Continued)

Condition	COC	P/R	POP	DMPA NET-EN	LNG/ETG Implants	Cu-IUD		LNG-IUD	
Liver tumor									
1. Benign (adenoma)	4	4	3	3	3	1		3	
2. Malignant (hepatoma)	4	4	3	3	3	1		3	
Drug interactions									
Drugs which affect liver enzymes									
1. Rifampicin	3	3	3	2	3	1		1	
2. Certain anticonvulsants (phenytoin, carbamazepine, barbiturates, primidone, topiramate, oxcarbazepine)	3	3	3	2	3	1		1	
Antibiotics (excluding rifampicin)									
1. Griseofulvin	2	2	2	1	2	1		1	
2. Other antibiotics	1	1	1	1	1	1		1	
Antiretroviral therapy						I	C	I	C
	2	2	2	2	2	2/3	2	2/3	2

COC, combined oral contraceptives; P/R, Patch/Ring; POP, progestin-only pills; DMPA/NET-EN, depot medroxyprogesterone acetate/norethisterone enantate; LNG/ENG implant, levonorgestrel/etonogestrel implants; Cu-IUD, copper intrauterine device; LNG-IUD, levonorgestrel intrauterine device; AIDS, acquired immunodeficiency syndrome; I, initiation; C, continuation. Modified from: Medical eligibility criteria for contraceptive use - 3rd edition, World Health Organization, Geneva, 2004.

Hemorrhagic Disorders. Hormonal methods are excellent choices for patients with hemorrhagic disorders. Hormonal contraceptives tend to diminish menorrhagia in women with coagulation disorders by limiting or eliminating menstrual flow. Combination hormonal contraceptives and progestin injections suppress ovulation and decrease the risk of hemorrhage with follicle extrusion.

Psychiatric Disease and Mental Retardation

Adolescents with psychiatric conditions frequently have their family planning needs overlooked. Their sexuality may be seen as acting out or a manifestation of their underlying disease. These patients may have difficulty in providing informed consent or in effectively using a contraceptive method. Many mentally ill patients have dual diagnoses, such as substance abuse and mental illness or epilepsy. Barrier methods provide needed reduction in the risk of acquiring an STD, but they may not be consistently used. IUDs are usually not appropriate because of the high risk of PID. Mentally retarded adolescents are vulnerable to exploitation and need additional sex education, which may be neglected. Mental retardation by itself usually does not constitute a medical contraindication to use of hormonal contraceptives, but studies show that long-term compliance with OCPs in noncontrolled environments is low. Satisfaction was highest with injectable contraception. Implants require patient cooperation for insertion and removal under local anesthesia; severely retarded patients may not be able to comply. Injections offer effective intermediate-term contraception, and the progestin injections usually offer the additional benefit of ultimate amenorrhea. Barrier methods and natural family planning (NFP) have no adverse effects in the mentally retarded, but the severely impaired patient may not be capable of understanding how to use them.

Connective Tissue Disease

Systemic Lupus Erythematosus (SLE). SLE has been closely related to hormones. Two recent studies suggested that the incidence of adverse events were similar among women with SLE, irrespective of type of contraceptive used. Another study showed that oral contraceptives do not increase the risk of flare among women with SLE whose disease is stable. Progestin-only methods appear safe in most women with lupus; Labeling for the LNG-IUS indicates that its use is not recommended if the SLE patient is immunocompromised by her condition or by corticosteroid use, but copper-bearing IUDs are allowed. Barrier methods have the least number of side effects and offer STD risk reduction. However, they have high failure rates, and pregnancy can pose serious hazards. NFP similarly has no direct adverse effects, but it is associated with significantly higher failure rates.

Rheumatoid Arthritis. Hormonal contraceptive methods are excellent choices for women with rheumatoid arthritis. Copper IUDs may be used by women who are able to check monthly for strings. Barrier methods are not contraindicated, but female barrier methods may not be appropriate if severe disabilities of the hands and hips are present.

Renal Disease

Hemodialysis. Most adolescents with chronic renal failure are infertile owing to hypothalamic-pituitary dysfunction. During dialysis therapy, some women resume ovulatory function. For sexually active adolescents with menstrual function, contraception is important. The major contraindications to OC use (estrogen-containing method) are hypertension and thromboembolic problems. Serum progestin concentrations from injections for patients undergoing hemodialysis are maintained within therapeutic levels.

Transplantation. Ovulation and fertility often return within 6 months after renal transplantation. Information regarding OC use in an adolescent with a renal transplant is limited. In teens without hypertension, low-dose estrogen-containing methods can be used with caution. Progestin-only methods are good choices, except the LNG-IUS because the women are immunosuppressed to prevent graft rejection. Other methods may be used as outlined earlier.

WEB SITES AND REFERENCES

http://www.itsyoursexlife.com/. Henry J. Kaiser Family Foundation site provides sexual health information for young adults and their parents.

http://www.sxetc.org/. This online teen newsletter examines love, sex, relationships, and health.

http://www.teenwire.com/. This teen site from the Planned Parenthood Federation of America provides information and news about teen sexuality, sexual health, and relationships.

http://www.youngwomenshealth.org/. The Center for Young Women's Health site, sponsored by Children's Hospital in Boston, provides information on health issues that affect teenage girls and young women.

http://www.guttmacher.org/index.html. Information and resources from the Alan Guttmacher Institute.

http://www.arhp.org/. Information and resources from the Association of Reproductive Health Professionals.

http://www.conrad.org/. Contraceptive Research and Development Program site provides general information on birth control methods, updates on ongoing research projects, and information on contraceptive technology workshops.

http://www.fhi.org/. Family Health International's site provides information on AIDS/HIV, STDs, family planning, reproductive health, and women's studies.

http://www.kff.org/. Henry J. Kaiser Family Foundation site provides information on adolescent sexual health.

Centers for Disease Control. Youth Risk Behavior Surveillance, United States, 2005. Surveillance Summaries June 9, 2006. *MMWR* 2006;55(No. SS-5).

CHAPTER 43

Combination Hormonal Contraceptives

Anita L. Nelson and Lawrence S. Neinstein

ORAL CONTRACEPTIVES

Oral contraceptives (OCs) are the most widely used method of reversible birth control in the United States.

Efficacy. The first-year failure rates in typical use for combined OCs is about 8%. In clinical trials, failure rates with perfect use are observed to be <1%; thus, most failures are attributed to incorrect pill taking. Recent studies have suggested a connection between heavier body weight and increased failure rates with OCs. However, a retrospective analysis of the 1997 National Health Interview Survey and the 1995 National Survey of Family Growth found that the increase in pregnancy rates in women with a BMI >30 was no longer significant after adjustments were made for age, marital status, education, poverty, ethnic/race, parity, and dual-method use. It is appropriate to counsel heavier women that they may be at higher risk for pregnancy than slender women.

Current Formulations. Pills with >50 μg of estrogen are no longer sold in the United States.

Estrogen Component. All combination OCs contain one of two synthetic estrogens, mestranol or ethinyl estradiol (EE). Mestranol must be hepatically cleaved into EE; 50 μcg of mestranol is equivalent to approximately 35 to 40 μg of EE. Most current combination pills contain 30 to 35 μg of EE, although formulations with 20 or 25 μg of EE are increasing in popularity. Formulations with 50 μg of EE are reserved for use with medications that induce hepatic enzymes.

Progestin Component. All pills in the United States today have one of eight synthetic progestins. Seven (norethindrone, norethindrone acetate, ethynodiol diacetate, norgestrel, levonorgestrel, norgestimate, and desogestrel) are derived from an androgen precursor; these progestins have progestational and androgenic metabolic effects. In many instances, the latter can be interpreted as antiestrogenic. The eighth progestin, drospirenone, is a derivative of spironolactone and has progestational, antiandrogenic and antimineralocorticoid properties.

An extensive array of formulations has evolved over the years in an attempt to meet the needs of women with individual sensitivities to particular sex hormone combinations.

Packaging. Most packs provide pills for only a single cycle. Some include only the active pills (generally 21), while others add additional (generally nonactive) pills to make a total of 28 pills in the pack. Active pills are packaged in one of three patterns: (1) *Monophasic packets:* Each of active pills has the same dose of estrogen and progestin. (2) *Multiphasic packets (biphasic or triphasic):* The active pills vary the dose of the estrogen and progestin throughout the active pill cycle. In most cases, the progestin progressively increases in dose; however, a few formulations hold the dose of progestin constant and increase the estrogen dose over the cycle. Some formulations vary both hormones. (3) *Progestin-only or minipill packets:* Each pill contains a small progestin dose. No estrogen or placebo pill is included.

Pill-free Intervals. The placebo pills have been the focus of much recent innovation in pills. Some formulations add iron supplements to placebo pills. The 7-day pill-free interval has been recognized to be excessively long with modern low-dose formulations. With modern formulations, endometrial support is lost within 2 days after taking the last active pill, so that ovarian follicular recruitment with the low-dose formulations begins early during the pill-free week. To reduce the 7-day hormone-free interval, one formulation (Mircette) replaced the last five placebo pills with five pills containing 10 μg EE. Two newer formulations (Yaz and Loestrin 24 Fe) include 24 active low-dose pills in their 28-day pill packet.

Extended-Cycle Pills. The most profound change has been the elimination or minimization of the numbers of withdrawal bleeding episodes each year. Early in OC development, women wanted regular menses to help reassure them that they were not pregnant. Currently, it is recognized that scheduled bleeding with OCs is not medically necessary and also inconvenient. Elimination of the pill-free interval also reduces breakthrough ovulation. Extended-cycle use of hormonal contraceptives is clearly the wave of the future for most women. Although extended-cycle use of any monophasic formulation is possible, the available FDA-approved extended cycle OCs (Seasonale) and (Seasonique) allow easier patient education and utilization, which is important for young women. Lybrel was approved in May 2007 and includes 365 active pills per year.

Drug Interactions. Drugs that induce hepatic enzymes can decrease serum levels of estrogen or progestin components of combination hormonal contraceptives, thus increasing failures (Table 43.1).

Anticonvulsants. Anticonvulsants are the most common class of drugs known to have this effect; they are also teratogens. The anticonvulsants that increase hepatic clearance include barbiturates (phenobarbital and primidone), phenytoin, carbamazepine, felbamate, topiramate, and vigabatrin; all of these are known to decrease serum steroid levels. Women using them may be better served by using progestin injections or intrauterine contraceptives. If a 3-month trial of 35-μg EE pills coupled with condoms yields continued

TABLE 43.1

Drug Interactions

Drugs that decrease contraceptive hormonal levels and/or efficacy

- Anticonvulsants that decrease ethinyl estradiol (EE) and progestins
  - Barbiturates (including phenobarbital and primidone)
  - Carbamazepine
  - Felbamate
  - Oxcarbazepine
  - Phenytoin
  - Topiramate
  - Vigabatrin (Listed on ACOG Committee on Practice Bulletins-Gynecology, 2000, but research and FFPRHC find no impact)
- Antibiotics/antifungals that reduce EE and progestins
  - Rifabutin
  - Rifampicin
  - Griseofulvin (pregnancies documented)
- Antiretrovirals that reduce EE and progestins
  - Protease inhibitors
    - Amprenavir
    - Atazanavir
    - Nelfinavir
    - Lopanavir
    - Saquinavir
    - Ritonavir
  - Nonnucleoside reverse transcription inhibitors
    - Efavirenz
    - Nevirapine
- Other agents that induce liver enzymes
  - Lansoprazole (no reduction in EE)
  - Tacrolimus (no published evidence of decreased efficacy)
  - Bosentan (no published evidence of decreased efficacy, but potent teratogen requiring monthly pregnancy testing)
  - Modafinil

Drugs whose effects may be altered by use of combination hormonal contraceptives

	Decreased clinical effect
• All antihypertensives	Hypotensive effect may be antagonized
• Antidiabetics	Hypoglycemic effects maybe antagonized
• Anticoagulants: *Phenidione, Warfarin*	Anticoagulant effect reduced[a]
• Tricyclic antidepressants	Antidepressant effects of tricyclics may be reduced, but side effects may increase because serum concentration increased. No evidence identified

(continued)

TABLE 43.1

(Continued)

	Increased clinical effect
• Immunosuppressants: *Cyclosporine*	Serum levels increased; potential toxicity
• Corticosteroid	Serum levels increased; no significant clinical effect
• Bronchodilators: *Theophylline*	Serum levels increased; potential toxicity[a]
• Dopaminergics: *Ropinirole*	Serum levels increased; no significant clinical effect
• Potassium-sparing diuretics	Drospirenone may lead to hyperkalemia[a]

FFPRHC, Faculty of Family Planning and Reproductive Health Care
[a]Measuring serum levels after contraceptive initiation may be appropriate.
Adapted from ACOG Committee on Practice Bulletins-Gynecology. ACOG practice bulletin. The use of hormonal contraception in women with coexisting medical conditions. Number 18, July 2000. *Int J Gynaecol Obstet* 2001;75(1):93.
Faculty of Family Planning and Reproductive Health Care Clinical Effectiveness Unit. FFPRHC Guidance (April 2005). Drug interactions with hormonal contraception. *J Fam Plann Reprod Health Care* 2005;31(2):139.

unscheduled spotting or bleeding, a 50-μg EE formulation may be necessary. However, no published data support the enhanced contraceptive efficacy of higher-dose (50 μg) EE pills or the effectiveness of nonoral delivery systems of combination hormonal contraceptives used with these drugs. It is advisable to shorten or eliminate the hormone-free interval when any of the combination hormonal contraceptives are used in women taking these anticonvulsants. Valproic acid, gabapentin, lamotrigine, and tiagabine do not affect sex steroid levels.

Antibiotics. The only two anti-infective agents that decrease steroid levels in women taking combination oral contraceptives are rifampin and griseofulvin. Isoniazid increases hepatic transaminase levels and may mask markers of an estrogen-induced hepatoma. Common anti-infective agents that do *not* decrease steroid levels in those taking combination oral contraceptives include tetracycline, doxycycline, ampicillin, metronidazole, and quinolones. Routine use of backup methods with these antibiotics is not warranted.

St. John's Wort. Studies have suggested that St. John's wort, which is sold over the counter to treat mild-to-moderate depression, may halve the serum levels of sex steroids.

Other Interactions. Some antiretroviral drugs induce hepatic enzymes and lower circulating steroid levels, while others decrease such activity and raise the steroid levels. Tobacco use also increases the metabolism of sex steroids.

Mechanisms of Action

Thickening of Cervical Mucus. The progestin component produces thick, viscous, scant cervical mucus that blocks sperm penetration into the upper genital tract. This is the most important mechanism of action common to all hormonal contraceptives.

Inhibition of Ovulation. The progestin-only pill contains a low dose of progestin such that ovulation is inhibited in only 40% to 60% of cycles. Combination pills, however, contain higher doses of progestin and suppress ovulation in 95% to 98% of cycles by inhibiting the surge in luteinizing hormone (LH).

Endometrial Changes. Although there are endometrial changes, contraceptive efficacy is undoubtedly minimal, since fertilization is so profoundly prevented by ovulation suppression and impenetrable cervical mucus.

Slowed Tubal Motility. The progestin in the pill slows tubal motility.

Workup Needed for Pill Initiation. A complete medical history is needed to identify contraindications requiring further evaluation. Blood pressure measurement is prudent prior to starting estrogen-containing contraceptives. Breast examination may also be needed. No other examinations are needed.

Pill Initiation

Quick Start/Same-Day Start. Teens are often in need of immediate contraception. The patient should be told to start with the first pill in the pack today and to abstain from intercourse or to use condoms for the next 7 days. If she has had unprotected sexual intercourse within the previous 5 days, administer two levonorgestrel emergency contraceptive pills immediately and have her start the first pill in her pack the next day. Urine pregnancy testing may be performed if there is anything in her history that raises suspicion of an ongoing pregnancy. The patient should be advised that her next scheduled bleeding will start during the placebo pills. If she fails to have a withdrawal bleed or has any symptoms of pregnancy, she should have pregnancy testing done as soon as possible. There is no concern that birth control pills are teratogenic, but early diagnosis of pregnancy is important. For women who are not having regular menses, the same Quick Start initiation rules apply.

First-Day Start. If Quick Start of OCs is not possible, then the first-day start is acceptable. The patient is given an interval method (condoms) to use until the *first* day of her next menses, when she should start her pills. No backup method is needed.

Sunday Start. The least attractive pill-initiation protocol is the Sunday start, since if a patient needs last-minute refills, she may have difficulty getting in touch with a provider during a weekend. However, sometimes the pill packets require a Sunday start.

Condoms and OCs. All teens should be given condoms and taught how to use them, as teens need dual methods to help reduce the risk of STDs. In addition, many will decide to discontinue the pill before they return. Since many women will forget to take all their pills, providing a prescription for emergency contraception in advance of need is an important part of OC initiation.

Prescription Length and Follow-up Appointments. When OCs are initiated, two other issues arise: how many cycles to dispense/prescribe, and how soon to see the patient in follow-up. One recent study showed that continuation rates are higher when women are given more patches or pills. The 3-month follow-up visit is still important for new-start adolescents, but in some situations it may be advisable to see the teen both 1 and 3 months after pill initiation.

Noncontraceptive Benefits Important to Adolescent Women

Decreased Menstrual Discomfort. Cyclically administered combination OCs significantly reduce monthly menstrual blood loss, the number of days of bleeding, and dysmenorrhea. Mittelschmerz is eliminated in most women because ovulation is inhibited in most cycles. Women with anovulatory cycles or dysfunctional uterine bleeding achieve predictable, controlled cycles with OCs. Women who are taking medications that increase menstrual blood loss (e.g., anticonvulsants, anticoagulants) or have bleeding disorders benefit from the use of OCs.

Dysmenorrhea is a particularly important problem faced by adolescent women (Chapter 50) and is the main cause of missed school and work in women <25 years. OCs significantly reduce dysmenorrhea, even when given in traditional cyclic fashion. Premenstrual tension syndrome may be reduced by use of combination OCs. One formulation (Yaz) has been proven to be an effective treatment for premenstrual dysphoric disorder.

Improvement in Acne, Hirsutism and Other Androgen Excess Problems. The FDA has approved three brands of oral contraceptives for the treatment of mild-to-moderate cystic acne in women wishing to use oral contraceptives (Ortho Tri Cyclen, Estrastep and Yaz). Maximal beneficial effects were seen at 6 months. Hair-shaft diameter is smaller in OC users, although this beneficial effect of OCs on hirsutism may take 12 months to become clinically apparent.

Treatment of Hypothalamic Hypoestrogenism. Many adolescents have eating disorders, excessive exercise programs, and/or stresses that suppress gonadotrophin production and create a hypoestrogenic state (Chapters 33 and 52). A lack of estrogen in a teen can compromise bone density and increase risk for osteoporosis and fracture. OCs have been the mainstay of therapy in treating women with the athletic triad, although the efficacy of OCs for enhanced bone density is still controversial.

Reduce the Risk of Ovarian and Endometrial Carcinoma. OCs are the only medical intervention with strong evidence for reducing the risk of developing ovarian cancer. Women who have used OCs for at least 1 year reduce their risk of developing epithelial ovarian cancer by 40%. Long-term users (>10 years) enjoy an 80% reduction in risk. OC use at any time during the reproductive years significantly reduces a woman's risk of developing any of the three major histologic forms of endometrial carcinoma by providing progestin. This protection increases with longer duration of use; women who use OCs for 12 years reduce their risk of endometrial carcinoma by 72%.

Other Health Benefits. Anemia is reduced by the reduction in menstrual blood loss. The thickened cervical mucus induced by OCs can block migration of bacteria into upper genital tract, which reduces a woman's risk of acquiring gonococcal-related pelvic inflammatory disease. Long-term OC use has also been associated with a reduction in benign breast changes.

Metabolic Impacts.
Both estrogen and progestin have important metabolic effects, with which clinicians should be familiar (Fig. 43.1). Differences among formulations may be helpful in selecting the optimal one for young women with different medical problems.

Coagulation Factors. Factors associated with the extrinsic clotting pathway (fibrinogen and factors I, V, VII, VIII, and X) are uniformly increased by estrogen-containing birth control pills in proportion to the estrogen dose.

Binding Globulins. Estrogen increases hepatic synthesis of carrier proteins such as albumin, sex hormone–binding globulin (SHBG), thyroxine-binding globulin (TBG), and corticosteroid-binding globulin (CBG).

Angiotensin. The estrogen component of the combination OCs increases angiotensin by increasing hepatic production of its precursor. Angiotensin can cause reversible hypertension.

Lipid Metabolism. Triglyceride levels are increased about 20% to 30% by exogenous estrogen use. Estrogen-induced triglycerides are composed of remnants that do not promote plaque formation, but they may pose a problem if a patient has baseline elevated triglyceride concentrations near the pancreatitis range (>500). Estrogen increases total cholesterol, high-density-lipoprotein (HDL) cholesterol, and triglycerides while decreasing low-density-lipoprotein (LDL) cholesterol. The androgenic component of the progestin has the opposite effect.

Glucose Metabolism. Estrogen may suppress insulin production and progesterone can increase peripheral insulin resistance. Most studies have found that current OCs cause no impairment in glucose tolerance in euglycemic women, but have some minor impact of insulin resistance. Even in high-risk patients, however, this is not clinically significant.

Contraindications.
Medical complications that are considered to be contraindications for estrogen-containing contraceptive use on the basis of current scientific evidence are listed on Table 43.2 as WHO category 4. The contraindications from product labeling are also listed. There are some profound differences between the two lists. For example, endometrial cancer is listed as an absolute contraindication to OC use on product labeling but is rated by WHO as category 1 (no restriction on use). Similarly, a history of cholestatic jaundice is a contraindication on labeling, but has been found to be only a relative contraindication by recent scientific evidence (WHO category 2). These differences underscore the need to be familiar with more than product labeling in addressing contraceptive needs.

TABLE 43.2

Absolute Contraindications to Estrogen-Containing Contraceptives

On Label	WHO Category 4
Exclusive breast-feeding	Breast-feeding ≤6 wk
History of thromboembolism	Current or history of DVT/PE
History of thrombophilia	Known thrombogenic mutation
Coronary artery disease	Current or history of ischemic heart disease
Cerebral vascular disease	Stroke (history of CVA)
Known or suspected cancer of the breast	Current breast cancer
Hepatic tumor (benign or malignant)	Liver tumors (benign or malignant)
History of cholestatic jaundice or jaundice with prior pill use	—
Known or suspected cancer of the endometrium or other estrogen-sensitive neoplasm	—
Unexplained abnormal vaginal bleeding	—
Known or suspected pregnancy	—
Postpartum (<3 wk)	—
	Age ≥35 years and smoking ≥15 cigarettes/d
	BP_S >160 or BP_D >100
	Hypertension with vascular disease
	Major surgery with prolonged immobilization
	Complicated vascular heart disease
	Migraine headaches with aura
	Active viral hepatitis
	Severe cirrhosis

WHO, World Health Organization; DVT/PE, deep vein thrombosis/pulmonary embolism; CVA, cerebral vascular accident; BP_S, systolic blood pressure; BP_D, diastolic blood pressure.

Health Issues and Risks with Combination Hormonal Contraceptive Use

Thromboembolism. Estrogen-containing combination hormonal contraceptives increase hepatic production of extrinsic clotting factors. Some women, such as those with anticardiolipin antibodies or factor V_{Leiden} mutation, are unable to compensate for this increase and have an increased risk for thromboembolic events. The overall relative risk (RR) of thrombosis is between 2.6 and 4.0; the absolute incidence of venous thrombosis is 15 to 30 per 100,000 woman-years for most of the low-dose OC formulations. The first-year relative risks of venous thromboembolism are higher, but rates are still lower than the incidence of venous thromboembolism in healthy pregnant women (approximately 60 per 100,000).

It is important to identify women at risk of venous thromboembolism by both personal and family history of prior thromboembolic events. Suspect histories are those with multiple family members who experienced multiple clots, often at an early age. Routine laboratory screening of all potential OC candidates for coagulopathies is inappropriate, but in high-risk women, testing should be considered.

Studies with low-dose formulations have detected no overall increased risk of hemorrhagic or ischemic stroke in healthy young women with OC use, but one study found that women reporting migraine headaches doubled their risk of stroke with OC use.

Cardiovascular Disease. Low-dose OCs (<50 μg EE) do not increase the risk of myocardial infarction (MI) in healthy, nonsmoking women. OCs do not increase plaque formation in adolescents; researchers reported a decrease in intimal thickness in new start OC users. However, there are clearly identified groups of at-risk women. Smoking cessation should be promoted with teens but smoking teens do not need to avoid pill use. Selection of a low-androgenic formulation may be prudent for smokers, as would shortening the pill-free interval.

Hypertension. Up to 3% of OC users experience increased blood pressure while on pills. Estrogen is largely responsible.

Liver and Gallbladder Effects. The risk of gallstones has been suggested with higher-dose pills, but it may still be seen with the lower-dose formulations.

Impact of Combination Hormonal Contraceptive Use on Neoplasia. The single largest concern women voice about OC use is the risk of cancer. Almost one third of all women believe that OCs cause cancer, but only a small minority is aware that OC use decreases the incidence of ovarian and endometrial cancer.

Leiomyoma. Historically, there has been concern that OC use might stimulate growth of leiomyomas (fibroids), but the risk of uterine fibroids decreases with duration of OC use. There is a slight increase in risk with early OC use, but this association may reflect an earlier age of menarche, which is itself a risk factor for fibroids. Women who have existing fibroids are often successfully prescribed OCs to reduce menorrhagia.

Cervical Cancer. More than 5 years of OC use causes a slight increase in risk of cervical dysplasia. However, the risk for squamous cell carcinoma does not appear to be affected by OC use. The risk of adenocarcinoma of the cervix may be increased, although this has not yet been conclusively demonstrated. OC users do not require any more intensive or more frequent Pap smears than their relevant risk factors would routinely dictate.

Breast Cancer. In contrast to the obvious benefits OCs have in reducing the risks of endometrial and ovarian cancer, the impact of OCs on breast cancer has been more controversial. In humans, there is no evidence that either estrogen or progestin initiates the development of abnormal mitotic figures in normal breast cells. Epidemiologic studies of present and past OC users have presented conflicting results, but virtually all the risk ratios for breast cancer calculated in these studies show either no increased risk or a small and reversible increased risk, especially with low-dose formulations, even in high risk women. One study of women age 35 to 64 found no increased risk of breast cancer in current/past OC users.

Based on all of these studies, it is not appropriate to deny any adolescent hormonal contraceptives. A strong family history of breast cancer, including one affected first-degree relative is at most, a relative contraindication for the use of modern, low-dose pills. Only a personal history of breast cancer is a contraindication.

Side Effects

As described earlier, the sex hormones in OCs have various degrees of progestogenic, estrogenic, antiestrogenic, and androgenic activities. These differences are important to understand, especially in responding to a patient's concerns about side effects.

Clinical studies conducted to evaluate the role of triphasic norgestimate-containing birth control pills in treating acne provided a unique opportunity to evaluate the incidence of side effects with modern low-dose pills. Over a 6-month period, the placebo group had the same incidence of headache, nausea, mastalgia, and other side effects generally attributed to OCs, as the OC group did. Even the incidence of excessive weight gain was identical.

Some women have particular sensitivity to sex steroids and may experience side effects as a result of the pharmacologic doses of hormone or because of hormonal imbalances. Many side effects are self-limited and resolve spontaneously in the first few cycles, but sometimes women require a change of pill formulation. When these side effects arise, it is important to analyze them by their constituent hormonal effects to select pills that meet the patient's needs.

Management of Common Side Effects

Unscheduled Bleeding or Spotting. Although irregular bleeding is quite common, other causes of vaginal spotting or bleeding must be considered, including chlamydial cervicitis and inconsistent pill use. Treatment for persistent spotting or bleeding due to OCs in the face of appropriate pill use depends on the timing of events within the woman's cycle. For women who have unscheduled spotting and/or bleeding at the end of their active pills, use a formulation with higher progesterone activity to support the endometrium during those days. Triphasic formulations, which progressively increase progestin dose, are particularly helpful in this situation. If the unscheduled spotting and/or bleeding occurs with the early pills, consider using formulations with higher estrogen in the early pills or those with lower progestin levels. This will allow the estrogen to induce endometrial proliferation and cover the denuded, bleeding areas left by menstrual shedding. Spotting and bleeding that occurs sporadically throughout the cycle is highly suspicious for inconsistent pill use, smoking, or drug-drug interactions. However, for women who do not have those problems but are still spotting, shortening the pill-free interval can reduce the frequency of that bleeding, especially if lower-dose formulations are being used.

Acne and Hirsutism. These symptoms are caused by free androgens. In order to cope, switch to a formulation with a higher estrogen content, which will increase SHBG and reduce the level of unbound testosterone, and/or switch to a formulation with a less androgenic progestin.

Chloasma or Melasma. Caused by estrogen stimulation of melanocytes, this should lead to decreasing or eliminating the estrogen content and advising the use of sunscreen and hats.

Weight Gain. Assess other potential causes. If the weight gain is concentrated in a woman's breasts, hips, and thighs, decrease the estrogen content of her pills. If the gain is accompanied by bloating and fluid retention, switch to a lower-dose pill or to a drospirenone-containing formulation. If the weight gain is slowly progressive (and not due to other factors), change to a less androgenic formulation.

Headaches. Rule out serious problems, such as hypertension and new-onset or worsening migraines, which would require OC cessation. Reduce the dose of estrogen or change to a progestin-only method. If the headache occurs only before or during menses (menstrual migraine), shorten or eliminate the pill-free interval.

Nausea. Have the patient take her pill at night. Reduce the estrogen dose if the first maneuver is not successful or if it will interfere with successful pill taking.

Mastalgia. Breast tenderness is usually self-limited, but if the problem persists, reduce the estrogen dose of the pill.

Coping with Missed Pills. Recommendations from WHO (Fig. 43.1) are based on number and timing of missed pills as well pill strength.

Increasing Adolescent Compliance

Methods to enhance adolescent compliance with contraceptive methods include the following: (1) Emphasizing the noncontraceptive benefits of OCs. (2) Demonstrating concretely how to use the pills. (3) Having the patient explicitly discuss her concerns about pill use so that they can be addressed. (4) Helping the teen plan for crucial logistics, such as where to store the pills and how to remember to take the pills each day. (5) Starting the pills immediately if pregnancy can be ruled out, simplifying instructions, and using a barrier method as backup for first cycle. (6) Shortening the pill-free interval. Start each new pack of pills on the first day of menses, or eliminate the pill-free interval for several packs ("bicycling," "recycling," or "combination continuous use"). (7) If the patient is unable to take daily pills, using a longer-acting product, such as the contraceptive patch or vaginal ring (see below).

Special Considerations in Adolescents

1. *When to start:* (a) *Young users:* If a young menarchal teen is sexually active, the risks of pregnancy exceed those of taking hormonal contraceptives. (b) *After pregnancy:* After a first-trimester therapeutic abortion or miscarriage, the pill should be started immediately to prevent ovulation. After a pregnancy, a 3- to 4-week delay should be allowed before starting OCs because of the

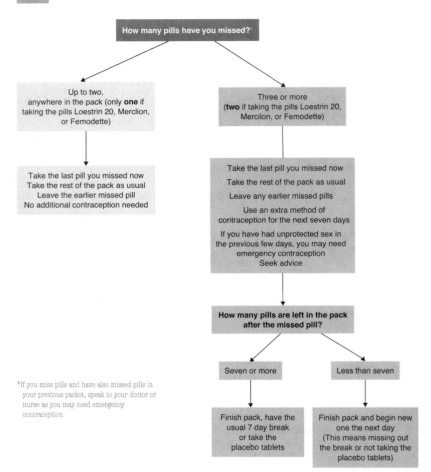

FIGURE 43.1 Missed pills. (Adapted from Family Planning Association. *How Many Pills Have You Missed? Contraception and Sexual Health Guide.* London: Family Planning Association.)

risk of thromboembolism. However, progestin-only methods can be initiated immediately.

2. *Irregular cycles:* Teen should be informed that her cycles are likely to be regular while she is using the pills but will return to their usual, irregular intervals when the pills are stopped.

3. *Initial examination:* (a) *History:* Menstrual history, past history, risk factors for STDs, history of problems that suggest contraindications for use of the pill, and sexual and family histories. (b) *Physical examination:* Only a blood pressure measurement and a breast examination are required to start hormonal contraceptives. The pelvic examination may be deferred for 3 to 6 months at least. (c) *Laboratory tests:* Screening for *Chlamydia* is

recommended for every sexually active teen but it is not needed prior to prescribing pills. (d) *Education:* Counseling is the most critical component.
4. *Follow-up:* It is preferable to see the teen at 1 month and again at 3 months after starting the pill, and then every 6 months. Blood pressure should be checked at 3 months and then as indicated for well-adolescent care.

PROGESTIN-ONLY PILLS

Progestin-only pills have traditionally been reserved for use by breast-feeding women. However, virtually every woman may be a candidate from a medical standpoint for use of progestin-only pills. The only condition that WHO rates as category 4 (do not use) for progestin-only pills is current breast cancer. Because the dose of progestin is significantly lower in progestin-only pills than it is in combination OCs, success requires consistent use. The progestin-only pill must be taken at the same time each day. Ovulation is suppressed in 40% to 60% of cycles. There are no placebo pills; a woman takes one active pill a day even while she is menstruating. The most common side effect from progestin-only pills is unscheduled spotting and bleeding or amenorrhea, just as is seen with other progestin-only methods. Whenever estrogen is contraindicated or undesired, the progestin-only pill is an excellent option.

TRANSDERMAL CONTRACEPTIVE PATCH

The Ortho Evra transdermal contraceptive system is composed of a 20-cm^2 tan-colored, thin patch containing ethinyl estradiol and norelgestromin. It is used once a week. The patch can be worn anywhere on the woman's trunk (except the breasts) or on her upper arms. The efficacy of the patch is at least equivalent to that of standard birth control pills for women weighing <90 kg. In the clinical trials, over 30% of the pregnancies occurred in those who weighed >198 pounds. In clinical studies, 87.7% of 18- to 19-year-old women in the patch arm used their patches correctly and consistently during the 1-year trial, compared to 67.7% of those who used OCs.

The first patch should be applied during the first 5 days of a cycle and is worn for 7 days, at which time another is applied in a different site. The third patch replaces the second patch at a different site 7 days later. After the last patch has been in place for 7 days, labeling instructs the patient to remove it and not use a patch the next week, during which she should start withdrawal bleeding. Provide guidance to patients about what to do if things go wrong, including (1) *If the patch detaches:* the teen should attempt to reattach it using its own adhesive; never anchor the patch in place with tape. If the patch will not reattach, have the patient place a new patch on a different site and replace that patch on her next regularly scheduled "change day," or change her change day to the current day. (2) *The patch was detached for >24 hours:* she should use a backup method for 7 days. Consider use of ECs (see Chapter 46). (3) *If late in changing her patch,* change it as soon as possible. If she is >2 days late, she should replace the patch and use a backup method for 7 days and consider whether she needs ECs.

Adolescents switching from pills to patches should place their first patch on the first day of withdrawal bleeding; they should not wait until they complete a pill pack. The patch should be started immediately after a first-trimester pregnancy loss or intrauterine contraception is removed or 13 weeks after the last DMPA injection. It takes 2 days to achieve therapeutic hormonal levels, so a backup method should be recommended if the patient is at risk. The safety and efficacy of quick start of the contraceptive patch has been demonstrated. However, compared with Quick Start with OCs, Quick Start with the patch did not increase short-term continuation rates.

The patch has virtually the same contraindications, precautions, and side effects as combination OCs. One exception is that the patch does not require GI absorption, so that conditions that limit GI absorption, such as diarrhea associated with irritable bowel syndrome (IBS), do not present any problems with patch use. Patches cannot be applied to irritated skin surfaces. The patch will not attach or may detach if oils or moisturizers, sun tan lotions, or other skin products coat the area. Women using the patch are more likely to report first-cycle mastalgia than are OC users, but by the second month, the frequency of this problem decreases to a level comparable to that of pill users.

The total daily estrogen exposure within the patch is 60% higher than with a 35-μg EE pill and 3.4 times higher than the vaginal ring. Product labeling acknowledges the higher estrogen exposure, although the clinical significance of this higher dose is unknown. The reason that higher doses of estrogen from the patch may not have the same thrombotic impact as higher-dose pills have is that the percutaneous route of administration bypasses the pill's first-pass effect. With the patch, the liver is not exposed to estrogen that does not appear in the bloodstream. Epidemiologic studies have yielded conflicting answers about the risk of thromboembolism with patch use.

VAGINAL CONTRACEPTIVE RINGS

Metabolism and Efficacy. NuvaRing contraceptive vaginal ring is a soft, flexible ring with an outer diameter of 54 mm and a cross-sectional diameter of 4 mm. The ring is impregnated with EE and etonogestrel (a metabolite of desogestrel). The ring is placed within the first 5 cycle days in a woman's vagina, where it releases a constant amount of contraceptive hormones for 21 days. Then it is removed and placed in its resealable pouch and discarded and a new ring placed 7 days later. Efficacy is comparable to that of OCs.

Advantages. The ring has features that are attractive to adolescent women. It is a once-a-month self-administered method with no external evidence of its use. Cycle control is impressive; tested against the best modern pill for cycle control (Nordette), ring users had fewer days of unscheduled spotting and bleeding than with pills. Since the ring releases estrogen directly into the vagina, it increases vaginal lubrication and has been reported to reduce recurrences of bacterial vaginosis. Women who need vaginal therapies, such as antifungal agents or spermicides, may use them without fear of adversely affecting vaginal ring efficacy.

Contraindications. The vaginal ring has the same contraindications as the transdermal patch except that there are no concerns about dermatologic conditions. The greatest barrier to acceptance of the vaginal ring is its placement and removal. Placement can be facilitated by loading the ring into an emptied tampon inserter with blunt opening. Removal of the ring requires only that the woman introduce a finger into her vagina, locate the ring with her fingertip, and withdraw it from her vagina.

Quick Start and Extended-Cycle Use. Clinical trials have now been published validating the safety of Quick Start for the vaginal ring and extended-cycle use of NuvaRing. In the extended-cycle study, some women changed rings every 3 weeks for up to a year without having a withdrawal bleed.

Other Formulations. Another estrogen-progestin ring that is to be used in 3-week cycles with 1 week out for up to 1 year is now undergoing clinical trials. Progestin-only vaginal rings are under development to provide the benefits of 1- to 3-month-duration vaginal rings without estrogen's side effects or contraindications. None are currently available in the United States.

WEB SITES

http://www.advocatesforyouth.org/youth/health/contraceptives/pill.htm. Advocates for Youth information on OCs with links to other contraceptive choices.

http://www.sex-ed101.com/oral.html. Sex Education 101 Web site on OCs and other contraceptives.

http://www.teenwire.com/index.asp. Teenwire from Planned Parenthood with information about reproductive health including contraception.

http://www.fhi.org/en/RH/FAQs/COC_faq.htm. Frequently asked questions sheet on combined OCs from Family Health International.

http://www.orthowomenshealth.com/orthowomenshealth/pages/pills_or_patch.jsp. Information from the Ortho Women's Health Web site.

http://www.arhp.org/healthcareproviders/resources/contraceptionresources/. Association of Reproductive Health Professionals.

CHAPTER 44

Intrauterine Contraception

Patricia A. Lohr

Intrauterine contraception (IUC) is one of the most effective forms of reversible birth control available in the United States. Candidates for IUC are multiparous and nulliparous women who desire long-term, highly effective reversible contraception. IUC is also an excellent choice of birth control for adolescents. Early studies on insertion in adolescents found high continuation and low complication rates. Recent data on the levonorgestrel-releasing intrauterine system (IUS) suggest that it is highly acceptable to young women. Types of IUC available in the United States are the copper T-380A intrauterine contraceptive device (IUD) and the levonorgestrel IUS.

The following contraindicate IUC use (ACOG, 2005): (1) Pregnancy or suspicion of pregnancy; (2) pelvic inflammatory disease (current or within the past 3 months); (3) acute and/or purulent cervicitis; (4) puerperal or postabortion sepsis (current or within the past 3 months); (5) undiagnosed abnormal vaginal bleeding; (6) malignancy of the genital tract; (7) uterine abnormalities that distort the cavity precluding proper insertion; (8) allergy to any component of the IUC or Wilson disease (for copper-containing IUDs).

COMMON MISCONCEPTIONS ABOUT INTRAUTERINE CONTRACEPTION

Issues Regarding Pelvic Infection

The Dalkon shield IUD was associated with PID and infertility. Its polyfilament tail allowed vaginal pathogens to ascend into the upper genital tract by wicking action. Modern IUCs have monofilament tails and do not facilitate infection. Infection is increased only in the first 20 days after insertion owing to endometrial contamination. This underscores the need to evaluate for cervicitis and to use meticulously sterile insertion technique. Antibiotic prophylaxis, including spontaneous bacterial endocarditis prophylaxis, is not warranted.

Actinomyces israelii is a gram-positive anaerobic bacterium normally found in the gastrointestinal tract. Colonization appears to increase with the duration of IUC use. The correlation between *Actinomyces* on a Pap smear and the development of pelvic actinomycosis, a very rare but serious condition, is unclear. Management of asymptomatic users should be based on clinical judgment.

Options include expectant management, oral antibiotics, and/or removal (ACOG, 2005).

Issues Regarding Ectopic Pregnancy

IUC reduces the risk of ectopic pregnancy. The ectopic pregnancy rate with the copper T-380A IUD and the levonorgestrel IUS are 0 to 0.5 per 1,000 woman-years compared with 3.25 to 5.25 per 1,000 woman-years among women not using contraception.

Issues Regarding Fertility

A large case-control study of nulligravid women with primary infertility found no increased risk of tubal infertility among previous users of copper-containg IUC (Hubacher et al, 2001). However, a significant association was demonstrated between antichlamydial antibodies and infertility. The fertility of women after IUC removal is comparable to that in the general population.

Issues Regarding Mechanism of Action

It is important to note that *IUC does not work by causing an abortion*. Serial beta human chorionic gonadotropin (beta-hCG) determinations obtained from IUC users over time failed to show the anticipated rise and fall characteristic of postimplantation (pregnancy) interruption. In addition, intrauterine flushing experiments have failed to yield blastocysts.

Lack of Knowledge about Intrauterine Contraception

A study of young pregnant women (ages 14 to 25) revealed that only 50% had heard of IUC. Of those, most were not aware of its safety (71%) or efficacy (58%). Younger women were less likely to have information about IUC, highlighting the need for education.

TYPES OF INTRAUTERINE CONTRACEPTIVE DEVICES

ParaGard Copper T-380A Intrauterine Device

Description of Device. The copper T-380A IUD is a flexible T-shaped polyethylene frame whose vertical stem is wrapped with copper wire coil and whose horizontal arms are each encased in a copper collar. The copper surface area totals 380 mm^2. Monofilament strings are threaded through the bulb at the end of the stem. Approval is for 10 years of use, but studies show that it is highly effective for 12 years.

Candidates for IUD Use. The prescribing label has been revised to explicitly include nulliparous and nonmonogamous women and those with a history of PID. The list also includes immunosuppressed women and those with non-infectious vaginitis, prior ectopic pregnancy, or an abnormal Pap smear not suggestive of cervical or endometrial carcinoma.

The IUD can be inserted at any time in the cycle if the patient is not pregnant. Immediate insertion after an uncomplicated first-trimester surgical abortion is safe and effective. A new IUD can be placed immediately after removal if the patient is still an appropriate candidate.

Effectiveness. The typical first-year failure rate of the copper T-380A IUD is 0.8%; the 10- and the 12-year cumulative failure rates are 2.2% respectively.

Mechanisms of Action. The best overall description of the copper T-380A IUD is a "functional spermicide." Copper ions interfere with sperm motility, transport, and capacitation and frequently cause sperm head-tail disconnection. The foreign-body inflammatory reaction induced by the device is also spermicidal.

Contraindications. The copper T-380A IUD should not be inserted if any of the previously listed contraindications exist (see page 418) or a uterine cavity <6 cm or >9 cm on sounding.

Relative Contraindications. Anemia, menorrhagia, and severe dysmenorrhea.

Advantages. Extremely effective, decreased risk of ectopic pregnancy, convenient (does not require regular method adherence), private, rapidly reversible, and can be used as emergency contraception (EC) within 5 days of unprotected intercourse.

Disadvantages. Professional assistance required for insertion and removal; no protection against STDs, *Actinomyces* colonization appears to increase with duration of use, there are some side effects (discussed later), and the initial cost is relatively high.

Side Effects
1. *Increased menstrual bleeding and cramping:* Menstrual blood loss increases by about 35%; dysmenorrhea can result. Prophylactic ibuprofen does not appear to reduce early removals due to bleeding and/or pain. An isolated episode of increased or untimely bleeding or cramping may indicate partial expulsion or failure and requires evaluation.
2. *IUD expulsion:* First-year rates range from 2% to 8%.
3. *Perforation or embedment:* Uterine perforation is rare (1 in 1,000 insertions) but increased with inexperienced inserters. An adherent IUD can often be removed in an office setting, but a deeply embedded IUD may require surgical removal.

Mirena Intrauterine System (Levonorgestrel IUS)
Description of Device. The levonorgestrel IUS has a flexible T-shaped frame with a steroid reservoir surrounding its vertical stem containing levonorgestrel and polydimethylsiloxane. Twenty micrograms of levonorgestrel are released daily. Two monofilament tail strings are threaded through a bulb at the base of the T. The IUS is approved for 5 years of use.

Efficacy. The typical first-year failure rates for the levonorgestrel IUS is 0.1%. The cumulative 5-year failure rate ranges from 0.5% to 1.1%.

Mechanisms of Action. The IUS renders cervical mucus impenetrable to sperm, produces an atrophic endometrium, and slows tubal motility. Ovulation is not consistently suppressed.

Contraindications. In addition to the general IUC contraindications (see page 418), an allergy to any IUS component precludes use. The uterus should sound to a depth of 6 to 9 cm.

Advantages. The levonorgestrel IUS reduces menstrual blood loss and dysmenorrhea. It may lower the risk of PID, and colonization by *Actinomyces*-like organisms.

Disadvantages. The disadvantages are similar to those of the copper T-380A IUD. The levonorgestrel IUS cannot be used as EC.

Side Effects

1. *Bleeding irregularities*: Most users experience unpredictable spotting or bleeding in the first 3 to 6 months after insertion. Subsequent amenorrhea or oligomenorrhea are common.
2. *IUS expulsion and perforation*: The expulsion rate in the first 1 to 2 years of use is approximately 4%, and the cumulative 5-year rate is about 11%. The risk of perforation is approximately 1/1000.
3. *Pain at insertion*: IUS insertion may be more uncomfortable than copper IUD insertion owing to a wider insertion tube. Cervical dilation or local anesthesia may reduce discomfort.
4. *Ovarian cysts*: Enlarged ovarian follicles can occur; intervention is not typically indicated.
5. *Progestin effects*: Systemic progestin effects (mastalgia, acne, headaches) can occur.

PREGNANCY WITH INTRAUTERINE CONTRACEPTION IN PLACE

The most common reason for pregnancy is undetected expulsion. When pregnancy occurs with IUC in situ, the location should be determined promptly; 8% of pregnancies with the copper T-380A IUD and 50% of those with the levonorgestrel IUS are ectopic. Remove IUC in the first trimester if the strings are visible because of an increased risk of spontaneous or septic abortion. Later in pregnancy, the IUC should not be removed. The risk of birth defects is not increased, but the chances of a premature birth may be increased. If a teen elects abortion, IUC can be removed for the procedure and a new one placed afterward if desired.

REFERENCES AND ADDITIONAL READINGS

American College of Obstetricians and Gynecologists. Intrauterine device. ACOG Practice Bulletin No. 59. *Obstet Gynecol* 2005;105:223.

Hubacher D, Lara-Ricalde R, Taylor DJ, et al. Use of copper intrauterine devices and the risk of tubal infertility among nulligravid women. *N Engl J Med* 2001;345:561.

Lippes J. Pelvic actinomycosis: a review and preliminary look at prevalence. *Am J Obstet Gynecol* 1999;180:265.

Sivin I. IUDs are contraceptives, not abortifacients: a comment on research and belief. *Stud Fam Plann* 1989;20:355.

Stanwood NL, Bradley KA. Young pregnant women's knowledge of modern intrauterine devices. *Obstet Gynecol* 2006;108:1417–1422.

UN Development Programme/United Nations Population Fund/World Health Organization/World Bank, Special Programme of Research, Development and Research Training in Human Reproduction. Long-term reversible contraception: twelve years of experience with the TCu380A and TCu220C. *Contraception* 1997;56:341.

WHO Scientific Group. *Mechanisms of action, safety and efficacy of intrauterine devices.* WHO Technical Report 753. Geneva: World Health Organization, 1987.

CHAPTER 45

Barrier Contraceptives and Spermicides

Patricia A. Lohr

MALE CONDOMS

Male condoms (Fig. 45.1) are made from latex, polyurethane, and lamb cecum (natural membrane or "skin" condoms). Shapes, colors, and textures vary, and they may be lubricated with silicone, water-based gel, or spermicide. Polyurethane condoms may be best reserved for couples who cannot tolerate latex, as polyurethane lacks elasticity, leading to higher slippage and breakage rates than latex. Condoms coated with the spermicide nonoxynol-9 are no longer advocated because of their increased cost, shorter shelf life, and association with urinary tract infections in women. Natural membrane condoms afford almost equal pregnancy protection as latex condoms but are more expensive and do not reduce STD risks.

Mechanism of Action
Condoms are sheaths that fit over the penis and block transmission of semen.

Effectiveness
The typical first-year failure rate of the latex male condom is 15%. The failure rate for correct and consistent use is 2%. Polyurethane condoms have higher breakage and slippage rates but similar pregnancy rates. Both are highly effective at preventing STDs, including HIV.

Improving Condom Success
Condom use by adolescents is increased when they believe that their peers use condoms and that condoms can prevent STDs. Other factors affecting use are when adolescents have easy access to condoms, know how to use a condom, and carry condoms with them. Providers should be responsive to patient complaints and apprehension, teach teens to use condoms effectively (Fig. 45.1), and practice placing condoms on models or over two fingers during office visits.

Patient Education
Adolescents should be counseled on condom types, failure rates, correct use and disposal, as well as what measures to take in the event of a condom break or slip (Fig. 45.1).

The male condom is a sheath of plastic or rubber that fits snugly over the erect penis. It blocks the man's sperm from entering the woman's body. It also covers the penis to help protect the man and the woman from getting sexually transmitted infections from each other. The male condom can be used with other contraceptives. It can be used with other birth control methods such as birth control pills, shots, implants, spermicide and diaphragms. It should not be used with the female condom. On average, if 100 couples use condoms for a year, 12 will become pregnant. Correct and more consistent use can reduce the risk of pregnancy even more.

- Use a condom every time you have sex. Keep a few handy.
- Put the condom on before there is any genital contact.
- Open the package carefully.
- Unroll the condom all the way to the base of the penis.
- Squeeze the air out of the top of the condom to make room for the ejaculate.
- Make sure your partner is well lubricated. Use spermicide or water-based or silicon-based lubricants. Do *not* use petroleum-based lubricants with latex condoms.
- If the condom tears or starts to slip off during sex, grasp the rim of the condom against the penis and withdraw the penis. The man should wash his hands and his penis. The woman should wash her hands and her labia (do *not* douche). If spermicide is available, the woman should insert spermicide into her vagina according to product directions. She should also use emergency contraception as soon as possible. If the couple wants to have sex again, use a new condom.
- Right after ejaculation, while the penis is still firm, the rim of the condom could be gently pressed against the penis as it is removed from the vagina.
- Check the used condom for any breaks or tears. If breaks or tears are noticed follow instructions above regarding spermicide and emergency contraception. Tie up the end and throw it away.

FIGURE 45.1   The male condom; patient information sheet.

Advantages
Readily available, inexpensive, portable, involves men in family planning, reduces STD risk.

Disadvantages
Requires use with each act of intercourse, requires cooperation of male partner, higher failure rate than hormonal methods or intrauterine contraception,

DOs and DON'Ts:

Do use a new condom each time you have sex	Don't reuse a condom
Do use a condom made of latex or polyurethane	Don't use lambskin or fake plastic condoms
Do change your condom if you have oral or anal sex before you have intercourse	Don't use the same condom for different sex practices or different sex partners
Do check the expiration date of the condom	Don't use a condom after the expiration date
Do place the condom before the penis touches her genitals	Don't let the penis touch her genitals before the condom goes on
Do use water-based lubricants if needed, such as spermicide, K-Y jelly	Don't use the petroleum-based products, such as Vaseline, oils, vaginal creams for infection treatment
Do hold the condom rim against the penis and pull them out together before the penis starts to soften or after ejaculation	Don't let the penis become soft inside her vagina – the condom can fall off
Do check the condom for tears, then tie it off and throw it away	Don't ever wash the condom and recycle it
Do keep emergency contraception and spermicide ready in case something happens and the condom does not work well	Don't wait until you need it, because emergency contraception works better the sooner you use it

FIGURE 45.1 *(Continued)*

may diminish the pleasure of intercourse due to decreased sensation, and side effects (see below).

Side Effects of Male Condoms

2% to 4% of couples using condoms have latex allergies and should use polyurethane condoms; the transition from mild reactions to anaphylaxis can develop rapidly.

FEMALE CONDOMS

The only female condom available in the United States is the FC Female Condom (Fig. 45.2). The device is a thin polyurethane sheath with flexible polyurethane rings at each end. The female condom provides a vaginal barrier and partially covers the introitus. At insertion, the inner ring is used to introduce the device. After insertion, the inner ring is rotated at the top of the vault to stabilize the device. The outer ring remains outside the vagina. The female condom should never be used with a latex male condom.

Efficacy
In 6-month clinical efficacy trials, a 12.5% typical failure rate was observed. This has been annualized to a typical first-year failure rate of 21%; perfect-use rates are 5%. The female condom is impermeable to HIV and other STDs.

Advantages and Disadvantages
Available over the counter, no known side effects, not sensitive to petroleum-based products, may be inserted up to 8 hours before intercourse, use may be challenging, the female condom is more expensive than the male condom.

Patient Education
Counselling should be performed on the correct insertion and removal of the female condom (Fig. 45.2). During intercourse, the penis should be manually guided into the device and the couple should remain attentive to the position of the outer ring to ensure that it does not ride up or get pushed into the vagina. Lubrication applied within the condom can help reduce breakage and noise from the device.

DIAPHRAGM

The diaphragm is a dome-shaped latex device that extends from the posterior fornix to the anterior vaginal wall to completely cover the cervix. The semi-rigid outer ring stabilizes the device and the dome holds spermicide against the cervix. The diaphragm must be professionally fitted and is obtained by prescription. Diaphragm users should be motivated, willing to touch their genitals, and must use device with every act of intercourse. Not recommended for women with a markedly anteverted or retroverted uterus (diaphragm tends to dislodge).

Types of Diaphragm
Diaphragms range in size from 50 to 105 mm and come in four styles: arcing spring rim, coil-spring rim, flat-spring rim, and wide-seal rim.

Contraindications to Use
History of toxic shock syndrome, allergy to latex or spermicidal agents, recent pregnancy (before renormalization of anatomy), and inability of patient to correctly insert and remove diaphragm.

The Female Condom

What is the female condom?

The female condom is a thin, soft, loose-fitting pouch with two flexible rings at either end. One ring helps hold the device in place inside the woman's vagina over the end of the womb (cervix), while the other ring rests outside the vagina.

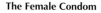

Outer ring lies against the labia (lips of the vulva)

Inner ring is used for insertion; helps hold female condom in place

How does it work?

The female condom is made of polyurethane, a type of plastic. The plastic condom covers the inside of the vagina, cervix, and area around the opening to the vagina. The device acts as a barrier to help prevent pregnancy and the transmission of germs that can cause sexually transmitted diseases (STDs), including human immunodeficiency virus (HIV) and acquired immunodeficiency syndrome (AIDS). The device can be inserted by the woman up to 8 hours before sex.

How to insert the female condom

1. Find a comfortable position. You may want to stand up with one foot on a chair, squat with knees apart, or lie down with legs bent and knees apart.
2. Hold the female condom with the open end hanging down. Squeeze the inner ring with your thumb and middle finger.
3. Holding the inner ring squeezed together, insert the ring into the vagina and push the inner ring and pouch into the vagina past the pubic bone.
4. When properly inserted, the outer ring will hang down slightly outside the vagina. During intercourse, when the penis enters the vagina, the slack will lessen.

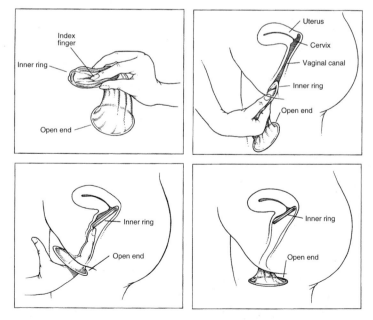

FIGURE 45.2 The female condom.

Remember:

The female condom may be hard to hold or slippery at first. Before you use one for the first time during sex, practice inserting one to get used to it. Take your time. Be sure to insert the condom straight into the vagina without twisting the pouch.

During Sex

1. It's helpful to use your hand to guide the penis into the vagina inside the female condom.
2. The ring may move from side to side or up and down during intercourse. This is OK.
3. If the female condom seems to be sticking to and moving with the penis rather than resting in the vagina, stop and add more lubricant to the inside of the device (near the outer ring) or to the penis.

How to remove the female condom after intercourse

1. Squeeze and twist the outer ring to close it.
2. Pull the female condom out gently.
3. Throw the condom away in the garbage. Do not flush down the toilet.
4. Do not wash out and use again.

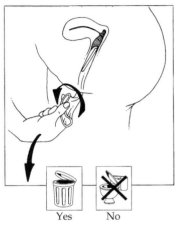

Special Reminders

- Use a new female condom with every act of intercourse.
- Use it every time you have intercourse.
- Read and follow the directions carefully.
- Do not use a male and female condom at the same time.
- Be careful not to tear the condom with fingernails or sharp objects.
- Use enough lubricant.

Yes   No

Latex condoms for men are highly effective at preventing STDs, including HIV infection (AIDS), if used properly. If your partner refuses to use a male latex condom, use a female condom to help protect yourself and your partner.

FIGURE 45.2 *(Continued)*

Effectiveness

The typical-use failure rate varies between 16% and 18%. The perfect-use failure rate is 6%.

Correct Fitting of Diaphragm

Measure the diagonal length of the vaginal canal from the posterior aspect of the symphysis pubis to the posterior vaginal by inserting the second and third fingers into the vagina until the tip of the middle finger touches the posterior vaginal wall. The point at which the index finger touches the symphysis pubis is marked with the thumb. The hand is withdrawn and the diaphragm is placed on the tip of the third finger with the opposite rim in front of the thumb to measure the correct size. The diaphragm is inserted and checked. It should touch the lateral vaginal walls, cover the cervix, and fit snugly between the posterior vaginal fornix and behind the symphysis pubis. Then the next larger size is fitted. The correct size is one size smaller than the first one perceived by the patient.

Patient Education
(1) Demonstrate and observe insertion and removal. (2) Spermicide should coat the inner surface of the diaphragm; one application is effective for 6 hours. Add additional spermicide into the vagina if intercourse is delayed beyond 6 hours or if additional acts of coitus are anticipated. The diaphragm should not be removed to add spermicide. (3) Wait at least 6 hours after the last episode of coitus to remove the device but remove before 24 hours of use to reduce the risk of toxic shock syndrome. (4) Wash device in soap and water, soaking not necessary after each application. Coat with cornstarch to prevent contamination or cracking, and store in a dry container. (6) Refit every 1 to 2 years, after every pregnancy, or after a 10% to 20% change in body weight.

Advantages
Most effective of the female barrier methods available; can reduce risk of STDs.

Disadvantages
Requires professional sizing; available only by prescription; requires education, preparation, and motivation for proper use; not an acceptable method if either partner is allergic to spermicide or latex; small risk of toxic shock syndrome with prolonged use; and increased risk of cystitis.

CERVICAL CAP AND CERVICAL SHIELD

The FemCap is a silicone cervical cap shaped like a sailor's hat with a dome, rim, brim, and removal strap. The cap covers the cervix and is held in place by a seal that forms between the brim and the vaginal wall. Sizes are determined by the diameter of the inner rim and based on parity. The smallest (22 mm) is intended for nulliparas, the medium size (26 mm) for parous women who have not had a vaginal delivery, and the largest (30 mm) for women who have had a full-term vaginal delivery. The cap can be only obtained by prescription.

Lea's Shield is a silicone cervical barrier that is held in place by its volume. The shield is oval in shape with a bowl that covers the cervix and fills the posterior fornix of the vagina. An anterior loop aids in insertion and withdrawal, and a flat, tubular flutter valve leading from the inner surface of the bowl through to the convex side prevents trapping of air. It is a one-size-fits-all device. The shield can be used with or without spermicide; however the addition of spermicide increases its contraceptive efficacy.

Contraindications to the cervical cap and shield include all those mentioned for the diaphragm with the exception of latex allergy. The cervical cap is not intended for use during menses. The shield may be used during menstruation, although none of the efficacy or safety trials included menstruating women.

Efficacy. The 6-month typical-use failure rate for the cap was 13.5%. Extrapolating to 12 months gives a probability of 22.8 pregnancies per 100 women. A 6-month efficacy trial of Lea's Shield found a typical-use pregnancy rate of 8.7 per 100 women among those who used the device with spermicide. There were no pregnancies among nulliparous women, but the unadjusted typical-use failure rate for parous women was 11 per 100 women.

Fitting the Cervical Cap. Neither the cap nor the shield require fitting; a clinician visit is required, however, as both require a prescription.

Patient Education

Insertion of the FemCap. Apply $1/4$ teaspoon of spermicide in the bowl, spread a thin layer over the outer brim, and insert $1/2$ teaspoon between the brim and the dome. Gently squeeze the cup and insert it into the vagina with the bowl facing upward and the longer brim entering first, then push the cap down toward the rectum and back as far as it can go. Check to make sure that the cap completely covers the cervix.

Removal of the FemCap. Squat and bear down then push the tip of a finger against the dome cap to break the suction. Grasp the removal strap with the tip of your finger and gently remove the device. Wash thoroughly with a mild soap, rinse, dry, and store.

Insertion of Lea's Shield. Apply a small amount of spermicide in the bowl of the device then gently squeeze the shield and insert into the vagina bowl-first as high as it will go. Check to make sure that the entire cervix is covered by the bowl.

Removal of Lea's Shield. Insert a finger into the vagina, grasp and twist the control loop to break the suction, and gently remove. The shield should be washed thoroughly with mild liquid soap for approximately 2 minutes, rinsed, dried, and then stored.

Advantages. Effective for up to 48 hours without additional doses of spermicide; may be placed several hours before coitus; usually is not detected by partner; may offer some reduction in STD risk.

Disadvantages. Requires a prescription and training in use, needs replacing every 1 to 3 years; must be refitted after pregnancy; insertion and/or removal may be difficult for some women.

CONTRACEPTIVE SPONGE

The contraceptive sponge (Today Sponge) is made of polyurethane foam and contains 1 g of nonoxynol-9. A concave depression on one side fits against the cervix and a woven polyester loop on the other side can be grasped for removal. After it is moistened with water, it is inserted into the vagina and is effective immediately. The sponge protects against pregnancy for 24 hours regardless of the number of acts of intercourse. The sponge comes in one size and does not require fitting by a physician or a prescription.

Mechanism of Action
The sponge releases 125 to 150 mg of the spermicide nonoxynol-9 slowly over a 24-hour period. The sponge also traps and absorbs semen and acts as a physical barrier.

Efficacy
The typical-use failure rate is 16% in nulliparous women and 32% in parous women. Perfect-use rates are 9% and 20% respectively.

Patient Education
Insertion. Remove the sponge from its package and hold it with the loop hanging down. Moisten and squeeze the sponge a few times until it becomes sudsy. Fold the sides upward with a finger on each side to support it, gently introduce sponge into the vagina, and push it upward as far as it will go. Run a finger around the edge to make sure that the entire cervix is covered.

Removal. Wait 6 hours after the last act of intercourse before removing the sponge. Insert one finger into the vagina until the loop is felt. If the loop cannot be felt, bear down, lie on your back on the bed with your knees up against your chest, squat down in a low position, or sit on the toilet and tilt your pelvis forward (so that the small of your back is rounded) to bring the sponge closer to the vaginal opening. Hook one finger into the loop then gently pull the sponge out, checking to make sure that it is intact. If it is torn, remove all pieces from the vagina and discard.

Contraindications
History of toxic shock syndrome, allergy or sensitivity to polyurethane foam, nonoxynol-9, or metabisulfite (the preservative used in the sponge; women or partners with an allergy to sulfa should consult with a health care provider), and current menstruation.

Advantages
Lack of hormonal side effects or medical contraindications, allows for spontaneity after insertion, available without a prescription, one size fits all, does not require partner participation, may be more comfortable to wear than other barrier methods such as the diaphragm, easy to use.

Disadvantages
Relatively high failure rate, teen must be comfortable touching genitals, spermicide may cause irritation, sponge can become discolored or malodorous in the presence of vaginitis, can be difficult to remove.

Side Effects
Approximately 4% of users will experience a sensitivity reaction to the sponge.

VAGINAL SPERMICIDES

Vaginal spermicides are available in a wide array of delivery systems and can be used alone or in combination with barrier methods. They can play an important role in contraception for the adolescent because they require neither a prescription nor a pelvic examination and are free from systemic side effects.

Types of Spermicides

The various spermicidal preparations differ in their onset and duration of action and mode of application. Table 45.1 displays the more commonly used products. Nonoxynol-9 is the active agent in all spermicides available in the United States. In general, each agent is active for approximately 1 hour. Encourage patients to choose a spermicide that will work well for them.

Efficacy

Typical first-year failure rates for spermicides used alone are estimated to be as high as 29%. The correct and consistent failure rate is 18%.

Mechanism of Action

All spermicides contain a base and the spermicidal agent. Spermicides destroy sperm by breaking down the outer cell membrane and act as a barrier to sperm.

Contraindications

Allergy or sensitivity to any component of the spermicidal product.

Advantages

No proven systemic side effects, readily available without prescription, convenient, easy to use, may be used with or without partner involvement, may provide lubrication, useful as a backup method for other contraceptives.

Disadvantages

Relatively high failure rate, must be used only a short time before intercourse is started, requires that woman be comfortable with touching her genitals, unpleasant taste if oral–genital sex is involved, may cause a local allergic reaction.

TABLE 45.1

Vaginal Spermicides

Base of Carrier	Onset of Action (min)	Duration of Action (min)	Concentration (%)
Aerosol foams	Immediate	60	8–12
Creams and gels[a]	Immediate	60	2–5
Suppositories and tablets	10–15	60	2.3–5.6
Film	15	60	28

[a]Creams and gels are usually used in conjunction with diaphragms or cervical caps but may be used as single agents.

Data from Hatcher RA, Trussell J, Stewart F, et al. *Contraceptive technology*, 17th rev. ed. New York: Ardent Media, 1998:358.

REFERENCES AND ADDITIONAL READINGS

Davis KR, Weller SC. The effectiveness of condoms in reducing heterosexual transmission of HIV. *Fam Plann Perspect* 1999;31:272.

Gallo MF, Grimes DA, Schulz KF. Nonlatex vs. latex male condoms for contraception: a systematic review of randomized controlled trials. *Contraception* 2003;68:319.

Mauck C, Glover LH, Miller E, et al. Lea's Shield: a study of a the safety and efficacy of a new vaginal barrier contraceptive used with and without spermicide. *Contraception* 1996;53:239.

Mauck C, Callahan M, Wiener DH, et al. A comparative study of the safety and efficacy of FemCap®, a new vaginal barrier contraceptive, and the Ortho All-Flex®diaphragm. *Contraception* 1999;60:71.

Trussell J. Contraceptive failure in the United States. *Contraception* 2004;70:89.

CHAPTER 46

Emergency Contraception

Lisa Johnson and Melanie A. Gold

Emergency contraception (EC) has the potential to prevent 1.7 million unplanned pregnancies and 800,000 abortions each year.

EMERGENCY CONTRACEPTION METHODS

Three types of EC are available in the United States, including (1) the Yuzpe regimen: two doses of 100 μg ethinyl estradiol and 0.5 mg levonorgestrel (or 1.0 mg norgestrel) taken 12 hours apart; (2) the progestin-only method: two single doses of 0.75 mg levonorgestrel taken 12 hours apart or a single dose of 1.5 mg of levonorgestrel taken once; and (3) the T-380A copper IUD (or ParaGard): inserted up to 5 days after unprotected coitus. Table 46.1 lists combination oral contraceptives (COCs) that can be used to make up the Yuzpe regimen and their appropriate doses. A dedicated progestin-only product (Plan B) contains two tablets each containing 0.75 mg of levonorgestrel. The FDA-approved instructions for Plan B are to take a single tablet as soon as possible after unprotected intercourse (up to 72 hours after coitus) and to take the second single tablet 12 hours later. However, the current standard is to prescribe levonorgestrel in a single dose of 1.5 mg taken up to 120 hours after unprotected intercourse because it is as effective as the split dose regimen without causing any increase in side effects. *A progestin-only EC product is the current product of choice.*

The progestin-only method of EC has several advantages over combination regimens, including superior efficacy (89% reduction in pregnancies versus 75%), virtually no contraindications to use, and fewer side effects (especially less nausea and vomiting).

EFFICACY

The expected pregnancy rate per single act of unprotected intercourse is estimated to be 8%. The Yuzpe regimen has a failure rate a little over 3.2% (a 75% reduction in expected pregnancies) compared to the levonorgestrel regimen failure rate of 1.1% and the copper IUD failure rate of 0.1%. A World Health Organization (WHO) trial demonstrated that the effectiveness of a hormonal EC depends on how soon it is initiated after intercourse (Table 46.2), with higher effectiveness rates the sooner the medication is taken. The 72-hour limit is

TABLE 46.1

Hormonal Emergency Contraception Regimens: Two Doses 12 Hours Apart

Brand	Manufacturer	Tablets/Dose
Progestin-only emergency contraceptive pills		
Plan B	Barr	1 white tablet[a]
Combination emergency contraceptive pills (Yuzpe regimen)		
Ogestrel	Watson	2 white tablets
Alesse	Wyeth-Ayerst	5 pink tablets
Aviane	Barr	5 orange tablets
Lessina	Barr	5 orange tablets
Levlite	Berlex	5 pink tablets
Levlen	Berlex	4 light-orange tablets
Levora	Watson	4 white tablets
Lo/Ovral	Wyeth-Ayerst	4 white tablets
Low-Ogestrel	Watson	4 white tablets
Nordette	Wyeth-Ayerst	4 light-orange tablets
Seasonale	Barr	4 pink tablets
Tri-Levlen	Berlex	4 light-yellow tablets
Triphasil	Wyeth-Ayerst	4 light-yellow tablets
Trivora	Watson	4 pink tablets

[a]Preferable to give both doses (two tablets) at once and can be given up to 120 hr after unprotected intercourse.

expandable to 120 hours, but there is controversy over whether later use is associated with diminished protection.

MECHANISMS OF ACTION

Hormonal methods of EC are approved by the FDA as *contraceptives*. The primary mechanism of action of hormonal methods of EC appears to be delaying

TABLE 46.2

Comparative Efficacy (Reduction in Pregnancy Rate) of Combination Emergency Contraceptive (EC) Pills versus Progestin-Only EC Pills over Various Time Periods

Time (hr)	Combination EC Pills (Yuzpe)	Progestin-Only EC Pills
<24 hr	77%	95%
25–48 hr	36%	85%
49–72 hr	31%	58%

or inhibiting ovulation. Other suggested mechanisms are suppressing or delaying the luteinizing hormone (LH) peak and inhibiting follicle rupture, alteration of tubal motility, decreasing progesterone production by the corpus luteum, and changing the composition of the endometrium to prevent implantation. EC is not an abortifacient. EC taken after a pregnancy has been established to have no effect, it will not cause a miscarriage, and it will not increase the risk of fetal malformations.

INDICATIONS

EC is indicated any time a woman of reproductive age wishes to lower her risk of becoming pregnant following unprotected intercourse or after inadequately protected sexual intercourse from failure or misuse of a contraceptive method.

CONTRAINDICATIONS

Yuzpe Method. Absolute contraindications to prescribing the Yuzpe regimen are current pregnancy, hypersensitivity to any component of product, and acute current migraine with neurologic deficits. A history of previous thrombosis is not a contraindication to a single course of the Yuzpe regimen, although if available, the progestin-only regimen would be preferable.

Progestin-Only Method. The three contraindications for progestin-only oral contraceptives (including Plan B) are current pregnancy, hypersensitivity to any component of the product, and undiagnosed abnormal genital bleeding. However, an adolescent with abnormal genital bleeding can be prescribed EC as long as pregnancy is ruled out. The progestin-only method is preferred for breast-feeding women, since estrogen in the Yuzpe regimen has the potential to decrease the production of breast milk.

Copper Intrauterine Device Method. The copper IUD, intended for long-term contraception, has several contraindications (see Chapter 44). Because short-term use cannot be ensured, these same contraindications have been applied to the use of the copper IUD for EC.

SIDE EFFECTS

Side effects of the Yuzpe regimen and progestin-only EC are largely hormone-related and can last for 2 to 3 days. The most common side effects are gastrointestinal. With the Yuzpe method, 30% and 66% of women report nausea and 12% to 22% vomiting. Gastrointestinal complaints can be reduced by routinely giving an antiemetic (such as meclizine 50 mg) 1 hour before the first EC dose. The progestin-only method has a lower incidence of gastrointestinal side effects; only 23% of users reported nausea, 6% vomiting, and 5% diarrhea; thus, antiemetics need not be routinely offered when prescribing progestin-only EC. Other hormone-related side effects of EC include breast tenderness, headache, abdominal bloating, fatigue, and dizziness. Nearly all women (98%) should have menstrual bleeding within 3 weeks of taking EC. A woman who does not menstruate within 21 days after taking EC should be tested for pregnancy. If she is pregnant, she should be reassured that taking EC will not adversely affect her fetus or the pregnancy. If she is not pregnant, watchful waiting for return to normal cycling is appropriate for up to 3 months, but contraception should be offered. Some adolescent health care providers recommend a routine pregnancy test 14 days after EC use, regardless of menses.

MANAGEMENT ISSUES

1. *Advance prescription and education:* The most effective way to provide EC is in advance of need. Advance provision of EC may increase immediate use and enhance efficacy.
2. *Assessment: history:* This should include (a) timing, duration, and quality of last menstrual period; (b) number and timing of any previous acts of intercourse (protected or not) during the cycle; (c) symptoms of pregnancy; (d) prior experience with EC or birth control pills; and (e) contraindications to EC. No physical examination is needed and no laboratory tests are mandatory, although a sensitive urine pregnancy test can be done if it is likely that the patient might already be pregnant. EC can be prescribed after telephone triage. Pharmacists in several states can provide EC without a prescription, and EC has been approved in the United States without a prescription in individuals who are 18 years of age and older (with proof of age).
3. *Multiple doses:* Women who experienced multiple episodes of unprotected intercourse can be provided EC for their last coital exposure if they are not pregnant. There is no absolute limit to the number of times EC can be used within one cycle if there is need. Women who are using EC frequently should receive counseling about effective ongoing contraception methods.
4. *EC is a standard of care:* Courts have ruled that EC is a community standard of care for women who have been exposed to potential unintended pregnancy (especially for victims of sexual assault).
5. *Contraception after EC:* For ongoing contraception using oral contraceptives, the Ortho-Evra patch or the NuvaRing can be initiated or restarted the same day that either the Yuzpe regimen or Plan B is taken or can be started 24 hours later. Prescribe a single cycle of contraception and have the patient return 2 weeks after her EC dose for a urine pregnancy test and for subsequent supply of contraception. Depot medroxyprogesterone acetate (depot medroxyprogesterone acetate, DMPA, or Depo-Provera) can be administered the same day EC is taken if the patient understands and accepts the uncertainty of the impact her contraceptive will have on her next menses and if she agrees to return for routine pregnancy testing in 10 to 14 days. Appropriate backup methods should be provided for the first cycle. Women who have a copper IUD inserted are provided with both EC and ongoing contraceptive protection.

PHARMACY ISSUES

Pharmacies in some areas of the country refuse to carry EC because of their confusion about its mechanisms of action. Other pharmacists and pharmacy chains claim that their decisions are based on economic factors—that the demand for EC is too low to justify the cost of the shelf space. If a patient presents after unprotected intercourse for EC and it is known that she may encounter problems filling a prescription for Plan B, it may be prudent to use one of the standard Yuzpe regimens (Table 46.1), with prescription instructions to "take as directed," while providing the patient with specific EC instructions. Patients can learn the names and addresses of local providers of EC by accessing the EC Hotline, either by telephone at 1-888-NOT-2-LATE or on the World Wide Web at http://www.NOT-2-LATE.com/. The FDA approved sales of Plan B in August 2006 without a prescription in individuals who are 18 years of age and older (with proof of age).

WEB SITES AND REFERENCES

http://www.go2planb.com
Information about EC and directory of providers on the Internet
• http://www.NOT-2-LATE.com
• http://ec.princeton.edu
Toll-free telephone information about EC and provider referrals
• 1-888-NOT-2-LATE (English and Spanish instructions)
American College of Obstetricians and Gynecologists. ACOG Practice Bulletin: clinical management guidelines for obstetricians-gynecologists: emergency contraception. No. 69, December 2005 (replaces No. 25, March 2001). *Obstet Gynecol* 2005;106(6):1443–1452.
Gold MA, Sucato G, Conard LE, Hillard P. Provision of emergency contraception to adolescents: position paper of the Society for Adolescent Medicine. *J Adolesc Health* 2004;35:66.
Trussell J, Ellertson C, Rodriguez G. The Yuzpe regimen of emergency contraception: how long after the morning after? *Obstet Gynecol* 1996;88:150.

CHAPTER 47

Long-Acting Progestins

Anita L. Nelson

INJECTABLE PROGESTINS

There are two different formulations of depot medroxyprogesterone acetate (DMPA) available in the United States: the traditional 150-mg formulation (Depo-Provera), injected intramuscularly every 11 to 13 weeks (DMPA-IM), and a newer formulation with different buffers (Depo-SubQ Provera 104), administered subcutaneously every 12 to 14 weeks (DMPA-SC). The formulations have similar labeling and side effect profiles.

Efficacy.   The failure rate with correct and consistent use of DMPA-IM is 0.3%. However, the first-year typical-use failure rate is 3%. One study compared DMPA and oral contraceptives (OCs) in postpartum adolescents and found that the repeat pregnancy rates by 15 months were lower in the DMPA users (15%) compared with OC users (36%). In clinical trials of DMPA-SC, there were no pregnancies and patient weight did not influence efficacy. Typical use failure rates are not yet available.

Mechanisms of Action.   DMPA is a contraceptive agent that has two primary mechanisms of action: thickening of cervical mucus to prevent sperm entry into the upper genital tract and suppression of gonadotropin levels to block ovulation.

Drug Interactions.   Aminoglutethimide increases hepatic DMPA clearance and, if administered with DMPA, may depress serum concentrations of medroxyprogesterone acetate. Some antiretroviral medications impact cytochrome P450 activity, but have not been reported to affect DMPA efficacy. Anticonvulsants do not detract from contraceptive protection provided by DMPA.

Contraindications.   The only condition rated in World Health Organization (WHO) category 4 (should not use) is current breast cancer (see Table 42.3).

Administration.   DMPA labeling advises that regularly cycling women receive DMPA in the first 5 days of a menstrual cycle. Often teens are in immediate need of contraception. WHO guidelines allow for DMPA injection at any other time in the cycle if it is reasonably certain that a woman is not pregnant. Beyond the first 7 days of her cycle, she should abstain from intercourse or use an

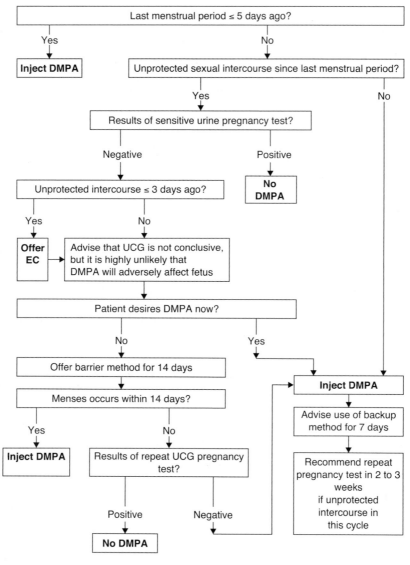

FIGURE 47.1   Quick Start DMPA.

additional contraceptive method for 7 days after her off-label injection time. If there has been recent unprotected intercourse, WHO also suggests that EC be offered. Reassuringly, one study found no fetal anomalies with intrauterine exposure to DMPA. An algorithm to expedite DMPA start/restart (Quick Start or Same-Day Start) is outlined in Figure 47.1. Avoid massaging the injection site after injection because early massage increases the surface area of the drug, allows faster absorption, and results in shorter effective life.

Advantages. (1) Extremely effective with excellent pregnancy protection. (2) Private. With DMPA, there is no external evidence of contraceptive use (no pill packs or condoms to hide). (3) Convenient and low-maintenance. This feature is "most important" or "likely important" to 89.3% of teens surveyed. (4) Cost-effective without high initial cost. (5) Intermediate-term method with built-in grace period. (6) No estrogen contraindications or side effects. (7) Amenorrhea common with long-term use. This is helpful for busy women; athletes; patients with anemia; those with HIV infection, coagulopathies, or renal failure; patients on anticoagulants; and mentally challenged women. (8) Reduced incidence of sickle cell crises. (9) Decreased risk of endometrial and perhaps epithelial ovarian cancer. (10) May be used off label by breast-feeding women after delivery. The provision of convenient and reliable contraception to teen mothers can make a significant contribution to reducing the rate of repeat pregnancies. (11) DMPA is also used to treat symptomatic endometriosis.

Metabolic Impacts. Because there is no estrogen component, DMPA causes no alterations in coagulation factors, angiotensinogen, or hepatic globulin production. Blood pressure measurements are unchanged. However, serum progestin levels with injections are higher than those seen with the implants or intrauterine contraceptives. DMPA has greater impact on glucose tolerance, insulin levels, and lipid profiles. For healthy, normal subjects, the changes in glucose tolerance are not clinically significant. Teens with glucose intolerance or overt diabetes must be monitored closely when using the DMPA injections. DMPA can lower total cholesterol and triglycerides; it has a negligible impact on low-density-lipoprotein (LDL) and high-density-lipoprotein (HDL) cholesterol.

Disadvantages. (1) Side effects (see later discussion). (2) Must continue to remind patients of the need for safer sex practices and provide a method to reduce the risk of sexually transmitted diseases (STDs). (3) Requires medical intervention (unless self-injection of subcutaneous DMPA becomes available). A hotline is available 24/7 in English and Spanish to answer patients' questions and remind patients about appointments for reinjection. [1-866-554 DEPO (3376)]. (4) Delays return to fertility: Average delay is 10 months after last injection, but there is considerable variation in that estimate. A higher body mass index (BMI) is associated with slower return to fertility. (5) Immediate anaphylactic reactions (rare).

Side Effects
Menstrual Changes. Missed menstrual periods and amenorrhea become more common over time with DMPA. After the first year of use, some 50% of DMPA users are amenorrheic; after 2 years, that number rises to 75%. With the initial one to three injections, many women experience significant unscheduled vaginal spotting and bleeding. Although there are no studies of effective interventions, clinicians often advise short courses of nonsteroidal anti-inflammatory drugs (NSAIDs) (e.g., ibuprofen 800 mg orally t.i.d. for 3 days) or low-dose estrogen supplementation to reduce immediate bleeding irregularities.

Changes in Bone Mineral Density. Controlled cross-sectional studies of older, long-term DMPA users found that, although the bone mineral density (BMD) of DMPA users was statistically significantly lower than that of controls, BMD normalized after DMPA discontinuation. In one study, the BMD of former DMPA users was almost identical to that of never users. DMPA may decrease BMD via suppression of estrogen, a critical issue as most of lifetime bone mineralization occurs during adolescence. Studies have shown that many adolescents on DMPA not only fail to increase their BMD, but experience bone loss compared with baseline (4% to 7% BMD decrease in one study compared to unprotected controls). At least partial BMD recovery was seen in many women in short-term follow-up after DMPA discontinuation.

The FDA issued a black box warning for both formulations of DMPA, advising "Depo-Provera Contraceptive Injection should be used as a long-term birth control method (e.g., >2 years) only if other birth control methods are inadequate." The labeling also advises that if prolonged use is contemplated, the patient's BMD should be evaluated. In response, the California Office of Family Planning sent clinicians recommendations that "Bone mineral density screening should not be recommended to a client for the sole purpose of evaluating appropriateness of DMPA usage." The American College of Obstetrics and Gynecology reviewed the evidence and concluded that "the current evidence on DMPA use and skeletal health indicates that concerns regarding BMD should not restrict initiation or continuation of DMPA use in adults or teens. All adolescents, whether they use DMPA or not, should be advised to consume at least 1,300 mg calcium and adequate vitamin D (minimum of 200 to 400 IU) to ensure maximal bone accretion." One study demonstrated that higher calcium intake by adolescents, even in pregnancy, protects against trabecular bone loss. Estrogen supplements are protective of bone in adolescent girls receiving DMPA and may be a prudent option for women who have a low bone mass.

Weight Changes. Despite widespread belief that DMPA use increases weight, clinical trials do not consistently support this assumption. Complicating the analysis is the fact that U.S. women gain an average >2 lb/year regardless of contraceptive method. Adolescents gain even more and individual weight changes vary considerably.

Breast Tenderness. Mastalgia is reported in 15% to 20% of women starting DMPA; this side effect usually decreases rapidly.

Mood Disturbances. Although there is no consistent evidence that DMPA use causes adverse psychological effects (e.g., nervousness, insomnia, somnolence, fatigue, dizziness, and depression), labeling mentions these as possible side effects. Many patients with chronic depression tolerate DMPA, but use in those cases must be individualized.

Other Changes. Acne, alopecia, hirsutism, fluid retention, headaches, libido changes, changes in cervical mucus, nausea, cholestatic jaundice, and local skin reaction to injection have been reported, but seldom have been serious enough to warrant a change in method.

Summary. DMPA-IM and DMPA-SQ are attractive contraceptive options for adolescents. They provide top-tier efficacy, are low maintenance and safe. The progestin-only side effect profile and need for periodic reinjection pose challenges for long-term continuation. Adolescents at risk for STDs need to use dual methods (male condoms) to meet all their reproductive needs.

Etonogestrel (ENG)-Releasing Implant

Subdermal implants provide long-acting, extremely effective, rapidly reversible contraception that requires little user effort. Progestin-only implants avoid estrogen side effects and can be used by virtually every woman. There are only a few medical conditions that were rated 3 (risks usually outweigh advantages) or 4 (unacceptable health risk) for implant use in the WHO 2004 Medical Eligibility Criteria for Contraceptive Use; they are listed in Table 47.1. The ENG implant (Implanon, NV Organon, Oss, the Netherlands) is available in >30 countries and has been used by >2 million women worldwide since 1999. The ENG implant was approved by the FDA in July 2006 and is becoming increasingly available in the United States.

Description of System. The ENG implant is a single rod (40 mm long and 2 mm in diameter) contraceptive implant made of a core and a releasing membrane. The core consists of steroid microcrystals containing 68 mg etonogestrel (3-ketodesogestrel) imbedded in a rod of ethylene vinyl acetate (EVA) copolymer covered by a thin, 0.06 mm, EVA copolymer membrane. The implant provides contraceptive protection for at least 3 years and comes individually packaged in the needle of a sterile, disposable, inserter, specifically designed inserter for subdermal placement.

Mechanisms of Action. The ENG implant was developed specifically to inhibit ovulation. It acts as a contraceptive by providing sustained release of a relatively low dose of contraceptive hormone. No ovulation was found in any test cycle until 30 months; two women (3.1% of subjects) ovulated at least once from months 30 to 36 of use. Progestin also makes the cervical mucus viscous and impenetrable by sperm, so fertilization does not take place. However, in contrast to DMPA, the ENG implant use does not cause hypoestrogenemia; 95% of the E2 measures were >110 pmol/L. ENG impacts on the endometrium are measurable. The mean value thickness of the endometrial stripe determined by transvaginal ultrasound was 4 mm.

Contraceptive Efficacy. No pregnancies were seen in users, while the implants were in place, but six pregnancies occurred within 2 weeks of removal. The FDA included those six pregnancies in its Pearl index of 0.38%. Efficacy in heavier women was not as well studied. However, none of the 365 women who weighed ≥70 kg reported in the literature experienced pregnancies.

Drug Interactions. Serum ENG levels are low. Concomitant use with other drugs which enhance cytochrome P450 activity reduces efficacy. WHO lists anticonvulsants and other drugs as a category 3 for this reason. See Table 47.1.

Insertion. The ENG implant comes packaged in a preloaded, sterile, disposable inserter. Health care providers must be trained and maintain their competency for insertion and removal. In clinical trials, the time for insertion from

TABLE 47.1

World Health Organization 2004 Medical Eligibility Criteria for Contraceptive Use

WHO Categories:

1. A condition for which there is no restriction for the use of the contraceptive method
2. A condition where the advantages of using the method generally outweigh the theoretical or proven risks
3. A condition where the theoretical or proven risks usually outweigh the advantages of using the method
4. A condition which represents an unacceptable health risk if the contraceptive method is used

Conditions with Category 3 and/or Category 4	Category		Clarifications/Evidence
	DMPA	LNG/ENG Implant	
Breast-feeding < 6 wk postpartum	3	3	Clarification: There is concern that the neonate may be at risk of exposure to steroid hormones during the first 6 wk postpartum. However, in many settings pregnancy morbidity and mortality risks are high, and access to services is limited. In such settings, POCs may be one of the few types of methods widely available and accessible to breast-feeding women immediately postpartum. Evidence: Studies have shown that among breast-feeding women < 6 wk postpartum, progestogen-only contraceptives did not affect breast-feeding performance, and infant health and growth. However, there are no data evaluating the effects of progestogen exposure through breast milk on brain and liver development.

Condition	I	C	I	C	Clarifications/Evidence
Multiple risk factors for arterial cardiovascular disease (such as older age, smoking, diabetes, and hypertension)	3		2		Clarification: When multiple major risk factors exist, risk of cardiovascular disease may increase substantially. The effects of DMPA may persist for some time after discontinuation.
Hypertension • Elevated blood pressure levels (properly taken measurements) systolic > 160 mm Hg or diastolic > 100 mm Hg • Vascular disease	3		2		Evidence: Limited evidence suggests that among women with hypertension, those who used progestogen-only injectables had a small increased risk of cardiovascular events compared with women who did not use these methods.
Deep venous thrombosis (DVT)/Pulmonary embolism (PE) Current DVT/PE	3		3		
Current and history of ischemic heart disease	3	3	1	2 3	
Stroke (history of cerebrovascular accident)	3		1	2 3	
Headaches	I	C	I	C	
Migraine with aura, at any age	2	3	2	3	

(continued)

TABLE 47.1

(Continued)

Conditions with Category 3 and/or Category 4	Category		Clarifications/Evidence
	DMPA	LNG/ENG Implant	
Unexplained vaginal bleeding (suspicious for serious underlying condition) Before evaluation	3	3	Clarification: If pregnancy or an underlying pathological condition (such as pelvic malignancy) is suspected, it must be evaluated and the category adjusted after evaluation.
Breast disease Breast cancer	4	4	
• Current			
• Past and no evidence of current disease for 5 years	3	3	
Diabetes	3	2	
• Nephropathy/retinopathy/neuropathy			
• Other vascular disease or diabetes of > 20 years duration			
Viral hepatitis Active	3	3	
Cirrhosis Severe (decompensated)	3	3	

Liver tumors	3	3	
Drugs which affect liver enzymes			Clarification: Although the interaction of rifampicin
• Rifampicin	2	3	or certain anticonvulsants with LNG/ENG
• Certain anticonvulsants			implants is not harmful to women, it is likely to
(phenytoin, carbamazepine,			reduce the effectiveness of LNG/ENG implants.
barbiturates, primidone,			Use of other contraceptives should be
topiramate, oxcarbazepine)			encouraged for women who are long-term users
			of any of these drugs.
			Evidence: Use of certain anticonvulsants decreased
			the contraceptive effectiveness of POCs.

I, initiation; C, continuation; POCs, progestogen-only contraceptives; DMPA, depot medroxyprogesterone acetate; LNG, levonorgestrel-releasing; ENG, etonogestrel-releasing.

the skin entry to complete insertion was 1 minute. There was a low complication rate with insertion in the clinical studies; only 10 per 1,710 (0.6%) of women reported complications. The most common were bleeding at insertion site or failure of the insertion device. No expulsions occurred, but 1% of women complained of pain at the insertion site at some time during the trial.

Removal. Removal of ENG implants is easier than the removal of the 6 Norplant (levonorgestrel (LNG)-capsules). In clinical studies, the ENG implant was removed in under 5 minutes in the majority of women.

Advantages. (1) Extremely effective. (2) Private. Implants are not generally visible, but the same factors that compromise DMPA privacy occur with implants. (3) Convenient and low-maintenance. One office insertion procedure provides 3 years of contraceptive protection. (4) Cost effective. (5) No estrogen contraindications or side effects.

Metabolic Impacts

Bone Mineral Density (BMD). Compared to concerns of low estrogen levels and decreased bone mineralization with DMPA, at least two studies have found that women using the ENG implant did not have suppressed estradiol levels and one demonstrated that the levels were similar to those individuals using a nonmedicated IUD. Even the ENG implant users with amenorrhea had no deleterious impact on their BMD. The authors concluded that ENG implant use would be safe in young women who had not achieved maximum bone density.

Carbohydrate Metabolism. Comparative trials of ENG implant versus LNG implant in 80 healthy volunteers, ages 18 to 40 for 24 months revealed a slight increase in insulin resistance. Area-under-the-curve analysis revealed significant increases in glucose (30% to 60%) and insulin levels (50%) by 6 months. Fasting HbA_{1c} levels also were increased throughout the study. Although each of these changes was statistically significant, it should be noted that virtually all the values remained in the normal range. No glucose intolerance or diabetes was induced.

Disadvantages. (1) Side effects (see below). (2) Provides no protection against STDs. Dual methods are needed for at-risk couples. (3) Requires medical intervention, including insertion and removal procedures performed by trained clinicians. (4) Expensive, with large up-front costs.

Side Effects

Changes in Bleeding Patterns. Menstrual bleeding changes are to be expected with progestin-only methods. There was no consistency or predictable trends in the bleeding patterns seen in individual women using ENG implants. Bleeding patterns are unpredictable both for individual women and for users as a whole. This is the most important point about when potential implant users need to be counseled. Hemoglobin levels of women in the studies were relatively unchanged. Normal menses returns within 3 months after removal of the implant capsules in almost all subjects.

Weight Changes. Weight increase was reported as an adverse event by 6.4% of all ENG implant users in a clinical trial, but was the reason for discontinuation for only 1.5% of users. Lighter women (<50 kg) were more likely to gain weight than those whose baseline weight was >50 kg.

Headaches. In clinical trials with ENG implant, the frequency of women complaining of headache generally was not excessive; 21% of the ENG implant users complained of headaches, but only 4.7% of women discontinued the method for this reason.

Acne. Acne was the most frequently reported drug-related adverse event in the ENG implant trials. Slightly over 15% of the women reported acne as an adverse event, but only 1% of users had the implants removed because of this problem. Interestingly, of the women who initiated implant use acne, nearly 60% had improvement or disappearance of that acne.

Mood Changes, Nervousness, and Depression. There are no estimates of attributable risks for these mood problems. Requests for removal for each of these complaints ranged from 0% to 2%.

Blood Pressure. Significant BP increases were defined as BP_S >140 or increased by 20 mm Hg over baseline or last visit or BP_D >90 or increase by 10 mg Hg over baseline or last visit. Such increases were observed in 0.7% of women (10 per 1,640) at any time during the 24 months of the studies. In comparative studies, 0.6% of ENG implant users and 0.7% of LNG implant users had significant increases.

Ovarian Cysts. Progestins are known to slow atresia of ovarian cysts. In the large clinical trials, ovarian cysts were found on physical exam in 2% to 3% of implant users. In Chile, 9% of ENG implant users were found at some time to have such cysts. In asymptomatic women, no action was needed.

Summary. ENG contraceptive implant provides unsurpassed contraceptive efficacy with very little metabolic impact in part because ovarian production of estradiol continues in the follicular range. Continuation rates have been encouraging and return to fertility is very rapid. Medical contraindications are rare. The bleeding patterns with ENG implant generally are better than with previous generations of implants, but are still unpredictable. Insertion and removal procedures have been greatly simplified and are more easily accomplished in a busy office practice. However, specific training is required.

Telephone Hotlines for Health Providers
DMPA hotline: 1-866-554-DEPO (3376)

WEB SITES AND REFERENCES

http://kidshealth.org/teen/sexual_health/contraception/contraception_depo.html. Teen site with information about DMPA-IM.

http://www.depoprovera.com/. Pfizer site on DMPA-IM.

http://www.depo-subqprovera104.com/. Pfizer site on DMPA-SC.

http://www.plannedparenthood.org/pp2/portal/files/portal/medicalinfo/ birthcontrol/pub-depo-provera.xml. Planned Parenthood information about DMPA-IM.

http://www.youngwomenshealth.org/femalehormone.html. Children's Hospital Boston Web site on contraception including DMPA-IM.

http://www.organon.com/products/contraception/Implanon.asp. Organon site for ENG implant (not yet approved in the United States).

World Health Organization, Department of Reproductive Health and Research. *Medical Eligibility Criteria for Contraceptive Use*, 3rd ed. Geneva: World Health Organization, 2004.

World Health Organization, Department of Reproductive Health and Research. *Selected Practice Recommendations for Contraceptive Use,* 2nd ed. Geneva: World Health Organization, 2005.

World Health Organization Expanded Programme of Research, Development and Research Training in Human Reproduction Task Force on Long-Acting Systemic Agents for Regulation of Fertility. Multinational comparative clinical evaluation of two long-acting injectable contraceptive steroids: norethisterone enanthate and medroxyprogesterone acetate. *Contraception* 1983;28:1.

CHAPTER **48**

Gynecologic Examination of the Adolescent Female

Merrill Weitzel and Jean S. Emans

The first pelvic examination can influence an adolescent's attitudes about reproductive health care for the rest of her life. A sensitive approach can aid in creating a positive and instructive experience.

OFFICE SETTING

1. Provide an office setting that is comfortable and friendly, with welcoming support staff.
2. Practices limited to adolescents can have posters, pamphlets, and website information directed at the concerns of teens.
3. Parents of adolescent patients should be included as much as possible in the history gathering and medical plan. However, the adolescent's need for medical privacy and confidentiality should be respected and time should be set aside for a private interview with the teen. The limits of confidentiality (conditions that are life-threatening or that require reporting by law) should also be discussed with the patient and her family.
4. During part of the gynecologic assessment, the adolescent should be interviewed privately in a comfortable environment about risk behaviors and health-promoting behaviors.
5. Be aware of the fears and worries of the adolescent about the pelvic examination.
6. Listening to the adolescent, rather than lecturing her, is essential. Dispelling myths and respecting cultural preferences about pelvic examinations is important.
7. Reassure the teen of her normality, as appropriate.

INDICATIONS FOR GYNECOLOGIC EXAMINATIONS

The indications for a pelvic examination vary with the patient complaint. Most professional organizations suggest that cervical cancer screening be initiated at 21 years of age or 3 years after the onset of sexual activity, whichever occurs first. Sexually active girls with episodic care or immunosuppression (e.g., HIV infection) should start screening earlier. It is important for patients (and their parents) to realize that a pelvic exam and Pap test are not the same. Aside from the above, other indications include:

1. Symptoms of vaginal or uterine infection
2. Menstrual disorders, including amenorrhea, dysfunctional uterine bleeding, severe dysmenorrhea, or mild-to-moderate dysmenorrhea unresponsive to therapy
3. Undiagnosed lower abdominal pain
4. Sexual assault (modified to collect the appropriate information and samples)
5. Suspected pelvic mass
6. Request by the adolescent

OBTAINING THE HISTORY

The history should include a gynecologic assessment, general health history, review of systems, and information on risk behaviors (see Chapter 3). The history should include the following:

1. Menstrual history
2. History and type of vaginal discharge
3. Sexual history
4. Family history (gynecologic problems, blood clotting disorders or stroke; and breast or gynecologic cancer)

GYNECOLOGIC EXAMINATION EQUIPMENT

Materials needed include the following:

1. Examination table with ankle supports
2. Gowns, sheet
3. Light source
4. Specula
5. Gonorrhea culture or nucleic acid amplification tests (NAATS) medium
6. *Chlamydia* screening test: NAATs
7. Spatula and cytobrush for Pap test, Pap slide containers and fixative, or kits for ThinPrep or other Pap systems
8. Cotton swabs and either tubes or slides for wet mounts
9. Potassium hydroxide (10% KOH) and saline for wet mounts, pH paper
10. Water-soluble lubricating jelly
11. Warm water source
12. Nonsterile gloves
13. Handheld mirror (optional)
14. Tissues
15. Tampons and sanitary napkins
16. Rapid pregnancy test kits

PELVIC EXAMINATION

A pelvic examination is generally performed annually for sexually active adolescents starting approximately 3 years after the initiation of sexual intercourse. Before the examination begins, it is helpful to explain to the teen, while she is fully clothed, the various parts of the examination: general physical, inspection of the genitalia, speculum, and bimanual examination. Each step is then explained again during the examination.

The steps are as follows:

1. Make sure that the patient has emptied her bladder.
2. Ask the patient to undress completely and put on a gown.
3. Perform a general examination.
4. Have the patient lie supine on the examination table, feet resting in the ankle supports. The drape or sheet should be positioned so that eye contact can be maintained with the patient.
5. Ask the patient to touch her knees to your hands, which are held out to the side. Do not try to pry her legs apart.
6. Inspect the external genitalia (Fig. 48.1).
   a. Note pubic hair distribution and sexual maturity rating (Tanner stage).
   b. Assess for signs of erythema, inflammation, or lesions over the perineum, thighs, mons, labia, and perianal region. Place the palms of both hands

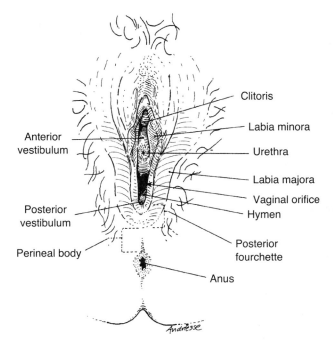

FIGURE 48.1 External genitalia of the pubertal female. (Reproduced from Fig 1-22 in Emans et al. *Pediatric and adolescent gynecology*, 5th ed. Philadelphia: Lippincott Williams & Wilkins, 2005, with permission.)

adjacent to the labia majora and gently separate them to examine the external structures. Check the size of the clitoris; a width of 5 to 10 mm is considered a possible sign of virilization, and >10 mm indicates definite virilization.

 c. Careful inspection of hymen for estrogen effect (light pink, thickened), congenital anomalies (septate, imperforate, microperforate), and transections that might result from consensual or nonconsensual sexual intercourse. For girls who are being evaluated for prior sexual abuse or assault, a saline-moistened cotton-tipped applicator can be used to run the edge of the hymen to look for transections.

 d. Obtaining samples: Saline-moistened or dry cotton-tipped applicators can be used to obtain samples.

7. *Speculum examination:* The correct size of speculum should be selected, and the speculum warmed, if possible, before insertion. It should be lubricated only with water if samples are being obtained. If the hymeneal opening is small, a Huffman (Huffman-Graves) speculum ($1/2 \times 4^{1}/_{2}$ in.) is used to visualize the cervix. For the sexually active teen, a Pederson speculum ($7/8 \times 4^{1}/_{2}$ in.) is appropriate. In the virginal teenager, a one-finger, gloved (water-moistened) examination demonstrates the size of the hymeneal opening and location of the cervix and allows subsequent easy insertion of the speculum. The speculum should be inserted posteriorly in a downward direction to avoid the urethra (Fig. 48.2). Applying pressure to the inner thigh at the same time the speculum is inserted into the vagina may be helpful.

 a. Observe the vaginal walls for signs of estrogenization, inflammation, or lesions.

 b. Inspect the cervix: The erythematous area of columnar epithelium surrounding the cervical os is called the ectropion. The junction between the squamous and columnar mucosa is called the squamocolumnar junction. Mucopurulent discharge from the cervix suggests cervicitis.

 c. To assess signs and symptoms of vaginitis, vaginal swabs for wet mounts and pH can be obtained and placed into one drop of saline on one slide (for *Trichomonas,* white cells, or "clue cells"), and one drop of 10% KOH (for pseudohyphae) on another slide. A swab should also be applied to pH paper; a pH <4.5 suggests normal physiologic discharge or *Candida* infection, and a pH >4.5 suggests bacterial vaginosis or *Trichomonas* infection.

 d. If indicated, obtain a Pap test of the cervix with a spatula and cytobrush, or a cytobroom. This should include at least a 360-degree rotation of the spatula in contact with the cervix, with care taken to sample the "transition zone" or squamocolumnar junction. Cytobrushes are used to ensure the collection of cells from the endocervical canal.

 e. Endocervical tests for sexually transmitted diseases (STDs): Tests for *Neisseriae gonorrhoeae* and *Chlamydia* include NAATs, DNA probes, and cultures. NAATs are preferred for Chlamydia screening from the cervix or urine.

8. *Bimanual examination:* This vaginal–abdominal examination involves the insertion of one or two gloved, lubricated fingers into the vagina while the other hand is placed on the abdomen. Remind the patient that you will be examining her uterus and ovaries and to communicate any feelings of discomfort she may be experiencing.

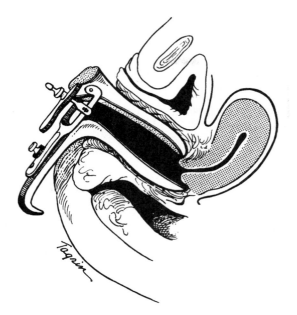

FIGURE 48.2 Speculum examination of the cervix. (From Clarke-Pearson D, Dawood M. *Green's Gynecology: essentials of clinical practice,* 4th ed. Boston: Little, Brown, 1990, with permission. Reproduced in Figure 1-27 Emans, et al. *Pediatric and adolescent gynecology,* 5th ed. Philadelphia: Lippincott Williams & Wilkins, 2005, with permission.)

    a. Palpation of the vagina and cervix.
    b. Palpation of the uterus: Assess the size and position of the uterus and any masses or tenderness.
    c. Gently explore the posterior fornix and the rectouterine pouch (pouch of Douglas) for masses, fullness, and tenderness.
    d. Palpation of the adnexa: Assess for masses, tenderness, or abnormalities of the ovaries or the adnexal area. To palpate these structures, insert the examining fingers into each lateral fornix, positioning them slightly posteriorly and high. Sweep the abdominal examining hand downward over the internal fingers. If there is a history of pelvic pain or an adnexal mass is felt, a rectovaginal–abdominal examination can help complete the evaluation of the adnexa or uterus and the rectum, anus, and posterior cul-de-sac. A rectovaginal–abdominal examination is performed with the index finger in the vagina, the middle finger in the rectum, and the other hand on the abdomen.
9. At the completion of the examination, offer the patient tissues to be used to remove the lubrication from her perineum after you leave the room. Return to the office for a discussion of your findings and plan and to answer any questions. The parent can be informed of the results of the examination and the treatment plan, and depending on confidential issues discussed.

WEB SITES

For Teenagers and Parents

http://www.youngwomenshealth.org/pelvicinfo.html. Information about your first pelvic examination from Boston Children's Hospital.

http://www.vaginitis.com/firstpelvic.html. Information about a first pelvic in question and answer format.

http://www.goaskalice.columbia.edu/0643.html. Questions and answers for college students about reproductive health and specifically about pelvic examination.

CHAPTER 49

Normal Menstrual Physiology

Sari L. Kives and Judith A. Lacy

For cyclic menses to occur, there must be a coordinated sequence of events beginning with the hypothalamic secretion of gonadotropin-releasing hormone (GnRH). In response to GnRH, the pituitary secretes follicle-stimulating hormone (FSH) and luteinizing hormone (LH), and the ovaries secrete, estrogen, progesterone, activin, and inhibins. Ultimately, the endometrium of the uterus responds to estrogen and progesterone with stimulation and withdrawal, culminating in menses.

The menstrual cycle is governed by positive and negative feedback. In the beginning of a cycle, low levels of estradiol perpetuate a positive feedback mechanism and subsequently stimulate FSH and LH secretion. At higher levels, estradiol and progesterone create a negative feedback effect and suppress FSH and LH thereby preventing further follicular recruitment. Although the gonadotropins act synergistically, FSH primarily affects follicular growth and LH stimulates ovarian steroid biosynthesis.

Hypothesized mechanisms for the onset of menses include the following:

1. A progressive decrease in the sensitivity of the hypothalamus to gonadal steroids
2. An increase in pulsatile secretion of GnRH, leading to increased sex steroids.
3. A critical body composition or percentage of body fat (about 17% body fat at menarche)

DEFINITION OF MENSTRUAL CYCLE

A menstrual cycle is defined as the time from the first day of flow to the first day of the next period. Based on current understanding, the menstrual cycle may be described by the response of the pituitary, ovary, and endometrium (Fig. 49.1).

FSH and LH are secreted in a pulsatile fashion, with FSH and LH secretions secondary to pulsatile hypothalamic secretion of GnRH. Secretion of GnRH can be modulated by estradiol and progesterone feedback and by neurotransmitters. The physiologic mechanisms of the menstrual cycle can be divided into the follicular, ovulatory, and luteal phases.

Follicular Phase

The duration of this phase is usually 14 days, but the length varies (range 7 to 22 days). This phase begins with the onset of menses and ends with

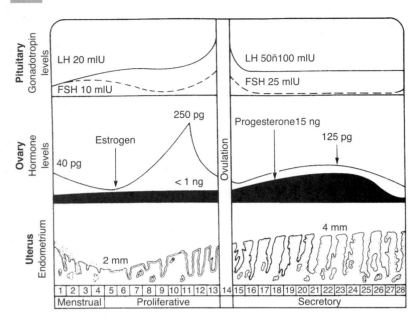

FIGURE 49.1 Normal menstrual cycle. (Reproduced from Neinstein LS. Menstrual disorders. *Semin Fam Med* 1981;2:184.)

ovulation. The duration of the follicular phase is the major determinant of cycle length.

1. During the end of the prior cycle, corpus luteum involution occurs, with resulting decreasing estradiol and progesterone levels. The low levels stimulate hypothalamic GnRH release, which, in turn, increases the pituitary's FSH and LH release.
2. FSH stimulates recruitment of ovarian follicles.
3. At present, it is believed that LH stimulates ovarian theca cells to produce androgens, which are then converted to estrogens in ovarian granulosa cells under the influence of FSH. Estradiol increases FSH binding to granulosa cell receptors, leading to amplification of the FSH effect and allowing one follicle to predominate.
4. Under the influence of estrogen, the proliferative phase of the endometrium occurs, increasing the endometrium from 1 mm at the time of menstruation to 5 mm at the time of ovulation.
5. Estrogen causes maturation of vaginal basal cells into superficial squamous epithelial cells and the formation of watery vaginal mucus, which can be strung out (spinnbarkeit) or dried into a ferning pattern.
6. In response to rising estradiol levels in the middle and late follicular phase, FSH levels fall.

Ovulatory Phase

1. A preovulatory estradiol surge leads to a midcycle LH surge, which initiates ovulation approximately 10 to 16 hours after the LH surge. A small preovulatory rise in progesterone is required to induce the FSH surge.

2. A mature follicle releases an oocyte and becomes a functioning corpus luteum.
3. At this stage, there are copious clear vaginal secretions.

Luteal Phase

This phase begins with ovulation and ends with menstrual flow. This phase is more constant; it lasts about 14 ± 2 days.

1. The corpus luteum produces large amounts of progesterone and estrogen. Rising levels of estrogen and progesterone lead to falling levels of FSH and LH.
2. Progesterone antagonizes the action of estrogen by reducing estrogen receptor sites and increasing conversion of estradiol to estrone, a less potent estrogen. Progesterone halts the growth of the endometrium and stimulates differentiation into a secretory endometrium. The secretory endometrium is prepared for implantation.
3. Local progesterone produced by the corpus luteum suppresses follicular development in the ipsilateral ovary, so that ovulation during the following month occurs in the contralateral ovary.
4. Cervical mucus becomes thick during the luteal phase, owing to the influence of progesterone.
5. Unless there is fertilization, the corpus luteum involutes after 10 to 12 days. Sloughing of the endometrium occurs secondary to a loss of estrogen and progesterone. Local prostaglandins cause vasoconstriction and uterine contractions.
6. The decreased levels of estrogen and progesterone lead to increased levels of FSH and LH, providing the positive feedback loop required to begin another menstrual cycle.

WEB SITES

http://www.fda.gov/fdac/reprints/ots_mens.html. U.S. Food and Drug Administration Web site for teenagers, abridged from *FDA Consumer,* December, 1993. Provides general information on menstruation for teens.

http://www.youngwomenshealth.org/menstrual.html. Boston Children's Hospital site, guide to puberty and menses.

CHAPTER 50

Dysmenorrhea and Premenstrual Syndrome

Paula K. Braverman

More than 50% of female adolescents experience some menstrual dysfunction. Dysmenorrhea and premenstrual syndrome are discussed in this chapter.

DYSMENORRHEA

Primary dysmenorrhea refers to pain associated with the menstrual flow with no evidence of organic pelvic disease. *Secondary dysmenorrhea* is pain associated with menses secondary to organic disease (e.g., endometriosis, outflow tract obstruction, or pelvic inflammatory disease).

Etiology. Pain is caused by myometrial contractions induced by prostaglandins from the secretory endometrium. $PGF_{2\alpha}$, considered the most important prostaglandin, is formed through the cyclooxygenase pathway. It is postulated that women with dysmenorrhea may be more sensitive to prostaglandins. The following have been noted: (1) Locally, prostaglandins cause uterine contractions; they also enter the bloodstream and cause associated symptoms (e.g., headache, nausea, vomiting, etc.). (2) Anovulatory cycles are associated with lower menstrual prostaglandin levels and usually no dysmenorrhea. (3) Patients with dysmenorrhea have higher levels of prostaglandins in the endometrium. (4) Most of the prostaglandins are released within the first 48 hours of menstruation, correlating with the most severe symptoms. (5) Prostaglandin inhibitors decrease dysmenorrhea.

Epidemiology. Dysmenorrhea is the greatest single cause of lost work and school hours in females, with >140 million hours lost per year. Various studies worldwide have shown that 43% to 93% of all postpubescent females have some degree of dysmenorrhea; between 5% and 42% of these females describe the pain as severe and are incapacitated for 1 to 3 days per month.

Clinical Manifestations. Primary dysmenorrhea usually begins within 1 to 3 years of menarche and is associated with the establishment of ovulatory cycles. Although the pain usually begins within hours of menses, it may start several days prior to the onset. Local symptoms include pain that is spasmodic in nature and is strongest in the lower abdomen, with radiation to the back and anterior thighs. In most cases, the pain resolves within 24 to 48 hours, but the symptoms sometimes persist for longer. Associated systemic symptoms may include nausea or vomiting, fatigue, mood changes, dizziness, diarrhea, backache, and headache.

Differential Diagnosis

Gynecologic Causes. Endometriosis, pelvic inflammatory disease, benign uterine tumors (fibroids), intrauterine devices, anatomic abnormalities (congenital obstructive müllerian malformations, outflow obstruction), pelvic adhesions, ovarian cysts or masses.

Nongynecologic Causes. Gastrointestinal disorders (inflammatory bowel disease, irritable bowel syndrome, constipation, lactose intolerance), musculoskeletal pain, genitourinary abnormalities (cystitis, ureteral obstruction, calculi), psychogenic disorders (history of abuse, trauma, psychogenic complaints).

Diagnosis

History

1. *Menstrual history:* Primary dysmenorrhea usually starts 1 to 3 years after menarche and usually decreases during the twenties and thirties. Secondary dysmenorrhea should be considered if the pain starts with the onset of menarche or after the age of 20 years. Adolescents should be asked about the degree of pain and the amount of impairment in daily activities. Any previous use of therapeutic modalities and their effectiveness should be ascertained.
2. *Other history:* Additional questions should include prior sexually transmitted diseases (STDs) and sexual activity; a review of systems related to the gastrointestinal, genitourinary, and musculoskeletal systems; and a psychosocial history to assess stress, substance abuse, and sexual abuse.

Physical Examination. Examine the pelvis for evidence of endometriosis, endometritis, fibroids, uterine or cervical abnormalities, or adnexal masses and tenderness. If the teen is not sexually active and the history is typical for dysmenorrhea, a pelvic examination is indicated only if the symptoms do not respond to standard medical therapy. Examination limited to a Q-tip inserted into the vagina can help rule out a hymenal abnormality or vaginal septum without performing a speculum exam. The musculoskeletal examination should focus on range of motion of the hips and spine to assess for tenderness and limitation in motion.

Laboratory Tests. A complete blood count and erythrocyte sedimentation rate should be performed if pelvic inflammatory disease or inflammatory bowel disease is suspected. Sexually active adolescents should be tested for STDs and pregnancy. A urinalysis and urine culture will help diagnose urinary tract problems. If a müllerian abnormality is suspected, pelvic ultrasound or magnetic resonance imaging will define the anatomy. If evaluation of the genitourinary, gastrointestinal, and musculoskeletal tracts fails to reveal a cause of the pain, and it is severe and intractable despite treatment with antiprostaglandins and oral contraceptives, then laparoscopy should be considered.

Therapy

The two most effective treatments for primary dysmenorrhea are nonsteroidal anti-inflammatory drugs (NSAIDs) and oral contraceptives. The patient should be educated and reassured that the problem is physiologic and can be helped.

Nonsteroidal Anti-inflammatory Drugs. NSAIDs are the primary modality of therapy; 80% of dysmenorrhea can be relieved with these medications. Many NSAIDs have been found effective in alleviating menstrual cramps. The two most useful subgroups are propionic acids (e.g. ibuprofen, naproxen, naproxen sodium) and the fenamates such as mefenamic acid. These medications should be started either as soon as symptoms occur (prior to the onset of menses) or should coincide with the first sign of menstruation. Usually these medications are needed for only 1 to 3 days and side effects are usually minimal.

Hormonal Therapies. If the patient wishes contraception or the pain is severe and not responsive to NSAIDs, oral contraceptives can be tried. The maximal effect may not become apparent for several months. Two recent studies demonstrate in randomized double-blind placebo controlled studies that currently available low-dose oral contraceptive pills (OCPs) are effective. Combined oral contraceptives inhibit ovulation and lead to an atrophic decidualized endometrium, resulting in decreased menstrual flow and prostaglandin release.

Oral contraceptives decrease symptoms in >90% of patients with primary dysmenorrhea. If cyclic hormonal contraception is ineffective, continuous combination hormonal therapy can be tried. Injectable depot medroxyprogesterone acetate has also been effective.

Other Hormonal Modalities. Other hormonal options include gonadotropin-releasing hormone agonists with utilization of add-back therapy to prevent side effects related to hypoestrogenic state, Danazol, and the levonorgestrel-releasing intrauterine system.

Other Nonhormonal Modalities Likely to Be Beneficial. Vitamin B1, magnesium, vitamin E, transcutaneous nerve stimulation

PREMENSTRUAL SYNDROME

The term *premenstrual syndrome* (PMS) is used to describe an array of predictable physical, cognitive, affective, and behavioral symptoms that occur cyclically during the luteal phase of the menstrual cycle, and resolve quickly near the onset of menstruation. It is characterized by a broad spectrum of symptoms and until recently had confusing definitions. The etiology of PMS is currently unknown, but there is some evidence that reduced serotonergic function in the luteal phase and alteration in the gamma-aminobutyric acid (GABA) receptor complex response may be among the mechanisms responsible. Evidence is accumulating that PMS is not a single condition, but a set of interrelated symptom complexes, with multiple phenotypes of subtypes and pathophysiologic events that begin with ovulation.

In the mental health field, criteria have been developed to define a syndrome called premenstrual dysphoric disorder (PMDD) as a distinct clinical entity.

Although PMS and PMDD overlap, in PMDD the focus is more on the problems with mood and the symptoms are more severe, leading to a higher level of dysfunction before the onset of menses. Some experts conclude that it is not useful to differentiate PMS from PMDD and agree that there is a broad spectrum of severity.

Epidemiology. The exact prevalence is unknown, but estimates are that up to 85% of menstruating women have some degree of symptoms before menses and that 3% to 8% are so severely afflicted that daily activities are hindered. This smaller subset of women meet criteria for PMDD. Studies in adolescents have shown similar rates among adolescents.

Risk Factors. Risk factors for PMS include advancing age (beyond 30 years) and genetic factors. There are no significant differences in personality profile or level of stress in women with PMS compared with asymptomatic women. However, women with PMS may not handle stress as well.

Pathophysiology. The exact mechanism is unknown, but is likely to involve an interaction between sex steroids and central neurotransmitters. Theories include the following: (1) Alterations in neurotransmitters: Endorphins, GABA, and serotonin have been implicated. Serotonergic dysregulation is the most plausible theory, although not all women respond to selective serotonin re-uptake inhibitors (SSRIs), implying that other factors must be involved. (2) Hormonal factors: Women with PMS/PMDD are felt to be more sensitive to normal cyclical hormonal fluctuations. (3) Vitamin deficiencies have not been documented.

Clinical Manifestations. More than 150 symptoms have been described in literature, ranging from mild symptoms to those severe enough to interfere with normal activities. These include emotional and physical symptoms such as irritability, depression, fatigue or lethargy, anger/argumentative, insomnia or hypersomnia, mood lability, anxiety, poor concentration, confusion, tearfulness, social withdrawal, headaches, swelling (legs or breasts), breast tenderness, increased appetite, food cravings, weight gain, sense of abdominal bloating, fatigue, muscle and joint aches and pain, hot flashes.

Diagnosis. The diagnosis relies on the history of cyclic symptoms. No specific physical findings or laboratory tests have proved useful. Although there are no universally accepted specific diagnostic criteria among the various sources defining PMS including the World Health Organization's International Classification of Diseases, the American College of Obstetrics and Gynecology (ACOG), the National Institute of Mental Health, and the *Diagnostic and Statistical Manual of Mental Disorders,* 4th ed., Text Revision (DSM-IV-TR), three important findings are usually needed to diagnosis PMS:

1. Symptoms must occur in the luteal phase and resolve within a few days after onset of menstruation. Symptoms should not be present in the follicular phase.
2. The symptoms must be documented over several menstrual cycles and not be caused by other physical or psychological problems.
3. Symptoms must be recurrent and severe enough to disrupt normal activities.

TABLE 50.1

Diagnosis of Premenstrual Dysphoric Disorder (DSM-IV-TR Criteria)

I. In most menstrual cycles in the past year at least 5 of these symptoms (including at least one of the symptoms in category A) were present for most of the time 1 week before menses, began to remit within a few days after the onset of the follicular phase (menses), and were absent in the week after menses.

A.
1. Markedly depressed mood, feelings of hopelessness or self-deprecating thoughts
2. Marked anxiety, tension
3. Marked affective lability (i.e., feeling suddenly sad or tearful)
4. Persistent and marked anger or irritability or increased interpersonal conflicts

B. Other symptoms
1. Decreased interest in usual activities, such as friends and hobbies
2. Subjective sense of difficulty in concentrating
3. Lethargy, easy fatigability, or marked lack of energy
4. Marked change in appetite, overeating, or specific food cravings
5. Hypersomnia or insomnia
6. A subjective sense of being overwhelmed or out of control
7. Other physical symptoms (e.g., breast tenderness, bloating, weight gain, headache, joint or muscle pain)

II. The symptoms markedly interfere with work, school, usual activities, or relationships with others.

III. Symptoms are not merely an exacerbation of another disorder, such as major depressive disorder, panic disorder, dysthymic disorder, or a personality disorder (although it may be superimposed on any of these disorders).

IV. Criteria I, II, and III are confirmed by prospective daily ratings for at least two consecutive symptomatic menstrual cycles.

Adapted from American Psychiatric Association. *Diagnostic and statistical manual of mental disorders,* text revision, 4th ed. Washington, DC. American Psychiatric Press, 2000.

A calendar can be helpful in the diagnosis and in monitoring teens after the start of any therapy. Prospective recording should be done for at least 2 to 3 months to document that symptoms are occurring cyclically in the luteal phase.

The DSM-IV-TR lists similar criteria for PMDD (Table 50.1). It is important to remember that the symptoms cannot represent exacerbation of an existing disorder such as major depression, anxiety disorders, panic, dysthymic disorder, or personality disorder, but they may be superimposed on one of these psychiatric disorders. Women may have psychiatric disorders that become exacerbated during menstruation (i.e., menstrual magnification). Certain medical disorders can also become worse during menses, including seizures, migraine headaches, irritable bowel syndrome, asthma, and allergies.

Therapy

No single treatment is universally acceptable as effective. Studies have yielded conflicting results with most therapies, and most trials have not been well controlled. Treatments have included the following: lifestyle changes, education, stress management, aerobic exercise, vitamin and mineral supplementation, herbal preparations, dietary manipulation, suppression of ovulation, SSRIs, and medications to suppress physical and psychological symptoms.

1. There have been some positive outcomes for complementary and alternative therapies. However, although some show definite promise, more research needs to be done to definitively recommend any of these therapies. Some of the more promising therapies have included calcium, magnesium, *Vitex agnus-castus* (chasteberry), *Gingko biloba* (gingko leaf extract), and carbohydrate supplements.
2. Because PMS appears to be a cyclic disorder of menses occurring in the luteal phase, suppression of ovulation has been used as a therapy, including combination oral contraceptives, medroxyprogesterone acetate (Depo-Provera), and gonadotropin-releasing hormone (GnRH). The current thinking is that oral contraceptive pills should be considered if the symptoms are primarily physical and not mood-related because OCPs appear to be more effective for the physical symptoms. Continuous hormonal therapy with combined hormonal contraceptives can also be considered to suppress cyclic changes and endogenous sex hormone variability.
3. Medications to suppress physical symptoms include prostaglandin inhibitors (NSAIDs) and spironolactone.
4. SSRIs are the drugs of choice and first-line therapy for *severe* PMS/PMDD. Placebo-controlled studies have shown that they are effective for severe PMS and PMDD and improve both physical symptoms and mood. Studies have shown that using these drugs intermittently only during the luteal phase (i.e., 14 days prior to onset of menses) rather than continuously is equally effective for symptom reduction.
5. Studies have shown some positive effects on somatic and affective symptoms by utilizing medications to suppress psychological symptoms, including anxiolytics and other antidepressants such as benzodiazepines (especially alprazolam), clomipramine, and buspirone. These medications can be given in the luteal phase rather than continuously. None of these would be recommended for routine use in adolescents but only for use in selected adolescents with severe symptoms unresponsive to other treatment modalities.

SUMMARY: STEPS IN THE TREATMENT OF SYMPTOMS OF PREMENSTRUAL SYNDROME

The following successive steps were outlined in the *ACOG Practice Bulletin* (2000) and in recent review by Johnson (2004):

Step 1: A. *If mild/moderate symptoms:* Supportive therapy with good nutrition, complex carbohydrates, aerobic exercise, calcium supplements, and possibly magnesium or chasteberry fruit

   B. *If physical symptoms predominate:* spironolactone, hormonal suppression with OCPs, medroxyprogesterone acetate, NSAIDs

Step 2: *When mood symptoms predominate:* SSRI therapy. An anxiolytic can be used for specific symptoms not relieved by the SSRI medication.

Step 3: *If there is no response to steps 1 or 2:* GnRH agonists.

WEB SITES AND REFERENCES

http://kidshealth.org/teen/sexual_health/girls/menstruation.html. Teen site on dysmenorrhea.

http://www.youngwomenshealth.org/menstrual.html. Information from Children's Hospital Boston on dysmenorrhea and PMS.

http://www.nlm.nih.gov/medlineplus/ency/article/001505.htm. Medical encyclopedia from the U.S. National Library of Medicine and National Institutes of Health. Information on PMS and dysmenorrhea.

American College of Obstetrics and Gynecology. *ACOG practice bulletin: premenstrual syndrome.* Washington, DC: ACOG, April 2000:15.

American College of Obstetrics and Gynecology. ACOG Committee on Adolescent Health Care. Committee Opinion No 310. Endometriosis in adolescents. *Obstet Gynecol* 2005;105:921.

American Psychiatric Association. *Diagnostic and Statistical Manual of Mental Disorders,* 4th ed, Text Revision (DSM-IV-TR). Washington, DC: American Psychiatric Association, 2000.

Johnson SR. Premenstrual syndrome, premenstrual dysphoric disorder, and beyond: a clinical primer for practitioners. *Obstet Gynecol* 2004;104:845.

CHAPTER 51

Dysfunctional Uterine Bleeding

Laurie A.P. Mitan and Gail B. Slap

Dysfunctional uterine bleeding (DUB) is irregular and/or prolonged vaginal bleeding due to endometrial sloughing in the absence of structural pathology.

DIFFERENTIAL DIAGNOSIS OF ABNORMAL BLEEDING

- Leading causes in adults, uterine fibroids and malignancy, are rare in adolescents.
- The leading cause in adolescents is anovulation secondary to physiologic immaturity of the hypothalamic-pituitary-ovarian axis.
- Other common causes include breakthrough bleeding of a proliferative endometrium produced by prolonged or excessive estrogen (e.g., use of the 90-day oral contraceptive); breakthrough bleeding of an atrophic endometrium produced by prolonged or excessive progesterone in the absence of adequate estrogen (e.g., use of depot medroxyprogesterone acetate); and withdrawal bleeding after a sudden drop in estrogen (e.g., discontinuation of the oral contraceptive) or progesterone (e.g., defective corpus luteum).
- Two important conditions to consider in adolescents are polycystic ovary syndrome (Chapter 52) and late-onset congenital adrenal hyperplasia (see Chapter 58).
- Less common are ectopic pregnancy; spontaneous, threatened, or incomplete abortion; placental polyp or mole; foreign body; sexually transmitted or iatrogenic infection; trauma; congenital anomaly of the outflow tract; bleeding diathesis; and hypo- or hyperthyroidism.

EVALUATION

- Assess hemodynamic stability (orthostatic vital signs).
  Pelvic examination is essential in all sexually active adolescents, but can be deferred in the adolescent with suspected anovulatory DUB who has never had sexual intercourse.
- Obtain the sexual history from the adolescent alone in most instances.
- Determine the sexual maturity ratings; look for hirsutism, acanthosis nigricans, acne, petechiae, purpura, ecchymoses; gum bleeding, epistaxis;

thyroid enlargement, tenderness, and nodules; galactorrhea; hepatospleno-megaly.

Laboratory Tests. May not be necessary with mild anovulatory DUB associated with physiologic immaturity. Other patients may require the following laboratory evaluation:

1. Pregnancy test if there is any question of past sexual intercourse.
2. Complete blood count.
3. Screening for sexually transmitted diseases (STDs) including tests for *Neisseria gonorrhoeae* and *Chlamydia*.
4. Erythrocyte sedimentation rate to evaluate for pelvic inflammatory disease (PID) or underlying systemic illness.
5. Thyroid function tests for all patients with moderate to severe menorrhagia.
6. Prothrombin time, partial thromboplastin time, and PFA-100 as a preliminary screen for a bleeding disorder. Patients with moderate to severe anemia, personal history of bleeding in addition to menorrhagia, or family history of significant bleeding should be evaluated with more specific diagnostic tests, such as von Willebrand factor antigen and ristocetin cofactor activity. Hematology consultation may be necessary.
7. Liver function tests and blood urea nitrogen if there is evidence of abnormal clotting factors or platelet function.
8. LH, FSH, testosterone (total and free), dehydroepiandrosterone sulfate, if polycystic ovary syndrome (PCOS) is suspected (see Chapter 52).
9. *Pelvic ultrasonography:* Transabdominal ultrasonography is essential in the virginal patient with possible structural pathology who cannot tolerate a bimanual examination.
10. Endometrial aspirate and/or biopsy are rarely indicated in adolescents.

THERAPY

The severity and cause of the bleeding guide its management. Bleeding secondary to a systemic problem, such as a clotting abnormality or thyroid dysfunction, may require short-term hormonal therapy identical to that for anovulatory bleeding until the systemic problem is brought under control.

Treatment of Anovulatory DUB

1. *Light to moderate flow, hemoglobin level of at least 12 g/dL:* Reassurance, multivitamin with iron, menstrual calendar, reevaluation within 3 months.
2. *Moderate flow, hemoglobin level of 10 to 12 g/dL:* Begin a 35-μg combined oral contraceptive pill every 6 to 12 hours for 24 to 48 hours until the bleeding stops, along with an NSAID and antiemetic if needed. Taper to one pill daily by day 5; continue for 21 days prior to the placebo pill week. The resulting withdrawal bleed should be heavy, but controlled. Continue the combined oral contraceptive for 3 to 6 months.
3. *Heavy flow, hemoglobin level <10 g/dL:* Outpatient management as above for the patient who is hemodynamically stable, tolerating oral therapy, and reliable. Otherwise, hospitalize for the above regimen (or a 50-μg combined pill if the bleeding does not slow). For persistent bleeding, add intravenous conjugated estrogen 25 mg every 6 hours up to six doses. Taper to one pill

daily by day 7. Persistent bleeding on intravenous therapy usually warrants cervical dilation with endometrial curettage.

Treatment of DUB Secondary to Hormonal Contraception

Persistent bleeding on hormonal contraception usually responds to the following measures:

1. Changing a 20-μg combined pill to a 30- to 35-μg combined pill.
2. Changing a 30- to 35-μg combined pill to either a 50-μg combined pill for one cycle or adding conjugated estrogen 0.625 mg daily to the 30- to 35-μg pill for one cycle.
3. Adding conjugated estrogen 1.25 to 2.50 mg daily for 5 to 7 days to progestin-only contraceptives. Spotting after discontinuation of the estrogen is common because of the consequent estrogen-induced endometrial proliferation.

Treatment of Bleeding Diathesis

Iatrogenic DUB is common in patients receiving chemotherapeutic or other interventions that alter bone marrow production, platelet function, or clotting factor synthesis. The following interventions decrease menstrual frequency or induce endometrial atrophy: (1) Combined pill daily for 3 monthly cycles and discontinue 1 week every 3 months to allow a withdrawal bleeding and prevent excessive endometrial proliferation; (2) DMPA, 150 mg intramuscularly every 12 weeks; (3) Progesterone, 10 mg orally daily for an unlimited number of months; (4) Gonadotropin-releasing hormone analog (e.g., leuprolide acetate) for up to 6 months. Low-dose estrogen may need to be added back to control symptoms of hypoestrogenemia. Treatment may be started 2 to 3 weeks prior to the onset of planned thrombocytopenia, as in bone marrow transplantation.

WEB SITES

http://www.youngwomenshealth.org. From Boston Children's Hospital.
http://www.nlm.nih.gov. The National Library of Medicine health information site.
http://www.acog.org. American College of Obstetricians and Gynecologists.
http://www.naspag.org. North American Society for Pediatric and Adolescent Gynecology (NASPAG).

CHAPTER 52

Menstrual Disorders: Amenorrhea and Polycystic Ovary Syndrome

Amy Fleischman, Catherine M. Gordon, and Lawrence S. Neinstein

AMENORRHEA

Definition

1. *Primary amenorrhea*
   a. No spontaneous uterine bleeding by age of 14 years and no secondary sex characteristics
   b. No spontaneous bleeding by age 16 years regardless of secondary sex characteristics
   c. No spontaneous bleeding despite having attained sexual maturity rating (SMR, Tanner stage) 5 for at least 1 year or the onset of breast development 4 years previously
   d. No spontaneous bleeding by age 14 with clinical or genotypic evidence of Turner's syndrome
2. *Secondary amenorrhea:* After previous menses, no subsequent bleeding for 6 months or length of time equal to three previous cycles

Etiology

1. *Primary amenorrhea without secondary sex characteristics (absent breast development) but with normal genitalia (uterus and vagina)*
   a. Genetic or enzymatic defects causing gonadal (ovarian) failure (hypergonadotropic hypogonadism): The most common genetic disorders are (i) Turner's syndrome; (ii) Turner's mosaicism or related genotypes (45,X, 45 XX/X, or 45 XY/X); (iii) structurally abnormal X chromosome; (iv) mosaicism: X/XX; (v) Pure gonadal dysgenesis (46,XX or 46 XX/XY with streaked gonads); (vi) 17α-hydroxylase deficiency with 46,XX karyotype
   b. Isolated pituitary gonadotropin insufficiency: Kallmann syndrome should be considered
   c. Hypothalamic failure due to inadequate gonadotropin-releasing hormone (GnRH) release
2. *Primary amenorrhea with normal breast development but absent uterus*
   a. Complete androgen insensitivity (formerly testicular feminization): The underlying defect is a mutation in the androgen receptor. Manifestations

include (i) 46,XY karyotype; (ii) female phenotype in complete androgen insensitivity (genital ambiguity often presents in incomplete forms); (iii) testes present in abdomen, pelvis, or inguinal canal; (iv) lack of axillary and pubic hair; (v) normal breast development; (vi) blind vaginal pouch with absence of ovaries, uterus, and fallopian tubes; (vii) normal or elevated male testosterone concentrations.

  b. Congenital absence of uterus: Manifestations include (i) 46,XX karyotype; (ii) ovaries are present, possible cyclic breast and mood changes; (iii) normal secondary sex characteristics; (iv) uterus absent or rudimentary cords; (v) absent or blind vaginal pouch; (vi) normal female testosterone level; (vi) possibly associated renal, skeletal, or other congenital anomalies.

3. *Primary amenorrhea with no breast development and no uterus:* The individual usually has a male karyotype, elevated gonadotropin levels, and testosterone values that are equal to or less than a normal female level. The causes include (i) 17,20-lyase deficiency; (ii) agonadism, including no internal sex organs; (iii) 17α-hydroxylase deficiency with 46,XY karyotype.

4. *Primary and secondary amenorrhea with normal secondary sex characteristics (breast development) and normal genitalia*

  a. Hypothalamic causes, including (i) idiopathic; (ii) medications and drugs (e.g., phenothiazines, contraceptives); (iii) endocrinopathies (e.g., thyroid dysfunction); (iv) stress; (v) strenuous exercise; (vi) weight loss; (vii) chronic illnesses; (viii) hypothalamic failure (e.g., idiopathic or mass) (ix) polycystic ovary syndrome (PCOS)

  b. Pituitary causes (e.g., idiopathic, tumors or nonneoplastic lesions such as Sheehan's syndrome, Simmonds disease, or empty sella syndrome)

  c. Ovarian causes such as premature ovarian failure (may be associated with autoantibodies or after chemotherapy or radiation therapy)

  d. Uterine causes: uterine synechiae (Asherman's syndrome)

  e. Pregnancy

Diagnosis

History. Including (1) systemic diseases; (2) family history (especially ages of parental growth and development, thyroid disease or diabetes mellitus); (3) past medical history; (4) pubertal growth and development; (5) emotional status; (6) medications, including illicit drugs; (7) nutritional status and recent weight changes; (8) exercise history; (9) sexual history, contraception, and symptoms of pregnancy; (10) menstrual history; (11) history of androgen excess suggesting PCOS or another ovarian or adrenal abnormality

Physical Examination

1. Signs of systemic disease or malnutrition
2. SMR: Important for evaluating progress in secondary sex characteristics as most adolescents are not menarchal until SMR 4 and 95% are menarchal by 1 year after SMR 5
3. Height and weight
4. Signs of androgen excess (e.g., acne, hirsutism)
5. Signs of thyroid dysfunction
6. Signs of insulin resistance such as acanthosis nigricans
7. Signs of gonadal dysgenesis: Webbed neck, low-set ears, broad, shield-like chest, short fourth metacarpal, and increased carrying angle

8. Test for anosmia in females with primary amenorrhea to evaluate for Kallmann's syndrome
9. Breast examination, including check for galactorrhea
10. Pelvic examination: Search for stenotic cervix, vaginal agenesis, imperforate hymen, transverse vaginal septum, absent uterus, or pregnancy; an external genital examination critical; full pelvic examination possibly not necessary if the teen is not sexually active.

Laboratory Evaluation

1. *Primary and secondary amenorrhea with normal secondary sex characteristics.*
   a. Pregnancy should always be considered and ruled out.
   b. If evidence of galactorrhea or androgen excess, adolescent should be evaluated.
   c. Diabetes mellitus and hypothyroidism should be considered and if clinically indicated, ruled out with blood sugar or thyroid function test measurements.
   d. Uterine synechiae, or Asherman syndrome, should be considered if there is a history of dilation and curettage or endometritis. This condition may cause partial or total uterine obliteration. If the problem is suspected, a gynecologic referral is indicated.

If the results of the evaluation are negative, the work-up should include (Fig. 52.1) administration of progesterone withdrawal test or "challenge."

Positive Response
A positive response to progesterone indicates adequate estrogen levels, seen with hypothalamic-pituitary dysfunction or PCOS. (1) Prolactin level should be measured, the most sensitive test for pituitary microadenomas; (2) Thyroid-stimulating hormone and T_4 should be measured to rule out primary or central hypothyroidism; (3) LH or LH:FSH ratios have been used to evaluate for PCOS, but these values lack sensitivity and specificity.

Negative Response
If there is no response to progesterone, hypothalamic–pituitary dysfunction or ovarian failure is likely. A high FSH level indicates ovarian failure, whereas a normal or low FSH level suggests a hypothalamic-pituitary disturbance. If ovarian failure is suspected, a karyotype, antiovarian antibodies, and screening for autoimmune endocrinopathies should be considered. If hypothalamic-pituitary failure is suspected, a magnetic resonance imaging (MRI) scan, visual fields, and pituitary stimulation tests should be considered.

Individuals with weight loss, anorexia nervosa, heavy substance abuse, or heavy exercise may or may not withdraw to progesterone. If they do not experience withdrawal bleeding within 10 to 14 days after discontinuing the progesterone, it is indicative of low E_2 levels.

2. *Primary amenorrhea with absent uterus or absent secondary sex characteristics (Fig. 52.2)*
   a. A physical examination will divide the teens into three groups: (i) absent uterus, normal breasts; (ii) absent breasts, normal uterus; (iii) absent breasts and uterus. Breast development should be at least at SMR 4 to be considered indicative of full gonadal function. A breast stage of SMR 2 or SMR 3 may indicate adrenal function without gonadal function.

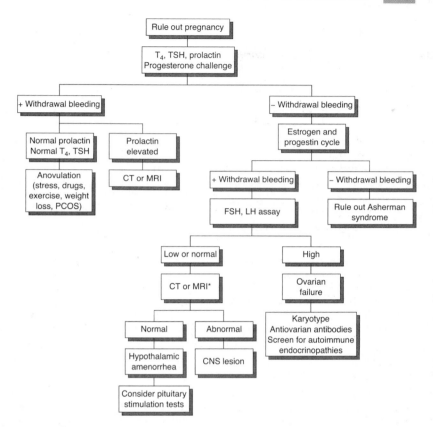

FIGURE 52.1 The evaluation of secondary amenorrhea. CNS, central nervous system; CT, computed axial tomography; TSH, thyroid-stimulating hormone.

b. If the examination reveals normal breast development, but absent uterus and blind vaginal pouch, a karyotype and serum testosterone concentrations are indicated.
  • XX karyotype plus female testosterone concentration: Congenital absence of uterus
  • XY karyotype plus male testosterone concentration: Androgen insensitivity
c. If examination reveals absent secondary sex characteristics, but normal uterus, measure serum FSH.
  • A low or normal FSH level suggests a hypothalamic or pituitary abnormality, and a careful neuroendocrine evaluation is in order.
  • A high FSH level and blood pressure within the reference range suggest a genetic disorder or gonadal dysgenesis. Order a karyotype.
  • A high FSH level and hypertension suggest 17α-hydroxylase deficiency. Confirmed by an elevated progesterone level (>3 ng/mL), low

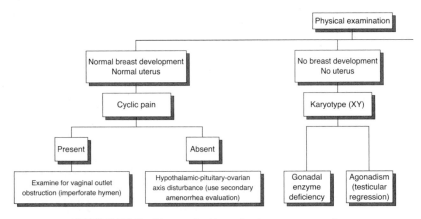

FIGURE 52.2 The evaluation of primary amenorrhea.

17α-hydroxyprogesterone level ($<$0.2 ng/mL), and an elevated serum deoxycorticosterone level.

d. Absence of both breast development and uterus or vagina is rare. These findings suggest gonadal failure and the presence of testicular muellerian inhibitory factor (MIF) secretion. This could arise from anorchia or an enzyme block, such as a 17,20-lyase defect. The evaluation includes LH, FSH, progesterone, 17-hydroxyprogesterone measurements, and a karyotype.

Treatment

Primary Amenorrhea

Hypothalamic Hypogonadotropic Hypogonadism (Hypothalamic Failure). Therapy should begin with estrogen therapy (0.3 mg/day or less if the adolescent is short to avoid premature epiphyseal closure). A transdermal patch can be used starting at 0.025 mg of estradiol/day, or half of the 0.3-mg conjugated estrogen (Premarin) pill. Patients with normal height can receive up to 0.625 mg/day of conjugated estrogen or 0.1 mg of estradiol via transdermal patch. High doses of estrogen and premature introduction of progesterone should be avoided early to avoid abnormal breast development (increased subareolar breast tissue and abnormal contours).

A typical maintenance schedule includes 0.625 to 1.25 mg/day of conjugated estrogens days 1 through 25 each month or twice weekly estrogen patch application at 0.1 mg of estradiol, with 10 mg of medroxyprogesterone acetate (Provera) on days 12 through 25. Schedule can be repeated the first of each month. The dose of estrogen may range from 0.625 to 2.5 mg/day, depending on the individual and the estrogen response (usually does not exceed 1.25 mg/day of conjugated estrogens).

Pituitary Defect. Hormonal therapy, as outlined.

Genetic Abnormalities Leading to Gonadal Defects. Hormonal therapy, as outlined. If a Y chromosome is present in an XX-karyotyped individual, gonadal removal is necessary owing to the risk of gonadoblastoma.

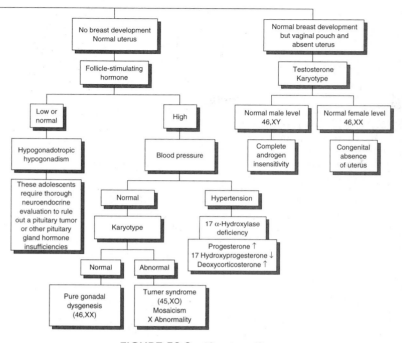

FIGURE 52.2 (*Continued*)

Enzyme Defects. For 17α-hydroxylase deficiency, both glucocorticoid and estrogen–progestin replacement are needed. For 17,20-lyase deficiency, prescribe estrogen-progestin replacement; remove gonads if Y chromosome is present.

Androgen Insensitivity
1. Gonadal removal: intra-abdominal gonads containing a Y chromosome have a high potential for malignancy and should be removed.
2. Maintenance estrogen therapy is needed.
3. The adolescent may require vaginoplasty for normal sexual function.
4. The adolescent should be informed that she cannot become pregnant.
5. Counseling: The adolescent should be informed that she has an abnormal sex chromosome and may require counseling regarding her identity, infertility, and sexual function.

Congenital Absence of the Uterus. Because these adolescents have normally functioning ovaries, they do not require hormonal replacement therapy. They may require a vaginoplasty for normal sexual function and an MRI or intravenous pyelogram to rule out renal anomalies. These adolescents cannot become pregnant; thus, they may require support and counseling.

Primary and Secondary Amenorrhea with Normal Secondary Sex Characteristics

1. PCOS
   a. Medroxyprogesterone acetate (10 mg) should be given for 10 days every 1 to 2 months to induce withdrawal bleeding, or estrogen and progestins can be given as oral contraceptive pills or patches with or without spironolactone.
   b. Insulin-sensitizing agents should be considered, particularly in adolescents with hyperinsulinism.
2. Hypothalamic-pituitary dysfunction
   a. Alleviate known precipitating causes
   b. Hormonal therapy with progestins to induce uterine bleeding every 1 to 2 months
3. Hypothalamic-pituitary failure
   a. The cause must be evaluated and corrected if possible.
   b. Replacement therapy with cyclic conjugated estrogens and progestins
4. Ovarian failure
   a. Cyclic estrogen/progestin therapy
   b. These adolescents are generally infertile and should be counseled accordingly.
5. Uterine synechiae: refer to a gynecologist

Amenorrhea Associated with Weight Loss

In young women with amenorrhea associated with weight loss, bone loss can occur. Treatment to prevent loss of bone mineral density or promote bone accretion should start after 6 months of amenorrhea. The efficacy of estrogen replacement therapy in this setting is controversial.

Female Athlete Triad

1. Regular menses and fertility should return with decreased activity.
2. Calcium intake should be increased to 1,500 mg/day.
3. Estrogen/progestin replacement therapy should be considered if estrogen levels are low.

POLYCYSTIC OVARY SYNDROME

PCOS is a disorder of hypothalamic–pituitary–ovarian axis giving rise to temporary or persistent anovulation and androgen excess. Key features include clinical or biochemical hyperandrogenism, menstrual dysfunction, and exclusion of congenital adrenal hyperplasia (CAH).

Etiology

Endocrine Findings. Menstrual irregularities including amenorrhea, oligomenorrhea, or dysfunctional uterine bleeding. Hyperandrogenism can lead to hirsutism, acne, and rarely mild virilization. The changes in gonadotropins and steroid hormones that cause these manifestations include the following:

1. Inappropriate gonadotropin secretion (IGS) characterized by (a) elevated serum LH level (>21 mIU/mL); (b) normal or low FSH level; (c) exaggerated response of LH, not FSH, to GnRH; (d) LH:FSH ratio often >3; (e) elevated bioactive LH

2. *Steroid hormones*
   a. Estrone (E_1): significantly elevated serum levels
   b. E_2: reference-range level of total E_2, but elevated unbound or free
   c. Androstenedione and dehydroepiandrosterone sulfate (DHEAS): elevated
   d. Testosterone: often minimally elevated total, with elevated free (unbound) testosterone
3. *Source of excess androgens:* May be secreted by ovaries, adrenals, or both in women with a primary diagnosis of PCOS.

Pathophysiology

Factors leading to the development of PCOS:

1. Insulin resistance
2. Increased ovarian androgen levels cause follicular atresia, impairing E_2 production.
3. The E_1 levels are elevated due to increased conversion of androstenedione to E_1 in adipose cells, which leads to suppression of FSH and tonic stimulation of LH, which further aggravate theca cell stimulation.
4. The combination of theca cell hyperplasia and arrested follicular maturation constitutes the typical histological features of PCOS.
5. Possible genetic factor

   Valproate can also induce menstrual disturbances, polycystic ovaries, and hyperandrogenism.

Clinical Consequences

1. Anovulation
2. Polycystic ovaries: A sign but not a disease entity.
3. Hyperandrogenism/hirsutism: Primarily ovarian in origin although adrenal androgens may contribute. The development of hirsutism depends on the concentration of androgens in the blood and sensitivity of hair follicles.
4. Obesity: About 40% to 50% of women with PCOS are obese.
5. Infertility: Increased risk due to anovulation.
6. Cancer risk: Increased risk for endometrial and potentially breast cancer.
7. Elevated lipoprotein profile: Abnormalities include elevated levels of cholesterol, triglycerides, and LDL-C, HDL-C, and apolipoprotein A-I.
8. Insulin resistance and hyperinsulinemia: Approximately 50% are insulin resistant.
9. Impaired glucose tolerance and diabetes: Increased risk for insulin resistance, impaired glucose tolerance and overt type 2 diabetes mellitus.
10. Cardiovascular disease: May be at long-term risk for increased cardiovascular disease.

Differential Diagnosis

1. Familial hirsutism and/or increased sensitivity to androgens
2. Androgen-producing ovarian or adrenal tumors
3. Cushing syndrome: Usually excluded by history and physical examination and, if needed, a 24-hour urine collection for free cortisol and an overnight dexamethasone suppression test.
4. CAH: A mild 21-hydroxylase deficiency can mimic PCOS. The diagnosis of CAH is based on elevated serum 17-hydroxyprogesterone level, particularly after a 0.25-mg single-dose injection of adrenocorticotropic hormone.

5. Stromal hyperthecosis: Probably represents a disorder related to PCOS. However, in this disorder, the testosterone levels are higher and may be as high as those in patients with androgen-producing tumors.

Diagnosis

Criteria include:

1. Irregular menses
2. Hyperandrogenism with or without skin manifestations: Serum testosterone level is the best marker for ovarian causes of hyperandrogenism and DHEAS, most helpful for adrenal sources.
3. Absence of other androgen disorders (adrenal hyperplasia or tumor).

The following are not needed for diagnosis but are supportive evidence:

1. Polycystic ovaries on ultrasonography
2. Increased body weight: BMI >30 kg/m^2 in adults or >85th percentile in children
3. Elevated LH and FSH levels
4. Prolactin: usually normal, but 20% have mildly elevated levels

Therapy

Hirsutism (see Chapter 58)

Menstrual Irregularities. With amenorrhea or oligomenorrhea, give medroxyprogesterone acetate (Provera) (10 mg daily for 10 days every 6 to 12 weeks) for withdrawal bleeding. However, the monthly use of medroxyprogesterone acetate has no significant effect on ovarian androgen production; it is not helpful if hirsutism is present. Oral contraceptive therapy helps to regulate menses.

Obesity. A major focus of preventive health care for women with PCOS.

Metabolic Changes. Because of the potential for abnormal glucose tolerance and hyperlipidemia, it can be important to measure these parameters. Many clinicians favor treatment of insulin resistance in women with PCOS. Studies have shown that the use of metformin in adolescents with PCOS may regulate menstrual cycling and reduce clinical hyperandrogenism and may also prevent the development of PCOS in girls with premature adrenarche. Adolescents and young women with PCOS should have their cholesterol, triglycerides, and both LDL-C and HDL-C measured. These patients should also be followed for impaired glucose tolerance and diabetes.

WEB SITES

http://www.youngwomenshealth.org/. Children's Hospital Boston Adolescent and Young Adult Program Web site

http://www.goaskalice.columbia.edu/0814.html. "Go Ask Alice" site for missed periods.

http://www.turner-syndrome-us.org. The Turner's Syndrome Society of the United States.

http://www.pcosupport.org/. The PCOS Association's Web site

http://www.obgyn.net/pcos/pcos.asp. PCOS Pavilion.

CHAPTER 53

Pelvic Masses

Paula J. Adams Hillard

CONGENITAL ANOMALIES

Anatomic genital anomalies are rare, but can have profound implications for future reproductive capability. The diagnosis can be suggested on the basis of a pelvic ultrasound. If a developmental anomaly is suspected, MRI is the best imaging technique, although laparoscopy may be required.

Women with uterovaginal agenesis—Mayer-Rokitansky-Kuster-Hauser syndrome—may have uterine remnants that contain functioning endometrium that cause pain and a mass, diagnosed by ultrasound or MRI.

Another class of anatomic congenital anomalies that can create pelvic masses arises from remnants of the mesonephric/müllerian duct system or mesovarium. Paraovarian cysts or paratubal and Gartner duct cysts are examples. These lesions are rarely symptomatic; however, torsion can occur, and they may be confused with neoplasms.

PREGNANCY PRESENTING AS PELVIC MASS

The possibility of an intrauterine or ectopic pregnancy must be considered in the differential diagnosis of every young woman with an adnexal mass and secondary sexual characteristics. A urine pregnancy test can reliably rule out pregnancy.

INFECTION AS A CAUSE OF A PELVIC MASS

As rates of sexually transmitted diseases (STDs) have increased, the incidence of upper tract involvement—with salpingitis or pelvic abscess—has also increased. After resolution of the acute infection, hydrosalpinges can form. Treated pelvic abscesses may also cause palpable masses from adhesions. An appendiceal abscess should also be considered.

ADNEXAL TORSION

Adnexal torsion involves the acute rotation of adnexal structures. Intense pelvic pain is seen, which may be accompanied by nausea and vomiting.

Findings on examination include peritoneal signs with rebound tenderness. Typical findings on ultrasound with Doppler flow studies include the presence of a mass, edema, adnexal asymmetry, and absent venous and/or arterial flow. Consultation with a gynecologist is essential.

UTERINE NEOPLASMS

In adolescents, uterine neoplasms are rare. Leiomyomas (fibroids) develop within the wall of the uterus (intramural myomas) and later extend toward the endometrium (submucosal myomas) or toward the external surface of the myometrium (subserosal myomas).

BENIGN OVARIAN MASSES

Benign ovarian masses (Table 53.1) include functional ovarian cysts, endometriomas, and benign ovarian neoplasms. In an adolescent or prepubertal child, every effort must be made to preserve fertility.

Physiologic (Functional) Ovarian Cysts

Functional ovarian cysts are benign and usually do not cause symptoms or require surgery. Functional cysts result from expansion of the cavity of a pre-ovulatory follicle (follicular cyst) or corpus luteum (corpus luteum cysts), and are associated with the disordered function of the pituitary–ovarian axis.

TABLE 53.1

Benign Ovarian Tumors

Functional
   Follicular
   Corpus luteum
   Theca lutein
Inflammatory
   Tuboovarian abscess or complex
Neoplastic
   Germ cell
   Benign cystic teratoma
   Other and mixed
Epithelial
   Serous cystadenoma
   Mucinous cystadenoma
   Fibroma
   Cystadenofibroma
   Brenner tumor
   Mixed tumor
Other
   Endometrioma

Follicular Cysts. Follicular cysts do not usually cause symptoms, and may be an incidental finding. Torsion or rupture may occasionally occur. In general, conservative management of cysts <8 cm in a premenopausal woman is recommended for up to 8 weeks. Persistent masses should prompt referral for possible surgical excision.

Corpus Luteum (CL) Cysts. CLCs are less common than follicular cysts, but are more significant because they can be associated with acute pain or rupture, leading to hemoperitoneum. Patients presenting with pain and an adnexal mass may require gynecologic consultation to differentiate an unruptured corpus luteum cyst, which should be managed medically, from a mass with an acute surgical emergency. Oral contraceptives reduce the risk of CL cysts and follicular cysts in a dose-dependent fashion. Depot medroxyprogesterone acetate (DMPA) also reduces the risk of functional ovarian cyst formation.

Polycystic Ovary Syndrome. Polycystic ovary syndrome (PCOS) is common among adolescents. Diagnostic criteria, include two of three of the following: (a) oligo- or anovulation; (b) clinical or biochemical evidence of hyperandrogenism; and (c) polycystic ovaries by ultrasound along with the exclusion of other causes of hyperandrogenism. The volume of the ovary may be increased. The lifelong metabolic implications of the condition should prompt management with lifestyle modification, oral contraceptives, and/or insulin-sensitizing agents.

Endometriomas and Endometriosis

The presenting symptoms of endometriosis include worsening dysmenorrhea, premenstrual or acyclic pelvic pain, and dyspareunia. On pelvic examination, findings of tenderness, particularly in the cul-de-sac posterior to the uterus, diminished uterine motility, cervical motion tenderness, and possibly an ovarian mass (endometrioma) are suggestive. Referral to gynecologist for laparoscopy is indicated for adolescents with pelvic pain or dysmenorrhea unresponsive to nonsteroidal anti-inflammatory drugs (NSAIDs) and oral contraceptives.

Benign Ovarian Neoplasms

Ultrasonographic characteristics of the mass dictate management. Adolescents with persistent cystic masses following 6 to 8 weeks of observation may have an ovarian neoplasm and should be referred to a gynecologist. Because benign cystic teratomas (dermoid cysts) are the most common ovarian neoplasm in adolescents, these adolescents should also be referred, along with those with solid masses of any size.

Benign Germ Cell Tumors. Benign cystic teratomas (dermoid cysts) are the most common benign ovarian neoplasm of adolescence. On examination, they are unilateral, mobile, anteriorly positioned, nontender adnexal masses and usually asymptomatic. The risk of torsion is approximately 15%, and it occurs more frequently than with ovarian tumors in general. An ovarian cystectomy is almost always possible, even if it appears that only a small amount of ovarian tissue remains. Adolescents with ultrasonography suggesting a dermoid should be referred to a gynecologist.

Benign Epithelial Neoplasia. Serous or mucinous cystadenomas comprise 10% to 20% of benign ovarian neoplasms during adolescence. These tumors are multiloculated, fluid-filled cystic masses. Surgical removal is necessary.

Sex Cord–Stromal Tumors. These tumors account for 10% to 20% of childhood ovarian tumors and may be hormonally active. Granulosa cell tumors and theca cell tumors produce estrogen while Sertoli-Leydig cell tumors produce androgens, with or without estrogen. Associated signs of acne, virilization, menstrual abnormalities, etc., should prompt diagnostic pelvic imaging. Pure granulosa cell tumors are highly malignant, while mixed tumors behave less aggressively.

MALIGNANT OVARIAN MASSES

Ovarian cancer is rare in adolescents and younger girls. Efforts to preserve fertility are important to consider in the management of ovarian malignancies in adolescents.

Malignant Germ Cell Tumors

In women <20 years, one half to two thirds of all ovarian tumors are of germ cell origin and one third of those tumors are malignant. Malignant germ cell tumors include dysgerminoma, mixed germ cell tumor, endodermal sinus tumor, immature teratoma, embryonal tumor, choriocarcinoma, and polyembryoma. Levels of serum tumor markers—including alpha-fetoprotein (AFP), human chorionic gonadotropin (hCG), carcinoembryonic antigen (CEA), and lactate dehydrogenase (LDH)—can be helpful in making a diagnosis and in following malignant tumors for recurrence and clinical response. Measurement of estradiol and testosterone levels can also be helpful.

Dysgerminomas. These comprise 50% of all ovarian germ cell malignancies. Some 5% to 10% of these tumors occur in phenotypically female patients with gonadal dysgenesis. The presence of a Y chromosome or antigen is associated with a high risk of malignancy; thus bilateral gonadectomy is recommended.

Immature Teratomas. About half of pure immature teratomas occur in adolescents. The amount of immature neural tissue is predictive of lethality.

Endodermal Sinus Tumors. Also known as "yolk sac tumors" of the ovary, these are rare.

Malignant Epithelial Tumors

These tumor types rarely develop in adolescents. Included in this group are serous cystadenocarcinoma, mucinous cystadenocarcinoma, and endometrial cystadenocarcinoma. In adolescents, about 7% of epithelial tumors will be borderline malignancies, which can be managed with conservative surgery and appropriate staging procedures. Less than 5% of ovarian epithelial tumors in adolescents are invasive. These patients require management by a gynecologic oncologist.

Other Carcinomas
In young women, the more common metastatic lesions to the ovary include lymphomas and leukemias.

Genetic Risk of Epithelial Ovarian Cancers
Approximately 5% of ovarian cancer before age 70 years is associated with mutations in the breast cancer gene-1 (BRCA-1). Families with multiple individuals with breast and or ovarian cancer should be offered referral to specific familial cancer centers.

Minimizing the Risks of Ovarian Masses and Malignancies
Oral contraceptive pills minimize the risks of functional ovarian masses in a dose-dependent fashion. Ultra-low-dose estrogen containing oral contraceptive pills may not prevent follicular cysts as well those providing higher estrogen doses.

Adolescents who have had an oophorectomy, an ovarian cystectomy, or an ovarian neoplasm may particularly benefit from the use of oral contraceptive pills to minimize the risks of developing a subsequent functional cyst. Combination oral contraceptives are associated with a 30% to 60% reduction in the risk of epithelial ovarian malignancies.

WEB SITES

http://www.nlm.nih.gov/medlineplus/ency/article/001504.htm. National Institutes of Health site with references and links on ovarian cysts.

http://familydoctor.org/handouts/279.html. American Academy of Family Physicians handout on ovarian cysts.

http://www.4women.gov/faq/ovarian_cysts.pdf. The National Women's Health Information Center. U.S. Department of Health and Human Services, Office on Women's Health

http://www.goaskalice.columbia.edu/0724.html. "Go Ask Alice" information on ovarian cysts from the Columbia University Student Health Center.

CHAPTER 54

Pap Smears and Abnormal Cervical Cytology

Anna-Barbara Moscicki

Approximately 3% to 14% of women <19 years have abnormal cervical cytology, most being low-grade squamous intraepithelial lesions (LSIL). This is consistent with the high rates of human papillomavirus (HPV) infection in this age group, ranging from 20% to 57%, with some 50% of adolescents acquiring an HPV infection within 5 years of starting sexual activity. In a study of 15- to 19-year-olds, 14% of smears were abnormal, with 7% having LSIL and 0.7% having high-grade squamous intraepithelial lesions (HSIL). These differences are important, since LSIL are considered relatively benign, whereas HSIL are considered more important precancerous lesions worthy of treatment. Because of this disproportionate rate between LSIL and HSIL in adolescents, most adolescents with abnormal cytology are unnecessarily referred to colposcopy.

VULNERABILITY OF THE CERVIX TO HPV

The typical histologic cervical changes associated with HPV infections generally occur within the transformation zone (T-zone). Neonates are born with an squamocolumnar junction (SCJ) located on the ectocervix, with a predominance of columar epithelium. Squamous metaplasia is a process whereby undifferentiated columar cells transform themselves into squamous epithelium. This process is relatively quiescent until puberty, resulting in little change to the SCJ during childhood. The area of columnar epithelium seen on the ectocervix is referred to as ectopy.

Transformation Zone (T-Zone). The T-zone is where conversion from the columnar epithelium to squamous epithelium has occurred. The T-zone represents the area between the original SCJ and the current SCJ. By their late 20s and early 30s, most women have had substantial replacement of columnar epithelium, resulting in little to no visible ectopy, with continued squamous metaplasia occurring inside the endocervical canal. The T-zone is the cervical area most prone to development of SILs and invasive squamous cell cancers. This vulnerability is most likely related to the process of squamous metaplasia and its vulnerability to HPV and SIL development. This association reflects the natural life cycle of HPV and its dependence on host cell proliferation and differentiation, both characteristics of squamous metaplasia. Viral replication and viral protein expression result in pathologic features referred to as SIL.

Features that are mild in nature, and restricted to the basal and parabasal areas, are referred to as LSIL. HSIL refers to changes that are more extensive and extend into the upper half of the epithelium.

CERVICAL DYSPLASIA

Impact of Cofactors. HPV infection is the causative factor for cervical SIL. However, because rates of HPV are 4 to 10 times higher than those for SIL and 100 to 700 times higher than those for invasive cancers, it is assumed that HPV is a necessary but, not sufficient precursor to the development of these lesions. In the case of cancer, numerous molecular events most likely are needed. HPV persistence is essential for the development of invasive cancers. An inadequate immune response to HPV is thought to be associated with persistence. Other factors associated with HSIL and cancer development include tobacco exposure, herpes simplex virus, and *Chlamydia trachomatis* infections, multiparity, and a prolonged history of oral contraceptive use.

Cervical Screening Tests. Current recommendations for Pap smear testing include the following: (1) Beginning Pap smear screening within 3 years of becoming sexually active or at age 21 years. (2) After a patient has had three consecutive annual tests whose results are read as normal, she may be screened at 1- to 2-year intervals, depending on risk behavior [i.e. multiple partners, older partners, and high rates of sexually transmitted diseases (STDs)]. Most cytologists in the United States have adopted the Bethesda reporting system (Fig. 54.1), which includes more descriptive reports of their findings. Smear tests that are considered unsatisfactory should be repeated. The follow-up evaluation required for benign Pap smear findings not associated with neoplastic changes is shown in Table 54.1.

Recommendations for abnormal Pap smear changes in adult women include the following:
1. Atypical squamous cells of undetermined significance (ASCUS)
   a. Repeat the Pap smear within 4 to 6 months; if the Pap smear results remain ASCUS or worsen, refer for colposcopy. If the second Pap smear result is normal, another Pap smear should be obtained within 6 months. After two consecutive smears, the patient may return to routine screening. A diagnosis of ASCUS that cannot rule out HSIL should be treated as HSIL.
   b. Alternatively, use the HPV DNA test, which is best performed in the situation of reflex testing. This currently refers to using a liquid cytologic method in which the sample obtained for cytology is also adequate to test for the presence of HPV DNA at a later date. Currently the Hybrid Capture II HPV Test (Digene Diagnostics) is the only FDA-approved commercially available test kit for clinical HPV DNA detection in the United States. ASCUS that are HPV high-risk–positive are referred to colposcopy.
2. LSIL: This category includes evidence of HPV infection, referred to as koilocytosis, and cervical intraepithelial neoplasia I (CIN1) lesions merged together; this is done to reflect the technical difficulties in artificially distinguishing between them and the fact that very few of these lesions have any progressive or oncogenic potential. Currently, it is recommended that all LSIL in adult women (not adolescents/young adults <21 years) be referred for

BETHESDA SYSTEM 2001

SPECIMEN TYPE: *Indicate conventional smear (Pap smear) vs. liquid-based vs. other*

SPECIMEN ADEQUACY
- ❑ Satisfactory for evaluation (*describe presence or absence of endocervical/transformation zone component and any other quality indicators, e.g., partially obscuring blood, inflammation, etc.*)
- ❑ Unsatisfactory for evaluation . . . (*specify reason*)
  - ❑ Specimen rejected/not processed (*specify reason*)
  - ❑ Specimen processed and examined, but unsatisfactory for evaluation of epithelial abnormality because of (*specify reason*)

GENERAL CATEGORIZATION (*optional*)
- ❑ Negative for intraepithelial lesion or malignancy
- ❑ Epithelial cell abnormality: See Interpretation/Result (*specify 'squamous' or 'glandular' as appropriate*)
- ❑ Other: See Interpretation/Result (*e.g., endometrial cells in a woman ≥ 40 years of age*)

AUTOMATED REVIEW
If case examined by automated device, specify device and result.

ANCILLARY TESTING
Provide a brief description of the test methods and report the result so that it is easily understood by the clinician.

INTERPRETATION/RESULT
NEGATIVE FOR INTRAEPITHELIAL LESION OR MALIGNANCY (*when there is no cellular evidence of neoplasia, state this in the General Categorization above and/or in the Interpretation/Result section of the report, whether or not there are organisms or other non-neoplastic findings*)

ORGANISMS:
- ➤ *Trichomonas vaginalis*
- ➤ Fungal organisms morphologically consistent with *Candida* sp
- ➤ Shift in flora suggestive of bacterial vaginosis
- ➤ Bacteria morphologically consistent with *Actinomyces* sp
- ➤ Cellular changes consistent with Herpes simplex virus

OTHER NON-NEOPLASTIC FINDINGS (*Optional to report; list not inclusive*):
- ➤ Reactive cellular changes associated with
  - inflammation (includes typical repair)
  - radiation
  - intrauterine contraceptive device (IUD)
- ➤ Glandular cells status post hysterectomy
- ➤ Atrophy

OTHER
- ➤ Endometrial cells (*in a woman ≥ 40 years of age*)
  (*Specify if 'negative for squamous intraepithelial lesion'*)

FIGURE 54.1 The Bethesda system for reporting cervical or vaginal cytologic diagnoses, 2001. (www.bethesda2001.cancer.gov/terminology.html.)

colposcopy. HPV testing is not recommended in the triage of LSIL. If no CIN 2/3 is found, follow-up cytology at 6 and 12 months OR HR-HPV testing at 12 months is recommended. ASCUS or worse or positive HR-HPV test is criteria for referral for colposcopy. This is based on data showing that HPV testing is more sensitive than cytology; hence the interval can be extended to 12 months.

3. HSIL: This category includes moderate and severe dysplasia, and carcinoma in situ. HSIL require colposcopic evaluation with directed biopsies and endocervical evaluation.

EPITHELIAL CELL ABNORMALITIES
SQUAMOUS CELL
➢ Atypical squamous cells
- of undetermined significance (ASCUS)
- cannot exclude HSIL (ASC-H)
➢ Low grade squamous intraepithelial lesion (LSIL)
encompassing: HPV/mild dysplasia/CIN 1
➢ High grade squamous intraepithelial lesion (HSIL)
encompassing: moderate and severe dysplasia, CIS/CIN 2 and CIN 3
- with features suspicious for invasion (*if invasion is suspected*)
➢ Squamous cell carcinoma

GLANDULAR CELL
➢ Atypical
- endocervical cells (NOS *or specify in comments*)
- endometrial cells (NOS *or specify in comments*)
- glandular cells (NOS *or specify in comments*)
➢ Atypical
- endocervical cells, favor neoplastic
- glandular cells, favor neoplastic
➢ Endocervical adenocarcinoma in situ
➢ Adenocarcinoma
- endocervical
- endometrial
- extrauterine
- not otherwise specified (NOS)

OTHER MALIGNANT NEOPLASMS: (*specify*)

EDUCATIONAL NOTES AND SUGGESTIONS (*optional*)
Suggestions should be concise and consistent with clinical follow-up guidelines published by professional organizations (references to relevant publications may be included).

FIGURE 54.1   (*Continued*)

Special Considerations
Adolescent Patients
Invasive cancer among adolescents is rare, whereas a diagnosis of LSIL is at its highest in this age group. The common nature of LSIL in adolescents is not surprising, given the high rate of HPV infections in teens. Fortunately, both these conditions are mostly transient in this age group, with more than 90% of HPV infections and LSIL showing regression in adolescents and young women within 3 years. Triage for ASCUS and LSIL differs for adolescents (defined as <21 years of age) as compared with that in adult women. The following are recommendations by the American Society for Colposcopy and Cervical Pathology, but they are always subject to the latest consensus recommendations available at their web site: www.asccp.org/consensus.shtml. Note that extensive algorithms for management are available at this site.

1. *HPV testing in triage or follow-up for ASCUS or LSIL is not recommended in this age group.* Detection of HPV in adolescents is reflective of a transient infection, whereas in adult women, HPV detection more likely reflects a persistent infection, which is a strong risk for HSIL development. Data support the use of HPV in triage for ASCUS in adult women and its use in primary screening in women 30 years of age or older, but not in adolescents.
2. *ASCUS and LSIL are both treated with identical follow-up strategies, which include annual cytology alone for up to 2 years.* It is recommended that adolescents with ASCUS/LSIL can be followed up with repeat cytology at 12-month intervals for 2 years without immediate referral for colposcopy. At the

TABLE 54.1

Follow-up Evaluation Recommendations for Abnormal Pap Smear Findings

Pap Smear Finding	Recommendation
Insufficient quantity	Repeat Pap smears in 2–3 mo
Poor specimen	Repeat Pap smears in 2–3 mo
Air-drying artifact	Repeat Pap smears in 2–3 mo
No endocervical cells	No need to repeat Pap smear if patient has had normal test results previously and is in compliant with therapy; if not, repeat in 2–3 mo
Endometrial cells	Normal if near menses or while using oral contraceptives or intrauterine devices; otherwise, recall and evaluate endometrium
Trichomoniasis	Recall patient, perform STD evaluations
Yeast	Review chart; if no symptoms, no need to follow-up
Inflammation	Consider recent coitus, infection
Reactive, reparative changes	Identify irritant, if possible; essentially normal

12-month follow-up, only adolescents with HSIL or greater on the repeat cytology should be referred to colposcopy. At the 24-month follow-up, those with an ASCUS or greater result should be referred to colposcopy.

HIV Infected and Other Immunosuppressed Patients
Because of the high rate of progression to HSIL, it is currently recommended to refer all HIV-infected adolescents with any SIL (LSIL or HSIL) and ASCUS suggestive of HSIL to colposcopy. In patients with ASCUS alone, pap smear for cytology can be repeated in 4–6 months. If ASCUS or greater is found on repeat cytology, referral to colposcopy is warranted. HPV testing is not recommended in either triaging these individuals or in follow-up.

Triage and Therapy for Cervical Intra-epithelial Neoplasia
The colposcopically directed biopsy and the endocervical test results determine the extent of the lesion and direct therapy. The principle in developing a treatment plan is that cervical dysplasia, specifically HSIL, is treated to prevent progression to cancer. One inappropriate practice to avoid, particularly in adolescents and young women, is to combine the diagnostic and treatment steps by performing colposcopic examination to rule out invasion and excising the T-zone by a loop electrocautery excision procedure (LEEP) without biopsy confirmation. Each of the major treatment modalities has minimal adverse impacts when used once (Table 54.2). Because recurrent lesions may develop and require further treatment, the cumulative effects of multiple treatments (particularly LEEP) must be considered. Screening for STDs before cryotherapy or LEEP is recommended to avoid the complications of PID. Additionally, the following is recommended:

TABLE 54.2

Cervical Dysplasia Treatment Regimen Response Rates

	Cryotherapy	LEEP
Response rate		
Single (%)	80	95
Repeated (%)	95	95
Advantages	Simple office-based procedure	SCJ on ectocervix
	Inexpensive	Can tailor to lesion
	Only mildly painful	Provides specimen for pathology
Disadvantages	Watery vaginal discharge for 4–6 wk	Expensive
		More painful
	May not be as effective for large lesions or those that extend well onto the ectocervix	Bleeding complications
		Premature rupture of membrane in future
	New SCJ on endocervix	
	No specimen for pathology	
	Stenosis	

LEEP, loop electrocautery excision procedure; SCJ, squamocolumnar junction.

Adults

1. If the biopsy reveals CIN 1 and is preceded by a ASCUS/HR-HPV or LSIL, follow-up with repeat cytology at 6 and 12 months or high risk HPV DNA testing at 12 months is recommended. Women with ASCUS or greater or positive HPV-HR should be referred back to colposcopy. If CIN 1 is persistent at two years, provider may continue observation or treat (see Table 54.2). Excisional methods are preferred if colposcopy is unsatisfactory or the ECC is positive or the patient was treated before. A cone biopsy using traditional cold-knife procedures is an alternative method for the treatment of endocervical canal disease. Complications after cone biopsy are common, so cold-knife cone biopsies in adolescents and young women are rarely recommended.

2. If the biopsy reveals CIN 1 and is preceded by HSIL or AGC-NOS. management includes diagnostic excisional procedure, observation with colposcopy and cytology at 6 month intervals for one year or review cytology and biopsies. If a change in diagnosis, manage per ASCCP guidelines. If HSIL is found at the 6 or 12 month cytology in the observation arm, a diagnostic excisional procedure is recommended.

3. If the biopsy reveals CIN 2,3, excision or ablation are recommended, if the colposcopy is satisfactory. If the colposcopy is unsatisfactory, a diagnostic excisional procedure is recommended. Follow-up post treatment can include either cytology at 6 month intervals, cytology and colposcopy at 6 month intervals or HPV DNA testing at 12 months. ASCUS or greater or + HPV-HR are indications for referral. After two negative cytology and normal colposcopy

examinations, or after a negative HPV test at 12 months, the woman may go back to routine screening. Response rates are listed in Table 54.2.

Adolescents and Young Women

1. Adolescents with CIN 1 preceded by ASCUS or LSIL, should have repeat cytology at 12 month intervals. If repeat cytology shows HSIL at any follow-up visit, repeat colposcopy is indicated. If at two years, ASCUS or LSIL are found to persist, repeat colposcopy is indicated. If colposcopy is unsatisfactory and ECC is benign or CIN 1, observation is still recommended.
2. Adolescents and young women with CIN 2,3 and satisfactory colposcopy can be managed by observation or treatment using excision or ablation. Observation is with colposcopy and cytology at 6 month intervals for up to 24 months. If colposcopy worsens or high grade cytology or colposcopy persists at 1 year, repeat biopsy recommended. If CIN 3 at any time, or CIN 2, 3 that persists at 24 months, treatment is recommended. If the examination is unsatisfactory, excisional treatment is recommended.
Note: Young woman is defined as a woman for whom the risks of pregnancy complications from treatment outweigh the risks of progression to cancer from observation. These recommendations are based on the observation that most young women do not experience progression to cancer during this age group and that excisional therapies may result in complications such as preterm labor. The decision should be carefully weighed between the patient and the provider.

All women with dysplasia who smoke should be encouraged to stop smoking as continued tobacco use increases susceptibility to cancer. Condom use has been shown to enhance LSIL regression, so condom use should be encouraged.

It is currently not recommended to screen male partners of women with CIN for HPV infections as few studies have demonstrated HPV disease in this group.

HIV Infected and Immunosuppresed Patients

Treatment for CIN should follow the same guidelines as outlined for adults and adolescents without HIV infections or immunosuppression.

WEB SITES

http://www.ashastd.org. American Social Health Association: Learn about STDs/ HPV.

http://www.youngwomenshealth.org/abpap.html. Center for Young Women's Health: information sheet for teens on abnormal Pap smears.

http://www.nccc-online.org/. National Cervical Cancer Coalition site.

http://www.4woman.gov/faq/pap.htm. National Women's Health Information Center: frequently asked questions sheet.

http://www.asccp.org. American Society for Colposcopy and Cervical Pathology: patient education.

http://www.asct.com. American Society for Cytotechnologists.

http://www.ascp.org. American Society of Clinical Pathologists.

http://www.bethesda2001.cancer.gov/terminology.html. Bethesda 2001 classifications.

CHAPTER 55

Vaginitis and Vaginosis

Loris Y. Hwang and Mary-Ann Shafer

Vulvovaginitis in Prepubertal Females

Most vulvovaginitis in this group is related to poor hygiene, tight clothing, or nonabsorbent underpants. Patients should be counseled regarding hygienic measures, and antibiotics should be prescribed only if a predominant organism is identified by culture. Any sexually transmitted disease (STD) should prompt an investigation for sexual abuse.

Vulvovaginitis and Vaginosis in Pubertal and Postpubertal Females: General Approach

Prevalence

The most common types of vaginitis are vulvovaginal candidiasis (VVC) (20% to 25%), trichomoniasis (15% to 20%), and bacterial vaginosis (BV) (40% to 45%). BV is not a true "vaginitis," as it does not cause major inflammation of the vaginal mucosa, but it is included here from a clinical standpoint.

Evaluation

1. *History:* should include type, duration, and extent of symptoms (i.e., discharge, pruritus, odor, dyspareunia, dysuria, rash, pain); relation of symptoms to menses; frequency, type, and number of sexual partners; previous STDs; contraceptive history; medications, especially antibiotics and steroids; use of deodorants, soaps, lubricants, or douches; history of immunosuppression; and history of exercise and stress.
2. *Examination:* should include inspection of color, texture, origin (vaginal or cervical), adherence, and odor of the vaginal discharge; inspection of the perineum, vulva, vagina, and cervix for erythema, swelling, lesions, atrophy, trauma, and foreign bodies; palpation of the introitus, uterus, and adnexa for tenderness or masses.
3. *Laboratory:* The pH value of vaginal secretions is sampled from the anterior vaginal fornix or lateral vaginal wall. A saline wet mount is prepared by placing a drop of saline on a glass slide, and then the swab of vaginal discharge is applied to the saline area. Alternatively, the swab is placed in a test tube together with 0.5 to 1 mL of saline, and then the suspension is swabbed onto the slide. Under dry high power, normal findings include <5 to 10 WBCs per high-power field or ≤1 WBC per epithelial cell, as well as lactobacilli. Abnormal findings include presence of "clue cells," defined as epithelial cells

covered with bacteria, and demonstrating indistinct borders and intracellular debris, as well as trichomonads. Motility of trichomonads decreases with time; thus immediate inspection is advised. A potassium hydroxide (KOH) slide is prepared similarly, but with an added drop of KOH 10% solution. An immediate fishy, amine odor is called a positive "whiff test." Under dry high power, abnormal findings are yeast buds and pseudohyphae. In women with discharge, testing for *Chlamydia trachomatis* and *Neisseria gonorrhoeae* is advised. Urinalysis, urine culture, and pregnancy test are performed as indicated.

Vulvovaginal Candidiasis
Etiology
VVC is caused by *Candida albicans* (85% to 90% of clinical cases) and occasionally by other *Candida* species, *Torulopsis* species, or other yeasts.

Clinical Manifestations
1. Patients may experience nonspecific symptoms of intense burning, vulvar pruritus, erythema, external dysuria, dyspareunia, and discharge. The discharge may worsen before menses and classically appears white, odorless, and "cottage cheese–like."
2. Examination may reveal the classic discharge and erythematous vulva with fissures, excoriations, edema, and satellite lesions.

Diagnosis
1. Diagnosis is supported by wet prep or KOH findings of yeast buds and pseudohyphae (sensitivity 40% to 80%) and a normal pH of <4.5. Cultures are not used for routine diagnosis.
2. VVC is further classified as "uncomplicated," defined as infrequent episodes with mild-to-moderate symptoms due to *C. albicans* in nonimmunocompromised women; or "complicated," defined as recurrent VVC consisting of four or more episodes in 12 months, or severe symptoms, or due to non-*albicans* species, or in immunocompromised pregnant women.

Therapy
1. Uncomplicated cases in nonpregnant patients are effectively treated by short-course topical formulations. Asymptomatic women do not need treatment. Topical azoles (80% to 95% cure) are more effective than nystatin (70% to 90% cure). Available regimens are butoconazole 2% cream 5 g intravaginally for 3 days; butoconazole 2% cream sustained-release, single intravaginal application; clotrimazole 1% cream 5 g intravaginally for 7 to 14 days; clotrimazole 100-mg vaginal tablet once a day for 7 days or two tablets a day for 3 days; miconazole 2% cream 5 g intravaginally for 7 days; miconazole 200-mg vaginal suppository once a day for 3 days; miconazole 100-mg vaginal suppository once a day for 7 days; miconazole 1,200 mg vaginal suppository single dose; nystatin 100,000-unit vaginal tablet for 14 days; tioconazole 6.5% ointment 5 g intravaginally in a single application; terconazole 0.4% cream 5 g intravaginally for 7 days; terconazole 0.8% cream 5 g intravaginally for 3 days; terconazole 80-mg suppository once a day for 3 days.
2. Some patients may prefer a single-dose oral agent, such as the fluconazole 150-mg oral tablet.

3. *Counseling:* The creams and suppositories listed here are oil-based and may weaken a latex condom or diaphragm. Partners are not routinely treated unless the male partner has symptoms and signs of balanitis. Follow-up is not necessary unless symptoms persist.
4. *Pregnancy:* Topical azole medications (preferably 7-day) can be used, but not oral agents.
5. *Severe VVC or immunocompromised host:* treatment with either 7 to 14 days of topical azoles or fluconazole 150 mg once and then again in 3 days is advised.
6. HIV-infected women may receive the same regimens as non-HIV-infected women.
7. Recurrent VVC (four or more episodes per year) is seen in <5% of women. Predisposing factors should be reduced and vaginal cultures obtained. For recurrent *C. albicans* VVC, prescribe the routine short courses above or 7 to 14 days of topical treatment or fluconazole 100 mg or 150 mg or 200 mg oral tablet once every 3 days for three total doses. For non-*albicans Candida* species, prescribe boric acid 600 mg oral gelatin capsule once daily for 14 days or flucytosine vaginal cream 5 g once nightly. A maintenance regimen may help: one fluconazole 150-mg oral tablet each week for 6 months, one clotrimazole 500-mg vaginal tablet each week for 6 months, one itraconazole 400-mg oral tablet once monthly, one 100 mg oral tablet once daily for 6 months, flucytosine vaginal cream 5 g once nightly for 6 to 8 weeks, or one ketoconazole 100-mg oral tablet once daily for 6 months. Oral ketoconazole requires monitoring for hepatotoxicity. Partner treatment has not been helpful. HIV testing can be considered if other HIV risk factors are present.

Trichomoniasis
Etiology
Trichomonas vaginalis infection of the vaginal epithelium is caused by a protozoan with four anterior flagella and one posterior flagellum.

Clinical Manifestations
1. Up to 25% to 50% of females are asymptomatic. Nonspecific symptoms include pruritus, dysuria, dyspareunia, lower abdominal pain, and postcoital bleeding. Discharge is seen in 50% of cases, and is classically diffuse, frothy, yellow or green, and occasionally (10%) malodorous.
2. Examination may reveal edema and excoriation of the external genitalia; frothy, foul-smelling vaginal discharge; erythematous, edematous, and granular vaginal walls; bartholinitis; and, rarely, pelvic inflammatory disease (PID). Cervicitis ("strawberry cervix") consists of erosions or petechiae of the cervix and is seen in only 2% of cases.

Diagnosis
1. Wet prep and KOH are the most available diagnostic tools, but sensitivity is 60% to 70% at best. Trichomonads appear as flagellated pear-shaped motile organisms similar in size to polymorphonuclear leukocytes. The whiff test is often positive and vaginal pH is >4.5. Cultures are less readily available, but traditionally considered as the "gold standard."
2. The FDA has approved two rapid methods, the OSOM Trichomonas Rapid Test and the Affirm VP III. Sensitivity is >83% and specificity >97% compared to culture. However, false positives occur in low-prevalence populations.

Polymerase chain reaction (PCR) tests demonstrate very high sensitivity and specificity, but have not been FDA-approved. Also, urine sediments can show trichomonads and can be useful in males.

Therapy

1. Nonpregnant patients should receive metronidazole 2 g orally in a single dose or tinidazole 2 g orally in a single dose. The alternative regimen is metronidazole 500-mg tablet twice a day for 7 days. Patients allergic to nitroimidazoles should receive desensitization, since no other medication classes are effective.
2. *Counseling:* Oral metronidazole can cause nausea, vomiting, and a metallic taste. Owing to disulfiramlike effects, alcohol should be avoided until 24 hours after medication completion. All partners should routinely be treated, with abstinence from sexual activity until symptoms are resolved.
3. For treatment failure, metronidazole 500 mg oral is given twice daily for 7 days. For persistent failure, metronidazole 2 g oral is given daily for 3 to 5 days. Suspected medication resistance should be reported to the Centers for Disease Control for further management.
4. *Pregnancy:* metronidazole 2-g oral single dose is recommended.
5. HIV-infected patients may receive the same regimens as non-HIV infected women.

Bacterial Vaginosis (BV)

Etiology

BV is a syndrome characterized by the presence of diverse bacteria. Vaginal lactobacilli are replaced by *Gardnerella vaginalis*, anaerobic bacteria (i.e., *Bacteroides* sp., *Mobiluncus* sp.), and *Mycoplasma hominis*, resulting in a higher pH level.

Clinical Manifestations

1. Up to 50% of cases are asymptomatic. Symptoms include vaginal pruritus and discharge, more noticeable after intercourse or after menses. The discharge is classically homogeneous, thin, and grayish-white, with a "fishy" odor. Recent evidence is linking BV to serious sequelae such as pelvic inflammatory disease (PID), increased HIV acquisition and transmission, and infertility. Obstetric complications include chorioamnionitis, premature rupture of membranes, preterm labor, postpartum endometritis, and postabortal infection.
2. Examination may reveal the typical discharge and odor.

Diagnosis

1. Variations of the Amsel criteria are used for clinical diagnosis. *Three* of the four clinical symptoms and signs are required: (1) homogeneous, grayish white discharge; (2) vaginal pH level >4.5; (3) positive whiff test; and (4) wet prep showing "clue cells," defined as epithelial cells appearing granular with indistinct cell borders owing to adherence of bacteria and debris between cells, that comprise at least 20% of the epithelial cells.
2. Gram's stain is also sometimes available and is classified according to the Nugent criteria.

Therapy

1. For nonpregnant patients, recommended regimens are metronidazole 500-mg oral tablet twice daily for 7 days, metronidazole 0.75% gel 5 g

TABLE 55.1

Vaginal Discharge in the Adolescent

Condition	Signs and Symptoms	Diagnosis	Treatment
Physiological discharge	Clear gray discharge No offensive odor No burning or itching	Wet prep: Epithelial cells with no or few polymorphonuclear cells; no pathogens	Reassurance and explanation
Vulvovaginal candidiasis (VVC)	Curd-like discharge Intense burning, pruritus Usually no odor Often associated vulvitis	KOH: Budding yeast and pseudohyphae	Numerous acceptable regimens listed in text
Trichomoniasis	Pruritus Malodorous, frothy, yellow-green discharge Dysuria Rarely, abdominal pain	Wet prep: Pear-shaped organism with motile flagella	Metronidazole: 2 g single dose or 500 mg b.i.d. for 7 days Treat and evaluate partner
Bacterial vaginosis	Homogenous, malodorous, gray-white discharge Usually mild or no pruritus or burning	Wet prep: Epithelial cells covered with gram-negative rods Few polymorphonuclear leukocytes pH >4.5	Metronidazole: 500 mg b.i.d. for 7 days, or metronidazole gel 0.75% one applicator b.i.d. for 5 days, or clindamycin cream 2% one applicator (5 g) intravaginally for 7 days Alternative regimens listed in text Evaluate female partners and treat accordingly

(continued)

TABLE 55.1

(Continued)

Condition	Signs and Symptoms	Diagnosis	Treatment
N. gonorrhoeae infection	Majority asymptomatic Gray-white cervical discharge	Culture Gram stain can be used, but a negative smear must be confirmed by culture	Ceftriaxone 125 mg IM once, or cefixime 400 mg once; plus azithromycin 1 g orally once, or doxycycline 100 mg orally b.i.d. for 7 days
C. trachomatis infection	Majority asymptomatic Yellowish cervical discharge Cervicitis	Nucleic acid amplification test or culture Exclusion of other organisms in a girl with cervicitis	Azithromycin 1 g once, or doxycycline 100 mg PO b.i.d. for 7 days
Retained tampon	Malodorous discharge Local discomfort	History and physical examination History of exposure to deodorant spray or scented tampons	Removal of tampon
Irritant vaginitis	Vaginal discharge, erythema	Other agents listed in text	Cessation of irritant agent

intravaginally once daily for 5 days, or clindamycin 2% cream 5 g intravaginally daily for 7 days. Cure rates for all these regimens are 75% to 85%. Side effects of therapy are listed above, under "Trichomoniasis." Also, clindamycin cream may weaken latex condoms. Alternative regimens are clindamycin 300 mg oral tablet twice daily for 7 days or clindamycin ovules 100 g intravaginally daily for 3 days.

2. Asymptomatic women with BV before surgical procedures or other interventions should also be treated. BV treatment has been shown to reduce postabortion PID rates.
3. *Counseling:* Patients should be advised to avoid douching and reduce the number of sex partners. Treatment of male partners is not helpful, but female sex partners should be evaluated for BV. Follow-up is not necessary unless symptoms persist.
4. Recurrent BV occurs in 20% to 30% of cases within 3 months. The etiology is poorly understood, and maintenance regimens are under study.
5. *Pregnancy:* Symptomatic pregnant women in any trimester should be treated with either a metronidazole 500-mg oral tablet twice a day for 7 days, metronidazole 250 mg orally three times daily for 7 days, or clindamycin 300 mg orally twice a day for 7 days. Asymptomatic pregnant women at high risk (i.e., those with history of premature delivery) may be screened during the early second trimester and treated if BV is present, although optimal screening practices are as yet undetermined. Screening of asymptomatic pregnant women at low risk is generally not recommended.
6. HIV-infected women may receive the same regimens as non-HIV-infected women.

Other Causes of Vaginal Discharge

1. *Physiologic discharge:* normal overall increase in vaginal secretions 6 to 12 months before menarche and just before each menses.
2. *Extravaginal lesions:* may cause staining of the underwear and perception of a discharge.
3. *Enterobius vermicularis* (pinworms)
4. *Irritant vaginitis:* related to tampons, pads, douches, deodorants, powders, scented toilet paper, bubble baths, laundry detergents, fabric softeners, swimming pools, spermicides, and others
5. *Foreign bodies:* forgotten tampons and others
6. *Vulvodynia or vulvar vestibulitis*: may cause dyspareunia; topical steroids may help
7. *N. gonorrhoeae* and *C. trachomatis*: described in other chapters

Table 55.1 outlines the treatment of vaginitis in adolescents.

WEB SITES

For Teenagers and Parents
http://kidshealth.org/teen/sexual_health/. Teen-oriented Web site from the Nemours Foundation, including information on STDs and vaginitis.
http://www.health.state.mn.us/divs/idepc/diseases/vaginitis/. Vaginitis information from the Minnesota Department of Health, includes patient handouts in various languages (pdf files).

For Health Professionals

http://www.cdc.gov/std/treatment. Updates from the CDC regarding STDs.

http://www2a.cdc.gov/stdtraining/self-study/default.asp. Self-study modules from the CDC that include vaginitis and STD topics.

CHAPTER 56

Ectopic Pregnancy and Other Complications of Pregnancy

Melissa D. Mirosh and Mary Anne Jamieson

Pregnancy should be a consideration when any adolescent presents with new-onset abnormal vaginal bleeding or abdominal/pelvic pain; ectopic pregnancy should be considered in the differential diagnosis.

Incidence. The risk of ectopic pregnancy in the United States is about 19 per 1,000 pregnancies. From 1991 to 1999, ectopic pregnancies were responsible for 6% of all pregnancy-related deaths in the United States, of which 93% were due to hemorrhage.

Etiology. The most common predisposing factor for adolescents is pelvic inflammatory disease (PID). The resulting salpingitis is responsible for some 45% of initial ectopics. Other tubal pathology associated with ectopic pregnancy includes damage or adhesions from previous pelvic surgery. Current intrauterine contraceptive devices (IUCDs) are no longer considered to increase the absolute risk of ectopic pregnancy. If a patient were to become pregnant with an IUCD in situ, however, the chance that the pregnancy will be outside of the uterus is 15% to 20%. Other factors that increase the risk of ectopic pregnancy include smoking, infertility, in vitro fertilization, and prior ectopic pregnancy (Table 56.1).

Differential Diagnosis. The differential diagnosis of acute abdominal or pelvic pain is best divided into obstetric, gynecologic, and nongynecologic categories:

1. Obstetric
   a. Normal intrauterine pregnancy
   b. Hemorrhagic corpus luteum
   c. Spontaneous or threatened abortion
2. Gynecologic
   a. Ovarian torsion
   b. Hemorrhagic ovarian cyst
   c. Symptomatic or ruptured ovarian cyst
   d. Pelvic inflammatory disease

TABLE 56.1

Risk Factors for Ectopic Pregnancy

	Adjusted OR (95% CI)	*OR (95% CI)*
Previous tubal surgery	4.0 (2.6–6.1)	4.7–21.0
Infertility (risk increases with length of infertility)	2.1–2.7	2.5–21.0
Previous genital infection confirmed	3.4 (2.4–5.0)	2.5–3.7
Previous miscarriage	3.0 (>2)	—
Previous induced abortion	2.8 (1.1–7.2)	—
Past or ever smoker	1.5 (1.1–2.2)	2.5 (1.8–3.4)
Current smoker (risk increases with amount smoked per day)	1.7–3.9	2.3–2.5
Age 40 years and older	2.9 (1.4–6.1)	—
Intrauterine device use (>2 years)	2.9 (1.4–6.3)	4.2–45.0
Previous intrauterine device	2.4 (1.2–4.9)	—
Sterilization[a]	—	9.3 (4.9–18.0)
Previous ectopic pregnancy	—	8.3 (6.0–11.5)
Documented tubal pathology	3.7 (1.2–4.8)	2.5–3.5
More than one sexual partner	—	2.1–2.5
Diethylstilboestrol exposure	—	5.6 (2.4–13.0)

OR, odds ratio; CI, confidence interval.
From Farquhar CM. Ectopic pregnancy. *Lancet* 2005;366(9485):583.

3. Nongynecologic
   a. Appendicitis
   b. Renal colic
   c. Inflammatory bowel disease
   d. Gastroenteritis
   e. Severe constipation

CLINICAL PRESENTATIONS

Acute Presentation: Classic Ruptured Ectopic Pregnancy

The classic triad of vaginal bleeding, delayed menses, and severe lower abdominal pain is associated with tubal rupture and hypovolemic shock; it is now fairly infrequent due to earlier diagnosis.

Symptoms. The patient with an acutely ruptured ectopic pregnancy would typically exhibit (1) pelvic pain and possible referred shoulder pain; (2) dizziness, light-headedness, or loss of consciousness; (3) history of abnormal menses; and (4) symptoms of pregnancy.

Classic Signs of a Ruptured Ectopic. (1) Vital signs: Patient may present with signs of hypovolemia or shock. (2) Abdominal tenderness, ± rebound.

(3) Bimanual exam: Cervical motion tenderness, with or without a pelvic mass.

Laboratory Tests. (1) Pregnancy testing: Urine qualitative (rapid) and serum quantitative β-hCG. (2) The "three Cs of hemorrhage": CBC, crossmatch, and coagulation factors. (3) Ultrasound: Not necessary if the patient is hemodynamically unstable. The ultrasound may show a pelvic mass and/or free fluid in the pelvis.

Therapy. (1) Fluids via one (preferably two) large-bore intravenous line(s). Fluid resuscitation (and blood transfusion if clinically indicated) immediately. (2) Emergency surgery is required: conservative treatment is the goal. (3) Rh status must be confirmed and Rh immunoglobulin given if Rh negative.

Subacute Presentations: Probable Ectopic Pregnancy and Possible Ectopic Pregnancy

An adolescent with a positive pregnancy test who presents with cramping, abnormal vaginal spotting or bleeding, and/or lower abdominal/adnexal pain should be suspected of having an ectopic pregnancy. The workup and treatment depend on the patient's risk factors and her pregnancy intentions.

The initial diagnosis of a suspected ectopic pregnancy in a hemodynamically stable patient begins with a complete history and physical examination, lab work, and transvaginal ultrasound. Last menstrual period can assist in dating the pregnancy, along with the date of the first positive pregnancy test and previous ultrasounds. The lab work should include a CBC (for WBC, Hgb, and hematocrit), group and screen to determine Rh status, and a serum quantitative β-hCG.

Investigations

β-hCG. β-hCG levels will double every 2 days in a normal first-trimester intrauterine gestation. Only 15% of normal pregnancies will fail to have this appropriate increase in β-hCG. Serial β-hCG measurements can be helpful in determining the fate of these pregnancies.

Ultrasound. Ultrasound studies at appropriate β-hCG levels are usually diagnostic and often the definitive method of pregnancy dating in adolescents. The β-hCG cutoff is generally 1,500 to 2,000 IU/L by transvaginal ultrasound. If no intrauterine gestation is seen, an ectopic pregnancy should be suspected. If transabdominal scanning is the only method available, the β-hCG cutoff should be 6,500 IU/L.

Outpatient Follow-up

Using Serial β-hCG Levels. Declining β-hCG levels must be followed until they are undetectable. If the β-hCG levels are increasing by at least 66% every 2 to 3 days, they should be followed until they reach the discriminatory zone for ultrasound. If the teen becomes increasingly symptomatic prior to reaching this zone, laparoscopic investigation may be considered. If the β-hCG levels are declining or rising at an inappropriate rate, the pregnancy (either intrauterine or ectopic) is likely nonviable.

Management. The majority of women diagnosed with an ectopic pregnancy will be treated surgically via laparoscopy or laparotomy. The precise method is up to the discretion of the surgeon. The most common surgical procedures are salpingostomy and salpingectomy. There are no randomized controlled studies that directly compare the two methods. It is not necessary to close the tubal defect after salpingostomy. Occasionally, salpingectomy is the procedure of choice.

Medical Therapy. Methotrexate has become an established method of treatment for patients diagnosed with an unruptured ectopic pregnancy. The main advantage of medical therapy over surgical therapy is that it is less invasive and less expensive.

Factors that predict successful methotrexate therapy include an initial β-hCG <4,000 and lack of fetal cardiac activity. Indicators predictive of failure include a visible extrauterine yolk sac on ultrasound and previous ectopic pregnancy. Patients must be counseled about the possibility of treatment failure, and the associated signs and symptoms.

Expectant Management. Expectant management is reasonable for a certain subset of women presenting with ectopic pregnancy. These patients are asymptomatic and generally have a β-hCG under 1,000 IU/L. They must also be reliable, as losing a patient to follow-up could be disastrous.

Follow-up
Surgical. Resolution of the ectopic pregnancy must be documented by following β-hCG levels until they reach nonpregnant levels. If β-hCG levels plateau or rise postoperatively, persistent disease is presumed.

Nonsurgical. Obviously, women treated with methotrexate or expectant management will require weekly (or more frequent) quantitative β-hCG determinations until the levels become undetectable. Table 56.2 outlines specific guidelines for following a patient treated with methotrexate. It is critically important to provide your patient with effective contraception during her recovery period.

Rh Considerations. Unsensitized Rh-negative women should be given an appropriate dose of Rh immunoglobulin (50 to 120 μg if gestational age is <12 weeks; 300 μg if it is >12 weeks).

Other Complications of Pregnancy in Adolescents
It remains difficult to state definitively that being a teenager increases your risk of adverse pregnancy outcomes. Studies are conflicting, and none are able to prove causality. Only associations have been shown.

Anemia. Pregnant adolescents are more likely to become anemic than pregnant adults. The definition of anemia in pregnancy is <11 g/dL in the first trimester, <10.5 g/dL in the second trimester, and <11 g/dL in the third trimester. The anemia is considered severe if the Hb is <7 g/dL. In North America, iron deficiency anemia may occur in up to 25% of all pregnant women, and teens 15 of age or younger have a 40% increase in anemia compared to adult pregnant women.

TABLE 56.2

Methotrexate Therapy for Ectopic Pregnancy—Exclusion Criteria

Patient characteristics:
  Hemodynamically unstable
  Unable to comply with follow-up visit schedule or to return if
    complications develop
  Immunocompromised (white blood cell count <3,000)
  Anemia (Hemoglobin <8 g/dL)
  Active pulmonary disease
  Renal compromise (creatinine clearance >1.3 mg/dL)
  Hepatic compromise (elevated liver function test results; aspartate
    aminotransferase >50 IU/L)
  Hematological dysfunction
  Thrombocytopenia
β-hCG characteristics:
  Most institutions exclude levels >10,000 mIU/ng
Ultrasonography findings:
  Gestational sac (maximum density of entire mass) >3.5–4.0 cm[a]
  Fetal cardiac motion[a]
  Excessive fluid in cul-de-sac consistent with hemorrhage

[a]Relative contraindication.

Preterm Delivery, Low-Birth-Weight and Small-for-Gestational Age (SGA) Infants. Adolescents are more likely to give birth prematurely and tend to have smaller babies than adults. This effect remains even when controlling for gestational age at delivery. Poor weight gain and low maternal body-mass index (BMI) at the first visit has been associated with low-birth-weight babies. Teen mothers who gained <20 lb during their pregnancy had a 13% chance of delivering a baby weighing <2,500 g, compared with <1% of mothers who gained more than 20 lb.

Preeclampsia in Teens. Adolescents are probably at increased risk of developing preeclampsia compared with the general obstetrics population, but this may be entirely attributable to their primigravid state. Smoking has been associated with a decrease in preeclampsia, while increased BMI doubles the risk.

Late Presentation. One of the challenges in caring for teens is that they tend to present late for prenatal care. In many cases, they have been unwilling or unable to admit to their parents or caregivers that they were sexually active, let alone pregnant. Thus, the opportunity is lost for appropriate counseling regarding pregnancy termination, accurate pregnancy dating, and appropriate antenatal screening and testing. There is also the possibility of the Rh-negative patient becoming isoimmunized.

Substance Use and Abuse. The pregnant teen may engage in substance use, alcohol consumption, and cigarette smoking. Most pregnant adolescents decrease or discontinue such use during pregnancy, but often resume it postpartum. Pregnant adolescents who continue to smoke may be motivated to quit if told that babies of smokers are more likely to have asthma and/or die of sudden infant death syndrome (SIDS). Although there are no data on the safety or efficacy of pharmaceutical smoking cessation products in pregnancy (e.g., nicotine patch, gum, etc.), the health care provider and patient may feel that the benefits outweigh the possible risk.

Pregnant teens may combine their smoking with other substances, usually alcohol, although overall, teens are less likely to drink during pregnancy than are adults. Patients who use one substance in pregnancy are more likely to use others, including nicotine, alcohol, marijuana, "ecstasy," and cocaine. Pregnant teens require additional follow-up postpartum, especially if they have a history of substance abuse before or during pregnancy. These teens tend to resume substance use after delivering their infants, which has obvious implications for parenting.

Pregnancies complicated by drug use are associated with low-birth-weight infants, preterm delivery, and admission to the neonatal intensive care unit. Cocaine use is associated with spontaneous abortion, placental abruption, and fetal death. Marijuana does not appear to have any detrimental effect on fetal morbidity or mortality. This is the type of information that should be provided to pregnant teens.

Sexually Transmitted Diseases and Teen Pregnancy. Somewhere between 20% and 30% of American adolescents presenting for pregnancy care are positive for chlamydial infection, gonorrhea, trichomoniasis, or syphilis. Many of these patients are asymptomatic; thus routine antenatal screening in each trimester should be offered and strongly encouraged in caring for pregnant teens.

There are both maternal and fetal consequences to untreated sexually transmitted diseases (STDs) in pregnancy. The most recent guidelines should be followed for the treatment of chlamydial infection, gonorrhea, and syphilis in pregnancy. Herpes simplex virus (HSV) in pregnancy is most concerning when it is a primary infection and, therefore, the fetus/neonate is not protected by placental transfer of maternal IgG antibodies. Any patient with an active HSV infection (either primary or recurrent) at the time of delivery should be offered a cesarean section.

Human papilloma virus (HPV) is common among adolescents, but the development of infantile laryngeal papillomatosis is uncommon. The Centers for Disease Control and Prevention and Health Canada both recommend testing in the first trimester for chlamydial infection, gonorrhea, syphilis, rubella, hepatitis B, and HIV. Patients at risk should also be offered hepatitis C screening. If a pregnant adolescent tests positive for a treatable STD, a test for cure should be performed. Pregnant teens should be offered repeat screening in the third trimester, even if the first-trimester, screens were negative. Teens are also at risk for reinfection postpartum.

Violence and Victimization. Teenagers of reproductive age face the dangers of violence from several angles. Females in abusive or manipulative relationships are at risk for unwanted pregnancy, as their partners may dictate contraception use or insist on conceiving. Sex may be used as a bargaining tool or punishment, and it may be unplanned. Becoming pregnant increases the chance that an adolescent may be abused, and pregnant teens are more likely to be abused than their adult counterparts. Pregnant teens who are abused are more likely to be abused postpartum, which is the time period associated with the highest rates of abuse for all ages.

Repeat Pregnancy. Although the majority of primigravid adolescents become pregnant "accidentally," second pregnancies are more likely to be planned and wanted. Approximately 10% of patients in a multidisciplinary clinic in Utah had repeat pregnancies within a 5-year period.

Advantages to Pregnancy before Age 18. There are some advantages to having a baby before age 18. During pregnancy, adolescents have a lower risk of gestational diabetes than older women. They are more likely to have a spontaneous vaginal delivery, thus avoiding an operative delivery or cesarean section. They also undergo fewer inductions of labor.

PRACTICAL STRATEGIES TO MODIFY ANTENATAL CARE FOR TEENS: REDUCING THE RISK

- More frequent visits
- Multidisciplinary team: dietician, social worker, public health nurse
- Test routinely (and retest) for sexually transmitted infections
- Counsel for postpartum contraception and follow-up for satisfaction and compliance
- Be flexible with appointments wherever possible
- Adolescent-friendly staff and clinic
- Make private time routine
- Follow-up postpartum (preferably with both physician and social worker)
- Counsel about substance use and other risk-taking behaviors
- Offer and counsel regarding smoking cessation

WEB SITES

http://www.rxmed.com/b.main/b1.illness/b1.illness.html. RxMed Web page providing basic information on ectopic pregnancy.

http://emedicine.com/emerg/topic478.htm. eMedicine Web page on ectopic pregnancy.

http://www.aafp.org/afp/20051101/1719ph.html. American Academy of Family Physicians article on ectopic pregnancy.

http://www2.mc.duke.edu/depts/obgyn/ivf/ectopic.htm. Information on ectopic pregnancy from Duke University.

http://www.cmaj.ca/cgi/content/full/173/8/905. Review article on diagnosis and management of ectopic pregnancy from the Canadian Medical Association Journal.

CHAPTER 57

Galactorrhea

Norman P. Spack and Sandra Loeb Salsberg

Galactorrhea is the discharge of milk or a milklike fluid from the breast in the absence of parturition or beyond 6 months postpartum in a non–breast-feeding woman. This discharge may be spontaneous or expressed.

Elevated prolactin levels are a major cause of galactorrhea in women. Prolactin is secreted from the anterior pituitary under hypothalamic regulation (Fig. 57.1) and levels increase during pregnancy, allowing normal lactation to occur.

DIFFERENTIAL DIAGNOSIS OF GALACTORRHEA

The most common etiologies are medication-induced and prolactinomas.

Associated with hyperprolactinemia:

1. Medications (see Table 57.1)
2. Hypothalamic and infundibular lesions that inhibit dopamine release
3. Hypothalmic-pituitary dysfunction
   a. Prolactinomas—benign anterior pituitary neoplasms that secrete prolactin
   b. Primary hypothyroidism (excess thyrotropin-releasing hormone secretion)
   c. Acromegaly
   d. Cushing disease
   e. Empty-sella syndrome
4. Idiopathic
5. Extracranial
   a. Spinal cord stimulation
   b. Renal failure
   c. Cirrhosis
   d. Adrenal insufficiency

Associated with normal prolactin levels:

1. Women with an unexplained hypersensitivity to prolactin
2. Acromegaly

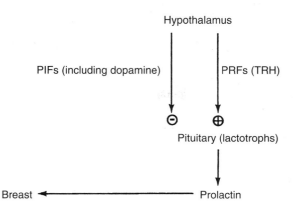

FIGURE 57.1 Medications causing hyperprolactinemia. PIFs, prolactin-inhibiting factors; PRFs, prolactin-releasing factors; TRH, thyrotropin-releasing hormone.

DIAGNOSIS

1. The work-up should start with a serum prolactin concentration.
2. Prolactin should be drawn in the morning in a fasting, nonexercised state, without prior breast manipulation. Abnormal results should be repeated.
3. The level of prolactin elevation may be helpful in predicting diagnosis.
   a. *Normal:* <25 ng/mL in females and <20 ng/mL in males
   b. *25 to 150 ng/mL:* non–prolactin-secreting tumor or dysfunction in the dopaminergic pathway
   c. *150 to 250 ng/mL:* microprolactinoma
   d. *>250 ng/mL:* macroprolactinoma

TABLE 57.1

Medications Causing Hyperprolactinemia

Antipsychotics	*Antihypertensive Agents*
Risperidone	Verapamil
Butyrophenones (haloperidol)	α-Methyldopa
Benzamines	Reserpine
Sulpiride	
Thioxanthenes	*Gastrointestinal Medications*
Phenothiazines	Metoclopramide
	Domperidone
Antidepressants	
Tricyclic antidepressants	*Others*
Monoamine oxidase inhibitors	Opiates
Elective serotonin reuptake inhibitors	Estrogens

4. Pregnancy, hypothyroidism, estrogen use, and renal failure should always be evaluated with a blood test for TSH, β-hCG, BUN, and creatinine.
5. With persistent prolactin elevation in a patient on a medication known to cause hyperprolactinemia, the offending drug should be changed or discontinued.
6. Any patient with persistent hyperprolactinemia with no underlying etiology or a prolactin >200 ng/mL, requires a cranial MRI.

PROLACTINOMAS

1. Treatment of microadenomas is optional and should be based on severity of symptoms and the woman's desire to conceive. Serum prolactin levels should be followed closely and an MRI repeated if the prolactin levels increase.
2. Macroadenomas have a large, significant potential for growth. Treatment with dopamine agonists and an annual MRI is recommended. There is a 26% chance of enlargement during pregnancy.

SPECIFIC THERAPEUTIC OPTIONS

Dopamine agonists decrease prolactin secretion and synthesis; they are usually the first and main option in therapy. Transsphenoidal surgery is rarely required.

Medications

1. Bromocriptine
   a. Starting dose is 1.25 mg at bedtime; this may be increased to 2.5 to 5 mg twice a day.
   b. Side effects (e.g., dizziness, nausea) are intolerable in 12% of patients.
2. Cabergoline
   a. Cabergoline is at least as effective as bromocriptine. It is the drug of choice in large tumors invading vital spaces (e.g., cavernous sinus) or compressing optic nerves, where fast action is required.
   b. Therapy should be started at 0.25 mg twice a week and titrated according to a patient's prolactin level to a maximum of 1 mg twice a week.
   c. 3% of patients cannot tolerate the drug because of side effects.

WEB SITES

http://pituitary.mgh.harvard.edu/Prolactinomas.htm. Massachusetts General Hospital Reproductive Endocrine Program's Web site containing patient information on prolactinomas.

http://familydoctor.org/673.xml. American Academy of Family Physicians Web site about galactorrhea.

http://www.emedicine.com/med/topic1915.htm. E-medicine article dicussing prolactinomas.

CHAPTER 58

Hirsutism and Virilization

Catherine M. Gordon and Lawrence S. Neinstein

Hirsutism is increased growth of terminal hair in a young woman in an amount more than is cosmetically acceptable. The term commonly refers to an increase in length and coarseness of the hair in a male pattern. Virilization implies the development of male secondary sex characteristics in a woman and may include a deepened voice, increased libido, increased muscle mass, clitoromegaly, temporal balding, and acne.

Hypertrichosis implies the predominance of excessive vellus hair on the body.

Hyperandrogenism results in appearance changes in a young woman and can be associated with abnormal menstrual patterns, infertility, and metabolic disturbances that include decreased high-density-lipoprotein cholesterol level, insulin resistance, and decreased sex hormone–binding globulin (SHBG).

ANDROGEN PHYSIOLOGY

Androgens are synthesized from the ovary or adrenals from steroidogenic pathways.

1. *Circulating androgens in females*
   a. 17-Ketosteroids (17-KSs): dehydroepiandrosterone sulfate (DHEAS), dehydroepiandrosterone (DHEA), androstenedione
   b. 17β-Hydroxysteroids: testosterone, dihydrotestosterone (DHT), androstenediol, 3β-androstenediol
2. *Metabolism:* Androgens originate in the adrenals and ovaries via direct secretion or peripheral conversion of precursors. DHEAS, DHEA, and androstenedione, which are mainly produced in the adrenal gland, exert their androgenic activity after peripheral conversion to testosterone or its metabolites.
   a. Adrenal: Androgens are by-products of cortisol synthesis.
   b. Ovarian: Androgens secreted by the ovary include testosterone and androstenedione.
   c. Peripheral conversion: About 50% of testosterone is derived from peripheral conversion of androstenedione in liver, fat, and skin.
   d. Testosterone is 95.5% bound to SHBG in females; the free portion is active.

DIFFERENTIAL DIAGNOSIS

1. *Idiopathic hirsutism:* Represents between 4% and 15% of hirsute women and is a diagnosis of exclusion.
2. *Ovarian causes:* (a) Polycystic ovary syndrome (PCOS)—or functional ovarian hyperandrogenism (see Chapter 52); (b) tumor—Sertoli-Leydig cell, lipoid cell, hilar cell; (c) pregnancy—luteoma
3. *Adrenal causes:* (a) congenital adrenal hyperplasia—21-hydroxylase or 11-hydroxylase deficiency; (b) tumors; (c) Cushing syndrome.
4. *Nonandrogenic causes of hirsutism:* (a) genetic—racial, familial; (b) physiologic—pregnancy, puberty; (c) endocrine—hypothyroidism, acromegaly; (d) porphyria, hamartomas; (e) drug-induced—testosterone, DHEA, danazol, corticotropin, high-dose corticosteroids, metyrapone, phenothiazine derivatives, anabolic steroids, androgenic progestin, acetazolamide, cyclosporine, phenytoin, diazoxide, triamterene-hydrochlorothiazide, minoxidil, hexachlorobenzene, penicillamine, psoralens, valproate; (f) CNS lesions—multiple sclerosis, encephalitis; (g) congenital lesions—Hurler syndrome, de Lange syndrome.

DIAGNOSIS

Indications for Evaluation. (1) Rapid onset of signs and symptoms; (2) virilization; (3) onset of hirsutism or virilization that is not peripubertal; (4) symptoms suggesting Cushing syndrome (e.g., weight gain, weakness, hypertension).

History. (1) Menstrual history—amenorrhea or oligomenorrhea; (2) drug history; (3) ethnic background and family history of hirsutism, irregular menses, infertility, miscarriages, or type 2 diabetes mellitus; (4) rapidity of androgenizing or virilizing symptoms and signs (rapid progression suspicious for androgen-producing ovarian or adrenal tumor).

Physical Examination. (1) Extent of hirsutism—systems are available that enable a clinician to quantitate the degree of hirsutism. One method is based on grading nine areas of the body from 1 to 4. The Ferriman-Gallwey hirsutism scoring system is another frequently used system. (2) Stigmata of Cushing syndrome (e.g., truncal obesity, striae, posterior fat pad, etc.); (3) Signs of virilization—A clitoral diameter >5 mm is abnormal. The clitoral index is the product of the vertical and horizontal dimensions of the glans. The normal range is 9 to 35 mm^2; a clitoral index >100 mm^2 suggests a serious underlying disorder. (4) Presence of ovarian or adrenal masses; (5) Evidence of insulin resistance.

Laboratory Evaluation

1. *Measuring androgen excess:*
   a. Plasma testosterone is the most important measurement, although this is a subject of debate in the diagnostic work-up. Levels >150 to 200 ng/dL suggest significant hyperandrogenism.
   b. Other important indicators: (i) DHEAS—levels >700 μg/dL suggest significant adrenal androgen production; (ii) 17-hydroxyprogesterone

(17-OHP)—should be measured in the morning (ideally between 7 and 9 A.M.). This is characteristically elevated in patients with congenital adrenal hyperplasia due to 21-hydroxylase deficiency. One can also measure 11-deoxycortisol in the morning to rule out 11-hydroxylase deficiency and determine the level of free testosterone. Free testosterone may be elevated in the presence of normal total testosterone.

   c. Prolactin and thyroid-stimulating hormone should be measured and a pregnancy test performed.

2. *Locating the source of androgen excess*

   a. If male levels of testosterone are obtained or a mass is felt on examination, perform an ultrasound or CT scan of adrenal glands and ovaries. Markedly elevated serum testosterone and DHEAS levels suggest an adrenal tumor and the need for a CT scan, whereas markedly elevated serum testosterone and normal DHEAS levels suggest an ovarian source; thus order the ultrasound.

   b. If androgens are elevated or signs suggest hypercortisolism, perform a dexamethasone suppression test.

- An ovarian source is suggested by cortisol suppression but a lack of androgen suppression. An ultrasound of the ovaries is helpful.
- Both adrenogenital syndrome and idiopathic hirsutism are suggested by suppression of cortisol and androgens after dexamethasone administration.
- Cushing syndrome or adrenal tumor is suggested by lack of cortisol suppression.

   c. If 17-OHP is elevated, perform an adrenocorticotropic hormone (ACTH) stimulation test. This is helpful in differentiating normal and idiopathic hirsute females from those with late-onset congenital adrenal hyperplasia.

- To perform the test, measure 17-OHP at baseline 17-OHP and 60 minutes after 0.25 mg of intravenous ACTH. A positive result is an increase in the serum level to >30 ng/mL, whereas in normal or idiopathic hirsute females, the levels are usually <5 ng/mL. This test can also be used to rule out less common forms of late-onset congenital adrenal hyperplasia.

3. *Specific diagnoses:* (a) Idiopathic hirsutism (these women generally ovulate regularly and have normal levels of androgens); (b) ovarian tumors (palpable adnexal mass, testosterone level >200 ng/mL, and nonsuppression of androgens after dexamethasone); (c) PCOS (hirsutism, infertility, menstrual irregularities, obesity, elevations in androgen levels, increase in LH:FSH ratio (ratio >3:1), and severe acne; (d) congenital adrenal hyperplasia— elevated 17-OHP with a large increase after ACTH administration is diagnostic of incomplete 21-hydroxylase deficiency. Elevated 11-deoxycortisol or DHEAS and 17-hydroxypregnenolone levels are found in 11-hydroxylase and 3β-hydroxysteroid dehydrogenase deficiencies. (e) Adrenal tumors— associated with rapid defeminization; adrenal mass—palpable in many individuals; elevated 17-KS, DHEAS, and DHEA levels; subnormal suppression with dexamethasone administration and mass on ultrasound, intravenous pyelogram, or CT scan. (f) Drug-induced hirsutism; (g) anabolic steroid abuse. (h) HAIR-AN syndrome—*h*yper*a*ndrogenism, *i*nsulin *r*esistance, and *a*canthosis *n*igricans. Insulin receptor mutations, circulating antibodies to the insulin receptor, and postreceptor signaling defects have been described in variants of this syndrome.

THERAPY

1. *Tumor:* Remove the androgen source.
2. *Drug-induced:* Stop medication.
3. *Congenital adrenal hyperplasia:* Replace cortisol and suppress adrenal androgen precursors with oral hydrocortisone or prednisone. Rarely, use low-dose dexamethasone (0.25 mg qd). Oral contraceptives may also be used.
4. *Functional ovarian hyperandrogenism (e.g., PCOS):* Multifaceted treatment directed at individual problems.
5. *Specific therapies (hyperandrogenism).*
   a. Hirsutism: cosmetic approaches; topical therapy—eflornithine hydrochloride 13.9% cream; weight loss; estrogen/progestins; antiandrogenic agents—e.g., spironolactone; combination therapy with low-dose oral contraceptives plus spironolactone
   b. Menstrual abnormality: Cyclic progestin; combined oral contraceptives

WEB SITES

http://www.obgyn.net/pcos/articles/hairissue_article.htm. OB-GYN net handout on hirsutism.

http://www.pcosupport.org. PCOS Association Web site.

http://www.pcossupport.com. PCO Teenlist home page is dedicated to teenagers with PCOS. Includes a chat room and bulletin board so teens can share their thoughts on the disease.

http://www.hormone.org/Polycystic/polycystic.cfm. A helpful overview of PCOS, including treatment options. Developed by the professional organization The Endocrine Society.

http://www.youngwomenshealth.org/pcosinfo.html. A teen-friendly Web site, developed at Children's Hospital Boston, that is written using terminology that adolescents can easily understand.

CHAPTER 59

Adolescent Breast Disorders

Heather R. MacDonald

To identify breast pathology, practitioners must command a detailed understanding of normal development, its variations, common breast complaints, and warning signs of serious disease. Table 59.1 lists common breast complaints in adolescence.

Normal Development. Breast development is arrested from birth until puberty; it is identical in boys and girls until puberty. Various conditions can lead to self-limited swelling of one or both breast buds in prepubertal patients, and this does not require intervention. Surgical removal can remove the breast bud entirely, leading to underdevelopment or complete developmental failure at puberty.

History. The history should ideally be taken with the patient dressed. A history of symptoms can give clues to a patient's underlying diagnosis. Key questions include pain, timing of pain, and relationship to trigger [e.g., menses], change in size (growth or shrinkage), recent medication changes or trauma.

Past medical history should include the patient's pubertal development and factors that increase the risk of malignancy (i.e., chest wall radiation) or history of malignancy that can metastasize to the breast (e.g., lymphoma, rhabdomyosarcoma). It should be noted that the majority of patients with cancer have no identifiable risk factors. Patients with strong family histories of breast cancer, especially of bilateral disease or in conjunction with ovarian cancer, should be referred for genetic counseling.

Physical Examination of the Breast

During the exam, a clinician must be sensitive to feelings of embarrassment or modesty. Before the exam, the teen should be informed of its components and given the opportunity to be accompanied by a parent or friend. If he or she declines, a chaperone should accompany the examiner, especially if the provider is of the opposite gender. The optimal time for a breast exam is within a week of completion of menses, when the breast is most quiescent and least tender. If an exam is indeterminant, repeat it at a different point in her menstrual cycle. The breast exam should include the following: (1) Inspection (arms outstretched, overhead, and resting at the waist). Look for skin changes, distortion and symmetry. (2) Palpation: sitting and standing. Cover each breast from the clavicle to inframammary fold and from the sternum to the midaxillary line. Include

TABLE 59.1

Common Breast Complaints in Adolescents

Congenital Anomalies	Disorders of Development	Benign Breast Disease
Polythelia	Asymmetry	Mastalgia
Polymastia	Macromastia	Nipple discharge
Supernumerary	Hypoplasia	Mastitis
breast	Tuberous breast	Abscess
Amastia	deformity	Mass
Inverted nipple	Gynecomastia	

the axillae and supraclavicular fossae. (3) Notation of nipple discharge: color, which and how many ducts it involved, and palpation of which quadrant of the breast elicited it. Use the clock-face analogy to describe its location. (4) Notation of breast mass: mobility, texture, and location. Only dominant masses with texture distinct from the surrounding tissue should be identified as masses; areas of nodularity without discrete masses should be identified as such. A discrete mass implies underlying pathology, while nodularity is often a variant of normal.

In examining a patient complaining of an ill-defined or deep mass or nipple discharge not elicited by the examiner, lotion, gel soap or lubrication on the examiners fingers can assist in deep or repeated palpation, with less discomfort to the patient.

Breast Imaging. Breast imaging is indicated when a clinician appreciates an abnormality on physical exam. Physical exam alone is not enough to rule out malignancy, despite its rarity in this age group.

Mammography is rarely indicted in an adolescent patient owning to high breast density.

Ultrasound is ideally suited to evaluating masses in the adolescent population. It is superior in characterizing masses and differentiating a cystic mass from a solid one. However, it cannot distinguish a benign solid from malignant mass. Hallmarks of benign lesions in adults, smooth regular borders, multiple masses, and homogeneous solid masses, can also be seen in metastatic lesions to juvenile breasts. Abscesses carry the same characteristics of malignant adult lesions: irregular borders and heterogeneous contents.

Breast Biopsy

Because of the limitations of physical exam and imaging, consideration should be given to obtaining a biopsy of any mass. A fine-needle aspiration (FNA) obtains important histologic evidence without causing much discomfort. FNA in pediatric patients has been demonstrated to have a sensitivity of 90% and specificity of 100% in diagnosing carcinoma. If an aspiration obtains nonbloody cyst fluid, the lesion can be diagnosed and treated with the same diagnostic test: it is a benign cyst. Cytology on the cyst fluid is not indicated unless it is bloody. If the cyst fails to resolve, it must be biopsied.

If, despite a reassuring FNA result, doubt remains regarding the benign nature of a mass, further tissue must be obtained for diagnosis. The preferred method is a minimally invasive core biopsy rather than an operative biopsy that will leave a scar.

Once cytologic or core biopsy results have been obtained, all three pieces of the diagnostic triad must be reviewed: physical exam, imaging and biopsy. If all three concur that the mass is benign, the practitioner may be 99% certain the mass is benign. The patient may then safely decline further intervention. She should be followed with serial exams and ultrasounds, every 6 months to a year, to establish stability of the lesion. Any sudden growth should raise suspicion of malignant transformation. If any one piece of the diagnostic triad is not in concordance, the lesion must be excised.

Common Breast Complaints

Gynecomastia. Uni- or bilateral breast development in males. This usually coincides with the onset of puberty and typically resolves within 2 years. The differential diagnosis includes medications (e.g., tricyclic antidepressants, hormonal agents such as estrogens and testosterone, insulin, anabolic steroids, alcohol, and illicit drugs, such as marijuana), endocrinopathies (hypogonadism, Klinefelter syndrome, or congenital adrenal hyperplasia), or underlying malignancy (pituitary, thyroid, adrenal gland, or testes). The work-up involves a history (medications, illicit drug or alcohol use, events of puberty) and physical exam, especially focusing on sexual maturity ratings, as well as a testicular exam. Management includes treating underlying causes; surgery is reserved for severe disfigurement only.

Congenital Anomalies

Aberrant Breast Tissue. This is failure of regression of the primordial milk crest and includes (1) *polythelia,* or accessory nipple (the most common congenital breast anomaly), (2) *polymastia,* or the presence of accessory breast tissue along the milk line, and (3) *supernumerary breast,* or the presence of an accessory nipple and underlying breast tissue.

The prevalence is about 2% to 6% of females. The condition usually presents with a soft tissue mass along the primordial milk line. It can be rarely associated with a carcinoma in the accessory breast tissue, and 10% to 15% of patients with supernumerary breast tissue may have major structural renal anomalies if two or more other phenotypic anomalies are present. The evaluation in these women should include a physical examination, ultrasound, and/or biopsy as needed. Excision is necessary only if the mass is bothersome or enlarging.

Amastia. Absence of breast tissue related to an iatrogenic cause (removal of breast bud usually in evaluation of a pseudomass in a pediatric breast) or congenital etiology (Poland syndrome). Poland syndrome typically presents with unilateral amastia, ipsilateral rib anomalies, webbed fingers, and radial nerve palsies. Treatment usually involves plastic surgery.

Nipple Inversion. This involves uni- or bilateral retraction of the nipple that is not reversible. It is common in newborns. The condition generally resolves within a few days of birth; if persistent from birth, patients can be reassured that this is a normal variant. Treatment involves reassurance; surgery is needed only for chronic infections.

Breast Asymmetry. Normally, some adolescents and adults exhibit moderate asymmetry of breast tissue. It is also normal for one breast to develop at a different rate than the other. Extremes of these normal variants can present as disorders. If the physical exam reveals breast asymmetry with normal breast tissue and no dominant masses, the appropriate treatment is reassurance. If the adolescent is pubertal, 75% of breast asymmetry will resolve completely by adulthood. If the asymmetry is marked and causes psychological distress, plastic surgical intervention may be an appropriate intervention. Breast asymmetry may also be caused by a large mass that distorts normal breast tissue or by pseudoasymmetry from deformities of the rib cage (e,g., pectus excavatum).

Macromastia. Another extreme of normal development includes *macromastia*, its further extreme is *gigantomastia,* or *virginal/juvenile hypertrophy*. In patients with juvenile hypertrophy, pendulous breasts can reach 30 to 50 pounds. This disorder includes unilateral or bilateral excessive breast growth. While the etiology is unknown, the condition may represent an abnormal response of breast tissue to normal hormonal stimulation. There is a strong association with family history and obesity. Adults usually present with complaints of back and shoulder pain and limited activity, while adolescents tend to focus on the issues related to self-image and social and athletic limitations. No definite therapeutic guidelines have been developed. Although it is preferable to delay surgery until the breasts have fully matured, this may not be practical in some adolescents if their breast size is unbearable. Treatment options include surgery with reduction mastopexy. Other approaches include hormonal treatment with medroxyprogesterone, dydrogesterone, danazol, or a combination of medications and surgery.

Breast Hypoplasia. This condition involves unilateral or bilateral breast underdevelopment secondary to iatrogenic injury, trauma, malnutrition, or as an idiopathic condition. It may also occur with aggressive weight loss or athletic activity. Teens should be screened for eating disorders, as breast underdevelopment may be a presenting symptom of anorexia or bulimia. Other disorders in the differential diagnosis include premature ovarian failure, androgen excess, and chronic diseases that lead to weight loss. Work-up consists of a careful physical examination exploring for any conditions listed above. Treatment is targeted at the underlying primary disorder. Idiopathic breast hypoplasia can be addressed by a plastic surgeon.

Tuberous Breast Deformity. A rare disorder presenting with long narrow ptotic breasts that appear to be an overdevelopment of the nipple–areolar complex with an underdevelopment of the breast mound. Treatment of choice is plastic surgery; reassurance is also an option for the milder cases.

Benign Breast Disease

Mastalgia/Mastodynia. *Mastalgia* is cyclic pain, versus *mastodynia,* which is noncylic pain. Both must be distinguished from the physiologic tenderness and swelling that occurs with normal menses due to proliferative lobular changes induced by hormonal stimulation. A thorough physical exam, with imaging and biopsy studies if abnormalities are found, is indicated to rule out underlying pathology. Other causes of breast pain include breast pathology, costochondritis, rib fracture, and gastritis, among others. Treatment includes analgesics (NSAIDs), good bra support, and reassurance that the pain is not a symptom of a more serious illness. Most breast pain resolves spontaneously within 3 to 6 months. Bromocriptine and tamoxifen, medications used to treat severe pain in adults, have not been studied in teens.

Nipple Discharge

Galactorrhea (See Chapter 57). Egress of milky fluid from one or both nipples spontaneously or during examination. Causes include physiologic factors, pregnancy/postpartum, prolactinoma, and medications. The evaluation should include a history including menstrual irregularities and headaches; a physical exam with visual field testing; serum prolactin levels; and a brain MRI. Management involves treating the underlying primary cause if identified, while a prolactinoma can be treated either medically with bromocriptine or surgically. If the condition is physiologic, treatment is reassurance and the condition is self-limiting.

Nonmilky Nipple Discharge. This usually indicates an underlying breast or nipple problem. Exam may reveal a local contact dermatitis of the nipple that can give rise to serous, purulent, or bloody discharge. Culprits include soap, clothes, clothing detergent, or lotion. Treatment is identification and discontinuation of the offending agent, with topical steroid cream for symptom relief. *Purulent discharge* usually indicates and infection and should be cultured and the patient treated with appropriate antibiotics and warm compresses. *Serous or bloody discharge* from a single duct may be due to an intraductal papilloma and should be examined by ductogram, and any abnormality should be excised. Cytologic analysis has not been shown to be cost effective in teens. Usually, *serous discharge* is a self-limiting condition and may be related to fibrocystic change. A *bloody nipple discharge*, while concerning in adults, is usually not related to underlying carcinoma in teens owing to the extremely low incidence of breast cancer in this population.

Montgomery Tubercles. Enlarged sebaceous glands around the areola associated with lactiferous ducts; these present as soft papules that may enlarge with pregnancy and lactation and elicit an episodic thin clear or brown discharge. Exam may reveal a soft mass beneath the areola. The condition resolves spontaneously within several months.

Breast Infection. May present with an acute history of a red, inflamed breast. Associated conditions include pregnancy, lactation, history of recent cessation of breast-feeding, pre-existing cyst, and breast trauma. Physical examination shows an edematous erythematous breast, with or without purulent discharge. Any discharge should be sent for culture and sensitivity. Treatment consists of warm compresses and antibiotics. Lactating mothers should continue milk expression from the affected side; if an abscess is present, it should be drained in the office with a large-bore needle, or referred for surgical incision and drainage. Patients should be reexamined within several days to confirm response to therapy.

Breast Masses

The presence of a dominant breast mass in a female patient of any age causes concern; in adolescence, however, breast masses are overwhelmingly benign

TABLE 59.2

Breast Masses in Adolescence

Benign Breast Masses—Common	Benign Breast Masses—Rare	Malignant Breast Masses—Extremely Rare
Fibroadenoma	Intraductal papilloma	Adenocarcinoma
Cyst	Juvenile papillomatosis	Cystosarcoma
Abscess	Tubular/lactational adenoma	Rhabdomyosarcoma
	Cystosarcoma phyllodes (benign)	Angiosarcoma
		Lymphoma
		Cystosarcoma phyllodes (malignant)
		Adenocarcinoma

(Table 59.2). Surgical studies show 86% of excisional biopsies reveal fibroadenomas (68%) or fibrocystic change (18%). Malignancies comprised <1% of excisional biopsies performed. A review of the adolescent literature in 1994 found 0.89% of breast masses excised to be primary adenocarcinoma.

Work-up of a Breast Mass. Every breast mass that feels benign should be confirmed with imaging and biopsy. Mammography is of low yield in adolescents and young women, as the breast density of these patients obscures pathology. Management seeks to establish a diagnosis with a minimally invasive breast biopsy, FNA or core needle, without surgical excision, saves patients with benign lesions an unnecessary operation. Studies of FNA in teenagers and adults have shown 99% correlation between excisional histology and the diagnostic triad of concordant physical exam, biopsy, and imaging.

Fibroadenomas. These are well-circumscribed fibroepithelial lesions that on exam feel like a round or oval firm mass, distinct from the rest of the breast and may be multiple and bilateral. On ultrasound these are hypoechoic lesions with smooth, round, distinct borders, wider than tall. Subtypes include *complex fibroadenoma,* which incorporate fibrocystic change, epithelial hyperplasia, sclerosing adenosis and other complex changes within a fibroadenoma and may confer an elevated risk of primary breast cancer in later life. *Giant fibroadenoma,* a lesion 8 cm or larger, is a distinction that has no clinical significance. The evaluation includes the exam, ultrasound, and biopsy (FNA or core needle). Treatment is either expectant with exam and ultrasound every 6 months; surgical excision for noncondordant or symptomatic lesions; minimally invasive surgery (cryoablation or removal by repeated core needle biopsy is available for lesions ≤3 cm); and surgical excision with plastic surgery consultation for giant fibroadenoma.

Cysts. A dominant breast mass may be a cyst and can present as one or multiple masses that increase in size and tenderness with menses. On examination, these are firm, well-circumscribed masses distinct from the breast. On ultrasound, these are round, well-demarcated hypoechoic structures with increased shine through transmission due to fluid content. Treatment is with FNA of fluid and resolution of the mass. The yellow, green, or brown fluid can be discarded. Bloody fluid should be sent for cytology and should raise concern regarding malignancy. A persistent solid mass after FNA expression of fluid implies a complex cyst, and the patient should be referred for image-guided core biopsy. Simple cysts can recur and can be reaspirated. Symptomatic cysts that recur after multiple aspirations should be referred for simple excision.

Fibrocystic Changes. These comprise proliferative changes of ducts and lobules, duct dilatation and elongation, and terminal duct cyst formation. Teens present with multiple masses or nodularity and with pain increasing with menses. Exam shows nodularity commonly in the upper outer quadrant of one or both breasts, decreased mobility of masses, and no distinct masses. On ultrasound, there is no dominant mass, with or without areas of increased fibrous tissue or microcysts. Treatment consists of mild analgesics, well-supporting bras, and oral contraceptives for more severe symptoms.

Tubular and Lactating Adenoma. This is rarely found at biopsy of a solitary mass in an adolescent, and is a well-circumscribed collection of uniform tubular structures spaced closely together, with or without lactational changes and hyperplastic lobules. No further treatment is required.

Juvenile Papillomatosis. This lesion presents as a unilateral solitary painless breast mass similar to a fibroadenoma. Some 50% of patients are <20 years of age. The mass includes multiple cysts separated by fibrous septa and, on histologic inspection, consists of simple cysts with cuboidal epithelial cells, papillary ductal hyperplasia, and apocrine metaplasia. There is controversy over whether this lesion is a preneoplastic condition. Local recurrence after diagnosis does occur; thus treatment is wide surgical excision and close follow-up.

Breast Malignancy. The incidence is rare in adolescents, with 18 cases in a 25-year review of one tertiary care center and 5 primary adenocarcinomas of 1,791 adolescent breast excisions in another large review. Types have included primary breast cancer: rhabdomyosarcoma, angiosarcoma, cystosarcoma phyllodes, lymphoma, and metastatic breast cancer. Risk factors have included history of chest wall irradiation and familial genetic risk factors. Treatment depends on the underlying pathology.

Cystosarcoma Phyllodes. Benign or malignant fibroepithelial lesions that make up 1% of breast neoplasms and 2.5% of fibroepithelial lesions. They represent the most common breast sarcoma during adolescence, but are most commonly found in later in life. Treatment involves wide local resection. The tumors do not metastasize to axillary nodes; no axillary procedure is indicated, but metastases to lung and bone can occur.

WEB SITES

http://www.puberty101.com. This Web site focuses mainly on teen sexuality.
http://www.youngwomenshealth.org look for breast section and glossary of terms.
http://www.womenshealth.about.com. Contains a section on teen breast complaints as well as question and answers.

http://www.goaskalice.Columbia.edu. Frank answers to common and uncommon teen questions.

http://www.teenshealth.com. Detailed discussions regarding plastic surgery in teens; excellent breast section.

http://www.cancer.org/docroot/home/index.asp. American Cancer Society.

http://www.acog.org. American College of Obstetrics and Gynecology.

CHAPTER **60**

Overview of Sexually Transmitted Diseases

J. Dennis Fortenberry and Lawrence S. Neinstein

Diagnostic possibilities for many sexually transmitted diseases (STDs), particularly gonorrhea and chlamydial infection, have been revolutionized by nucleic acid amplification (NAATs) and hybrid capture (HC) techniques. NAATs and HC have superior sensitivity and specificity compared with culture or other diagnostic tests such as direct fluorescent antibody (DFA) or DNA probe tests. NAATs and HC also allow use of urine and vaginal specimens, in addition to cervical or urethral specimens. Higher initial costs compared with other tests may be offset by reductions in morbidity.

In view of the fact that most adolescents complain of a particular set of symptoms and not a specific organism, a list of presenting symptoms for the STDs is also included (Table 60.1). As a broad overview, the appendix to this chapter summarizes the clinical features and treatments of many of the well-known STDs. The remaining chapters in Section 13 focus on individual STDs in more detail.

WEB SITES

http://www.niaid.nih.gov/publications/stds.htm. National Institute of Allergy and Infectious Diseases fact sheet on STDs.

http://www.ashastd.org. The American Social Health Association home page. Lots of information and hotline access.

http://www.cdc.gov/std/training/. CDC site with a variety of training resources related to STDs.

TABLE 60.1

Sexually Transmitted Diseases by Presenting Symptom

1. Urethral discharge/dysuria: (a) *Neisseria gonorrhoeae;* (b) *Chlamydia trachomatis;* (c) *Ureaplasma urealyticum:* (d) Herpes genitalis; (e) *Trichomonas vaginalis*
2. Vaginal discharge
   Vaginal site of infection: (a) *Candida* species; (b) *T. vaginalis;* (c) Bacterial vaginosis
   Cervical site of infection: (a) *N. gonorrhoeae;* (b) *C. trachomatis;* (c) H. genitalis
3. Genital ulcer/lymphadenopathy: (a) Herpes genitalis; (b) *Treponema pallidum;* (c) *Haemophilus ducreyi;* (d) *C. trachomatis* (LGV types); (e) *Calymmatobacterium granulomatis*
4. Genital growths: (a) Human papillomavirus (genital warts); (b) Molluscum contagiosum; (c) Condyloma latum (secondary syphilis)
5. Abdominal/pelvic pain: Pelvic inflammatory disease
6. Anorectal pain/discharge/bleeding: (a) *N. gonorrhoeae;* (b) *C. trachomatis;* (c) *Shigella* species; (d) *Campylobacter* species; (e) *Entamoeba histolytica;* (f) *Giardia lamblia*
7. Epididymitis: (a) *N. gonorrhoeae;* (b) *C. trachomatis;* (c) Coliform/enteric bacteria
8. Hepatitis: (a) Hepatitis A and B; (b) Cytomegalovirus; (c) *T. pallidum*
9. Arthralgia/arthritis: (a) *N. gonorrhoeae;* (b) Hepatitis B
10. Pruritus: (a) *Pthirus pubis;* (b) *Sarcoptes scabiei;* (c) *T. pallidum*
11. Flulike or mononucleosis syndrome: (a) Cytomegalovirus; (b) Herpes genitalis; (c) Hepatitis A and B; (d) Human immunodeficiency virus

APPENDIX 60.1: SEXUALLY TRANSMITTED DISEASES SUMMARY

Note: Adapted from the Centers for Disease Control and Prevention, Department of Health and Human Services. 2006 guidelines for treatment of sexually transmitted diseases. *MMWR Morb Mortal Wkly Rep* 2006;55(RR-11). For a copy of this publication, write to CDC, Technical Information Services, Atlanta, GA 30333. Copies, updates, downloadable PDA versions and slide show summaries are available online at http://www.cdc.gov/STD/treatment/.

Nongonococcal Urethritis (NGU)
Etiologic Agents

Chlamydia trachomatis (15% to 40%), *Ureaplasma urealyticum* (10% to 40%), *Mycoplasma genitalium* (5%–15%), *Trichomonas vaginalis* (2% to 5%), and HSV on occasion.

TYPICAL CLINICAL PRESENTATION

Dysuria, frequency, and mucoid-to-purulent urethral discharge.

PRESUMPTIVE DIAGNOSIS

Mucopurulent or purulent discharge.
Absence of gram-negative intracellular diplococci and ≥5 polymorphonuclear neutrophils (PMNs) per oil immersion field on a smear of an intraurethral swab specimen.
Positive leukocyte esterase test (LET) results on first-void urine or microscopic examination of first-void urine demonstrating ≥10 PMNs per high-power field. Should be confirmed with a Gram stain of a urethral swab specimen and/or testing for *Neisseria gonorrhoeae* and *Chlamydia*.
Asymptomatic men with negative gonorrhea test results are presumed to have NGU if they have ≥5 PMNs per oil immersion field on an intraurethral smear.

DEFINITIVE DIAGNOSIS

An agent etiologically associated with NGU is recovered from the male urethra.
Note that coinfection by multiple organisms is common, although specific testing only for *N. gonorrhoeae* and *Chlamydia* are done routinely.

THERAPY
Recommended Regimen:
Azithromycin (1 g PO in a single dose), OR
Doxycycline (100 mg PO BID for 7 days).

Alternative Regimens:
Erythromycin base, 500 mg PO QID for 7 days, OR
Erythromycin ethylsuccinate, 800 mg PO QID for 7 days, OR
Ofloxacin, 300 mg PO BID for 7 days, OR
Levofloxacin 500 mg PO once a day for 7 days.

For Apparent Treatment Failures or Recurrences: Metronidazole 2 g PO in a single dose, PLUS Azithromycin 1 g PO in a single dose (if not used in initial therapy). Note: Now that quinolones are not recommended for gonorrhea treatment, testing with culture or NAAT for gonorrhea is essential when treating chlamydial infection or NGU.

Management of Sex Partners: Sex partners should be referred for evaluation and treatment.

HIV Infection: Patients with HIV infection should receive the same treatment as patients without HIV.

EPIDIDYMITIS
Etiologic Agents

Chlamydia trachomatis, Neisseria gonorrhoeae, coliform/enteric bacteria.

TYPICAL CLINICAL PRESENTATION

Scrotal, inguinal, or flank pain and scrotal swelling. Most have accompanying dysuria, urethral discharge, or both.

PRESUMPTIVE DIAGNOSIS

Requires ruling out testicular torsion. Gram stain of urethral secretions may show PMNs and gram-negative intracellular diplococci. Urinalysis is often positive for white blood cells (WBCs).

DEFINITIVE DIAGNOSIS

Positive *Chlamydia* test result or a positive gonorrhea test result.

THERAPY

For epididymitis most likely caused by gonococcal or chlamydial infection:
Ceftriaxone, 250 mg IM in single dose, PLUS
Doxycycline, 100 mg PO BID for 10 days.
For epididymitis most likely caused by coliform/enteric organisms, or for patients allergic to cephalosporins or tetracyclines:
Ofloxacin, 300 mg PO BID for 10 days, OR
Levofloxacin 500 mg PO once a day for 10 days.

OTHER CONSIDERATIONS

Follow-up: Failure to improve within 3 days requires reevaluation.

Management of Sex Partners: Sex partners should be managed as appropriate for the identified STD.

HIV Infection: Patients with HIV infection should receive the same treatment as patients without HIV infection. Fungal and mycobacterial causes are more common among immunosuppressed patients.

MUCOPURULENT CERVICITIS (MPC)
Etiologic Agents
N. gonorrhoeae
C. trachomatis

In most cases, neither is isolated.

TYPICAL CLINICAL PRESENTATION

Most patients are asymptomatic. Symptomatic patients may complain of yellow vaginal discharge or abnormal vaginal bleeding (e.g., after coitus).

PRESUMPTIVE DIAGNOSIS

MPC is not a sensitive and specific predictor of infection by C. trachomatis or N. gonorrhoeae. The presence of yellow mucopurulent endocervical discharge suggests infection. Diagnosis based on presence of increased numbers of PMNs in endocervical mucus is not recommended.

DEFINITIVE DIAGNOSIS

Definitive diagnosis is made by a positive Chlamydia test result or a positive gonorrhea test result.

THERAPY

Treatment is based on the results of testing for Chlamydia and N. gonorrhoeae. If the patient is unreliable in a high-prevalence area, treat presumptively for both gonorrhea and Chlamydia.

OTHER CONSIDERATIONS

Management of Sex Partners: Sex partners should be managed as appropriate for the identified STD. Partners of presumptively treated patients should be notified, evaluated, and treated for infections identified or suspected in the index patient.

HIV Infection: Patients with HIV infection should receive the same treatment as patients without HIV.

GONORRHEA
Etiologic Agent
N. gonorrhoeae

TYPICAL CLINICAL PRESENTATION

When symptomatic, men complain of dysuria, urinary frequency, and purulent urethral discharge. Variable degrees of edema and erythema of the urethral meatus are often present.

Many infections in women are asymptomatic. Symptoms in women include abnormal vaginal discharge, intermenstrual bleeding, menorrhagia, or dysuria.

Symptoms of rectal gonococcal infection include mild anal pruritus, painless mucopurulent discharge, and mild bleeding. Symptoms of severe proctitis sometimes occur. Pharyngeal infections are usually asymptomatic.

PRESUMPTIVE DIAGNOSIS

Identification of typical gram-negative intracellular diplococci on smear of urethral discharge (men) or endocervical mucus (women). Gram stain is insufficiently sensitive for diagnosis in women and should be supplemented by culture, DNA probe, or NAAT confirmation.

DEFINITIVE DIAGNOSIS

Growth on selective medium demonstrating typical colonial morphology, positive oxidase reaction, and typical Gram stain morphology. Nucleic acid probes and NAATs are highly sensitive and specific for the diagnosis of gonorrhea. Tests based on several methods are FDA-approved and commercially available. Approved specimen sources include urethral and cervical discharge/mucus and urine. Urine is generally less sensitive for diagnosis of gonococcal infections in women. Provider and self-obtained vaginal swabs show high sensitivity and specificity in research settings but are FDA-approved specimen sources for only one of the commercially available tests. False-positive tests may be due to other nonpathogenic bacterial species and should be considered if screening patients with low probability of infection.

THERAPY

Uncomplicated Urogenital or Anorectal Gonococcal Infections (See "Other Considerations," below): Ceftriaxone, 125 mg IM at one time, OR
Cefixime, 400 mg PO in a single dose, OR
Treatment of coinfection by *C. trachomatis* should be added unless appropriate diagnostic test results are negative for *Chlamydia*.

Uncomplicated Pharyngeal Infections (See "Other Considerations," below): Ceftriaxone, 125 mg IM at one time. Concomitant treatment for chlamydial infection is recommended, although coinfection is unusual.

Alternative Regimens:

Spectinomycin, 2 g IM a single dose (*Potential shortage; see "Other Considerations," below*).

Injectable cephalosporin regimens such as ceftizoxime (500 mg IM in a single dose), cefotaxime (500 mg IM in a single dose), cefotetan (1 g IM in a single dose), and cefoxitin (2 g IM in a single dose). These regimens have no advantage over ceftriaxone.

Azithromycin 2 g PO is effective against uncomplicated gonococcal infection but is expensive and causes gastrointestinal distress and thus is not recommended for treatment for gonorrhea. Azithromycin 1 g PO is not recommended because of concerns regarding the possible rapid emergence of antimicrobial resistance.

OTHER CONSIDERATIONS

Note about spectinomycin: With the discontinuation of spectinomycin in the United States, patients allergic to cephalosporins may need desensitization treatment by a specialist.

Pregnant Women: Should not be treated with tetracycline or quinolones.

Follow-up: No test of cure is needed for appropriately treated patients.

Management of Sex Partners: Sex partners should be referred for evaluation and treatment. Sexual intercourse should be avoided until both patient and partner are cured.

HIV Infection: Patients with HIV infection should receive the same treatment as patients without HIV infection.

CHLAMYDIA
Etiologic Agent
C. trachomatis

TYPICAL CLINICAL PRESENTATION

Many patients are asymptomatic. Symptomatic women complain of dysuria or abnormal vaginal discharge. Symptomatic men usually have dysuria, urinary frequency, and a mucopurulent urethral discharge.

PRESUMPTIVE DIAGNOSIS

Women: Sexual contact with a partner with diagnosed nongonococcal or chlamydial urethritis.

Men: Sexual contact with partners with urogenital chlamydial infection. NGU (i.e., typical clinical symptoms and ≥5 PMNs per oil immersion field on a smear of an intraurethral swab specimen).

DEFINITIVE DIAGNOSIS

Definitive diagnosis is made with a positive *Chlamydia* test result (culture, DFA, nucleic acid probe or NAAT).

THERAPY

Recommended Regimens:
Azithromycin, 1 g PO in a single dose, OR
Doxycycline, 100 mg PO BID for 7 days.

Alternative Regimens: Ofloxacin, 300 mg PO BID for 7 days, OR
Levofloxacin 500 mg PO once a day for 7 days, OR
Erythromycin base, 500 mg PO QID for 7 days, OR
Erythromycin ethylsuccinate, 800 mg PO q.i.d. for 7 days.

OTHER CONSIDERATIONS

Pregnant Women: Doxycycline, ofloxacin, and levofloxacin are contraindicated for use during pregnancy. Azithromycin is a Class B drug, so its safety for pregnant and lactating women is not known. However, there is now extensive clinical experience with azithromycin treatment during pregnancy.
Recommended Regimen for Pregnant Women
Azithromycin 1 g PO in a single oral dose, OR
Amoxicillin, 500 mg PO TID for 7 days.
Alternative Regimens
Erythromycin base, 250 mg PO QID for 14 days, OR
Erythromycin base, 500 mg PO QID for 7 days, OR
Erythromycin ethylsuccinate, 800 mg PO QID for 7 days, OR
Erythromycin ethylsuccinate, 400 mg PO QID for 14 days

Follow-up: No need for retesting after completing treatment with doxycycline or azithromycin. Retesting at 3 weeks after completion of therapy may be useful for pregnant women because none of the regimens are highly efficacious and erythromycin side effects may prevent compliance. Reinfection is common in women with *C. trachomatis* and rescreening within 3 to 4 months after treatment is recommended, particularly in adolescents.

Management of Sex Partners: Sex partners should be referred for evaluation and treatment.

HIV Infection: Patients with HIV infection should receive the same treatment as patients without HIV infection.

PELVIC INFLAMMATORY DISEASE
Etiologic Agents

In most cases, sexually transmitted organisms, especially *N. gonorrhoeae* and *C. trachomatis,* are implicated.

TYPICAL CLINICAL PRESENTATION

The spectrum of PID includes any combination of endometritis, salpingitis, tuboovarian abscess (TOA), and pelvic peritonitis. The patient may present with pain and tenderness involving the lower abdomen, cervix, uterus, and adnexa. Fever, chills, elevated WBC count, and elevated erythrocyte sedimentation rate (ESR) are often absent.

PRESUMPTIVE DIAGNOSIS

No combination of symptoms, signs, or laboratory findings is both sensitive and specific for PID. Because delay in treatment increases the potential for damage to the reproductive health of the woman with PID, a low threshold for the diagnosis of PID is necessary.

Minimum Criteria: Adnexal tenderness, OR uterine OR cervical motion tenderness
Empiric treatment of PID should be initiated in sexually active young women and others at risk for STDs if the minimum criteria are present and no other cause(s) for the illness can be identified. Although PID occurs during pregnancy, patients with positive pregnancy tests require careful evaluation for ectopic pregnancy as a cause for pelvic pain.

Additional Criteria: Additional criteria may increase the specificity of the diagnosis. The likelihood of PID is reduced if all of these criteria are normal or negative.
Routine Criteria: (1) Oral temperature >38.3°C; (2) abnormal cervical or vaginal discharge; (3)

Presence of WBCs on saline microscopy of vaginal secretions; (4) elevated ESR; Elevated C-reactive protein; (5) laboratory documentation of cervical infection with *N. gonorrhoeae* or *C. trachomatis.* If the cervical discharge appears normal and no WBCs are observed on the wet prep of vaginal fluid, the diagnosis of PID is unlikely and another diagnosis should be explored.
Elaborate Criteria: (1) Histopathologic evidence of endometritis on endometrial biopsy; (2) TOA on sonography, (3) laparoscopic abnormalities consistent with PID.

DEFINITIVE DIAGNOSIS

Direct visualization of inflamed (edema, hyperemia, or tubal exudate) fallopian tube. A culture of tubal exudate establishes the etiology.

THERAPY

Hospitalization of patients with PID is particularly recommended in the following circumstances: (1) The diagnosis is uncertain, and surgical emergencies, such as appendicitis and ectopic pregnancy, cannot be excluded. (2) A pelvic abscess is suspected. (3) The patient is pregnant. (4) The patient has HIV infection. (5) Severe illness or nausea and vomiting preclude outpatient management. (6) The patient is unable to follow or tolerate an outpatient regimen. (7) The patient has failed to respond to outpatient therapy. (8) Clinical follow-up within 72 hours of starting antibiotic treatment cannot be arranged.

ORAL TREATMENT

If patients do not respond within 72 hours to outpatient regimens, they should be hospitalized to confirm diagnosis and receive parenteral treatment.

Ceftriaxone, 250 mg IM once, OR Cefoxitin, 2 g IM, plus probenecid, 1 g concurrently, OR Other parenteral third-generation cephalosporin such as ceftizoxime or cefotaxime, PLUS Doxycycline, 100 mg PO BID for 14 days; WITH or WITHOUT Metronidazole, 500 mg PO BID for 14 days.

PARENTERAL TREATMENT

Regimen A: Cefoxitin, 2 g IV q6h, or cefotetan, 2 g IV q12h, PLUS Doxycycline, 100 mg IV or PO q12h. Oral and IV doxycycline have similar bioavailability. Oral administration should be used when possible due to pain of IV administration.

Regimen B: Clindamycin, 900 mg IV q8h, PLUS Gentamicin loading dose, IV or IM 2 mg/kg of body weight, followed by a maintenance dose, 1.5 mg/kg q8h. These regimens should be continued for at least 24 hours after the patient demonstrates improvement. Thereafter, doxycycline (100 mg PO BID) or clindamycin (450 mg PO QID) should be continued for 14 days. When TOA is present, many health care providers use clindamycin for continued therapy, rather than doxycycline, because clindamycin provides more effective anaerobic coverage.

Alternative Parenteral Regimens: Ampicillin/sulbactam 3 g IV q6h PLUS Doxycycline 100 mg IV or PO q12h.

OTHER CONSIDERATIONS

Pregnant Women: Should be treated as inpatients.

Follow-up: Hospitalized patients should show substantial clinical improvement within 3 to 5 days or require further diagnostic workup. Some experts recommend retesting for *N. gonorrhoeae* and *C. trachomatis* 4 to 6 weeks after completing therapy.

Management of Sex Partners: Sex partners should be referred for evaluation and treatment. Treatment should include coverage for both *N. gonorrhoeae* and *C. trachomatis* infections.

HIV Infection: Patients with HIV infection should be managed aggressively, including hospitalization.

VAGINITIS
Etiologic Agent

The three diseases most frequently associated with vaginal discharge are Bacterial vaginosis (sometimes incorrectly called nonspecific vaginitis or *G. vaginalis*–associated vaginitis); *Trichomoniasis (T. vaginalis); Candidiasis* (vulvovaginal candidiasis, or VVC); and vaginitis caused by other infectious, chemical, allergenic, and physical agents).

TYPICAL CLINICAL PRESENTATION

Presentations vary from no signs or symptoms to erythema, edema, and pruritus of the external genitalia. Excessive or malodorous discharge is a common finding. Symptoms and clinical findings do not reliably distinguish among etiologies.
Male sex partners may develop urethritis, balanitis, or cutaneous lesions on penis.

PRESUMPTIVE DIAGNOSIS

The diagnosis of vaginitis is made by vaginal pH and microscopic examination of fresh samples of the discharge.

T. vaginalis **Vaginitis:** Small, punctate cervical hemorrhages called "colpitis macularis" or "strawberry cervix" are highly specific for the diagnosis of vaginal trichomoniasis. Vaginal pH level is almost always >4.5 and wet mount examination often shows many WBCs.

Bacterial Vaginosis: The clinical criteria include three of the following: (1) A homogenous gray or white noninflammatory discharge that adheres to vaginal walls; (2) Vaginal pH level >4.5; (3) A fishy odor from vaginal fluid before or after addition of 10% potassium hydroxide (KOH);

(4) Presence of "clue cells" on microscopic examination.

Vulvovaginal Candidiasis: The presumptive criteria are the typical symptoms of vaginitis or vulvitis and microscopic identification of yeast forms (budding cells or hyphae) in Gram stain or KOH wet mount preparation of vaginal discharge.

DEFINITIVE DIAGNOSIS

T. vaginalis **Vaginitis:** A vaginal culture, or commercially available tests (e.g., detection of *T. vaginalis* DNA or rapid antigen tests) or is positive for *T. vaginalis*, OR Typical motile trichomonads are identified in a saline wet mount of vaginal discharge (only 60% to 70% sensitive).

Bacterial Vaginosis: Gram stain demonstration of few or no lactobacilli, with a predominance of *G. vaginalis* plus other organisms resembling gram-negative *Bacteroides* sp., anaerobic gram-positive cocci, or curved rods.

Vulvovaginal Candidiasis: Culture may be useful when signs and symptoms are suggestive but when the fungus cannot be identified by direct microscopy. Therapy of apparent treatment failures is best guided by culture.

THERAPY

T. vaginalis Vaginitis:
Recommended regimen:
Metronidazole, 2 g PO in a single dose, or tinidazole 2 g PO in a single dose
Alternative regimen: Metronidazole, 500 mg BID for 7 days.
Both regimens have cure rates of approximately 95%.

Bacterial Vaginosis: *Recommended Regimen*
Metronidazole, 500 mg PO BID for 7 days, OR
Metronidazole gel 0.75%, one applicator (5 g) intravaginally QD or BID for 5 days.
Clindamycin cream 2%, one applicator (5 g) intravaginally at bedtime for 7 days.
Note: clindamycin cream is oil-based and may damage latex condoms
Alternative Regimens
Clindamycin, 300 mg PO BID for 7 days, OR
Clindamycin ovules, 100 mg intravaginally at bedtime for 3 days.

Vulvovaginal Candidiasis:
Intravaginal Agents
Clotrimazole, miconazole nitrate, terconazole, or butoconazole creams or vaginal tablets are recommended. Regimens range from 1 to 14 days of treatment. Several are available for over-the-counter purchase. Some contain oils that may weaken latex condoms.

Oral Agent
Fluconazole, 150-mg tablet in a single dose.

OTHER CONSIDERATIONS

Pregnant Women Metronidazole may be used during pregnancy in a single dose of 2 g, or 250 mg TID for 7 days.
Tinidazole is pregnancy category C and its safety during pregnancy has not been well evaluated.
Clindamycin vaginal cream should be avoided during pregnancy.
Vulvovaginal candidiasis should be treated with topical azole therapies during pregnancy. Many experts recommend 7 days of therapy.

Follow-up: *Bacterial vaginosis:* No follow-up visits are necessary.
Trichomoniasis: Follow-up is unnecessary for patients who become asymptomatic after treatment.
Vulvovaginal candidiasis: Follow-up is unnecessary for patients who respond to therapy.

Management of Sex Partners:
Bacterial Vaginosis: Treatment of partners is not recommended.
Trichomoniasis: Sex partners should be treated.
Vulvovaginal candidiasis: Treatment of sex partners is not routinely warranted unless male sex partner has balanitis.

HIV Infection: Bacterial vaginosis, trichomoniasis, and vulvovaginal candidiasis: patients with HIV infection should be managed in the same manner as patients without HIV infection.

CONDYLOMATA ACUMINATA (GENITAL WARTS)
Etiologic Agent

Human papillomavirus

TYPICAL CLINICAL PRESENTATION

Condylomata acuminata present as single or multiple soft, fleshy, papillary or sessile, painless growths around the anus, vulvovaginal area, penis, urethra, or perineum.

PRESUMPTIVE DIAGNOSIS

A diagnosis is made on the basis of the typical clinical presentation. Colposcopy may also aid in the diagnosis of certain cervical lesions.
Condylomata lata can be excluded by dark-field microscopy or a serologic test for syphilis.

DEFINITIVE DIAGNOSIS

A biopsy, although usually unnecessary, can make a definitive diagnosis. Atypical lesions, in which neoplasia is a consideration, should be biopsied before initiating therapy.
A Papanicolaou (Pap) smear of cervical lesions shows typical cytologic changes of koilocytosis. Direct DNA immunofluorescence staining techniques can diagnose certain types of HPV.
A hybrid capture test for detection of high-risk HPV types is now FDA-approved for triage of atypical squamous cells of undetermined significance (ASCUS). Women with ASCUS by Pap smear and a positive hybrid capture test result can be further evaluated by colposcopy. This test is not approved for routine screening for infection with high-risk HPV.

THERAPY

The goal of therapy is removal of exophytic warts and alleviation of signs and symptoms.

External Genital Warts: *Patient-Applied*
Podofilox 0.5% solution or gel: Apply to visible warts BID for 3 days, followed by 4 days without therapy. Repeat as necessary up to four cycles. Total area treated should not exceed 10 cm^2 and total volume should not exceed 0.5 mL/day.
Imiquimod 5% cream: Apply to visible warts at bedtime, three times per week. Treatment area should be washed with soap and water 6 to 10 hours after application.
Provider-Applied
Cryotherapy with liquid nitrogen or cryoprobe: for vaginal warts, do not use cryoprobe (to avoid perforations), OR
Podophyllin 10% to 25% in compound tincture of benzoin: wash off in 1 to 4 hours to reduce irritation, OR
Trichloroacetic acid (TCA) or bichloracetic acid 80% to 90%: weekly for maximum of 6 weeks, OR
Electrodesiccation or electrocautery.

Cervical Warts: Cervical dysplasia must be excluded before treatment is begun. Management should be carried out in consultation with an expert.

Vaginal Warts: Cryotherapy with liquid nitrogen, TCA, or podophyllin. Podophyllin treatments should be limited to ≤2 cm^2 and the treated area should be dry before speculum removal.

Anal or Oral Warts: Cryotherapy with liquid nitrogen or TCA or surgical removal.

OTHER CONSIDERATIONS

Prevention/Immunization: An effective vaccine against four HPV types (1, 6, 16, 18) is available for women 9 to 26 years of age (see Chapter 66).

Pregnancy: The safety of podophyllin, podofilox, and imiquimod during pregnancy is not established.

Follow-up: Not necessary after warts have responded to therapy.

Management of Sex Partners: Routine referral of partners for examination and treatment is not recommended. Use of condoms reduces but does not eliminate transmission to uninfected partners.

HIV Infection: Patients with HIV may not respond to therapy for HPV as well as persons without HIV. Cervical dysplasia may progress more rapidly among HIV-infected persons.

HERPES GENITALIS
Etiologic Agents

Herpes simplex virus (HSV) types 1 and 2

TYPICAL CLINICAL PRESENTATION

Single or multiple vesicles appear anywhere on the genitalia. Vesicles spontaneously rupture to form shallow ulcers that may be very painful. Lesions resolve spontaneously without scarring. The first occurrence is termed initial infection (mean duration, 12 days). Subsequent, usually milder, occurrences are termed recurrent infections (mean duration, 4 to 5 days). The interval between clinical episodes is termed *latency*. Viral shedding occurs intermittently and unpredictably during latency.

PRESUMPTIVE DIAGNOSIS

Clinical diagnosis of genital herpes is both insensitive and nonspecific. However, when typical genital lesions are present or a pattern of recurrence has developed, herpes infection is likely. The clinical diagnosis of genital herpes should be confirmed by laboratory testing. Both virologic and type-specific serologic tests for HSV should be available in the clinical setting. Several sensitive and specific type-specific relatively rapid screening tests are commercially available. These test results are usually negative until 3 weeks after initial infection. Repeat or confirmatory tested may be indicated, especially if the patient has low risk of genital herpes or if recent acquisition is suspected.

DEFINITIVE DIAGNOSIS

An HSV tissue culture demonstrates the characteristic cytopathic effect after inoculation of a specimen from the cervix, the urethra, or the base of a genital lesion.

THERAPY

First Clinical Episode of Genital Herpes: Acyclovir, 400 mg PO TID for 7 to 10 days, OR
Acyclovir, 200 mg PO 5 times daily for 7 to 10 days, OR
Famciclovir, 250 mg PO TID for 7 to 10 days, OR
Valacyclovir, 1 g PO BID for 7 to 10 days.
Treatment may be extended if healing is incomplete after 10 days of therapy.

First Clinical Episode of Herpes Proctitis: Acyclovir, 400 mg PO 5 times a day for 10 days or until clinical resolution is attained. Famciclovir and valacyclovir may also be effective, but clinical experience is lacking.

Episodic Treatment of Recurrent Episodes of Genital Herpes and Herpes Proctitis: When treatment is started during prodrome or within 1 day of onset of lesions, many patients experience shortened duration of symptoms. Acyclovir, 400 mg PO TID for 5 days, OR
Acyclovir, 800 mg PO BID for 5 days, OR
Acyclovir, 800 mg TID for 2 days, OR
Famciclovir, 125 mg PO BID for 5 days, OR
Famciclovir 1,000 mg PO BID for 1 day, OR
Valacyclovir, 500 mg PO bid for 3 to 5 days, OR
Valacyclovir, 1.0 g PO once a day for 5 days.

Daily Suppressive Therapy of Genital Herpes and Herpes Proctitis: Daily suppressive therapy reduces HSV recurrences by at least 75% and reduces risk of transmission to partners. Acyclovir, 400 mg PO BID, OR Famciclovir, 250 mg PO BID , OR Valacyclovir, 500 mg PO QD, OR Valacyclovir 1 mg PO QD. The valacyclovir 500-mg-QD regimen may be less effective for patients with >10 recurrences annually.

COMPLICATIONS AND SEQUELAE

Neuralgia, meningitis, ascending myelitis, urethral strictures, and lymphatic suppuration may occur.

Neonates: Virus from an active genital infection may be transmitted during vaginal delivery, causing neonatal herpes infection, which has a high case fatality rate, and many survivors have ocular or neurologic sequelae.

OTHER CONSIDERATIONS

Pregnant Women: The safety of systemic acyclovir, valacyclovir, and famciclovir during pregnancy has not been established. Available data do not indicate increased risk of birth defects among women receiving acyclovir during the first trimester.

Counseling: All persons with HSV should be encouraged to inform their partners. Individuals need to be aware of asymptomatic shedding, about potential decreased risk of transmission through the use of antivirals, the protective effects of condoms, the possibility of acquisition by partners (even without symptoms), and the risk of neonatal transmission.

Management of Sex Partners: Sexual transmission of HSV can occur during periods without evidence of lesions. The use of condoms should be encouraged during all sexual contact.

HIV Infection: HSV lesions are common among HIV-infected patients. Intermittent or suppressive therapy with oral acyclovir, valacyclovir or famciclovir may be required.

SYPHILIS
Etiologic Agent
Treponema pallidum

TYPICAL CLINICAL PRESENTATION

Primary: The classic chancre is painless, indurated, and located at the site of exposure. Genital chancres are often accompanied by tender inguinal lymphadenopathy.

Secondary: Patients may have a macular, maculopapular, or papulosquamous skin rash. Other signs include mucous patches and condylomata lata.

Tertiary: Patients have cardiac, neurologic, ophthalmic, auditory, or gummatous lesions.

Latent: Patients are without clinical signs.

PRESUMPTIVE DIAGNOSIS

Presumptive diagnosis relies on both nontreponemal serologic tests for syphilis (STS) (e.g., Venereal Disease Research Laboratories or rapid plasma reagin) and treponemal tests (fluorescent treponemal antibody-absorbed (FTA-ABS, *T. pallidum* (TP-PA) particle agglutination and enzyme immunoassays). Nontreponemal test antibody titers usually correlate with disease activity, and decline with therapy.

Primary: Patients have typical lesions and either a newly positive STS or STS titer at least fourfold greater than the last, or syphilis exposure within 90 days of lesion onset.

Secondary: Patients have the typical clinical presentation and a strongly reactive STS.

Latent: Patients have serologic evidence of untreated syphilis without clinical signs.

HIV-infected patients: When clinical findings suggest syphilis is present, but serologic test results are negative, alternative tests, such as biopsy, dark-field examination, and DFA staining of lesion material, should be employed.

DEFINITIVE DIAGNOSIS

Demonstration of characteristic spirochetes with dark-field microscopy of serous transudate from genital lesions. DFA of material from a chancre, regional lymph node, or other lesion.

THERAPY

Primary and Secondary Syphilis: Penicillin G benzathine, 2.4 million units IM in a single dose.
Penicillin-allergic Patients
Doxycycline, 100 mg PO BID for 2 weeks, OR
Tetracycline, 500 mg PO QID for 2 weeks.
Ceftriaxone 1 g IM or IV daily for 8 to 10 days.
Note: the optimal dose and duration of treatment has not been established. Some penicillin-allergic patients are also allergic to ceftriaxone.
Azithromycin 2.0 g PO in a single oral dose.
Note: Some areas have noted rapid emergence of resistant *T. pallidum* strains, suggesting need for careful clinical and serologic follow-up if this regimen is used.

Latent Syphilis: *Early latent (<1 year) syphilis:* Penicillin G benzathine, 2.4 million units IM in a single dose.

Late latent (>1 year) syphilis or latent syphilis of unknown duration: Penicillin G benzathine, 7.2 million units total, administered as three doses of 2.4 million units IM each at 1-week intervals.

Neurosyphilis: *Recommended regimen:* Aqueous crystalline penicillin G, 18 to 24 million units daily, administered as 2 to 4 million units IV q4h for 10 to 14 days. *Alternative regimen:* 2.4 million units procaine penicillin IM daily, plus probenecid 500 mg PO QID, both for 10 to 14 days.

OTHER CONSIDERATIONS

Pregnant Women: Pregnant women should receive the same therapy as listed earlier except that tetracycline, doxycycline, and erythromycin should not be used. Pregnant women with a history of penicillin allergy should be skin-tested, desensitized if allergy is documented, and then treated with penicillin.

Follow-up: Patients should be reexamined clinically and serologically at 3 and 6 months for primary and secondary syphilis and 6 and 12 months for latent syphilis. STS results become negative or reactive only in low titers (<1:8) in most successfully treated patients.

Management of Sex Partners: Persons exposed to a patient with primary, secondary, or early latent syphilis within 90 days should be treated presumptively. Those exposed >90 days should be treated presumptively if serologic tests are not available immediately or follow-up is uncertain. Partners considered at risk are those exposed within 3 months plus duration of symptoms for primary syphilis, within 6 months plus duration of symptoms for secondary syphilis, and within 1 year for early latent syphilis.

HIV Infection: Unusual serologic response may occur in HIV-infected persons. Penicillin regimens should be used whenever possible. Some authorities recommend cerebrospinal fluid examination or treatment with a regimen appropriate for neurosyphilis for all patients coinfected with syphilis and HIV. Patients should be followed clinically and serologically at 1, 2, 3, 6, 9, and 12 months after therapy.

CHANCROID
Etiologic Agent
Haemophilus ducreyi

A gram-negative bacillus with rounded ends, commonly observed in small clusters along strands of mucus.

TYPICAL CLINICAL PRESENTATION

Usually a single (but sometimes multiple), superficial, painful ulcer surrounded by a erythematous halo. Ulcers may also be necrotic or severely erosive with ragged serpiginous borders. Accompanying adenopathy is usually unilateral. A characteristic inguinal bubo occurs in 25% to 60% of cases.

PRESUMPTIVE DIAGNOSIS

(Warrants full treatment and follow-up.)
Chancroid is the third most common sexually transmitted cause of genital ulcer in the United States, although it is far less frequently seen than genital herpes or primary syphilis. Presumptive diagnosis depends on a clinically consistent lesion, a negative dark-field examination of lesion fluid, and absence of serologic evidence of syphilis.

DEFINITIVE DIAGNOSIS

Culture identification of *H. ducreyi*. No FDA-cleared PCR test of *H. ducreyi* is available in the United States, but such testing can be performed by clinical laboratories that have developed their own PCR test and conducted a CLIA verification study.

THERAPY

Recommended Regimens:
Azithromycin, 1 g PO in a single dose, OR

Ceftriaxone, 250 mg IM in a single dose, OR
Ciprofloxacin, 500 mg PO BID for 3 days, OR
Erythromycin base, 500 mg PO TID for 7 days.

COMPLICATIONS AND SEQUELAE

Systemic spread is not known to occur. Lesions may become secondarily infected and necrotic. Buboes may rupture and suppurate, resulting in fistulae. Ulcers on the prepuce may cause paraphimosis or phimosis.

OTHER CONSIDERATIONS

Pregnant Women: Safety of azithromycin during pregnancy has not been established. Ciprofloxacin is contraindicated during pregnancy.

Follow-up: Successfully treated ulcers are clinically improved by 7 days after institution of therapy. If the condition does not improve, the clinician should consider whether antimicrobials were taken as prescribed; the *H. ducreyi* is resistant to the prescribed antimicrobial; the diagnosis is correct; there is a coinfection with another STD; or the patient is infected with HIV.

Management of Sex Partners: Partners who had contact within 10 days before the onset of symptoms should be examined and treated.

HIV Infection: Patients with HIV infections should be closely monitored and may require longer courses of therapy.

Lymphogranuloma Venereum (LGV)
Etiologic Agent
C. trachomatis

An obligate intracellular organism of serovars L1, L2, or L3.

TYPICAL CLINICAL PRESENTATION

The primary lesion of lymphogranuloma venereum (LGV) is a 2- to 3-mm painless vesicle or nonindurated ulcer at the site of inoculation. Patients commonly fail to notice this primary lesion. Regional adenopathy, typically unilateral, follows a week to a month later and is the most common clinical presentation. Sensation of stiffness and aching in the groin, followed by swelling of the inguinal region, may be the first indications of infection for most patients. Adenopathy may subside spontaneously or proceed to the formation of abscesses that rupture to produce draining sinuses or fistulae.

PRESUMPTIVE DIAGNOSIS

(Warrants full treatment and follow-up.)
The LGV complement-fixation test result is typically positive, with titers of 1:64 or higher. Cross-reactions due to other chlamydial infections may be misleading. Because the sequelae of LGV are serious and preventable, treatment should be provided pending laboratory confirmation.

DEFINITIVE DIAGNOSIS

A definitive diagnosis requires isolation of *C. trachomatis* from an appropriate specimen and confirmation of the isolate as an LGV immunotype.

THERAPY

Recommended regimen:
Doxycycline, 100 mg PO BID for 21 days.

Alternative regimen:
Erythromycin, 500 mg PO QID for 21 days.

COMPLICATIONS AND SEQUELAE

Dissemination may occur with nephropathy, hepatomegaly, or phlebitis. Large polypoid swellings of the vulva, anal margin, or rectal mucosa may occur, and rectal strictures may occur.

OTHER CONSIDERATIONS

Pregnant Women: Pregnant patients should be treated with the erythromycin regimen.

Follow-up: Patients should be followed clinically until signs and symptoms have resolved.

Management of Sex Partners: Persons having had sexual contact with a patient who has LGV within 30 days before onset of the patient's symptoms should be examined and treated.

HIV Infection: Patients with HIV infection are managed in the same manner as patients without HIV infection.

MOLLUSCUM CONTAGIOSUM
Etiologic Agent

Molluscum contagiosum virus

TYPICAL CLINICAL PRESENTATION

Lesions are 1 to 5 mm in diameter, smooth, rounded, shiny, firm, flesh-colored to pearly white papules with umbilicated centers, most commonly seen on the trunk and anogenital areas. Most patients are asymptomatic. Extensive skin involvement is seen in advanced HIV disease.

PRESUMPTIVE DIAGNOSIS

Usually diagnosed on the basis of the typical clinical presentation.

DEFINITIVE DIAGNOSIS

Microscopic examination of lesions shows pathognomonic molluscum inclusion bodies.

THERAPY

Lesions resolve spontaneously; most within 2 months.

Caustic chemicals (podophyllin, TCA, silver nitrate) and cryotherapy (liquid nitrogen) have been used successfully. Self-applied podophyllotoxin may also be effective. Recurrence is reported in 15% to 35% of cases.

OTHER CONSIDERATIONS

Pregnant Women: Podophyllin should be avoided during pregnancy.

Follow-up: Patients should return for evaluation 1 month after treatment so any new lesions can be removed.

Management of Sex Partners: Sex partners should be examined.

HIV Infection: Patients with HIV infection should be managed in the same manner as patients without HIV infection.

PEDICULOSIS PUBIS
Etiologic Agent

Pthirus pubis (pubic or crab louse)

TYPICAL CLINICAL PRESENTATION

Symptoms range from slight discomfort to intolerable itching. Erythematous papules, nits, or adult lice clinging to pubic, perineal, or perianal hairs are often noticed by patients.

PRESUMPTIVE DIAGNOSIS

A presumptive diagnosis is made when a patient with a history of recent exposure to pubic lice has pruritic, erythematous macules, papules, or secondary excoriations in the genital area.

DEFINITIVE DIAGNOSIS

A definitive diagnosis is made by finding lice or nits attached to genital hairs.

THERAPY

Permethrin 1% creme rinse applied to affected areas and washed off after 10 minutes, OR
Pyrethrins with piperonyl butoxide applied to the infested area and washed off after 10 minutes.
Alternative Therapies:
Malathion 0.5% lotion applied for 8 to 12 hours and washed off, OR
Ivermectin 250 μg/kg PO in a single dose, repeated in 2 weeks.
Owing to increased risk of neurotoxicity, lindane should be used only if other treatments are not tolerated or have failed. The recommended regimens should not be applied to the eyes. Involvement of the eyelashes should be treated by applying occlusive ophthalmic ointment to the eyelid margins BID for 10 days. Clothing and linen should be disinfected by washing in hot water, by dry-cleaning, or by removal from human exposure for at least 72 hours.

COMPLICATIONS AND SEQUELAE

Secondary excoriations; lymphadenitis; pyoderma

OTHER CONSIDERATIONS

Pregnant Women: Lindane is contraindicated in pregnant or lactating women.

Follow-up: Patients should be evaluated after 1 week if symptoms persist. If lice are found or if eggs are observed at the hair–skin junction, retreatment is necessary. Increasing resistance of lice to permethrins may account for treatment failures.

Management of Sex Partners: Sex partners within the last month should be treated.

HIV Infection: Patients with HIV infection are managed in the same manner as patients without HIV infection.

SCABIES

Etiologic Agent

Sarcoptes scabiei

TYPICAL CLINICAL PRESENTATION

Symptoms include itching, often worse at night, and the presence of erythematous, papular eruptions. Excoriations and secondary infections are common. Reddish-brown nodules are caused by hypersensitivity and develop 1 or more months after infection has occurred. The primary lesion is the burrow. When not obliterated by excoriations, burrows are usually seen on the fingers, penis, and wrists.

PRESUMPTIVE DIAGNOSIS

The diagnosis is often made on clinical grounds alone. Exposure to a person with scabies within the previous 2 months supports the diagnosis.

DEFINITIVE DIAGNOSIS

Definitive diagnosis is made by microscopic identification of the mite or its eggs, larvae, or feces in scrapings from an elevated papule or burrow.

THERAPY

Recommended Regimen:
Permethrin cream 5% applied to all areas of the body from the neck down and washed off after 8 to 14 hours, OR
Ivermectin 200 μg/kg PO, repeated in 2 weeks.
Lindane (1%) 1 ounce of lotion or 30 g of cream applied thinly to all areas of the body from the neck down and washed off thoroughly after 8 hours. Lindane should not be used after a bath and should not be used by persons with extensive dermatitis, pregnant or lactating women, and children <2 years. Not recommended for pregnant or lactating women or infants and young children. Lindane should be used only if other treatments fail or are not tolerated.

COMPLICATIONS AND SEQUELAE

Secondary bacterial infection occurs, particularly with nephritogenic strains of streptococci. Norwegian or crusted scabies (with up to 2 million adult mites in the crusts) is a risk for patients with neurologic defects and the immunologically compromised.

OTHER CONSIDERATIONS

Pregnant Women: Lindane is contraindicated in pregnant or lactating women.

Follow-up: Pruritus may persist for several weeks. Retreatment should be considered in patients who are symptomatic after 1 week, particularly if live mites are observed.

Management of Sex Partners: Sex partners and close personal or household contacts within the last month should be examined and treated.

HIV Infection: Patients with HIV infection are managed in the same manner as patients without HIV infection.

ENTERIC INFECTIONS
Etiologic Agent

Proctitis: *N. gonorrhoeae, C. trachomatis, T. pallidum,* and HSV; Proctocolitis: *Campylobacter* sp. *Shigella* sp. *Entamoeba histolytica,* and rarely *C. trachomatis;* Enteritis: *Giardia lamblia;* Among HIV-infected patients, others include cytomegalovirus (CMV), *Mycobacterium avium-intracellulare, Salmonella* sp., *Cryptosporidium,* microsporidia, and *Isospora.*

TYPICAL CLINICAL PRESENTATION

Infections are frequently asymptomatic or minimally symptomatic. Symptoms include the following:

Proctitis: Anorectal pain, tenesmus, and rectal discharge.

Proctocolitis: Symptoms of proctitis plus diarrhea or abdominal cramps.

Enteritis: Diarrhea and abdominal cramping.

PRESUMPTIVE DIAGNOSIS

The finding of WBCs on direct microscopy of a suspension of fresh stool or the finding of occult or grossly bloody stools supports the diagnosis.

DEFINITIVE DIAGNOSIS

Definitive diagnostic tests vary according to the agent and site of infection involved.

THERAPY

Treatment of proctitis and enteritis should be based on etiologic diagnosis. Some asymptomatic infected individuals for whom anal–oral contact is a sexual practice should be treated in accordance with recommendations for symptomatic individuals, as should persons whose work or social situation is associated with a likelihood of transmission (e.g., food handlers, hospital workers, day-care center employees). Until laboratory test results are available, persons with acute proctitis who have recently practiced receptive anal intercourse and have either anorectal pus on examination or PMNs on a Gram stain should receive treatment for anogenital gonorrhea and doxycycline (100 mg PO BID for 7 days).

COMPLICATIONS AND SEQUELAE

Complications and sequelae vary with the disease agent, health of the host, therapy, and other factors. Spontaneous cures are common. Morbidity may be severe, requiring hospitalization and intravenous hydration. Infections may become systemic (such as gram-negative septicemia) or distantly localized (amebic hepatic cyst). Some infections may rarely be fatal (hepatitis A, disseminated bacterial disease).

OTHER CONSIDERATIONS

Follow-up: Follow-up should be based on severity of clinical symptoms and specific etiologic agent involved.

Management of Sex Partners: Sex partners should be evaluated for any diseases diagnosed in the index patient.

HIV Infection: Patients with HIV infection should be managed in the same manner as patients without HIV infection. HIV-infected patients are at risk for infections not commonly found in non-HIV-infected patients.

HIV Infections and Acquired Immunodeficiency Syndrome
Etiologic Agent

Human immunodeficiency virus (HIV) 1 or 2

TYPICAL CLINICAL PRESENTATION

The range of symptoms associated with HIV infection extends from an acute illness shortly after infection to the full clinical acquired immunodeficiency syndrome (AIDS). Acute HIV infection includes a mononucleosislike syndrome consisting of headache, myalgia, sore throat, rash, diarrhea, fever, and lymphadenopathy. The acute HIV retroviral syndrome is reported 1 to 3 weeks after initial infection and resolves within a few weeks. This is a period of high levels of viral replication and viremia, with great potential for transmission. A latent or asymptomatic stage, lasting from a year to a decade or more, often follows. Disease progression appears inevitable, with ongoing destruction of the host immune system, followed by wasting and weight loss, symptoms specific to opportunistic infections (e.g., shortness of breath and cough from *Pneumocystis carinii* pneumonia [PCP] infection), or purple to bluish skin lesions associated with Kaposi sarcoma. Virtually all organ systems are affected by advanced HIV disease.

PRESUMPTIVE DIAGNOSIS

Presumptive diagnosis of HIV infection is made usually by clinical evidence, supported by tests for antibodies to HIV infection. Screening tests are based on enzyme immunoassay, with positive results confirmed by immunoblot (Western blot). Rapid serologic tests are now available that provide results within 15 to 30 minutes, although these tests always require confirmation by immunoblot. Screening may also be done with whole blood, saliva, or urine. These tests increase the ease of screening, but their results should be confirmed by immunoblot. Clinicians and patients should keep in mind that the median time between infection and confirmed seropositivity is 3 months and may be as long as 6 months. Retesting is recommended when suspicion is high, particularly when the clinical presentation is consistent with the acute HIV syndrome.

DEFINITIVE DIAGNOSIS

Currently, isolation of the virus from body fluids is the most highly specific means to make a definitive diagnosis of HIV infection. Results from reactive enzyme immunoassay tests, confirmed by immunoblot (Western blots) or other confirmatory tests, are considered diagnostic. Indeterminate tests are usually resolved by retesting, combined with examination of the pattern of the indeterminate Western blot and a careful risk-assessment interview.

THERAPY

A number of antiretroviral drugs are used to limit viral replication, restore immunocompetence, and delay onset of AIDS-related illness.

Acute Retroviral Syndrome: Immediate initiation of antiretroviral treatments improves prognosis of HIV-related infection. The optimal regimen is not known. Single-drug therapy with zidovudine may be effective, but many experts recommend two nucleoside reverse-transcriptase inhibitors and a protease inhibitor. Antiretroviral therapy is central to the treatment of HIV disease. Three classes of antiretroviral agents are available and are typically used in combination. Therapy can be monitored with highly sensitive viral load assays. Tuberculin skin testing, review of vaccination status, provision of pneumococcal and influenza vaccines, and serologic tests for syphilis are all important aspects of comprehensive therapy. PCP prophylaxis with trimethoprim/sulfamethoxazole, dapsone, or aerosolized pentamidine should be instituted for adolescents and adults with <200 CD4-positive T cells per milliliter or after an initial episode of PCP. Prophylaxis should be continued for the lifetime of the patient. Prophylaxis for individuals seropositive for *Toxoplasma gondii* and CD4+ counts <100 T cells per milliliter includes trimethoprim/sulfamethoxazole or dapsone with pyrimethamine.

COMPLICATIONS AND SEQUELAE

Most people with HIV will eventually have symptoms related to the infection. Aggressive antiretroviral therapy improves diseasefree survival, but relapse is expected when therapy is stopped.

OTHER CONSIDERATIONS

Management of Sex Partners: Sex partners should be notified either by their partners or through a referral to health department partner-notification programs. Partners should receive counseling and testing.

CHAPTER 61

Gonorrhea

Margaret J. Blythe

Gonorrhea is an important sexually transmitted disease (STD) in teens because of its incidence and potential for complications.

Etiology

Gonorrhea is an STD caused by *Neisseria gonorrhoeae,* described as small gram-negative intracellular organisms that are oxidase-positive diplococci. There are >70 different strains.

Epidemiology

1. *Incidence:* Gonorrhea is the second most frequently reportable disease in the United States, with approximately 358,366 cases in 2006 thought to represent <50% of cases.
2. *Trends:* Rates of gonorrhea declined 73.8% between 1975 and 1998 to 122.4 per 100,000 and continued decrease in 2005 to 115.6 per 100,000, although there was an increase to 120.9 in 2006. www.cdc.gov/STD/stats/tables/table1.htm.
3. *Risk groups:*
   a. Some 60% of reported cases occur in 15- to 24-year-olds and 20% in those between 25 and 29 years of age.
   b. African Americans had the highest (629.6 per 100,000) incidence and Asian/Pacific Islanders had the lowest (22.6 per 100,000).
   c. The highest rates are found in the South (159.2 per 100,000) and the lowest in the Northeast (73.8 per 100,000).
   d. Gender: 122.7 per 100,000, women; 115.3 per 100,000, men.
4. *Prevalence:* depends on population and location.
   a. *Nationally representative sample, 18 to 26 years of age, males and females:* 0.43%.
   b. *STD clinics:* males, range 8% to 25%.
   c. *Family planning clinics:* median rate 0.88% (range 0.1% to 4.2%).
   d. *Job Corps:* female, median 2.4% (0.0% to 6.4%); males, median 3.7% (1.0 to 5.7%).
   e. *University and college student health centers:* <1% to 2% positive for gonorrhea.
   f. *Juvenile detention facilities:* males, median gonorrhea rate 0.8% (0% to 18.2%); females, median rate 4.5% (0% to 16.6%).

g. *Adolescent clinics:* Approximately 3% to 9% positive for gonorrhea.

h. *Urban emergency departments (EDs):* 1% to 7%.

5. *Reasons for the high incidence in 15- to 19-year-olds:* biological factors (cervical ectopy); psychosocial factors, including number of sexual partners; frequency of sexual intercourse; early age of first intercourse; low rates of consistent, appropriate use of barrier methods; lack of accessible, confidential clinical services for teens; lack of screening by health care providers in a variety of health care settings.

Host

Humans are the only natural host for *N. gonorrhoeae.*

Transmission

Virtually exclusively through oral, vaginal, or anal sexual contact with the exception of gonococcal ophthalmia in newborns.

PATHOPHYSIOLOGY

N. gonorrhoeae causes disease by direct invasion and spread on mucosal and glandular structures lined by columnar or cuboidal, noncornified epithelium. *Chlamydia trachomatis* and *N. gonorrhoeae* occur frequently together in the same individual, causing similar clinical manifestations.

Virulence

The virulence of the infection may be related to certain characteristics of the organism: pili, colony morphology and autotyping (nutritional requirements of the organism).

Clinical Manifestations

The spectrum of gonococcal infections includes the following:

1. *Asymptomatic infections:* may persist for months if untreated and represent the majority of infections in women and vary in presentation for young men. Sites possibly involved: urethra, male and female; endocervix; rectum; pharynx.

2. Symptomatic uncomplicated infections may result in urethritis, cervicitis, proctitis, pharyngitis, bartholinitis, conjunctivitis.

3. Complicated disease includes pelvic inflammatory disease (PID), epididymitis, Bartholin gland abscess, penile edema, periurethral abscess, abscess of bulbourethral glands (Cowper glands) or sebaceous glands of the prepuce or foreskin (Tyson glands), prostatitis, perihepatitis: complication of salpingitis (Fitz-Hugh-Curtis syndrome), seminal vesiculitis.

4. Systemic complications might include disseminated gonococcal disease (DGI); arthritis-dermatitis syndromes; gonococcal meningitis, and endocarditis.

Genitourinary Infections

Most common clinical manifestation of gonorrhea.

Males

1. Urethritis

a. *Incubation period:* most symptomatic 2 to 5 days (range 1 to 14 days) after exposure

b. *Symptoms:* dysuria, meatal pruritus
c. *Clinical findings:* profuse purulent urethral discharge, with 25% presenting with scanty, minimally purulent discharge.
d. *Risk of infection:* 20% to 50% after a single exposure with an infected female.

2. Infection can spread and cause epididymitis, prostatitis, seminal vesiculitis, and infection of Cowper and Tyson glands.
   a. *Epididymitis:* 10% to 30% of *untreated* men develop this complication, which is manifest by the following:
   - Urethral discharge and dysuria
   - Scrotal pain and tenderness, usually unilateral
   - Scrotal swelling and erythema
   - Pain in the inguinal area and flank pain in severe cases
   - Pain, tenderness, or swelling of the lower pole of the epididymis, which can spread to the head of the epididymis
   - Swelling and pain of the spermatic cord
   b. *Prostatitis:* rare complication of gonorrhea, with the following signs and symptoms:
   - May be asymptomatic
   - Chills, fever, malaise, myalgia
   - Rectal pain and discomfort
   - Lower back pain
   - Lower abdominal pain, suprapubic discomfort
   - Dysuria, urinary frequency, and occasionally acute urinary retention

Females
Signs and symptoms are less specific in females than in males, with following common problems:

1. Endocervicitis, including increased vaginal discharge, often purulent; dyspareunia; erythema, edema, and friability of cervix resulting in spotting; risk of infection: 60% to 90% for female after single exposure to infected male.
2. Urethritis including dysuria; urinary frequency; exudate from urethra or periurethral glands (Skene gland); and suprapubic pain.
3. *Bartholinitis:* purulent exudate from Bartholin gland
4. *Bartholin gland abscess:* labial pain and swelling
5. Spread of infection can extend into endometrium (endometritis), fallopian tubes, upper abdomen (perihepatitis, Fitz-Hugh-Curtis syndrome) and ovaries (tubo-ovarian abscess).

Extragenital Sites
1. Pharyngitis
   a. Usually asymptomatic in >90% of infected individuals.
   b. Presents with a sore throat in 3 to 7 days, occasionally fever, cervical adenopathy.
   c. Fellatio more effective mode of transmission than cunnilingus.
   d. Infected individuals at risk for dissemination of gonorrhea.
2. Rectal gonorrhea
   a. Rectal cultures are positive in 35% to 50% of females with genital infection and in males with gonorrhea who have sex with men.

b. Rectal gonorrhea can produce symptoms of distal proctitis including mucopurulent anal discharge, rectal bleeding, anorectal pain or pruritus ani, tenesmus and constipation.
  c. Differential diagnosis for infections involving the first 5 to 10 cm of the rectum (proctitis) is *Chlamydia*, herpes, cytomegalovirus (CMV) infection and syphilis; other infections are caused by *Shigella, Campylobacter, Entamoeba histolytica,* or *Salmonella;* these may extend 15 cm into the rectum and colon (proctocolitis).
3. Conjunctivitis is usually severe, with high risk of sequelae.

Disseminated Disease. Less than 1% of those with gonorrhea develop disseminated gonococcal infection (DGI), which is more common in females, with a 4-to-1 ratio. DGI often follows asymptomatic urogenital infection or pharyngeal infection with other risk factors, including immune-altering disease states such as lupus erythematosus.

Arthritis-Dermatitis Syndrome
1. Arthritis
  a. The knee is the most common site of purulent arthritis, but it may also involve the wrist, metacarpophalangeal joints, and ankle (25% to 50% present with monoarticular septic arthritis).
  b. Presentation may include migratory polyarthralgias or asymmetric polyarticular arthritis. Any or all joints including the hip and shoulder may be involved, often with not enough fluid to aspirate. Sacroiliac, temporomandibular, and sternoclavicular joints are rarely involved.
  c. Tenosynovitis may affect the extensor and flexor tendons and sheaths of the hands and fingers but less likely the lower extremities.
2. Clinical presentation includes arthritis, arthralgias, rash, fever, chills, and leukocytosis (40% are afebrile). Symptoms occur usually within 1 month of exposure.
3. Approximately 90% will have a skin rash.
  a. *Variable presentations: hemorrhagic lesions* presenting as purpura and necrotic centers; others, *vesiculopapular lesions* on an erythematous base. All lesions begin as *erythematous papules.*
  b. Painful, asymmetric over extremities near the joints, palms, soles of feet, and occasionally on trunk and rarely face.
4. *Diagnosis:* Positive blood cultures occur in 20% to 30%; joint cultures are rarely positive with polyarticular presentation; for monoarticular presentation, positive joint cultures in <50% of cases; polymerase chain reaction (PCR) has been used on joint fluid to make the diagnosis; Gram stain results and cultures are usually negative from skin; gonococci are found on mucosal surfaces such as the cervix and pharynx 80% of the time despite negative blood, skin, and joint fluid cultures.
5. Differential diagnosis of gonococcal arthritis
  a. *Infections:* meningococcemia, bacteremias, endocarditis, infectious arthritis, and infectious tenosynovitis
  b. *Seronegative arthritides:* Reiter syndrome, ankylosing spondylitis, psoriatic arthritis, rheumatoid arthritis, rheumatic fever, Lyme disease, bacterial endocarditis

c. Lupus erythematosus
d. Allergic reaction to drugs

Sexually Acquired Reactive Arthritis (Reiter Syndrome) (See Chapter 62)

Table 61.1 compares gonococcal arthritis and acute Reiter syndrome.

Other types of dissemination include the following: perihepatitis, mild hepatitis, gonococcal meningitis, rare cardiac manifestations (myopericarditis, heart block, endocarditis), osteomyelitis and pneumonia.

DIAGNOSIS

Gonococcal Urethritis: Males and Females

1. Gram-negative intracellular diplococci on smear of male urethral exudates.
2. If Gram stain result is negative or not done or urethral exudate is not present, culture a specimen from male anterior urethra, inoculate on Thayer-Martin medium, and transport in 36- to 37-degree environment with 5% to 10% carbon dioxide.
3. NAATs of urethral site for males may be used (Table 61.2).
4. An alternative to urethral swab would be urine testing with NAATs for males or females *except PCR for gonorrhea on female urine* (Table 61.2).
5. Homosexual male adolescents should also have *cultures* obtained from the rectum and pharynx, as NAATs methods *are not approved* for those sites.
6. In *asymptomatic* males, the urinary leukocyte esterase dipstick test (LET) on first-catch urine can be a valuable screening technique in certain situations.

Gonococcal Endocervicitis: Females

1. Cultures obtained from the endocervical canal should be inoculated on Thayer-Martin medium and transport in 36- to 37-degree environment with 5% to 10% carbon dioxide. If anorectal sex has occurred, a separate swab can be used in the anal canal (Table 61.2).
2. Gram stain smears from the endocervix *are not* recommended.
3. Nucleic Acid Amplification Tests (NAATs) methods (polymerase chain reaction [PCR], transcriptional mediated amplification [TMA], and strand displacement amplification [SDA]) can be used on *endocervical specimens.* PCR, TMA, and SDA are approved for first-void *urine specimens* in females for *Chlamydia* but only TMA, SDA for gonorrhea in females on urine. PCR[*] and SDA tested on *vaginal swabs* and show similar or superior results to cervical specimens (Table 61.2).

Anorectal Gonorrhea. Positive cultures from the rectum are required for diagnosis of anorectal gonorrhea. NAATs have not been adequately studied for this site.

Gonococcal Pharyngitis. Diagnosis requires a positive culture from the pharynx. NAATs and Gram stains are not considered appropriate.

---

[*] Cross-reacts with other nonpathogenic *Neisseria* species found in the vagina.

TABLE 61.1

Comparison of Acute Gonococcal Arthritis and Acute Reiter Syndrome

Characteristic	Acute Gonococcal Arthritis (%)	Acute Reiter Syndrome (%)
Back pain	0	20
Urethritis	28	76
Migratory arthralgias	83	10
Chills	33	0
Temperature >39.4°C	27	39
Skin lesions	Isolated papules and pustules on extremities and trunk	Circinate balanitis; keratoderma of shaft of penis. Asymptomatic oral macular lesions on palate, buccal mucosa.
Sacroiliac involvement	3	30
Wrist involvement	67	30
Heel involvement	7	67
Antigen HLA-B27	Usually negative	>90 positive

TABLE 61.2

Comparison of Nucleic Acid Amplification Tests (NAATS) for *Neisseria gonorrhoeae*

	PCR	SDA	TMA	Culture
Test	COBAS Amplicor	Probe Tec	Aptima	
Company	Roche	Becton Dickinson	Gen Probe	
Gender/site				
Male/urethra				
Sensitivity	97.3%–99.0%[a]	98.5%–100%	73.1%–98.1%	80%–95%[b]
Specificity	98.8%–99.9%	91.9%–100%	95.9%–97.5%	100%
Male/urine				
Sensitivity	94.1%–100%[c]	97.9%	95.2%	Not available
Specificity	99.2%–99.9%	92.5%–100%	98.2%	
Female/cervix				
Sensitivity	92.4%–100%	95.6%–99.6%	83.7%–96.1%	76.6%–84.8%
Specificity	99.5%	99.3%–99.6%	98.1%–99.6%	100.0%
Female/urine[d]				
Sensitivity	64.8%–94.4%	98.5%–100%	86.5%–97.4%	Not available
Specificity	95.9%–99.5%	99.3%–99.6%	99.1%–99.5%	
Vaginal swab			FDA approved	Not available

PCR, polymerase chain reaction: COBAS Amplicor (Roche); TMA, transcriptional mediated amplification: Aptima Combo (Gen Probe); Aptima Ct and Aptima N. *gonorrhoeae* (Gen Probe); SDA, strand displacement amplification: Probe Tec (Becton Dickinson).

[a] Asymptomatic, 73.1%.
[b] Asymptomatic, 46.2%.
[c] Asymptomatic, 42.3%.
[d] All sites for all tests FDA approved except for female urine N. *gonorrhoeae* PCR; only TMA FDA approved for vaginal swabs (Martin et al., 2000; Wheeler et al., 2005; Chernesky et al., 2005; Crotchfelt et al., 1997; Cook et al., 2005; Cosentino et al., 2003; Schachter et al., 2003).

553

Systemic Infection

1. Positive cultures from the urethra, endocervix, pharynx, rectum, conjunctiva, or positive NAATs from urethra and/or endocervix/vagina
2. Positive cultures from skin lesions, synovial fluid, or blood

THERAPY

Treatment of gonorrhea should take into account that strains of *N. gonorrhoeae* resistant to traditional treatment are rising, that chlamydial infections often coexist with gonorrhea, and that serious complications can arise from both gonococcal and chlamydial infections (see Chapter 60 as well as CDC guidelines, available at: www.cdc.gov/STD/treatment/).

Resistance

In 2004, all isolates were susceptible to spectinomycin, ceftriaxone, and cefixime, while 6.8% demonstrated resistance to ciprofloxacin. Most of the "resistant" samples are from West Coast states such as Hawaii, California, and Washington. Resistance to ciprofloxacin was 23.8% in 2004 in males who have sex with males compared to 2.9% in heterosexuals. Therefore, the recommendation as of April 13, 2007 in the CDC update to the 2006 STD Guidelines is to no longer use fluoroquinolones for the treatment of gonococcal infections and associated conditions such as pelvic inflammatory disease.

Coinfection. In a variety of populations, prevalence of *Chlamydia* in those with diagnosed or contact of gonorrhea varies from 20% to 54%.

Treatment Recommendations

1. See Chapter 60 for treatment of uncomplicated infections and CDC guidelines (www.cdc.gov/STD/treatment/).
2. *Treatment of sex partners:* Sex partners of patients diagnosed with gonorrhea should be evaluated and treated empirically for both *Chlamydia* and gonorrhea if *Chlamydia* was not ruled out. Instructions should include avoidance of sexual intercourse until treatment is completed and symptoms are gone. Partner-delivered treatment may be considered.
3. *Acute salpingitis:* See Chapters 60 and 63.
4. *Acute epididymitis:* See Chapters 28 and 60.
5. *Disseminated gonococcal infection:* Hospitalization for intravenous treatment is recommended for initial therapy: ceftriaxone 1 g IM or IV every 24 hours.

Alternative. Cefotaxime 1 g IV every 8 hours *or* ceftizoxime 1 g IV every 8 hours *or* spectinomycin 2 g IM every 12 hours. All of the preceding regimens should be continued for 24 to 48 hours after improvement begins, at which time therapy may be switched to one of the following regimens to complete at least 1 week of antimicrobial therapy:

Cefixime[†] 400 mg orally twice daily
Cefixime suspension 500 mg twice daily orally (25 mL twice daily)
Cefpodoxime 400 mg orally twice daily

[†] The tablet formulation of cefixime is currently not available in the United States.

6. *Meningitis and endocarditis:* The recommended initial regimen is 1 to 2 g of ceftriaxone IV every 12 hours. Although the optimal duration is not known, most authorities treat gonococcal meningitis for 10 to 14 days and endocarditis for at least 4 weeks.
7. Adolescents with documented gonorrhea but "no history" of sexual activity should be carefully evaluated for sexual abuse.
8. *Prevention:* If *male latex condoms* are used consistently and correctly, they are effective in preventing the sexual transmission of genital gonorrhea.

WEB SITES AND REFERENCES

http://www.cdc.gov/STD/treatment/. Centers for Disease Control and Prevention. Sexually Transmitted Diseases Treatment Guidelines, 2006. *MMWR* 2006;55(RR-11):42. (Accessed 04/21/07). Updated recommended treatment regimens for gonococcal infections and associated conditions—United States, April 2007. *MMWR* 2007;56 (14):332.

http://www.cdc.gov/std/treatment/2006/updated-regimens.htm.

http://www.cdc.gov/std/Gonorrhea/. CDC link to gonorrhea fact sheets, 2004 surveillance statistics, and 2006 treatment guidelines.

http://www.niaid.nih.gov/factsheets/stdgon.htm. National Institutes of Health (NIH) fact sheet on gonorrhea. (Accessed 02/2/2007).

http://www2a.cdc.gov/stdtraining/self-study/gonorrhea.asp. Web-based training course designed to guide clinicians in the diagnosis, treatment, and prevention of gonorrhea, based on STD curriculum developed by the National Network of STD/HIV Prevention Training Centers.

Cook RL, Hutchinson SL, Ostergaard L, et al. Systematic Review: non-invasive testing for Chlamydia trachomatis and Neisseria gonorrhoeae. *Ann Intern Med* 2005;142:914.

Spigarelli MG, Biro FM. Sexually transmitted disease testing: evaluation of diagnostic tests and methods In Braverman PK, Rosenfeld WD, eds. Sexually transmitted infections. *Adolesc Med Clin* 2004;15:287.

CHAPTER 62

Chlamydia Trachomatis

Catherine Miller and Mary-Ann Shafer

Genital infections caused by *Chlamydia trachomatis* represent the most prevalent bacterial sexually transmitted disease (STD) in the United States and the most frequently reported infectious disease. These infections pose a major public health threat because of associated damaging sequelae in women; the most serious include pelvic inflammatory disease (PID), ectopic pregnancy, and infertility.

ETIOLOGY

The genus Chlamydia is divided into four species: C. psittaci, C. pecorum, C. pneumoniae, and *C. trachomatis. C. trachomatis* contains 18 serologically distinct variants known as serovars. Chlamydial genital disease and neonatal disease (pneumonia and conjunctivitis) are caused by serovars B, D, E, F, G, H, I, J, and K.

DEVELOPMENTAL CYCLE AND PATHOGENESIS

1. *C. trachomatis developmental cycle:* Cycle lasts 48 to 72 hours and is characterized by transformation between infectious and reproductive forms. The infectious form attaches to a susceptible epithelial cell and is ingested. Within an endocytotic vesicle, transformation to the reproductive form occurs. After 48 hours of replication, new infectious bodies are released from the cell.
2. *Predilection for columnar epithelium:* An important factor in female adolescent infections, as columnar epithelium is commonly found on the cervix of young women and involutes with increasing age.

EPIDEMIOLOGY

National rates reported by the Centers for Disease Control (CDC) in 2006 are as follows:

1. *Overall rate in the United States:* 347.8 cases per 100,000 population.

2. Adolescent girls ages 15 to 19 years had the highest rates of reported *C. trachomatis* infection (2,862.7 per 100,000).
3. The rate is 1,275 per 100,000 African Americans, more than eight times the rate among whites (153.1 per 100,000).
4. Median *Chlamydia* test positivity was 6.3% (3.2% to 16.3%) in women aged 15 to 24 years screened during visits to selected family planning clinics in all states and outlying areas in 2004.

Risk Factors

C. trachomatis infection is associated with a number of factors, including younger age, presence of cervical ectopy, female gender, prior history of STDs, new sexual partner, multiple sexual partners, living in a community with a high background prevalence, oral contraceptive use, douching, nonwhite race/ethnicity (African American predominance), unmarried, and young age at sexual debut.

Transmission

Transmitted during vaginal, anal, or oral sex and to infant during vaginal childbirth. Male-to female and female-to-male transmission after multiple sexual encounters appears equivalent. Correct and consistent condom use is protective for *C. trachomatis* transmission.

CLINICAL MANIFESTATIONS

The clinical manifestations of *C. trachomatis* are similar to those of *Neisseria gonorrhoeae* (see Table 62.1).

MALE INFECTIONS

There is some evidence, though still controversial, that *C. trachomatis* infection can affect male fertility.

Urethritis. Urethral infection is the most common problem associated with *C. trachomatis* in men and is more often asymptomatic than gonococcal urethral infection. There is a 7- to 21-day incubation period from infection to development of symptoms.

Epididymitis. *C. trachomatis* is responsible for 70% of epididymitis cases in adolescent and young men. Men will usually complain of unilateral testicular pain and tenderness, and a hydrocele or swelling of the epididymis is usually present (see Chapter 28).

Prostatitis. *C. trachomatis* has been isolated from prostatic secretions of some patients with prostatitis.

Proctitis. Either the lymhogranuloma venereum (LGV) strains or the genital strains D through K are responsible for the development of proctitis, producing a range of symptoms from no symptoms to rectal bleeding, diarrhea, rectal discharge, and ulceration.

TABLE 62.1

Comparison of Clinical Manifestations of *C. trachomatis* and *N. gonorrhoeae*

Site of Infection	Resulting Clinical Syndrome	
	Neisseria gonorrhoeae	*Chlamydia trachomatis*
Males		
Urethra	Urethritis	Nongonococcal urethritis
Epididymis	Epididymitis	Epididymitis
Rectum	Proctitis	Proctitis
Conjunctiva	Conjunctivitis	Conjunctivitis
Systemic	Disseminated gonococcal infection: Arthritis-dermatitis syndrome	Reiter syndrome
Females		
Urethra	Acute urethral syndrome	Acute urethral syndrome
Bartholin gland	Bartholinitis	Bartholinitis
Cervix	Cervicitis	Cervicitis
Fallopian tube	Salpingitis	Salpingitis
Conjunctiva	Conjunctivitis	Conjunctivitis
Liver capsule	Perihepatitis	Perihepatitis
Systemic	Disseminated gonococcal infection: Arthritis-dermatitis syndrome	Reiter syndrome

FEMALE INFECTIONS

Cervicitis. Approximately 70% of women infected with *C. trachomatis* are asymptomatic, while others have mild symptoms such as vaginal discharge, vaginal spotting, mild abdominal pain, or dysuria. On examination, the cervix may appear edematous and may bleed easily when touched by a swab. There may be a mucopurulent discharge from the cervical os.

Urethritis. Screening studies in STD clinics suggest that >50% of women infected with *C. trachomatis* have coinfections at both the urethra and endocervix. The acute urethral syndrome of chlamydial urethritis is characterized by the finding of "sterile" pyuria for urine pathogens in the face of symptoms of dysuria and urinary frequency.

Pelvic Inflammatory Disease. Infections can ascend through the cervical os causing endometriosis and infection of the fallopian tubes. When the infection extends to the ovaries and peritoneal cavity, it can result in abscess formation. The symptom spectrum of PID ranges from acute, severe disease to asymptomatic or "silent" disease. Women with a history of PID can experience serious reproductive sequelae, including infertility, ectopic pregnancy, and chronic pelvic pain (see Chapter 63).

Perihepatitis (Fitz-Hugh-Curtis Syndrome). This syndrome can occur in up to 25% of women with PID and may be associated with chlamydial (70% of cases) and gonococcal salpingitis. Signs and symptoms include right-upper-quadrant pain and tenderness, fever, nausea, and vomiting. Women may also have signs of PID.

Pregnancy-Related Chlamydial Infections. Associated with adverse outcomes such as spontaneous miscarriage and premature delivery. Infected women can develop PID after vaginal delivery or after therapeutic abortion. Two thirds of infants born to infected mothers become colonized during delivery and may develop conjunctivitis or pneumonia.

Other Infections and Complications, Male and Female

Pharyngeal Colonization. *C. trachomatis* is isolated from the pharynx but causes few problems.

Conjunctivitis. Direct contact with infectious secretions during sexual activity or from autoinoculation can result in conjunctivitis. Symptoms usually include unilateral eye discharge, hyperemia, and pain.

Cardiac Complications. Rare cardiac complications include endocarditis and myocarditis.

Reiter Syndrome. The syndrome of conjunctivitis, dermatitis, urethritis, and arthritis occurs most frequently after a bacterial infection of the genital tract or gastrointestinal tract. Most individuals who develop Reiter syndrome are HLA-B27–positive and male.

DIFFERENTIAL DIAGNOSIS

Women

In women, mucopurulent cervicitis (MPC) or urethritis can also be caused by the following:

1. Infections such as *N. gonorrhoeae, Trichomonas vaginalis,* herpes simplex, human papillomavirus and other organisms such as *Escherichia coli*
2. Intrauterine device (IUD)
3. Allergic reaction to contraceptive foam, gel, or film
4. Idiopathic disease, such as local irritation due to feminine hygiene products, perfumes, or sexual activity

Men

The most common problem is urethritis, which can also be caused by the following:

1. Infections such as *N. gonorrhoeae, Ureaplasma urealyticum, T. vaginalis,* human papillomavirus, and herpes simplex

2. Allergic reaction to contraceptive foam, gel, or film
3. Idiopathic disease (see earlier description)

In men presenting with symptoms of acute epididymitis or orchitis, it is important to consider the following in the differential diagnosis:

1. Epididymitis can also be due to *N. gonorrhoea,* and gram-positive cocci.
2. Another important cause of an acute painful scrotal swelling in the sexually active male adolescent is torsion of the spermatic cord, which is a surgical emergency. Therefore, the workup for a painful scrotum should include both torsion and infectious etiology and must be done with urgency.

DIAGNOSIS

The introduction of nucleic acid amplification technology (NAATs) for the diagnosis of *C. trachomatis* now provides readily available, highly sensitive, inexpensive, and noninvasive screening tests. The newer testing technology allows noninvasive sampling of first-void urine and self-administered vaginal swabs to collect specimens. The focus for testing has broadened from testing symptomatic individuals to also screening at-risk asymptomatic individuals.

Collection of Specimens

Correct specimen collection and handling is essential for all testing methods. The preferred method of collection is dictated by the particular test's manufacturer's directives. Collection sites include endocervical, urethral, urine specimen, vaginal, rectal, conjunctival, and pharyngeal. See Table 62.2 for collection site comparisons based on test type.

1. All testing techniques can be applied to the endocervical and urethral specimens.
2. *To optimize the urine sample:* First-catch "dirty" sample (first 15 to 20 mL of micturition) should be used with specimen collection delayed until more than 1 hour after prior urination.
3. The U.S. Food and Drug Administration (FDA) recently approved the transcription-mediated amplification assay for chlamydial testing of vaginal samples.
4. For conjunctival samples, culture is preferred because of high sensitivity and specificity. Enzyme immunoassay (EIA), nucleic acid probe, and direct fluorescent antibody (DFA) tests are also FDA-cleared for use with conjunctival specimens.
5. Rectal specimens have not proved to be amenable to NAATs owing to inhibitors present in rectal specimens. Culture isolation is acceptable for detecting *C. trachomatis* in rectal or pharyngeal swab specimens. DFA can also be performed on rectal or pharyngeal swabs.
6. In general, urine specimen testing has lower sensitivity than cervical, urethral, or vaginal swab samples.

Laboratory Diagnosis

Chlamydia-Specific Tests. Testing technologies are summarized in Table 62.2.

TABLE 62.2

Comparison of C. trachomatis Testing Technologies

	Test Types	Preferred Test	Collection Site	Sensitivity	Specificity
Nucleic acid amplification technology (NAAT)	Ligase chain reaction (LCR) Polymerase chain reaction (PCR) Transcription-mediated amplification (TMA) Strand displacement amplification (SDA)	Yes	Male and female urine, endocervical and urethral swabs Vaginal swab (TMA)	80%–90%	>98%
Cell culture		No	Endocervical, urethral, rectal, conjunctival, nasopharyngeal	60%–80%	>99%
Direct fluorescent antibody (DFA)		No	Endocervical, urethral, rectal, conjunctival, nasopharyngeal	65%–75%	97%–99%
Enzyme immunoassay (EIA)		No	Endocervical, urethral, conjunctival	60%–75%	97%–99%
Nucleic acid probe	DNA probe hybridization Hybrid capture with signal amplification	No	Endocervical, urethral, conjunctival	65%–75%	98/99%

From Centers for Disease Control and Prevention: Screening Tests To Detect *Chlamydia trachomatis* and *Neisseria gonorrhoeae* Infections–2002. MMWR 2002:51.

California STD/HIV Prevention Training Center: Sexually transmitted chlamydial infections: A primary care clinician's guide to diagnosis, treatment and prevention, http://www.stdhivtraining.org/pdf/chlamydia.screen.pdf, Dec 2003.

Chlamydia-Nonspecific Tests

1. *Leukocyte esterase urine dipstick test (LET):* A nonspecific but inexpensive test that can be used as a first step to screen asymptomatic male patients. An LE dipstick reading of at least 1+ when applied to a first-catch urine is suggestive of infection and should be followed by more definitive testing.

2. *Serology:* There is no use for the application of serology in acute genital infection, as previous chlamydial infection frequently elicits long-lasting antibodies that cannot be easily distinguished from the antibodies produced in a current infection.

Who Should Be Tested for Chlamydial Infection?

Screening. According to national guidelines, all sexually active female adolescents aged 25 years and younger should be screened for *C. trachomatis* at least once a year. National guidelines do not yet specify a screening recommendation for male adolescents, but screening programs for male patients are currently being explored in high-prevalence populations.

Testing. In addition to the obvious teenage male or female patient who has genitourinary symptoms, adolescents on the street, in detention, who are paid for sex, who use intravenous drugs, who are pregnant, who are victims of sexual assault, who have chosen to have a therapeutic abortion, who have had prior STDs, who have new and multiple partners, and who do not use barrier contraception consistently should be considered for screening.

TREATMENT

Treatment guidelines and recommendations were derived from the 2006 CDC guidelines (see Chapter 60 and www.cdc.gov/STD/treatment/). Now that quinolones are not recommended for gonorrhea treatment, testing with culture or NAAT for gonorrhea is essential in treating *Chlamydia.*

Sex Partners. The CDC recommends that sex partners should be evaluated if they had sexual contact with the patient during the 60 days preceding onset of symptoms in the patient or diagnosis of *C. trachomatis.* The most recent sex partner should be treated even if the time interval is more than 60 days. Patients and their partners should avoid sexual contact until 7 days after completing single-dose treatment or following a 7-day antibiotic course. Partner-delivered treatment may be considered.

For pelvic inflammatory disease, see Chapters 60 and 63. For epididymitis, see Chapters 60 and 28.

WEB SITES AND REFERENCES

http://www.emedicine.com/emerg/topic925.htm. E-medicine article on *Chlamydia.*

http://www.cdc.gov/std/chlamydia/. CDC link to *Chlamydia* facts, 2004 surveillance statistics, and 2006 treatment guidelines.

http://www.niaid.nih.gov/factsheets/stdclam.htm. National Institutes of Health (NIH) fact sheet on *Chlamydia.*

Hwang L, Shafer MA. *Chlamydia trachomatis* infection in adolescents. *Adv Pediatr* 2004;51:379.

Centers for Disease Control and Prevention. Sexually Transmitted Diseases Treatment Guidelines, 2006. *MMWR* 2006;55 (No. RR-11):40. www.cdc.gov/STD/treatment/.

Olshen E, Shrier LA. Diagnostic tests for chamydial and gonorrheal infections. *Semin Pediatr Infect Dis* 2005;16:192.

CHAPTER 63

Pelvic Inflammatory Disease

Lydia A. Shrier

Pelvic inflammatory disease (PID) is an ascending polymicrobial infection of the female upper genital tract and includes endometritis, parametritis, salpingitis, oophoritis, tuboovarian abscess (TOA), peritonitis, and perihepatitis. *Neisseria gonorrhoeae* and *Chlamydia trachomatis* are usually the causative agents of PID, but vaginal and enteric microorganisms also contribute to its pathogenesis. Nearly 20% of women with PID experience at least one long-term consequence, such as chronic pelvic pain, ectopic pregnancy, or infertility.

Etiology

Risk Factors. These include (1) age; (2) cervical ectropion (transition zone is highly susceptible to sexually transmitted diseases (STDs)); (3) lower levels of cervical secretory immunoglobulin A; (4) cervicitis with *N. gonorrhoeae* or *C. trachomatis;* (5) sexual and other risk behaviors (unprotected intercourse, frequent intercourse, multiple sex partners, intercourse during menses, smoking, alcohol and other drug use, and douching); (6) young age at first intercourse; (7) previous PID (increases the risk 2.3-fold); (8) nonwhite race; (9) contraceptive methods—decreased risk of PID (consistent condom use, spermicides and probably oral contraceptives); increased risk of PID (women who have a STD at the time of the insertion of an intrauterine contraceptive device (IUCD) have a greater, although still low, risk of PID than women who are free of infection); (10) bacterial vaginosis (may facilitate ascension to the upper genital tract of organisms pathogenic for PID); (11) menses.

Microbiology

Polymicrobial infection that usually begins with a sexually transmitted organism such as *N. gonorrhoeae* or *C. trachomatis* but involves other organisms as well, such as *Bacteroides* species and other anaerobes; *Escherichia coli, Streptococcus* species, and other facultative bacteria; *Mycoplasma hominis* and *Ureaplasma urealyticum.*

Pathogenesis

1. Lower tract infection with *N. gonorrhoeae* or *C. trachomatis.*
2. Normal vaginal lactobacilli are supplanted by anaerobes, facultative bacteria, and genital mycoplasmas.

3. Inflammatory disruption of the cervical barrier facilitates ascension of the inciting sexually transmitted pathogens and other microorganisms from the vagina into the normally sterile uterus.
4. Decreased tubal motility secondary to inflammation results in collection of fluid (hydrosalpinx) or pus (pyosalpinx) within the tube.
5. Spillage of infected contents from the tubal fimbriae into the peritoneal cavity may result in peritonitis, perihepatitis (Fitz-Hugh-Curtis syndrome), TOA, and adhesions.

Presenting Signs and Symptoms

The classic presentation is seen in only about one in five laparoscopically verified cases of PID: (1) lower abdominal or pelvic pain; (2) abnormal vaginal and/or cervical discharge; (3) fever and chills; (4) leukocytosis; (5) increased erthrocyte sedimentation rate (ESR).

Subclinical infection likely accounts for most cases of PID.

Other history, signs, and symptoms compatible with a diagnosis of PID include (1) abnormal, painful vaginal bleeding; (2) onset of symptoms within 1 week of menses; (3) gastrointestinal symptoms; (4) dysuria or urinary frequency; (5) dyspareunia; (6) a sexual partner with recent urethritis.

Findings on Physical Examination

1. *Vital signs:* Fever and tachycardia
2. *Abdomen:* Lower abdominal tenderness with or without rebound and guarding
3. *Pelvic examination:* (a) abnormal vaginal or cervical discharge; (b) friable, inflamed cervix; (c) cervical motion tenderness; (d) adnexal tenderness (unilateral or bilateral); (e) palpation of an adnexal mass; (f) uterine tenderness

Laboratory and Radiological Evaluation

No single test is diagnostic of PID. The following tests should be considered:

1. *White blood cell (WBC) count:* Elevated
2. *ESR (or C-reactive protein (CPR)):* Elevated
3. *Neutrophils on saline wet mount of vaginal secretions:* The absence of any leukocytes in the secretions suggests a diagnosis other than PID.
4. *Microbiological tests for N. gonorrhoeae and C. trachomatis:* Presumptive diagnosis and treatment of PID should not await microbiological test results. Positive results for *N. gonorrhoeae* or *C. trachomatis* support but does not confirm the diagnosis of PID and negative results do not eliminate the diagnosis.
   a. Collect samples and send to the laboratory before initiating antibiotic therapy.
   b. Because a pelvic examination is required for the diagnosis of PID, endocervical, rather than vaginal or urine samples, are preferred.
   c. The preferred test for *N. gonorrhoeae* in patients with suspected PID is either endocervical cell culture or a nucleic acid amplification test (NAAT).
   d. The preferred test for *C. trachomatis* in patients with suspected PID is a NAAT.
5. *Urinalysis and urine culture*
6. *Urine pregnancy test.* If positive, an ectopic pregnancy must be considered.
7. *Human immunodeficiency virus (HIV) testing*

8. *Pelvic ultrasonography:* If the clinician cannot adequately assess the adnexa, palpates an adnexal mass, or questions the presence of an ectopic pregnancy or TOA.
9. *Laparoscopy:* Indicated diagnostically in the patient whose pain does not respond to antibiotic therapy and therapeutically in the patient with a persistent TOA.

Diagnosis

The timely and accurate diagnosis of PID is essential in preventing sequelae. The differential diagnosis is broad (Table 63.1).

The Centers for Disease Control and Prevention (CDC) criteria for the diagnosis of PID are listed in Table 63.2. PID should be considered as a likely

TABLE 63.1

Differential Diagnosis of Pelvic Inflammatory Disease

Gastrointestinal
  Appendicitis
  Cholecystitis
  Cholelithiasis
  Constipation
  Diverticulitis
  Gastroenteritis
  Hernia
  Inflammatory bowel disease
  Irritable bowel syndrome
Gynecological
  Corpus luteum cyst
  Dysmenorrhea
  Ectopic pregnancy
  Endometriosis
  Mittelschmerz
  Ovarian
    Cyst
    Torsion
    Tumor
  Pregnancy
    Ectopic
    Spontaneous, septic, or threatened abortion
    Postabortion endometritis
Urological
  Cystitis
  Nephrolithiasis
  Pyelonephritis
  Urethritis
Musculoskeletal
Rheumatologic/autoimmune
Psychiatric

TABLE 63.2

Centers for Disease Control and Prevention Diagnostic Criteria for Pelvic Inflammatory Disease

Minimum criteria (initiate treatment in females at risk for STDs and
  complaining of lower abdominal pain when one or more clinical sign is
  present and no other diagnosis is apparent)
  Cervical motion tenderness, OR
  Uterine tenderness, OR
  Adnexal tenderness
Additional criteria (support a diagnosis of PID)
  Oral temperature >101°F (>38.3°C)
  Abnormal cervical or vaginal mucopurulent discharge
  Presence of abundant numbers of white blood cells on saline
  microscopy of vaginal secretions
  Elevated erythrocyte sedimentation rate
  Elevated C-reactive protein level
  Laboratory documentation of cervical infection with *N. gonorrhoeae* or
    C. trachomatis
Definitive criteria (warranted in selected cases)
  Endometrial biopsy with histopathological evidence of endometritis
  Transvaginal sonography or magnetic resonance imaging techniques
    showing thickened, fluid-filled tubes with or without free pelvic fluid or
    tuboovarian complex, or Doppler studies suggesting pelvic infection
    (e.g., tubal hyperemia)
  Laparoscopic abnormalities consistent with PID

diagnosis in any woman with pelvic tenderness and signs or symptoms of lower genital tract inflammation. Empiric treatment should be initiated in young women at risk for STDs if any of the minimum criteria are present and no other cause(s) for the illness can be identified.

The CDC urges that clinicians maintain a low threshold for the diagnosis and empiric treatment of PID. However, because incorrect diagnosis and management can cause unnecessary morbidity, more elaborate diagnostic criteria may be used to enhance the specificity of the minimum criteria.

Therapy

Refer to treatment guidelines in Chapter 60 and www.cdc.gov/std/treatment. Fluoroquinolones are no longer recommended for the treatment of PID owing to increased prevalence of gonococcal resistance. CDC criteria for hospitalization include (1) surgical emergencies such as appendicitis; (2) pregnancy; (3) poor response to oral antimicrobial therapy; (4) inability to follow or tolerate an outpatient oral regimen; (5) severe illness, nausea and vomiting, or high fever; (6) TOA (at least 24 hours inpatient followed by outpatient antimicrobial therapy for a total of 14 days); (7) immunodeficiency.

Other reasons to consider hospitalization of the adolescent with suspected PID include age <15 years, abortion or other gynecologic surgery procedure within previous 14 days, a history of a previous episode of PID, and other extenuating medical or social circumstances that may preclude receipt of appropriate treatment as an outpatient. Among women with mild-to-moderate PID, there does not appear to be any difference in reproductive outcomes between inpatient and outpatient treatment.

Consequences

(1) Recurrence; (2) TOA; (3) infertility; (4) ectopic pregnancy; (5) chronic abdominal pain

WEB SITES AND REFERENCES

http://www.cdc.gov/STD/treatment 2006. CDC STD Treatment Guidelines.

Centers for Disease Control and Prevention. Sexually transmitted diseases treatment guidelines, 2006. *MMWR Recomm Rep* 2006;55(RR11).

http://www.emedicine.com/med/topic1774.htm. eMedicine Web site.

Shrier LA. Bacterial sexually transmitted infections: gonorrhea, chlamydia, pelvic inflammatory disease, and syphilis. In: Emans SJ, Laufer MR, Goldstein DP, eds. *Pediatric and Adolescent Gynecology,* 5th ed. Philadelphia: Lippincott Williams & Wilkins, 2005:565.

Trent M, Ellen JM, Walker A. Pelvic inflammatory disease in adolescents: care delivery in pediatric ambulatory settings. *Pediatr Emerg Care* 2005;21:431.

CHAPTER 64

Syphilis

J. Dennis Fortenberry and Lawrence S. Neinstein

ETIOLOGY

The agent causing syphilis is *Treponema pallidum,* a motile, spiral microorganism. The organisms do not stain well, are best visualized by dark-field microscopy, and do not grow in artificial media. Most infections are contracted during sexual contact, including kissing and sexual intercourse. Rare cases occur from direct contact with infectious cutaneous or mucous membrane lesions. Rashes are not infectious if the skin is intact. Other modes of transmission include congenital and transfusion-related transmission. The estimated rate of transmission after sexual exposure to a person with a chancre is 30%. The risk of transmission persists during the first 4 years of untreated syphilis. Latent syphilis, neurosyphilis, and tertiary syphilis are rare in adolescents.

CLINICAL MANIFESTATIONS

Primary Syphilis

Syphilis should be considered in the differential diagnosis of any ulcerating lesion of the anogenital or oral areas and occasionally of the breasts, face, and fingers. Syphilis is characterized by a chancre at the point of inoculation 9 to 90 days (mean 21 days) after contact.

1. *Location:* (a) Ninety-five percent are on the external genitalia. (b) Single lesions are typical but multiple lesions are common. (c) They may appear as "kissing lesions."
2. The ulcer typically has a punched-out (1- to 2-cm), clean appearance, with elevated, firm margins.
3. *Regional adenopathy:* firm, nonsuppurative, and bilateral and may be painless.
4. *Healing:* The chancre heals in 3 to 6 weeks.

The primary infection may manifest itself with an inconspicuous lesion, particularly in women. Infection may occur with no papule or ulcer at all, particularly in previously infected patients.

Secondary Syphilis

Develops approximately 6 to 8 weeks (maximum 6 months) after exposure and 4 to 10 weeks after the onset of the chancre. During this stage, *T. pallidum* can be identified in lesions and body fluids (i.e., lesions are infectious). The signs and symptoms of secondary syphilis usually disappear after weeks or months. Up to 25% of patients with untreated secondary syphilis develop relapses of secondary disease, with about one fourth of these having multiple relapses. Signs and symptoms include the following:

1. *General skin eruption (90%):* (a) seen on the trunk and extremities; (b) palms and soles may be scaly and hyperkeratotic and the last to clear; (c) lesions appear on skin as well as mucous membranes; (d) lines of cleavage are noted; (e) lesions are bilateral and symmetric; (f) individual lesions are sharply demarcated, 0.5 to 2.0 cm, with a reddish-brown hue; (g) most commonly they are macular, papular, or papulosquamous—rarely follicular, vesicular, and pustular rashes; (h) typically eruptions are nonpruritic but sometimes pruritic; (i) they last a few weeks to 12 months; (j) almost any type of rash may be seen, including acneform, herpetiform, and psoriatic. Lesions in intertriginous areas may erode and fissure, especially in the nasolabial folds and near the corners of the mouth and moist areas; hypertrophic granulomatous lesions (condylomata lata) occur.
2. *General or regional lymphadenopathy (about 70%):* (a) nonpainful nodes; (b) rubbery, hard-feeling, discrete, with no suppuration; (c) occasional hepatosplenomegaly.
3. *Flulike syndrome (about 50%):* (a) sore throat and malaise most common; (b) headaches; (c) lacrimation; (d) nasal discharge; (e) arthralgias and myalgias; (f) weight loss; (g) fever.
4. *Syphilis alopecia (uncommon):* moth-eaten alopecia of the scalp and eyebrows.
5. *Other rare manifestations:* (a) arthritis or bursitis; (b) hepatitis; (c) iritis and anterior uveitis; (d) glomerulonephritis.

DIFFERENTIAL DIAGNOSIS

Primary Syphilis

Sexually Transmitted Causes of Genital Ulcers. The most common sexually transmitted genital ulcers in the United States are herpes, syphilis, and chancroid, in that order. Lymphogranuloma venereum and Donovanosis (granuloma inguinale) are rare in the United States.

1. *Herpes simplex:* Usually painful, multiple lesions beginning as vesicles on an erythematous base. Primary lesions are usually bilateral, extensive, and associated with tender adenopathy.
2. *Chancroid:* Usually painful lesions with a deep purulent base and often erythematous borders. Local lymph nodes are often fluctuant and tender.
3. *Lymphogranuloma venereum:* The primary lesion may be a nonindurated, herpetiform ulcer that heals rapidly. Many patients present with advanced disease, including fever and massive regional adenopathy.

Non–Sexually Transmitted Causes of Genital Ulcers. The most common nonsexually transmitted cause is trauma: (1) traumatic lesions; (2) fixed drug reaction; (3) *Candida* balanitis; (4) Behçet syndrome; (5) psoriasis; (6) lichen planus; (7) erythema multiforme; (8) cancer (rare).

Secondary Syphilis. (1) psoriasis; (2) pityriasis rosea; (3) drug eruptions; (4) tinea versicolor; (5) alopecia areata; (6) lichen planus; (7) viremia; (8) lupus erythematosus;(9) scabies; (10) pediculosis; (11) rosacea; (12) infectious mononucleosis; (13) keratoderma blennorrhagica; (14) condyloma acuminatum. A Venereal Disease Research Laboratory (VDRL) or rapid plasma reagin (RPR) test should be performed in these conditions whenever doubt exists.

DIAGNOSIS

Adolescents should also be screened during pregnancy or when diagnosed with other sexually transmitted infections. In certain lower-risk groups, such as college students, the criteria for screening syphilis serology will have to be re-evaluated as prevalence rates fall.

Laboratory Findings

Dark-Field Examination. The dark-field examination is used in evaluating moist ulcers and lesions such as a chancre or condyloma lata. Technique is as follows: (1) Clean lesion with saline and gauze. (2) Abrade gently with dry gauze. Avoid inducing bleeding, which makes dark-field examination more difficult. (3) Squeeze lesion (with gloves) to express serous transudate. (4) Place a drop of transudate on a slide. (5) Place a drop of saline on the transudate and cover with a cover slip. (6) Examine under dark-field microscope. (7) For internal lesions, a bacteriologic loop can be used to transfer the fluid to a slide. (8) For lymph node aspirations, Clean the skin, inject 0.2 mL or less of sterile saline, and aspirate the node. Place the fluid on a slide.

Direct Fluorescent Antibody. Specimens from primary lesions can also be sent to reference laboratories or some state health departments for direct fluorescent antibody (DFA) staining. These specimens can be collected as described previously; however, saline should not be added to the slides, and they should be allowed to air-dry. Sensitivity depends on technique, age of lesions, and experience of laboratory personnel.

Serologic Tests

1. *Nontreponemal antibody tests:* Tests for a nonspecific anticardiolipin antibody that forms in response to surface lipids on the treponeme.
   a. *Types:* (1) agglutination: RPR; (2) floculation: VDRL.
   b. *Use:* Nontreponemal tests should be used for screening and to monitor treatment success. Nontreponemal test titers correlate with disease activity and fall after treatment. A fourfold change in titer, equivalent to a change of two dilutions (e.g., from 1:8 to 1:32 or 1:16 to 1:4), demonstrates substantial change of the same test.
2. *Specific treponemal antibody tests.*
   a. *Types:* (1) Immunofluorescence: FTA-ABS is used to confirm a positive result from RPR or VDRL. (2) Microhemagglutination: The *T. pallidum*

particle agglutination (TP-PA) test has replaced the FTA-ABS test as the specific treponemal test to confirm a positive result from VDRL. (3) Enzyme-linked immunosorbent assay (ELISA): used by some blood banks for donor screening.

b. *Use:* Treponemal tests are specific and sensitive, but because of their expense and more difficult technical requirement, they are used to confirm positive results from a screening test. Once positive, the patient usually remains positive for life. Titers are unrelated to disease activity or treatment. Treponemal antibody titers should be recorded as reactive, nonreactive, or minimally reactive. A minimally reactive test result may represent a false-positive finding and should be repeated.

3. *Sensitivity*

a. The sensitivity of nontreponemal tests (RPR and VDRL) in primary syphilis ranges from 60% to 90%, depending on the duration of infection and the population under study. Results are positive at the following times: (i) onset of primary chancre (About 25% of individuals are positive); (ii) 2 weeks after chancre appearance (50% are positive); (iii) 3 weeks after chancre appearance (75% are positive); (iv) 4 weeks after chancre appearance (100% are positive).

b. Treponemal tests (TP-PA and FTA-ABS) are positive in 80% to 100% of primary syphilis. Sensitivity of nontreponemal and treponemal tests approaches 100% in secondary syphilis.

4. *False-positive serology test results:* About 20% to 40% of all positive nontreponemal test results are false-positive results, as shown by a nonreactive treponemal test. Most false-positive nontreponemal test results show a low titer (dilution <1:8), and the probability of a false-positive finding decreases with increasing titer. The causes of false-positive test results include the following: (a) acute infection: viral infections, chlamydial infections, Lyme disease, *Mycoplasma* infections, nonsyphilitic spirochetal infections, and various bacterial, fungal, and protozoal infections; (b) autoimmune diseases; (c) narcotic addiction; (d) aging; (e) Hashimoto thyroiditis; (f) sarcoidosis; (g) lymphoma; (h) leprosy; (i) cirrhosis of the liver; (j) HIV infection: can lead to unusually high, unusually low, or fluctuating titers.

5. *Tests most commonly used:* (a) RPR (screening and quantitative measurement of clinical activity); (b) VDRL (quantitative measurement to assess clinical activity and response to therapy or qualitative test for screening); (c) TP-PA or FTA-ABS (to confirm diagnosis in a patient with a positive result from VDRL or RPR); (d) Other tests under development are based on PCR or enzyme-linked Immunospot testing for treponeme-specific antibody-secreting cells.

Diagnosis by Stage

Primary Syphilis. (1) Definitive diagnosis of early syphilis requires a positive dark-field examination or DFA test of lesion transudate or tissue. (2) Presumptive diagnosis relies on a positive nontreponemal test (VDRL or RPR) with a high titer (1:8 or higher) or rising titer (more than two dilutions) *and* a positive treponemal test result (e.g., FTA-ABS or MHA-TP). Adolescents with a positive dark-field examination should be treated, as should those with a typical lesion and a positive serologic test result. Sexual partners (within the previous 90 days) of persons with documented infection should also be treated. If the initial serologic test result is negative, it should be repeated 1 week, 1 month, and 3 months later in suspected cases. Lumbar puncture is not recommended for routine evaluation of primary syphilis unless clinical signs and symptoms of neurologic involvement are present.

Secondary Syphilis. (1) Dark-field examination of material from lesions or lymph nodes. (2) VDRL or RPR. An adolescent should be treated if the dark-field examination result is positive or if the patient has typical findings of secondary syphilis and a positive result from VDRL or RPR. Adolescents with atypical findings or a quantitative nontreponemal titer <1:16 should have a second quantitative nontreponemal test and an FTA-ABS or MHA-TP test.

Syphilis in Pregnancy. All pregnant adolescents should be screened early in pregnancy, during the third trimester, and again at delivery in areas or populations with a high prevalence of syphilis. A woman delivering a stillborn infant after 20 weeks' gestation should also be tested for syphilis.

Syphilis and HIV. Ulcerative lesions such as syphilitic chancres increase the risk of transmission of HIV. There is also evidence that infection with HIV alters the serologic response to syphilis. There have been reports of patients who were coinfected with HIV and syphilis and had unusual serologic responses, such as higher than expected serologic titers, but false-negative serologic test results have also been reported. Most treponemal and nontreponemal serologic tests for syphilis are accurate for the majority of individuals with both syphilis and HIV infection. If serologic tests are not consistent with clinical findings, alternative tests, such as biopsy and DFA staining of lesion material, should be considered. HIV-infected individuals with neurologic disease should be evaluated for neurosyphilis, but lumbar puncture in the routine evaluation of primary syphilis is controversial.

Treatment of Primary and Secondary Syphilis

See Chapter 60 and www.cdc.gov/STD/treatment/. Adolescents treated for gonorrhea or chlamydial infection with ceftriaxone, doxycycline, and azithromycin are probably covered for incubating syphilis. If a different regimen is used, a second serologic test for syphilis should be performed in 3 months.

1. *Other considerations:* (a) All patients with syphilis should be tested for HIV initially and at 3 months. (b) Those individuals with signs or symptoms that suggest neurologic or ophthalmic disease should be evaluated by cerebrospinal fluid (CSF) analysis or slit-lamp examination, respectively. Routine lumbar puncture is not recommended for individuals with primary or secondary syphilis unless clinical signs and symptoms suggest neurologic involvement.
2. *Follow-up:* (a) Infected individuals should be reexamined clinically and serologic test results should be rechecked at 3 and 6 months. Quantitative nontreponemal tests should be used because the FTA-ABS results usually remain positive throughout the individual's life. If signs or symptoms persist or nontreponemal antibody titers have not decreased fourfold by 6 months, the patient should have a CSF examination and HIV test and be retreated. By 1 year, 75% to 95% of individuals with secondary syphilis are seronegative. The drop in titers for primary and secondary syphilis applies only to first episodes of primary or secondary syphilis; those with reinfections have less

predictable serologic drops. (b) Individuals are at risk for treatment failure if their nontreponemal titers have not declined fourfold by 3 months after treatment for primary or secondary syphilis. HIV testing should be performed at 3 months in these individuals. (c) Retreatment should probably include three weekly injections of benzathine penicillin G 2.4 million units IM unless neurosyphilis is present.

3. *Infants should be followed closely:* (a) Seropositive infants untreated during the perinatal period: These infants must be observed closely at 1, 2, 3, 6, and 12 months after therapy. Nontreponemal titers should decline by 3 months of age and be absent by 6 months. If antibody titers do not follow this pattern, the child should be reevaluated, including a CSF examination, and treated. (b) Treated infants must be monitored closely every 2 to 3 months. The titers should become nonreactive by 6 months of age, but they may fall more slowly in infants treated after the neonatal period. Infants with cells in the CSF on initial examination should have a second CSF examination at 6 months or until the cell count is normal. The infant should be retreated if the cell count does not show a downward trend or is not normal by 2 years. The CSF-VDRL should also be checked at 6 months and the infant retreated if the test is still reactive.

HIV-Infected Individuals. Among HIV-positive individuals, there have been reports of higher rates of neurologic complications and treatment failures with traditional regimens for syphilis. There have also been cases in HIV-positive patients of rapid progress of syphilis into secondary and tertiary stages. However, no treatment regimens have yet been demonstrated to be more effective in treating HIV-infected individuals than those used in patients without HIV infection. HIV-positive patients with syphilis require careful evaluation, including CSF evaluation, for late and unusual manifestations of syphilis.

Jarisch-Herxheimer Reaction. A dramatic reaction occurs within 2 hours after treatment in 50% of patients with primary syphilis, 90% of those with secondary syphilis, and 25% of those with early latent syphilis. The reaction consists of the following: (1) fever and chills, (2) myalgias, (3) headache, (4) elevated neutrophil count, (5) tachycardia. The duration of symptoms is 12 to 24 hours, and treatment is reassurance, bed rest, and aspirin. The reaction can induce transient uterine contractions in pregnant women; during the second half of pregnancy, it can lead to premature labor or fetal distress.

WEB SITES

http://www.cdc.gov/std/Syphilis/STDFact-Syphilis.htm. CDC site on syphilis.

http://www.drkoop.com/ency/93/001327.html. Dr. Koop's site on syphilis.

http://www.cdc.gov/STD/treatment/. The CDC Web site with recent statistics and treatment guidelines.

http://www.ashastd.org. The American Social Health Association home page—lots of information and hotline access.

http://www.niaid.nih.gov/factsheets/stdsyph.htm. National Institute of Allergy and Infectious Diseases fact sheet from National Institutes of Health.

CHAPTER 65

Herpes Genitalis

Gale R. Burstein and Kimberly A. Workowski

Genital herpes is a chronic, lifelong viral disease. Herpes genitalis lesions are caused by a large DNA virus, herpes simplex virus (HSV), with two serotypes, herpes simplex type 1 (HSV-1) and herpes simplex type 2 (HSV-2). These viruses have the ability to become latent and recur.

EPIDEMIOLOGY

Incidence and Prevalence

1. HSV is the most common cause of genital ulcerative disease in the United States, but most people with serologic evidence of infection are asymptomatic.
2. HSV-2 prevalence varies by age, gender, and race.
   a. An estimated 1.6% of 14- to 19-year-olds and 11% of 20- to 29-year-olds are HSV-2–seropositive.
   b. Estimated HSV-2 seroprevalence rates are higher among women and blacks.

Recurrences. Symptomatic recurrent episodes and asymptomatic viral shedding are more likely following primary HSV-2 infection than after HSV-1.

Transmission. Transmission is through sexual contact, either genital–genital or oral–genital, and by mucosal contact with infected secretions. Viral shedding is highest in the presence of genital lesions. Most HSV-2 sexual transmission occurs on days without source partner genital lesions.

SEROLOGIC TYPES

1. *HSV-1:* Infection typically manifests as oral–labial lesions, but the frequency of HSV-1 genital infection is increasing. Recurrences and subclinical shedding are much less frequent than with genital HSV-2 infection.
2. *HSV-2:* Infection typically manifests as anogenital lesions.

CLINICAL MANIFESTATIONS

Definition of Terms

1. *Primary infection:* Genital herpes in a patient seronegative for antibody to HSV-1 or HSV-2.

2. *First clinical episode:* First episode of clinical manifestations due to HSV-1 or HSV-2 infection. This term includes both nonprimary first episodes (i.e., positive serology) and primary infections.
3. *Recurrent clinical episode:* Recurrence of genital HSV lesions in a patient with a previously documented symptomatic genital herpes episode.
4. *Atypical clinical episode:* Episode of clinical manifestations due to HSV-1 or HSV-2 infection that do not include classic genital lesions.

Classic Primary Infection

1. Involves both systemic and local symptoms.
2. Clinical manifestations begin approximately a week following initial infection.
3. Systemic symptoms may include fever, headache, malaise, and myalgias.
4. Local symptoms may include painful lesions, dysuria, pruritus, vaginal or urethral discharge, and tender inguinal adenopathy.
   a. Herpetic lesions usually begin as small papules or vesicles on an erythematous base that rapidly spread over the genital area. Multiple small pustular lesions coalesce into large areas of ulceration. Pain and irritation from lesions usually peak between days 7 and 11 of disease and heal over the second week. Crusting and re-epithelization occurs in the penile and mons area, but there is no crusting on mucosal surfaces. New crops of lesions can form. Lesions typically are healed by the end of the third week of disease.
5. CNS complaints may occur.
6. Median duration of viral shedding is 12 days.

Recurrent Episodes

1. Clinical manifestations are localized to the genital region and are comparably mild to moderate.
2. Episode usually last from 6 to 12 days.
3. Prodromal symptoms can occur.
4. Lesions are often fewer and unilateral, involving a much smaller area in predominantly nonmucosal skin and healing by the second week of disease.
5. In untreated patients, viral shedding lasts approximately 4 days.
6. After the first year, recurrences typically decrease in frequency.

Atypical Episodes

1. Atypical episodes may occur as either a primary infection or a recurrent episode.
2. Episodes may present with genital pruritus, nontender papules, or fissures, dysuria, urethritis, or cervicitis.

DIFFERENTIAL DIAGNOSIS

Herpes genitalis lesions must be differentiated from early syphilis, chancroid, lymphogranuloma venereum, granuloma inguinale, excoriations, allergic and irritant contact dermatitis, and Behçet syndrome lesions.

DIAGNOSIS

Genital herpes is the most prevalent cause of genital ulcers in the United States. Clinical diagnosis should be confirmed by laboratory testing.

Laboratory Evaluation

Virologic Tests. Isolation of HSV in cell culture is the preferred virologic test. Sensitivity of culture may be low in recurrent lesions and declines rapidly as lesions begin to heal. Polymerase chain reaction (PCR) HSV DNA assays are more sensitive and may be used instead of viral culture; however, PCR tests are not FDA-cleared for testing of genital specimens. As viral shedding is intermittent, lack of HSV detection does not indicate lack of HSV infection. Both PCR and viral culture should be typed to identify HSV-1 or HSV-2. Cytologic detection of cellular changes of herpes virus infection both in genital lesions (Tzanck preparation) and cervical Pap smears should not be used.

Type-Specific Serologic Tests. HSV antibodies develop during the first several weeks following infection and persist indefinitely. Accurate type-specific assays for HSV antibodies must be based on the HSV-specific glycoprotein G2 for the diagnosis of HSV-2 infection and glycoprotein G1 for diagnosis of HSV-1 infection. Older assays that do not accurately distinguish HSV-1 from HSV-2 antibody remain commercially available.

Currently, the FDA-approved laboratory gG-based type-specific tests include HerpeSelect-1 ELISA IgG, HerpeSelect2 ELISA IgG and HerpeSelect1 and 2 Immunoblot IgG (Focus Diagnostics, Inc., Cypress, CA); and CAPTIA HSV 1 IgG Type Specific EIA and CAPTIA HSV 2 IgG Type Specific EIA (Trinity Biotech, Bray, Ireland). The FDA-approved point-of-care tests include the BiokitHSV-2 Rapid Test (Biokit USA, Lexington, MA) and SureVue HSV-2 Rapid Test (Fisher HealthCare, Houston, TX). The sensitivities of these tests for detection of HSV-2 antibody vary from 80% to 98%, and the specificities are $\geq$96%. Type-specific HSV serologic assays may be useful in the following situations: (1) recurrent or atypical genital symptoms with negative HSV cultures, (2) a clinical diagnosis of genital herpes without laboratory confirmation, and (3) a sex partner with genital herpes. Some experts believe that HSV serologic testing should be included in a comprehensive sexually transmitted disease (STD) evaluation, for persons with multiple sexual partners, for HIV-infected persons, and for men who have sex with men at high HIV-risk. HSV-1 or HSV-2 screening in the general population is not indicated.

Additional Laboratory Workup. Additional genital ulcer evaluation should include a syphilis test; in settings where chancroid is prevalent, a *Haemophilus ducreyi* culture; and a gonorrhea, *Chlamydia, Trichomonas,* and HIV test.

THERAPY

See Chapter 60 and www.cdc.gov/STD/treatment.

Principles of Genital Herpes Management. Systemic antiviral chemotherapy is the mainstay of management. Topical antiviral therapy for genital HSV is not recommended. Counseling regarding the natural history of genital herpes, sexual and perinatal transmission, and methods to reduce transmission is integral to clinical management.

First Clinical Episode of Genital Herpes. See Chapter 60 for CDC Treatment Guidelines and http://www.cdc.gov/STD/treatment.

Established HSV-2 Infection. Treatment options (see Chapter 60) should be discussed with all patients regardless of recurrent outbreak severity or frequency. Recurrent genital herpes antiviral therapy can be administered either episodically, to diminish or shorten the duration of lesions, or continuously, as suppressive therapy to reduce the frequency of recurrences and possibly decrease the risk of transmission to susceptible partners.

Suppressive Therapy for Recurrent Genital Herpes. Suppressive therapy (see Chapter 60) reduces the frequency of genital herpes recurrences. Since recurrent outbreak frequency may diminish over time, continued therapy should be discussed periodically.

Episodic Therapy for Recurrent Genital Herpes. Effective recurrent herpes episodic treatment (see Chapter 60) requires therapy initiation within 1 day of lesion onset or during the prodrome. In those with known genital infection, a supply of drug or a prescription can be provided with instructions to self-initiate treatment immediately when symptoms begin.

Severe Disease. Intravenous acyclovir therapy should be provided for patients who have severe disease or complications that necessitate hospitalization. The recommended regimen is acyclovir 5 to 10 mg/kg body weight IV every 8 hours for 2 to 7 days or until clinical improvement is observed, followed by oral antiviral therapy to complete at least 10 days total therapy.

HIV Infection. Lesions caused by HSV are common among HIV-infected patients and may be severe, painful, and atypical. HSV shedding is increased in HIV infected persons. Subclinical mucosal HSV is associated with higher loads of mucosal HIV. Oral antiviral agent suppressive or episodic therapy is effective in decreasing HSV clinical manifestations of among HIV-seropositive persons. HIV-infected persons are likely to be more contagious; the extent to which suppressive antiviral therapy will decrease HSV transmission is unknown. Some experts suggest that type-specific serologies should be offered to HIV infected persons during their initial evaluation and suppressive antiviral therapy be considered. (See CDC Treatment Guidelines and www.cdc.gov/STD/treatment.)

Management of Sex Partners. The sex partners are likely to benefit from evaluation and counseling.

PREVENTION

Sexual transmission of HSV can occur during asymptomatic periods. Persons with active lesions or prodromal symptoms should abstain from intercourse with uninfected partners until the lesions are clearly healed. Providers should recommend consistent and correct condoms use to any patient who has had a genital herpes episode. Male latex condoms may reduce the risk of HSV acquisition and infection. Treatment with valacyclovir 500 mg daily decreases the rate of HSV-2 transmission in discordant heterosexual couples in which the source partner has a history of genital HSV-2 infection.

COMPLICATIONS

1. Significant psychological distress.
2. Local: Extragenital lesions, secondary bacterial infection of lesions, phimosis (men) or labial adhesions (women), urinary retention, constipation, and impotence. Sacral radiculopathy can also occur, causing paresthesias in the lower extremities.
3. Others complications may include proctitis, herpes keratitis, encephalitis and meningitis, disseminated disease, and neonatal herpes.

WEB SITES AND REFERENCES

http://www.ashastd.org/. American Social Health Association Herpes Resource Center.

http://www.cdc.gov/std/Herpes/default.htm. CDC Web site for statistics, fact sheets and treatment.

http://plannedparenthood.org/. Planned parenthood site.

http://www.cdc.gov/STD/treatment. Centers for Disease Control and Prevention. Sexually transmitted diseases treatment guidelines 2006. *MMWR* 2006;55(RR11):16.

Wald A, Langenberg AGM, Krantz E, et al. The relationship between condom use and herpes simplex virus acquisition. *Ann Intern Med* 2005;143:707.

Xu F, Sternberg MR, Kottiri BJ, et al. Trends in herpes simplex virus type 1 and type 2 seroprevalence in the United States. *JAMA* 2006;296:964.

CHAPTER 66

Human Papillomavirus Infection and Anogenital Warts

Jessica A. Kahn

Human papillomavirus (HPV) is the most prevalent sexually transmitted disease (STD) in the United States and may cause anogenital warts, oral warts, recurrent respiratory papillomatosis (RRP), abnormal Pap tests, cervical intraepithelial neoplasia, and cervical cancer.

HPV Genotypes and Clinical Sequelae

Human papillomaviruses are small, nonenveloped, double-stranded DNA viruses of the Papillomaviridae family. Approximately 40 mucosal types that cause diseases of the anogenital and aerodigestive tracts have been identified. Low-risk HPV types (e.g., types 6 and 11) cause anogenital warts and also may cause mild vulvar intraepithelial neoplasia (VIN), vaginal intraepithelial neoplasia (VAIN), cervical intraepithelial neoplasia (CIN), penile intraepithelial neoplasia (PIN), and anal intraepithelial neoplasia (AIN). Vertical transmission of low-risk types from mother to child during delivery rarely may cause RRP in young children. High-risk HPV types (e.g., types 16 and 18) may cause mild, moderate, or severe VIN, VAIN, CIN, PIN, and AIN as well as cervical cancer. Persistent infection with high-risk types is a key risk factor for development of CIN and cervical cancer.

Epidemiology

Prevalence and Transmission. At least 75% of sexually active adult men and women in the United States are exposed to genital HPV types at some point in their lives; the prevalence is highest during adolescence and young adulthood (25% to 64%). In a sample of U.S. women, 20% of 14- to 17-year-olds, 38% of 18- to 21-year-olds, and 42% of 22- to 25-year-olds were HPV-positive. The majority of women had at least one high-risk type. The estimated prevalence rate of symptomatic anogenital warts among U.S. adults is 1% to 5%, but prevalence rates up to 40% are reported in STD clinics. Sexual transmission occurs primarily through genital–genital or oral–genital contact. Adolescents often acquire HPV infection within a few months after sexual initiation. About 7 of 1,000 children born to mothers with genital warts will develop RRP.

Risk Factors. Multiple sexual partners; early age of sexual initiation; inconsistent condom use; cigarette smoking; immunosuppression (e.g., HIV infection and organ transplantation); cervical ectopy; oral contraceptive use (although some studies of adolescents show that oral contraceptive use is inversely associated with HPV infection, other studies in adults suggest that it may be a cofactor in cervical carcinogenesis); and history of genital warts and other STDs, including genital herpes.

Pathophysiology and Natural History of HPV Infection

Although HPV infection is extremely common in adolescents, infections usually are subclinical and transient: >90% of adolescents with subclinical HPV infection become HPV-negative within 9 to 12 months.

Clinical Manifestations

Types of Anogenital Warts. Condylomata acuminata (cauliflower-shaped growths), papular warts (smooth, skin-colored), keratotic warts (thick and horny), and flat-topped papules. Warts may be pink, red, tan, brown, or gray.

Location. In women, warts may occur on the cervix, vagina, vulva, urethra, and anus. In men, they may occur on the inner surface of the prepuce and on the frenulum, corona, penile shaft, glans, scrotum, and anus.

Symptoms. Usually these lesions are asymptomatic but they may cause pruritus, burning, pain, urethral or vaginal discharge, urethral bleeding, or postcoital bleeding.

Exacerbating Factors. Pregnancy, skin moisture, vaginal or urethral discharge

Clinical Course. Lesions usually appear 2 to 3 months after infection (range 3 weeks to 8 months). Warts may regress spontaneously, persist, or increase in size or number. They often recur after therapy, but over a period of months to years most anogenital warts resolve.

Differential Diagnosis. Micropapillomatosis labialis of labia minora, pearly penile papules (in men), seborrheic keratoses, other benign genital lesions (skin tags, fibromas, lipomas, hidradenomas, and adenomas), condylomata latum (due to secondary syphilis), molluscum contagiosum, granuloma inguinale (verrucous type), high-grade intraepithelial lesions, and cancer (Bowen disease, Bowenoid papulosis, dysplastic nevi, VIN, VAIN, PIN, AIN, and squamous cell carcinoma).

Diagnosis

Subclinical HPV Infection. The Hybrid Capture II assay is a hybridization and signal amplification technique that detects 13 different high-risk HPV types. Currently, HPV DNA testing is recommended routinely only in the context of cervical cancer screening in women (see Chapter 54).

Genital Warts. Genital warts are usually diagnosed using direct visual inspection with a bright light and, if necessary, magnification. A speculum examination is helpful in women to evaluate for vaginal and cervical warts. Patients with anogenital warts that are not responsive to therapy or have features suggestive of neoplasia (e.g., blue or black discoloration, increased pigmentation, rapid growth, or fixation to underlying structures) should be referred to a specialist.

Treatment

General Considerations. The goal of therapy is to eradicate or reduce the size of clinically apparent anogenital warts. If a patient prefers, it is reasonable to begin treatment only if warts persist or enlarge. Treatment includes eliminating or minimizing any predisposing factors and treating coexisting vaginitis or cervicitis. Treatment should be guided by the patient's preferences, extent and type of lesion, the provider's experience, and available resources. If one treatment strategy fails, another may be tried.

Specific Treatment Recommendations. Refer to Chapter 60 for treatment guidelines and to www.cdc.gov/std/treatment.

Counseling. Counseling should include education about the following topics: HPV infection, transmission, clinical consequences of infection, available treatment options, prognosis, strategies to prevent HPV-related disease and other STDs, abstinence, limiting number of sexual partners, avoiding tobacco, and using condoms consistently. HPV infection or genital warts may cause anxiety, distress, and fear of social stigmatization. Clinicians should provide support and, when necessary, may refer patients to support groups or for counseling. Clinicians should recommend that adolescents with genital warts undergo Pap testing according to published guidelines (not more frequently) and screen all sexually active adolescents for other STDs.

HPV Vaccines. Prophylactic HPV vaccines in development prevent primary HPV infection by inducing virus-neutralizing antibody and are most effective if given prior to sexual initiation. The vaccines do not contain viral DNA, so cannot cause infection, genital warts, or cancer. Clinical trials have shown that they are highly immunogenic, safe, well tolerated, and effective in preventing HPV infection, abnormal Pap tests, and CIN. The HPV-6, 11, 16, 18 vaccine (Gardasil, Merck & Co., Inc.)—which is designed to prevent genital warts, cervical cancer, and other HPV-associated malignancies—was approved by the FDA in June 2006 for use in girls and women 9 to 26 years of age. The Advisory Committee on Immunization Practices (ACIP) has recommended that the vaccine be given routinely to 11- and 12-year-old girls, with catch-up immunization of 13- to 26-year-old girls and women and immunization of 9- and 10-year-old girls at the discretion of the health care provider. The HPV-16, 18 vaccine Cervarix, (GlaxoSmithKline Biologicals), which is designed to prevent cervical cancer and other HPV-associated malignancies, was submitted for regulatory review in Europe and to the FDA in the United States for approval. Both vaccines are given as three intramuscular injections, Gardasil at 0, 2, and 6 months and Cervarix at 0, 1, and 6 months. Antibody levels appear to remain high for at least 4 to 5 years after initial vaccination.

In recommending HPV vaccines, providers should (a) address any specific parental or adolescent concerns; (b) reinforce prevention messages (i.e., because HPV vaccines do not protect against all HPV types or other STDs, adolescents should still postpone sexual initiation, limit the number of sexual partners, and use condoms consistently); and (c) reinforce the importance of continued Pap screening after vaccination. This is because 30% of cervical cancer is caused by types not contained in the vaccines and because vaccine efficacy may be compromised if women have been infected previously with HPV types contained in the vaccines or if they do not receive all three immunizations.

WEB SITES AND REFERENCES

http://www.emedicine.com/derm/topic454.htm. E-medicine chapter on genital warts.

http://www.obgyn.net/femalepatient/default.asp?page=warts_tfp. From *The Female Patient* on management of warts.

http://www.cdc.gov/std/hpv.default.htm. CDC Web site with excellent fact sheets about HPV for both providers and patients.

http://www.cdc.gov/STD/treatment 2006. CDC STD treatment guidelines.

Beutner KR, Reitano MV, Richwald GA, et al., and the AMA Expert Panel on External Genital Warts. External genital warts: report of the American Medical Association consensus conference. *Clin Infect Dis* 1998;27:796.

Centers for Disease Control and Prevention. 2006 Guidelines for treatment of sexually transmitted diseases. *MMWR Morb Mortal Wkly Rep* 2006;55[No. RR-11].

Kahn JA, Bernstein DI. Human papillomavirus vaccines and adolescents. *Curr Opin Obstet Gynecol* 2005;17:476.

Kahn JA, Lan D, Kahn RS. Sociodemographic factors associated with high-risk HPV infection. *Obstet Gynecol* 2007;110:87–102.

Villa LL, Costa RL, Petta CA. Prophylactic quadrivalent human papillomavirus (types 6, 11, 16, and 18) L1 virus-like particle vaccine in young women: a randomised double-blind placebo-controlled multicentre phase II efficacy trial. *Lancet Oncol* 2005;6:271.

CHAPTER 67

Other Sexually Transmitted Diseases Including Genital Ulcers, Pediculosis, Scabies, and Molluscum

Wendi G. Ehrman, M. Susan Jay, and Lawrence S. Neinstein

The first three minor sexually transmitted diseases (STDs) outlined below are uncommon but share an increased risk of associated HIV infection.

CHANCROID

Etiology. Gram-negative coccobacillus *Haemophilus ducreyi*.

Epidemiology. Uncommon in the United States, although probably under-diagnosed, with the highest prevalence in southern, central, and eastern Africa and other developing countries. A higher incidence in African American and Hispanic patients and a male/female ratio of >10.1 in outbreaks. Some 10% of patients with chancroid acquired in the United States are coinfected with *Treponema pallidum* or herpes simplex virus (HSV).

Clinical Manifestations
1. *Incubation period:* 3 to 10 days.
2. *Presentation:* Tender inflammatory papule on the genitalia.
3. *Progression:*
   a. Erosion within 1 to 2 days to an extremely painful, friable, nonindurated, shallow ulcer with ragged margins and a granulomatous base.
   b. Development of a foul-smelling yellow or gray necrotic purulent exudate.
   c. Multiple lesions may be present, especially in women.
   d. Lesions may remain pustular ("dwarf chancroid"), coalesce to form giant ulcers, or resemble folliculitis or a pyogenic infection.
   e. Within 1 to 23 weeks, a painful unilateral inguinal lymphadenitis ("bubo") may develop, which may become suppurative, rupture, and ulcerate if not aspirated and drained. Autoinoculation may also occur.
   f. Women may be asymptomatic or develop nontender ulcers associated with dysuria, dyspareunia, vaginal discharge, pain with defecation, and rectal bleeding.

4. *Pregnancy:* No known adverse effects
5. *HIV-infected patients:* may have increased numbers of genital ulcers that heal more slowly and require longer courses of therapy.

Treatment
See Chapter 60 and also CDC guidelines at http://www.cdc.gov/std/treatment.

1. Treatment of buboes includes aspiration of fluctuant buboes for symptomatic relief and prevention of rupture and incision and drainage of buboes with wound packing
2. Other testing includes HIV and syphilis testing with repeat testing in 3 months if negative, and gonorrhea, *Chlamydia,* hepatitis B and other STD testing.
3. *Follow-up:* (a) 3 to 7 days after initiation of therapy and then weekly until resolution of signs and symptoms. Subjective improvement occurs within 3 days and objective improvement is seen within 7 days. (c) Large ulcers may take more than 2 weeks to resolve, and fluctuant lymphadenopathy heals more slowly than ulcers. (d) Lack of improvement may signal misdiagnosis or need for other treatments. (e) Abstinence is essential while clinical disease is present.

LYMPHOGRANULOMA VENEREUM

Etiology. A systemic STD caused by the obligate intracellular organism *Chlamydia trachomatis,* with 18 serologic variants (serovars). Three (L_1, L_2, and L_3) cause lymphogranuloma venereum (LGV) and three (B, D, and K) are associated with nongonococcal urethritis and cervicitis.

Epidemiology. Very rare in the United States and probably underreported and misdiagnosed. Has not been nationally notifiable since 1995. Endemic in parts of Africa, India, South America, and the Caribbean. Peak incidence occurs between 15 and 40 years with a male-to-female predominance as high as a 5:1. Prevalence is higher among men having sex with men, especially when HIV-positive.

Clinical Manifestations
1. *Incubation period:* 3 to 30 days (usually 7 to 12 days)
2. *LGV occurs in three separate stages:*
   a. *Primary stage:* small, painless papule or pustule at the site of inoculation that can erode into an asymptomatic herpetiform ulcer. Lesions may be associated with diarrhea, rectal discharge, tenesmus, mucopurulent cervicitis, and urethritis.
   b. *Secondary or inguinal stage:* Occurs 2 to 6 weeks after the primary lesion and involves painful inflammation and infection of the inguinal and femoral lymph nodes. The "groove" sign (enlarged inguinal nodes above Poupart ligament and femoral nodes below it) is pathognomonic for LGV. Nodes can become matted and fluctuant, producing a bubo. Constitutional symptoms may occur with the inguinal buboes and be associated with systemic spread of chlamydial infection.

c. *Tertiary stage or genitoanorectal syndrome:* Uncommon but occurs more often in previously asymptomatic women and in homosexual men who have receptive anal intercourse. Patients develop proctocolitis with fever. Later manifestations include perirectal abscesses, rectovaginal and anorectal fistulas, rectal strictures and rectal stenosis. Chronic untreated LGV can lead to repetitive scarring and the formation of fistulous tracts in the genital region, leading to elephantiasis, destruction of the genitals, and infertility.

Diagnosis. Based on clinical findings owing to lack of available laboratory services, difficulty of culturing the organism, and cross-reactivity of serology between several serotypes. Available laboratory services can be located at www.cdc.gov/std/lgv-labs.htm.

Treatment
See Chapter 60 and also CDC guidelines at www.cdc.gov/std/treatment.

1. *Surgical intervention:* Aspiration of a fluctuant node or incision and drainage of an abscess may be required for prevention of ulcer formation or relief of inguinal pain.
2. *Follow-up:* Patients should be monitored clinically until signs and symptoms have resolved.

GRANULOMA INGUINALE

Granuloma inguinale, also known as Donovanosis, is a rare STD in the United States but should be considered in the differential diagnosis of chronic progressive genital ulcers.

Etiology. Caused by *Calymmatobacterium granulomatis,* a nonmotile, obligate-intracellular, encapsulated, gram-negative coccobacillus.

Epidemiology. Indigenous granuloma inguinale is no longer present in the United States or most other developed countries. Incidence is extremely rare except in Papua, New Guinea, Southeast India, South Africa, central Australia, Brazil, and the Caribbean, where it is considered endemic. A higher prevalence is seen in men, with the majority of cases occurs between the ages of 20 and 40. Transmission occurs primarily through sexual contact, most commonly from a person with an active infection but possibly also from a person with an asymptomatic rectal infection. Granuloma inguinale is thought to be only mildly contagious, requiring several exposures for clinical disease to develop.

Clinical Manifestations
1. *Incubation period:* 8 to 80 days
2. Variety of presentations and atypical lesions.
   a. *Ulcerovegetative or ulcerogranulomatous forms:* Large, extensive, nonindurated ulcerations with beefy-red, friable granulation tissue
   b. *Nodular form:* Soft red nodules or plaques that erode to form ulcerations
   c. *Hypertrophic or verrucous form:* Dry, vegetative masses with raised irregular edges that resemble a walnut or condyloma acuminata

   d. *Necrotic form:* Painful, foul-smelling, deep ulcer that produces rapid and extensive tissue destruction

   e. *Sclerotic or cicatricial form:* Rare, dry, nonbleeding ulcers that expand into plaques with band-like scarring

Diagnosis. Identification of intracytoplasmic inclusion bodies known as Donovan bodies within histiocytes of granulation tissue smears or biopsy specimens. Polymerase chain reaction tests and immunofluorescence are available on a research basis.

Treatment
See CDC guidelines at www.cdc.gov/std/treatment.

1. Doxycycline 100 mg orally twice a day for a minimum of 3 weeks or until healing of lesions. Erythromycin, azithromycin, ciprofloxacin, and trimethoprim/sulfamethoxazole are alternatives. Erythromycin and azithromycin are alternatives in pregnancy and lactation.
2. *HIV:* Same regimen as for HIV-negative patients although the addition of an aminoglycoside may be considered.
3. *Follow-up:* Follow patients until complete resolution of clinical signs and symptoms. Relapses can occur in 6 to 18 months after treatment, especially if antibiotics are stopped prematurely.
4. *Sexual partners:* Sexual partners should be examined and offered treatment if they had contact with the patient during the 60 days before the onset of symptoms or if they are clinically symptomatic.

PEDICULOSIS PUBIS

Etiology. Pubic or crab louse, *Pthirus pubis,* an obligate human parasite.

Epidemiology. Transmission via close bodily contact (mainly sexual contact), but can be potentially transmitted by infected clothing, towels, and bedding. Infestations most common among adolescents and young adults. Clustering of infections seen in school children, homeless people, hospital staff, and immunocompromised persons. Condoms do not prevent transmission, and frequently infestations coexist with other sexually transmitted diseases (STDs). Can be found on eyelashes of younger children and may be an indicator of sexual abuse.

Epidemiology. Lives on skin and feeds on blood. Dies in about 24 hours off its human host. Females lay about three or four eggs per day, which hatch into nymphs in 6 to 10 days and mature into adult lice within 10 to 14 days. Adult life expectancy is about 1 month.

Clinical Manifestations
1. Symptoms occur 2 weeks or more after contact.
2. Pruritus is related to the louse bite and is probably a hypersensitivity reaction. Secondary infections can occur from scratching.
3. Symptoms occur more rapidly if the patient experienced a prior infestation.

4. *Common areas of infection:* Pubic hair, hairs of abdomen, chest, thighs, axillae, and perianal area. Occasionally eyebrows and lashes are involved in young children and beards in men.
5. After prolonged infestation, small blue spots called maculae caeruleae may appear on thighs and abdomen. These are uncommon but specific for pubic lice and represent feeding sites.

Diagnosis. Direct visualization of lice or nits (eggs) on the hair shafts.

Treatment
See Chapter 60 and also CDC guidelines at www.cdc.gov/std/treatment. Residual nits not responding to treatment should be removed with a fine comb. For nits that are difficult to remove, a solution of vinegar and water can be used to loosen them.

SCABIES

Etiology. A highly contagious ectoparasitic infection caused by the mite *Sarcoptes scabiei* var. *hominis*. Host-specific for humans.

Epidemiology. One of the most widespread infestations in the world, with about 300 million cases worldwide each year. Transmitted via prolonged skin-to-skin contact and/or sexual activity and less often through infected clothes, bedding, and fomites. Can be transmitted before the patient is symptomatic and throughout the infestation as long as it remains untreated. Commonly seen in institutional settings and epidemics associated with poverty, overcrowding, sexual promiscuity, travel, waning immunity, and other factors. Highest prevalence in preschool and adolescents in underdeveloped countries.

Clinical Manifestations
1. *Incubation:* Symptoms occur 3 to 6 weeks after first exposure and 1 to 4 days after reexposure.
2. *Lesions:* Intensely pruritic, papular eruption associated with eczematous lesions and areas of excoriation. Pruritus is often worse at night or after a hot bath. When seen, burrows appear as short wavy lines a few millimeters to 1 cm in length.
3. *Involved areas:* In between finger webs, flexor surfaces of the wrists, axillary folds, nipples, waist, umbilicus, buttocks, thighs, knees, ankles, penis, and scrotum. Scabies usually spares the face, neck, and scalp except in children.
4. *Crusted or Norwegian scabies:* Rare and aggressive form of scabies most often associated with immunodeficient, debilitated, or malnourished patients. Characterized by hyperinfestation of the mite with a concomitant inflammatory and hyperkeratotic reaction. Numerous scaling lesions that are heavily infested with mites and more contagious than typical scabies. Treatment failures occur frequently and septicemia is a common complication.

Diagnosis. Based on the body distribution of lesions along with a history of intense itching and similar symptoms in family members or sexual partners. Definitive diagnosis requires microscopic identification of mites, eggs, or feces from skin scrapings of papules or burrows. Burrows are virtually pathognomonic for human scabies but are often difficult to demonstrate.

Treatment
See Chapter 60 and also CDC guidelines at www.cdc.gov/std/treatment. Alternative regimens also include crotamiton 10% (Eurax) applied for 24 hours once daily for 2 consecutive days followed by bathing 48 hours after the final application. Appears to work better as an antipyretic agent but is associated with higher treatment failures, irritation, and allergic reactions.
 Other considerations:

1. Bedding and clothing worn during the 3 days preceding treatment should be machine-washed, machine-dried using hot cycle, dry-cleaned, or removed from body contact and set aside in a sealed plastic bag for at least 72 hours. Fumigation is not necessary.
2. *Follow-up:* Pruritus may persist for up to 2 weeks after treatment. Consideration can be given to retreatment with a different regimen after 1 to 2 weeks, although some specialists recommend this only with the confirmation of live mites.
3. *Pregnancy/lactation:* Permethrin or crotamiton regimens.
4. Oral antipruritics such as hydroxyzine (Atarax) or topical corticosteroids can be used to relieve itching.
5. *Crusted scabies:* Difficult to treat and may require combined treatment with Ivermectin and topical scabicides and keratolytic therapy or multiple doses of ivermectin. Ivermectin is not FDA- licensed for this use.

MOLLUSCUM CONTAGIOSUM

Etiology. Self-limited, benign, viral skin disease caused by a large DNA poxvirus.

Epidemiology. Humans are the only known host of this worldwide virus, which is especially prevalent in warm, humid climates. Transmission is by direct person-to-person contact, fomites, or autoinoculation and anecdotally has also been associated with swimming pools. Sexual contact is believed to be the most common form of transmission among adolescents. The incubation period varies from 2 weeks to 6 months.

Clinical Manifestations
1. *Location:* Face, trunk and extremities. In sexually active adolescents, the lesions are commonly seen on the genital and pubic areas and inner thighs.
2. *Appearance:* Smooth, firm, flesh-colored, dome-shaped papules that can become soft, waxy or pearly gray and semitranslucent with central umbilication. Immunocompetent hosts typically have <20 lesions that grow up to 5 mm in diameter over a period of a couple weeks. HIV-positive and immunocompromised patients may develop hundreds of lesions that may present in clusters.
3. *Symptoms:* Typically asymptomatic; however, approximately 10% of patients will have an encircling eczematoid reaction.

Treatment

See Chapter 60 and also CDC guidelines at www.cdc.gov/std/treatment.

1. Owing to the benign nature and self-limiting course, nontreatment is an option for nongenital lesions. Individual lesions may resolve in 2 to 6 months, but untreated infections can last as long as 5 years.
2. *Mechanical ablation: All of the following are considered safe in pregnancy.*
   a. Curettage or needle extraction of the central molluscum core with/ without a local anesthetic such as EMLA. Cauterization of the lesion base with electrodesiccation or application of TCA or podophyllin to the base may be of added benefit.
   b. Cryotherapy via application of liquid nitrogen to the lesions and surrounding area for 5 to 10 seconds. Treatment may need to be repeated in 2- to 4-week intervals. Blistering and scarring are potential side effects.
   c. Electrodesiccation with a local anesthetic.
   d. Pulse dye laser for recalcitrant lesions. Laser treatment been associated with transient hyperpigmentation and development of new lesions after eradication of the old ones.
   e. Duct tape occlusion therapy over a course of months.
3. Chemical cytotoxic agents
   a. Podophyllin 25% applied to individual lesions and washed off 1 to 4 hours later. Applied weekly for 4 to 6 weeks; may be associated with significant irritation. Best used when limited numbers of nonfacial lesions are present. Alternatively, patients can self-apply Podofilox twice daily for 3 consecutive days followed by 4 days without treatment in 4 to 6 cycles. May be associated with pain, irritation, and mild scarring and has a low efficacy and potential toxicity. *Not approved for use in pregnancy.*
   b. Trichloroacetic acid (80% to 90%) applied to the lesion(s) once a week for 4 to 6 weeks. May result in mild pain, irritation and scarring. *Safe in pregnancy.*
   c. Cantharidin (0.7% to 0.9%) carefully applied to lesions and washed off within 2 to 6 hours. May be repeated in 2 to 4 weeks. Not FDA-approved or recommended for face or genitalia secondary to significant blistering.
   d. Topical 0.5% Tretinoin cream or gel applied to lesions daily for 2 to 3 months. Local irritation and dryness are side effects. No controlled clinical trials have been done and it is not recommended in pregnancy.
4. Immunomodulators
   a. Topically applied 5% imiquimod cream applied overnight 3 times per week and washed off in the morning for 4 to 12 weeks. Not FDA-approved currently for this use. May be associated with mild pain and erythema. *Not for use in pregnancy.*
5. *HIV/immunosuppressed patients:* 5% Imiquod may have some benefit and experimental treatments utilizing the antiviral drug cidofovir (topically or intralesionally) and alpha-interferon (intralesionally) may be of benefit.

Follow-up. Watch for the development of new lesions after several weeks that may have been incubating at the time of the initial treatment. Patients should refrain from sharing clothing or towels with others. Swimming in pools should be discouraged. Partners should be examined and treated for lesions, although the benefits of this are unknown.

WEB SITES AND REFERENCES

http://www.cdc.gov/std/lgv

American Academy of Pediatrics. Summaries of Infectious Diseases. In: Pickeing LK, ed. *Red Book: report of the Committee of Infectious Diseases,* 27th ed. Elk Grove Village, IL: American Academy of Pediatrics; 2006.

Centers for Disease Control and Prevention. Sexually transmitted diseases: treatment guidelines 2006. *MMWR* 2006;55(RR-11).

Holmes KK, Sparling PF, Mårdh PA, et al., eds. *Sexually transmitted diseases,* 3rd ed. New York: McGraw-Hill, 1999.

Orion E, Matz H, Wolf R. Ectoparasitic Sexually transmitted diseases: scabies and pediculosis. *Clin Dermatol* 2004;22:513.

Ting PT, Dytoc MT. Therapy of external anogenital warts and molluscum contagiosum: a literature review. *Dermatol Ther* 2004;17:68.

Trager J. Sexually transmitted diseases causing genital lesions in adolescents. *Adolesc Med Clin* 2004;15:323.

CHAPTER **68**

Adolescent Substance Use and Abuse

Robert E. Morris and Alain Joffe

Adolescents' use of alcohol, tobacco, and other illicit drugs (ATOD) continues to be a major public health problem. Drug use is associated with significant morbidity and mortality, and early use strongly predicts problems and lifelong use. Alcohol, tobacco, and marijuana are most abused by adolescents, while younger adolescents use inhalants. Drugs wax and wane in popularity, following a predictable pattern. Drug X becomes popular in part because it is presumed safe; as use becomes more widespread, its negative effects become known and its use is perceived as risky. The popularity of drug X wanes, to be replaced by another, presumably safer drug. Later, owing to the phenomenon known as "generational forgetting," drug X again becomes popular. Recently, the abuse of over-the-counter and prescription medications has emerged as a problem.

Advances in neuroimaging techniques and research using animal models of human puberty demonstrate the vulnerability of the developing adolescent brain to the effects of alcohol and other drugs, leading to changes that may become permanent. Research on the brain's reward circuitry finds that drugs of abuse share common pathways and exert their effects through similar mechanisms. Drug addiction is best viewed as a chronic disease with recurring relapses, and treatment can be effective.

EPIDEMIOLOGY

1. *Middle and high school youth:* The best data on adolescent substance abuse come from the Monitoring the Future (MTF) study, conducted by the Institute for Social Research at the University of Michigan

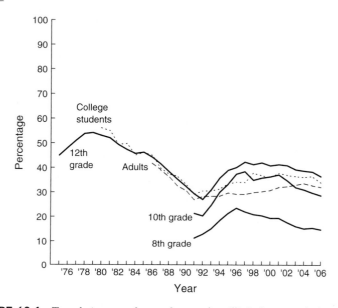

FIGURE 68.1 Trends in annual prevalence of an illicit drug use index across five populations. Source: Johnston LD, O'Malley PM, Bachman JG, et al. (2006). Monitoring the Future: national survey results on drug use, 1975–2005: Volume I. Secondary school students (NIH Publication No. 06-5883). Bethesda, MD: National Institute on Drug Abuse, page 58. Available at: http://monitoringthefuture.org/new.html

(www.monitoringthefuture.org). Volume I each year has data on secondary school students, while volume II is devoted to college students and adults (full volumes available as pdf files). This school-based survey began in 1975, utilizing a nationally representative sample of 12th graders, with the later addition of 8th- and 10th-grade students. The sample consists of approximately 50,000 youth. The anonymous surveys are conducted in schools and do not reflect drug use by out-of-school youth, whose use is typically higher. Trends in the annual prevalence of illicit drug use across five populations from this survey are shown in Figure 68.1. The most important findings from the 2006 MTF surveys are as follows:

- Drug use among 8th graders has decreased by approximately one third since 1996, while use among 10th and 12th graders was down by 25% and 10% respectively.
- Lifetime use: Use of illicit drugs by 12th graders peaked in 1980 to 1982, declined until 1992, and then increased again. Lifetime illicit drug use among 8th-grade students peaked in 1996 and then declined, while among 10th graders the peak was in 1999, after which use declined.
- Annual use: In 2006, 14.8% of 8th graders, 28.7% of 10th graders, and 36.5% of 12th graders reported having used an illicit substance during the previous year.
- Alcohol continues to be the drug most abused by adolescents. In 2006, approximately 33.6% of 8th graders, 55.8% of 10th graders, and 66.5% of

12th graders had used alcohol in the previous year. In 2006, some 10.9% of 8th graders, 21.9% of 10th graders, and 25.4% of 12th graders reported binge drinking (five or more drinks in a row) in the 2 weeks prior to the survey. Although boys drink more heavily than girls, the gap is narrowing.

- Marijuana: Among 8th graders, inhalants (16.1%) and marijuana (15.7%) had a lifetime use that was almost equal. In 2006, some 6.5% of 8th graders, 14.2% of 10th graders and 18.3% of 12th graders reported having used marijuana or hashish in the previous 30 days.
- "Ecstasy" (methylenedioxymethamphetamine, or MDMA) use climbed steeply from 1998 to 2001 and then, as perceived risk increased, began to decline in 2002, with a small increase in 2006.
- Methamphetamine: Generally, annual use has decreased.
- Steroids: Since 2000, steroid use declined among 8th graders, although it was stable from 2004 to 2006; use among 10th graders declined since 2002; while that among 12th graders declined from 2.5% in 2004 to 1.8% in 2006.
- Rohypnol/GHB: Use among 12th graders was 1.1% in 2006.

1. *Nonmedical use of prescription medications:* A worrisome new trend is nonmedical use of prescription medications. According to the National Survey on Drug Use and Health (NSDUH), 11.4% of 12- to 17-year-olds surveyed in 2004 had ever abused prescription pain relievers. (www.oas.samhsa.gov/NSDUH/2k4nsduh/2k4tabs/Sect1peTabs1to18.pdf). Approximately 28% of teens in this survey indicated that prescription drugs were "very easy" to get, compared with 48% for marijuana and 14% for ecstasy as reported at the Web site below. (www.drugfree.org/Files/Full_Report_PATS_Teens_7th-12th_grades_2004).

   Over-the-counter cough or cold medications: There is an increase in the use these medications; because they are accessible without a prescription, teens may not fully realize the dangers of use.

2. *College students and their noncollege peers:* Most college-aged youth cannot legally purchase alcohol, but 82% of college students and 79% of noncollege peers report that they used alcohol in the previous year. Binge drinking by college students has attracted considerable attention because of its association with poor academic performance, violence, sexual assault, and unprotected sexual intercourse. Past-year use of illicit drugs among college-aged youth reached a low point in 1991, peaked in 2001, and then remained constant for college students, but it increased for noncollege teens since then. After alcohol, marijuana is the drug most often used.

LONG-TERM OUTCOMES OF DRUG USE

Studies suggest that exposure to drugs, especially in early to midadolescence, causes long-term adverse consequences.

1. *Marijuana:* Various controlled studies of marijuana smokers indicate that there is an increased risk of anxiety, depression, suicidal thoughts/attempts, developing schizophrenia, and participation in violent crimes, especially among students who began to use before age 16.
2. *Alcohol:* Adolescent binge drinking as well as frequent alcohol or marijuana use are associated with later binge drinking and alcohol problems.

RISK AND PROTECTIVE FACTORS FOR DRUG USE

1. *Perception of risk:* There is a strong and inverse link between perceptions of the risk of drug use and the prevalence of use. In contrast, measures of availability and disapproval bear little relation to use patterns.
2. *Race/ethnicity:* Race and ethnicity are protective factors in drug use. Since 1975, drug use among African American 12th graders was lower than among white youth, with rates for Hispanic youth falling in between.
3. *Other risk/protective factors:* Decisions regarding drug use are complex; no single risk factor accurately predicts that an adolescent will use drugs or develop an abuse problem, nor does a single protective factor militate against use. These factors are outlined in Table 68.1.

ADOLESCENT BRAIN DEVELOPMENT AND SUSCEPTIBILITY TO DRUG USE AND DRUG ASSOCIATED BRAIN DAMAGE

Imaging techniques demonstrate significant brain development during adolescence. In a longitudinal study of 145 healthy children, the following changes were noted: (1) Linear increases (12.4%) in white matter (myelinization) volume in all brain regions. (2) Gray matter volume changes varied by lobe, indicating possible pruning of synapses. (3) Changes in the frontal cortex coincide with neuropsychological studies showing that frontal lobes mediate emotional regulation, planning, organizing, and response inhibition (i.e., "executive functioning"). Rat studies show that mesolimbic dopamine (DA) synthesis in the nucleus accumbens increases from preadolescence through the adult years, along with increased dopaminergic and noradrenergic transmitter systems. The mesolimbic system plays a large role in the reward circuitry fueling drug addiction. New memory formation in the hippocampus is a critical process in learning and reinforcing drug addiction. Given these changes, it is logical that adolescents may be especially susceptible to the harmful effects of drug use.

1. *Alcohol:* (a) Compared with adult rats, adolescent rats are less sedated by alcohol, suggesting that adolescents would be less likely to curtail their intake because of sedation. (b) In contrast with other ages, adolescent rats do not alter dopamine and 3,4-dihydroxyphenylacetic acid metabolism with repeated exposure to ethanol, suggesting a failure to adapt to alcohol use or to develop increased reactivity to ethanol. (c) After two or three drinks, young adults' immediate and delayed recall (learning) is more impaired than that of younger children. (d) Compared with binging in adult rats, binging in adolescent rats causes greater brain damage, including microglia and long-term changes in serotonergic innervation in adulthood compared to controls. (e) Adolescents display less motor impairment from alcohol than adults despite the fact that adolescents have higher peak brain ethanol levels.
2. *Nicotine:* (a) Compared with nonsmokers, adolescents, especially younger adolescents who smoke daily, have impairments in working memory that worsen with abstinence. (b) Rats exposed to nicotine in the periadolescent but not the postadolescent period become more sensitive to nicotine reinforcement as adults as a result of neurotransmitter changes. (c) In preadolescent rats, nicotine profoundly activates the midbrain catecholaminergic

TABLE 68.1

Risk and Protective Factors for Drug Use

Domain	Protective Factors	Risk Factors
Individual	High intelligence	Untreated mental health/behavioral problems (e.g., depression, anxiety, conduct disorder, aggressive behavior, impulsivity)
	Achievement oriented	School problems (including old for grade)
	Positive self-esteem	Genetic vulnerability (family history of alcoholism; "sensation-seeking" personality)
	Optimistic view of future	Early pubertal development
	Good coping skills	Rebelliousness
	Prosocial orientation	Perception that most peers use drugs
	Perception that most peers do not use drugs	Undiagnosed/untreated ADHD
	Treated ADHD	Low religiosity
	High religiosity	Drug use perceived as low risk
	Perception that drug use has risks	After school employment (middle–high income families)
Family	Clear messages about no use	Families expect children will try drugs or expectations about drug use not clear
	Parents model appropriate alcohol/drug use	Familial substance abuse
	Strong family–youth attachment	Alienated from family
	Moderate to high levels of parental monitoring	Permissive parenting
	Supportive parents	Coercive parenting
		Familial conflict

(continued)

TABLE 68.1

(Continued)

Domain	Protective Factors	Risk Factors
Peers	Peers do not use drugs Peers have prosocial/conventional values	Peers use drugs Peers alienated from community
Schools	Offer opportunities for success and involvement Students feel connected to school School personnel perceived as fair and caring	Poor quality Students feel alienated from school School personnel perceived as uncaring
Community	Good quality with adequate recreational activities Strong community institutions Media realistically portrays harms associated with drug use; counter marketing (media used to demonstrate how advertising manipulates youth)	Lack of recreational opportunities Community institutions lacking Lack of community norms about drug use Substance abuse common in community Drugs easily available Socioeconomic deprivation and social disorganization Media portrays drug use as normative and promotes positive expectancies associated with drug use

ADHD, attention-deficit hyperactivity disorder.

pathways, followed by a loss of response. With later exposure to nicotine, catecholaminergic pathways are again significantly activated. Adolescent female rats exposed to nicotine showed significant late-onset hippocampal cell damage and loss.

3 *Marijuana, cocaine, and amphetamines:* In rats, repeated exposure to the cannabinoid agonist WIN55212.2 (WIN) produced tolerance. Adolescent but not adult rats exposed to WIN displayed long-lasting cross-tolerance to morphine, cocaine, and amphetamines, suggesting a heightened sensitivity to psychoactive substances during a period of brain immaturity.

STAGES OF DRUG USE

Adolescent substance abuse proceeds from stage to stage, sometimes skipping a stage (adapted from MacDonald DI. *Drugs, Drinking, and Adolescents*. Chicago: Year Book Medical, 1984).

Stage 0—No drug use: There are no substance abuse health risks, although drug-using friends engaging in risky activities can create a risk. Counseling focuses on safety, praising and normalizing abstinence, and refusal skills.

Stage 1—Experimentation: Now drugs are tried out of curiosity or to fit in. Alcohol and tobacco are commonly used, but only marijuana may be used. There is risk of health problems or death even with occasional use. An unpleasant experience can revert youth to stage 0. Focus is the same as for stage 0.

Stage 2—Learning the mood swing: If available, drug experimentation continues on weekends in social settings without a concerted effort to obtain drugs, but the variety used will increase. Positive/pleasurable experiences outweigh negatives. Behavior change is slight but the adolescent may hide use. Clinician assesses for risk of progression and discusses the previously listed areas.

Stage 3—Seeking/preoccupation with the mood swing: Youth actively seek drugs and organize living around drugs. They seek out drug-use settings and avoid nondrug situations. They may buy or sell drugs to assure a supply and use a greater variety. Social networks consist of drug-using peers. Negative consequences and behavior changes cause the adolescent to be more vigilant in hiding drug use. The counseling focus is as above, plus challenging the adolescents' perception that they control their drug use (abstinence challenges/contracts), using motivational interviewing techniques. Careful follow-up is needed. Some will meet the criteria for substance dependence or abuse. Involvement of parents may be necessary.

Stage 4—Problem use/dependence: Drug use continues despite significant negative consequences. Drugs are used to feel normal. This stage requires a comprehensive evaluation and intensive treatment. This stage meets criteria for substance dependence or abuse.

PREVENTION

Early unsuccessful efforts at prevention assumed that use was driven by inadequate knowledge of the harm due to drugs. Authority figures delivering antidrug messages also failed. In the 1980s, more sophisticated prevention efforts recognized that multiple factors affect the use of drugs. Since 8th graders (or younger adolescents) begin use, prevention now targets youth before this age.

1. *Life skills approach:* Some successful programs, usually school-based, focus on life skills using the following components: (a) Information about the health risks of ATOD use; stressing the actual versus perceived prevalence of ATOD use by adolescents; discussing acceptability of ATOD use; refusal skills to resist use. (b) Personal self-management skills: improved decision making/problem solving; media analysis to resist protobacco/proalcohol media messages; teaching emotional coping for anxiety, frustration, and anger; all of which result in personal behavior change. (c) Social skills: improving students' social competence, including romantic/sexual relationships. The curriculum is highly structured and taught over 15 sessions by trained facilitators. Didactics plus role-playing, skills rehearsals, feedback, and homework are used and booster sessions occur in subsequent years.
2. *Risk-factor reduction:* Fifth-grade students in a high-crime area participating in a program that included teacher training, parenting classes, and social competence training for students had lower levels of heavy drinking at age 18.
3. *Community-based approaches, including policy changes and media campaigns:* These include strict enforcement of alcohol and tobacco laws, advertising campaigns countering substance abuse, and media criticism. Florida cigarette use dropped 6% among middle school and 5% among high school students after an antitobacco campaign.

WEB SITES AND REFERENCES

http://www.monitoringthefuture.org/. Home page for the MTF survey.
http://www.cdc.gov/HealthyYouth/yrbs/index.htm. Youth Risk Behavior Surveillance System.
http://www.oas.samhsa.gov/nhsda.htm. National Survey on Drug Use and Health.
http://www.whitehousedrugpolicy.gov/. Office of National Drug Control Policy (ONDCP).
http://ncadi.samhsa.gov/. National Clearinghouse for Alcohol and Drug Information.
http://www.nida.nih.gov/. National Institute on Drug Abuse.
http://www.erowid.org/. A Web site that contains information on a wide variety of drugs.
http://www.drugfree.org/. Partnership for a Drug Free America.
Faggiano F, Vigna-Taglianti FD, Versino E, et al. School-based prevention for illicit drugs' use. *The Cochrane Database of Systematic Reviews* 2005, Issue 2, Art. No.:CD003020.pub2. DOI: 10.1002/14651858.CD003020.pub2.

CHAPTER 69

Alcohol

Martin M. Anderson and Lawrence S. Neinstein

Alcohol is the most widely used drug in the United States. In 2006, some 45.3% of high school seniors had used alcohol in the preceding month and 66.5% had used it in the previous year. About 3.0% of high school seniors used alcohol daily in 2006. Twenty-eight percent of high school seniors reported that they had consumed more than five drinks in a row during the previous 2 weeks, and 60.3% of high school seniors said that they had been drunk. Trends in alcohol use for 8th, 10th, and 12th graders declined between 1991 and 2006 and are available at http://monitoringthefuture.org/.

MORBIDITY AND MORTALITY

Motor vehicle accidents caused by driving under the influence of alcohol are the leading cause of death in the 15- to 24-year-old age group. Almost 30% of students (28.5%) nationwide have ridden with a driver who had been drinking and 9.9% (8.1% female, 11.7% male) have driven a car after drinking. Some 40% to 50% of young males who drown were drinking when they died. Alcohol use is linked to the acquisition of sexually transmitted diseases (STDs). Higher alcohol taxes and higher minimum legal drinking ages are associated with a lower incidence of STDs among adolescents and young adults. There is evidence of alcohol's role in memory problems and in alterations in brain development.

RISK FACTORS FOR ADOLESCENT ALCOHOL USE

Many factors contribute to alcohol initiation, use and alcohol-related problem behaviors.

Reasons Teens Give for Drinking. (a) Curiosity; (b) peer conformity; (c) enjoyment; (d) escape; (e) parental encouragement to take first drink to celebrate a special occasion.

Genetic. The initiation of and use of alcohol result from a complex interplay between genes and environment. A twin study of alcohol use found that alcohol initiation arises from genetic, shared, and nonshared environmental contributions. Alcohol use in general is minimally influenced by genetics and is mainly influenced by environment. Problem use has a heritability component and is influenced by peer influences more than by family.

Ethnicity. Asian Americans and African Americans are less likely to drink than European Americans (white) or Native Americans. In general, white American adolescents start drinking earlier than nonwhite Americans with the exception of Native Americans. In the 2005 National Youth Risk Behavior Survey, Hispanic high school students and non-Hispanic white students had a higher percent of lifetime use (79.4% and 75.3%) than black students (69.0%). This was also true for current use of alcohol (46.8%, 46.4%, and 31.2% respectively).

Family Factors. Adolescents' perception of parental approval and parents' use of alcohol are predictive of teens' initiation of alcohol use. Teens with close relationships to their parents are less likely to initiate. Children of alcoholics are 4 to 10 times more likely to become alcoholic as compared with children whose parents were not alcoholic.

Peer Factors. Peer involvement in drugs or alcohol, delinquent behaviors, or the perception that there is a high prevalence of alcohol use among peers increases the likelihood that a teen will drink.

Behavioral Risk Factors. If teens have tolerant attitudes toward delinquent behavior or approve of alcohol use, they are at higher risk for drinking. Mood disorders, attention deficit hyperactivity syndrome (ADHD), conduct disorder, low school motivation, and low value placed on academic achievement are additional risk factors associated with the initiation of alcohol use in adolescence.

Risk Factors Predictive of Early Initiation
Early onset of alcohol use (before age 14) is often associated with escalated drinking during adolescence and the development of alcohol-related problems in adolescents and adults. Nearly a third of adolescents start drinking before age 13 and 10% of 9-year-olds have already started drinking. Youth who start drinking before age 13 are nine times more likely to binge-drink than high school students who begin later.

Factors Not Predictive of Initiation
• Gender
• Socioeconomic status

ALCOHOL AND ITS EFFECTS

Physiology and Metabolism. Alcohol is lipid-soluble and completely miscible in water. It is rapidly absorbed from the GI tract, is distributed throughout the total body water, and easily penetrates the CNS. It is a CNS depressant that also has the ability to increase brain activity in areas that produce endorphins and that activate the dopaminergic reward system. A shot of whiskey, a can of beer, and a glass of wine have approximately the same alcohol content. Women, because of their higher percentage of body fat and lower total body water per unit of weight, develop higher blood alcohol levels than men with the same alcohol intake.

Intoxication. Moderate doses of alcohol in the nontolerant individual induce sedation, euphoria, decreased inhibitions, and impaired coordination. As the dose and corresponding blood alcohol level increase, ataxia, decreased mentation, poor judgment, labile mood, and slurred speech occur. At higher doses, alcohol can induce unconsciousness, anesthesia, respiratory failure, coma, and death (Table 69.1).

Complications. Although alcohol can adversely affect many organ systems of the body, adolescent alcohol abusers are usually spared the complications of prolonged alcohol, use such as cirrhosis, alcoholic hepatitis, and pancreatitis. Acute withdrawal symptoms such as delirium tremens (DTs) or seizures also are unusual in adolescents. Acute alcohol intoxication can result in *blackouts,* which are caused by acute dysfunction of the hippocampus. Hangovers are a form of *subacute short-term withdrawal* and are mainly found in adults.

Hormonal Changes. Drinking can lower estrogen levels in girls and testosterone levels in boys. In both genders, acute alcohol intake reduces growth hormone levels.

Neurotoxicity. Alcohol is a neurotoxin. Adolescence is a time when the brain's efficiency is enhanced. The subcortical gray matter and limbic system increase in volume while the prefrontal cortex decreases in volume owing to synaptic pruning. These areas of the brain are responsible for planning, integrating information, abstract reasoning, problem solving, and judgment. Research to date demonstrates the following effects: (1) Adolescents are relatively resistant to the sedative effects of alcohol. They show less ataxia and social impairment and fewer acute withdrawal effects than adults. (2) Imaging studies of teens with significant alcohol use show a reduced volume of the hippocampus and abnormalities of the corpus callosum. Functional MRIs show decreased functional activity of the frontal and parietal areas of the right hemisphere—areas responsible for spatial memory. (3) Neurocognitive testing of long-term users shows decreased visuospatial motor speed and decreased reading recognition, total reading, and spelling subtests on IQ testing. (4) Increased consumption is associated with decreased memory, abstract thought, and language. Teens with over 100 drinking episodes showed decreased verbal and nonverbal retention when compared with nondrinking controls.

Fetal Alcohol Syndrome. Fetal alcohol syndrome is the most common cause of teratogenic mental retardation and also the most preventable. There is no known safe level of alcohol use during pregnancy. Characteristics of fetal alcohol syndrome include (1) abnormal facies: microcephaly; short, upturned nose; thin upper lip; short palpebral fissures; and hypoplastic maxilla; (2) cardiac abnormalities: especially atrial and ventricular septal defects; (3) renal abnormalities: deformed kidneys; (4) genital abnormalities: hypospadias and labial hypoplasia; (5) skeletal abnormalities: contractures of the extremities, pectus excavatum; (6) hirsutism; (7) CNS abnormalities: electroencephalographic changes, mental retardation; (8) abnormal size: small for gestational age; (9) behavior: irritability in infancy, hyperactivity in childhood.

TABLE 69.1

Effects of Alcohol Consumption in the Nontolerant Individual

Blood Alcohol Level (g/100 mL)	Effects
0.02	Reached after approximately one drink; light or moderate drinkers feel some effect—warmth and relaxation
0.04	Most people feel relaxed, talkative, and happy; skin may become flushed
0.05	First sizable changes begin to occur; light-headedness, giddiness, lowered inhibitions, and less control of thoughts may be experienced; both restraint and judgment are lowered; coordination may be slightly altered
0.06	Judgment is somewhat impaired; ability to make rational decisions about personal capabilities is affected (such as being able to drive)
0.08	Definite impairment of muscle coordination and slower reaction time occurs; driving ability becomes suspect; sensory feelings of numbness of the cheeks and lips occur; hands, arms, and legs may tingle and then feel numb (this constitutes legal impairment in Canada and in some U.S. states, e.g., California)
0.10	Clumsiness; speech may become fuzzy; clear deterioration of reaction time and muscle control (this level previously constituted drunkenness in most U.S. states)
0.15	Definite impairment of balance and movement
0.20	Motor and emotional control centers are measurably affected; slurred speech, staggering, loss of balance, and double vision can all be present
0.30	Lack of understanding of what is seen or heard occurs; individuals are confused or stuporous and may lose consciousness
0.40	Usually unconscious; the skin becomes clammy
0.45	Respiration slows and may stop altogether
0.50	Death occurs

From Morrison SF, Rogers PD, Thomas MH. Alcohol and adolescents. *Pediatr Clin North Am* 1995;42:371–387.

PROBLEM DRINKING AMONG ADOLESCENTS

Nationally in the year 2006, some 10.9% of 8th graders, 21.9% of 10th graders, and 25.4% of 12th graders were classified as heavy drinkers (five or more drinks in a row during the previous 2 weeks). In addition, 19.5% of 8th graders, 42% of 10th graders, and 57.5% of 12th graders said that they had been drunk. Daily alcohol use rates are 0.5% in the 8th grade, 1.4% in the 10th grade, and 3.0% in the 12th grade. In 2006, the percentage of high school students who had a history of being drunk daily was 0.2% in 8th grade, 0.5% in 10th grade, and 1.6% in 12th grade.

Binge-drinking adolescents are at higher risk for the harmful effects of acute intoxication. They are also more likely to engage in risk-taking behaviors. They are more likely to carry a gun, use marijuana and cocaine, earn lower grades (Ds and Fs), be injured in fights, attempt suicide, and have sex with multiple partners. The health care provider must be acutely aware of the differing patterns of use manifested in adolescence.

Characteristics of Alcoholism. (1) The disease is often progressive and may be fatal. (2) The individual has impaired control over drinking, progressive preoccupation with alcohol use despite significant adverse consequences, and distortions in thinking, most notably denial. (3) Adverse consequences include impairments in work or school functioning, negative influences on interpersonal relationships, and legal or health-status ramifications. (4) There is often a family history of alcoholism. (5) The biopsychosocial consequences of drug use during adolescence are often the same, whether or not addictions are present. (6) Further confounding diagnostic accuracy is the fact that adolescents who use large amounts of alcohol generally deceive the physicians with whom they come in contact.

DIAGNOSIS (SEE CHAPTER 73)

Behavioral Changes. Certain behavioral changes can arouse the suspicion of alcohol or other drug abuse (but none is an absolute indicator of excessive drinking). These include behaviors such as changes in activity; loss of interest in school, play, home, or work; changes in sleeping patterns; changes in eating patterns; and changes in personality. They may be reflected in mood changes, fighting with friends and family members, or truancy as well as manifestations of depression, trouble with the law enforcement system, multiple or frequent accident-related injuries, school failure, blackouts. Table 69.2 outlines developing signs of alcoholism in teens.

Screening Instruments. Determining the extent of alcohol abuse and diagnosing alcoholism in the adolescent is crucial. The HEEADSS psychosocial profile, as outlined in Chapter 3, is a helpful interview technique for eliciting a history of substance abuse. Several screening devices are also available to help make this diagnosis (see Chapter 73 for details). These include (1) CAGE (Fig. 69.1); (2) MAST (see The Michigan Alcoholism Screening Test: the quest for a new diagnostic instrument. *Am J Psychol* 1971;127:89 and http://ajp.psychiatryonline.org/cgi/reprint/127/12/1653); (3) CRAFFT (see Chapter 73); (4) AUDIT: The Alcohol Use Disorders Identification Test. AUDIT

TABLE 69.2

Developing Signs of Alcoholism in Teenagers

Social/Psychological Signs	Classroom Behavior	Physical Signs
Personality change when drinking	Attendance	A change in tolerance to alcohol, either an increase or a decrease
Blackouts or temporary amnesia during and after drinking episodes	Misses Monday mornings	Hangovers
Loss of control of drinking	Late after lunch	Marked weight gain or loss
Drinks more than peers and more often	Leaves school early on Fridays	Repeated minor injuries
Morning drinking to overcome hangover effects	Frequent absences	Sexual activity beyond standard of peer group
Drinking-related arrests	General	Characteristics of final phases— obvious and tragic:
Defensiveness about alcohol usage	Works below expected potential level	Extended binges
Obsession with consumption of next drink	Inconsistency in aggressiveness and passivity in classroom participation	Physical tremors
Mixing of alcohol with drugs for a better high	Drinks at school, hides alcohol in locker	Hallucinations
Need to drink before going to a party	Boasts about drinking	Deliria
Feeling of remorse about drinking	Alcohol on breath	Convulsions
Occurrence of fights when drinking	Change in peer group affiliation	
Development of elaborate system of lies, alibis, and excuses to cover up drinking	Sleeps during classes	
	General troubles in school	

Adapted from the National Council on Alcoholism of San Fernando Valley, California.

1. Have you ever felt you ought to Cut down on your drinking?
2. Have people Annoyed you by criticizing your drinking?
3. Have you ever felt bad or Guilty about your drinking?
4. Have you ever had a drink first thing in the morning to steady your nerves or to get rid of a hangover (Eye opener)?

FIGURE 69.1 CAGE questionnaire for alcoholism. (From Ewing JA. Detecting alcoholism: the CAGE questionnaire. *JAMA* 1985;252:14.)

is effective in identifying subjects with at-risk, hazardous, or harmful drinking (sensitivity, 51% to 97%; specificity, 78% to 96%). However, the CAGE questions proved better for discovering alcohol abuse and dependence (sensitivity, 43% to 94%; specificity, 70% to 97%). It should be noted that these tests were not specifically examined in adolescents. CRAFFT using two positive responses as the threshold for identifying alcohol use problems has a sensitivity of 76% and specificity of 94% and has been tested in primary care settings with adolescents (see Chapter 73).

Family History. A family history of alcoholism or addiction also places the adolescent at high risk for abuse of an addictive substance and subsequent addiction (see above).

TREATMENT

The American Medical Association *Guidelines for Adolescent Preventive Services* (GAPS), *Bright Futures*, and the American Academy of Pediatrics *Policy Statement on Substance Abuse* all recommend that every adolescent be screened during history taking for alcohol, tobacco, and other drug abuse (ATODA) as part of routine care. Research shows that brief interventions in physicians' offices can be effective in helping patients to change their behavior (see Chapters 72 and 73 for further discussion alcohol and drug abuse treatment interventions).

WEB SITES AND REFERENCES

http://www.nida.nih.gov. National Institute on Drug Abuse (NIDA).
http://www.nofas.org/about/programs.aspx. National Organization on Fetal Alcohol Syndrome.
http://www.niaaa.nih.gov/. National Institute on Alcohol Abuse and Alcoholism.
http://www.cdc.gov/ncbddd/fas/. CDC on Fetal Alcohol Syndrome.
http://www.healthfinder.gov/orgs/HR0027.htm. SAMHSA's National Clearinghouse.
http://www.ncadi.samhsa.gov. Prevention site for SAMHSA.
http://www.nida.nih.gov/TB/Clinical/Clinicaltoolbox.html. The NIDA Clinical Toolbox.
http://monitoringthefuture.org/. Monitoring the Future Site with statistics.
Al-Anon/Alateen Family Group Headquarters, Inc., P.O. Box 862 Midtown Station, New York, NY 10018-0862, telephone 1-212-302-7240 or 1-800-344-2666 (United States) or 1-800-443-4525 (Canada).

CHAPTER 70

Tobacco

Seth D. Ammerman

"Cigarette smoking is the chief, single avoidable cause of death in our society and the most important public health issue of our time." (C. Everett Koop, MD, as U.S. Surgeon General, 1981–1989.)

The World Health Organization (WHO) estimates that if current smoking patterns continue, tobacco use will cause 10 million deaths each year by 2020. In the United States, about 438,000 deaths each year—the equivalent of three 747 fatal airline crashes per day—can be attributed to cigarette smoking. This figure is almost triple the annual number of deaths due to illegal drugs, homicide, alcohol, AIDS, suicide, and motor vehicle accidents combined. The financial cost for smoking-related health care per year in the United States is about $75 billion, or about 10% of total medical expenditures, plus an additional $92 billion in productivity losses. Additionally, cigarettes are the leading cause of the roughly 1,000 fire-related deaths and many thousands of fire-related injuries each year, costing approximately $1/2 billion annually just in direct property losses. More than 80% of all cigarette smokers start before the age of 18 years; almost 5% of youth first began smoking by 8 years of age and another 15% before their 13th birthday. Estimates derived from current smoking rates indicate that about 250 million youth worldwide will die prematurely from a tobacco-related disease. Many youth who are daily smokers report that they want to quit smoking. Exposure to environmental tobacco smoke (ETS, or second-hand smoke) is also a serious problem. Clinicians can play an important role in preventing cigarette use by their patients and helping their patients who are already smoking to stop.

PREVALENCE

Use among Adolescents. Tobacco use by adolescents remains a serious problem, with more than 2,000 American teenagers becoming regular smokers each day. The tobacco industry needs an ongoing supply of new smokers to maintain profits. Prevalence data are available from the following websites: www.americanlegacy.org, www.cdc.gov/tobacco, www.monitoringthefuture.org, www.nida.nih.gov, and http://oas.samhsa.gov/nsduh.htm. The 2006 Monitoring the Future (MTF) data indicate that about 8.7% of 8th graders, 14.5% of 10th graders, and 21.6% of 12th graders reported current smoking (i.e., smoking one or more cigarettes during the previous 30 days). Also, 22.4% of 12th-grade boys were current smokers, as were 20.1% of 12th grade girls. Furthermore, 4.0% of 8th graders, 7.6% of 10th graders, and 12.2% of 12th graders were daily smokers in 2006. The MTF study has shown a decline in current and daily smoking from 1990 to 2006. Whites have the highest smoking rates, followed by Hispanics and then blacks. Smoking continues to be a problem among college students and young adults (for trends, see Chapter 84).

The 2004 National Youth Tobacco Survey examines the use of a variety of tobacco products including cigarettes, smokeless tobacco (snuff and chewing tobacco), cigars, pipes, bidis, and kreteks (Table 70.1). Adolescents used all of these products. Bidis, produced in India and other Southeast Asian countries, are handrolled cigarettes consisting of tobacco wrapped in a tendu or temburni leaf. Bidis are available in various flavors such as chocolate, cherry, and mango. Kreteks are cigarettes that contain 30% to 40% cut cloves; they are produced in Indonesia. Both bidis and kreteks are relatively new to the American market and are promoted as "safe" alternatives to cigarettes, as are "clove cigarettes." However, these products contain tobacco and may have even higher levels of nicotine, tar, and carbon monoxide than regular tobacco products.

WHY DO ADOLESCENTS USE TOBACCO?

Adolescent Development. Tobacco use in adolescence can be understood in terms of biopsychosocial development during adolescence. Cigarette smoking may, for example, be viewed as a means of attaining maturity and autonomy, since smoking is a legal adult behavior. Smoking may also be viewed as a social event and a means of fitting in with a peer group. Research has shown that peer influence (e.g., smoking status of best friends) is the most significant and consistent predictor of adolescent smoking. On the other hand, protective factors leading to less smoking among youth include giving clear messages against smoking, youth involvement in healthy activities such as sports and religious institutions, and limiting exposure to tobacco advertising, including magazines, movies, sporting events, etc. The price of tobacco products also correlates with adolescent tobacco use: a significant price increase leads to a decrease in use.

Psychosocial Factors. Psychosocial factors related to smoking initiation for both genders include low educational aspirations or attainment; low self-esteem or low self-image, or ongoing stress or depression; risk taking; minimizing perceived hazards of smoking; and favorable attitudes toward smoking or smokers. Other variables associated with adolescent smoking include parental or sibling smoking, perceived support for smoking by parents or peers, having lower socioeconomic status or parental educational attainment, or a history of abuse. There are also gender-specific factors associated with smoking. For example, adolescent girl smokers are more likely to be socially skilled, outgoing, and self-confident. In contrast, adolescent boy smokers may be more insecure in social settings. Teenage girls may use cigarette smoking as a method of weight control and maintenance of a thin appearance. Teenage boys may smoke for a sense of adventure and recreation as well as daring. Youth who identify themselves as gay, lesbian, or bisexual smoke at rates >50% higher

TABLE 70.1

Percentage of Students in High School (grades 9–12) Who were Current Users[a] of Any Tobacco Product, By Product Type, Sex, and Race/Ethnicity

Characteristic	Any Tobacco[b] %	(95% CI[c])	Cigarettes %	(95% CI)	Cigars %	(95% CI)	Smokeless Tobacco %	(95% CI)	Pipes %	(95% CI)	Bidis %	(95% CI)	Kreteks %	(95% CI)
High school, 2004														
Sex														
Male	31.5	(±3.0)	22.1	(±2.7)	18.4	(±1.8)	10.8	(±2.2)	4.6	(±0.9)	3.6	(±0.7)	3.2	(±0.8)
Female	24.7	(±3.1)	22.4	(±3.1)	7.5	(±1.4)	1.4	(±0.6)	1.6	(±0.6)	1.6	(±0.5)	1.5	(±0.5)
Race/Ethnicity														
White, non-Hispanic	31.5	(±4.1)	25.4	(±3.8)	13.6	(±2.1)	7.5	(±1.6)	2.9	(±0.8)	2.2	(±0.5)	2.3	(±0.7)
Black, non-Hispanic	17.1[d]	(±3.3)	11.4	(±3.1)	10.5	(±2.1)	1.7	(±1.2)	1.8[d]	(±0.8)	2.1	(±0.8)	1.3	(±0.5)
Hispanic	26.2	(±2.9)	21.6	(±3.1)	13.3[d]	(±1.7)	3.5	(±1.1)	5.0	(±1.0)	4.6	(±0.9)	3.3	(±0.7)
Asian	13.1	(±3.3)	11.2	(±2.6)	5.7	(±2.4)	2.1	(±1.7)	2.0	(±1.1)	2.1	(±1.2)	1.4	(±1.0)
Total	28.0	(±2.9)	22.3	(±2.7)	12.8	(±1.5)	6.0	(±1.2)	3.1	(±0.6)	2.6	(±0.5)	2.3	(±0.5)
High school, 2002														
Sex														
Male	32.6	(±2.3)	23.9	(±2.1)	16.9	(±1.4)	10.5	(±2.0)	5.0	(±0.9)	3.7	(±0.8)	3.5	(±0.7)
Female	23.7	(±1.8)	21.0	(±1.9)	6.2	(±0.9)	1.2	(±0.3)	1.4	(±0.4)	1.5	(±0.4)	1.8	(±0.5)
Race/Ethnicity														
White, non-Hispanic	30.9	(±2.0)	25.2	(±1.8)	11.8	(±1.0)	7.3	(±1.4)	2.8	(±0.6)	2.2	(±0.5)	2.7	(±0.6)
Black, non-Hispanic	21.7	(±2.9)	13.8	(±2.8)	12.0	(±1.9)	1.8	(±0.8)	3.7	(±1.2)	3.4	(±1.1)	1.9	(±0.8)
Hispanic	24.1	(±2.7)	19.8	(±2.5)	10.8	(±1.5)	3.3	(±1.1)	4.6	(±1.1)	3.5	(±0.9)	3.0	(±0.8)
Asian	14.6	(±3.8)	12.2	(±3.4)	5.4	(±2.3)	2.1	(±1.5)	2.7	(±1.5)	2.9	(±1.6)	2.1	(±1.7)
Total	28.2	(±1.7)	22.5	(±1.6)	11.6	(±0.9)	5.9	(±1.1)	3.2	(±0.6)	2.6	(±0.5)	2.7	(±0.4)

[a]Used tobacco on at least 1 day during the 30 days preceding the survey.
[b]Cigarettes, cigars, smokeless tobacco, pipes, bidis (leaf-wrapped, flavored cigarettes from India), or kreteks (clove cigarettes).
[c]Confidence interval.
[d]Significant difference ($p < 0.05$), 2004 versus 2002.
National Youth Tobacco Survey, United States, 2002 and 2004.

than those of their straight counterparts, and they are four times more likely to use smokeless tobacco products.

Advertising. Tobacco industry advertising plays an important role in inducing adolescents to smoke. The tobacco industry promotes its products in virtually every advertising medium, ranging from billboards and magazines to electronic media and movies. Studies have shown that >50% of the onset of youth tobacco use is due to smoking portrayed in the movies. The Smoke Free Movies campaign has proposed four measures to make sure that the U.S. film industry does not act as a marketing arm for the tobacco industry. The recommendations are as follows (see full details at www.smokefreemovies.ucsf.edu): **(1) Certify no payoffs. (2) Require antismoking ads. (3) Stop displaying brands. (4) Rate new smoking movies "R."** The tobacco industry spends more than $15 billion per year promoting tobacco products in the United States alone.

NICOTINE ADDICTION AND HEALTH CONSEQUENCES

Addiction. In addition to being a potent pesticide, nicotine is one of the most addictive substances known. Tobacco use by adolescents, which may have started primarily for psychosocial reasons, may over time become a serious drug addiction. Initial symptoms of nicotine dependence occur in some teens within days to weeks after onset of use.

Modes of Action. Nicotine seems to function as a positive reinforcer through its actions on nicotinic acetylcholine receptors in the mesocorticolimbic dopamine pathway. Stimulation of brain dopamine systems is of great importance for the rewarding and dependence-producing properties of nicotine. Abstinence from nicotine is associated with depletion of dopamine and other neurotransmitters, which may cause numerous withdrawal symptoms, including anxiety, irritability, and cravings (Fig. 70.1). Relapse rates for persons attempting to quit use of nicotine are comparable to those for quitting heroin. There are likely genetic factors [e.g., genetic variants in the dopamine D2 receptor (DRD2) gene] in an individual's susceptibility to tobacco addiction as well as to his or her response to the various pharmacologic treatments.

Effects of Other Compounds in Cigarettes. Besides nicotine, cigarettes contain tar, a toxic compound. Cigarettes usually contain literally thousands of other chemicals, many poisonous and cancer-causing, including ammonia, cadmium, carbon monoxide, cyanide, formaldehyde, nitrosamines, and polynuclear aromatic hydrocarbons.

Systemic Effects of Tobacco. The U.S. Surgeon General's report in 2004 updated the list of diseases related to tobacco use. Use of tobacco products can adversely affect virtually every organ system in the body. The report can be found at www.surgeongeneral.gov/reportspublications.html.

   Smokeless tobacco and exposure to environmental tobacco smoke (ETS) also have numerous serious and adverse health consequences.

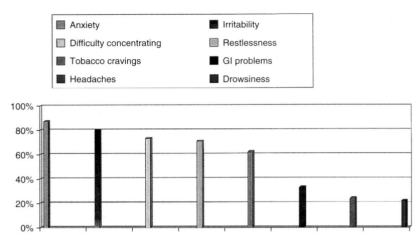

FIGURE 70.1 Nicotine withdrawal symptoms. (Adapted from National Center for Chronic Disease Prevention and Health Promotion, Office of Smoking and Health. *The health consequences of smoking: nicotine addiction. A report of the Surgeon General.* Washington, DC: U.S. Department of Health and Human Services, Public Health Service, Centers for Disease Control, 1988.)

PREVENTION AND TREATMENT

Brief Practitioner Interventions. Although smoking onset and maintenance by adolescents are complex psychosocial and biological phenomena, as noted earlier, research has demonstrated that 3-minute discussions of tobacco use *(brief interventions)* can have a significant impact on smoking prevention or smoking cessation. There are two types of 3-minute interventions: those directed toward *patients* (Fig. 70.2) and those directed toward *parents* (Fig. 70.3). Strong and direct language is purposefully used, and these kinds of messages have been found to be very helpful. Given the medical problems associated with ETS and given that parents are among the most important role models for adolescents, health care providers must also provide smoking cessation referrals and/or interventions for the parents of their patients. It is much more likely for an adolescent to start smoking, and much more difficult for an adolescent to successfully quit smoking, if he or she is living with siblings or parents who smoke. Therefore, siblings and parents need to be encouraged to quit too. Parents should be encouraged to maintain smokefree homes.

Antismoking Messages. The antismoking message should be varied according to the smoking status, age, and developmental stage of the patient. *Prevention* starts with the prenatal visit and continues throughout childhood (as noted earlier, children may start smoking by the age of 8 years) and during the preteen, teen, young adult, and adult years. Anticipatory guidance should always include tobacco use counseling.

U.S. Public Health Service Clinical Guidelines. In 2000, the clinical practice guideline for treating tobacco use and dependence was revised.

3-MINUTE CESSATION MESSAGES FOR TEEN PATIENTS

- Nicotine is an addictive drug. Do you want to be chained to a cigarette?

- There are thousands of chemicals in cigarettes. Many of these chemicals are toxic. Some cause cancer. Why pollute your body with these poisons?

- Cigarettes cost a lot of money. Wouldn't it be better to buy a compact disc, or go to a movie?

- Most teens are nonsmokers. Why is that?

- The tobacco companies have admitted that nicotine is addictive. But the tobacco companies think teens are stupid, because they make a lot of money off teen smokers.

- Smoking causes yellow teeth, bad skin and wrinkles, smelly clothes, and bad breath. Do you think that's attractive?

- Why not try to relax in a way that makes your body more fit, like sports, dancing, or exercise?

- Quitting may not be easy, but millions of people have successfully quit smoking. Remember, the average number of quit attempts before successful quitting is 7!

- There are medications to help you during the quit process, if you need them.

- Be smart. Don't let the tobacco companies manipulate you.

FIGURE 70.2 Patient 3-minute pointers. Adapted from Ammerman SD. Helping kids kick butts. *Contemp Pediatr* 1998;15(2):64.

The five "As"—**Ask, Advise, Assess, Assist, and Arrange**—are used for smoking cessation counseling. There are very few published (and even fewer methodologically sound) studies concerning smoking cessation in teens. Therefore, these treatment guidelines are based primarily on the adult literature.

1. ***Ask*** systematically about smoking at each visit. A simple and effective way to operationalize this is to add a yes/no question about tobacco exposure and use to the vital sign portion of the chart note (Fig. 70.4). Thus when vital signs are taken at every visit, the use of tobacco will be brought up. Smoking status can change quickly in teenagers, and a previous nonsmoker may be smoking by the time of the next visit—or a regular smoker who did not wish to quit in the past may now wish to quit smoking.
2. ***Advise*** all smokers strongly to quit. Advice that is clear and personally relevant is most effective. Physicians are looked on as authoritative figures, even by teens, and giving a consistent cessation message is important. Be sure that smokers understand that cigarettes labeled "light" or "ultralight" are not safer cigarettes. These cigarettes contain the same amount of nicotine, tar, and many other ingredients as regular cigarettes.

3-MINUTE CESSATION MESSAGES FOR PARENTS

- Second-hand smoke is dangerous to your child's health. Please do not smoke around your child.

- If your child is around smokers, he or she will have more respiratory infections and worsening of asthma.

- Smoking during pregnancy is associated with lower birth weights and sudden infant death syndrome (SIDS).

- Cigarettes are expensive: you waste approximately $1,000 a year if you smoke a pack a day. Aren't there better ways to spend that money?

- Your life insurance is much more expensive if you smoke.

- You are more likely to die at a younger age if you smoke; don't you want to see your children grow up, and be around for your grandchildren?

- If you smoke, your children are much more likely to smoke. Do you want your children to smoke?

- Most adults don't smoke. Why do you think you smoke?

- Quitting is easier sometimes if you use medications like the nicotine patch, or Zyban, during your quit attempt.

FIGURE 70.3 Parent 3-minute pointers. Adapted from Ammerman SD. Helping kids kick butts. *Contemp Pediatr* 1998;15(2):64.

3. **Assess** patient willingness to make a quit attempt. The more importance the patient attaches to quitting and the more self-confidence he or she has in successfully making a quit attempt, the more likely will the patient be successful.

4. **Assist** the patient in stopping smoking.

   a. *Motivational steps:* Setting a quit date has been shown to be an important and effective first step in smoking cessation. An actual calendar date should be chosen and agreed upon by the patient and physician. See Figure 70.5 for an example of a quit-date form. Once the quit date has been selected (usually 2 to 4 weeks away), the patient can prepare to become a nonsmoker. Psychosocial support has been shown to lead to more successful quit attempts. The patient should *actively elicit support from friends and family.* Going through the process with a "buddy" who is also willing to quit simultaneously can make the whole cessation process easier and should be encouraged. The clinician should provide "quit tips," as listed in Table 70.2.

   b. *Pharmacotherapy:* Pharmacotherapy includes nicotine replacement products (patch, gum, lozenge, inhaler, or nasal spray), and non-nicotine therapy (bupropion—Zyban and Varenicline—Chantix). These modalities may be very helpful for addicted smokers. Addiction is usually defined as

A Tobacco as a Vital Sign

For the Teen

Height _____ Weight _____ P_____ R_____ T _____ BP_____

Ask in a simple straightforward way:

"We now ask teens about tobacco use at each visit. This is confidential. Do you ever use any tobacco products? Are you around tobacco smoke at home or with friends?"

Teen tobacco exposure? Yes_____ No_____ Advice given_____

Teen tobacco use? Yes_____ No_____ Advice given_____

B Tobacco as a Vital Sign

For the Parent

Height _____ Weight _____ P_____ R_____ T _____ BP_____

Ask in a simple straightforward way:

"We now ask parents about their child's exposure to tobacco at each visit. Is your child ever exposed to tobacco smoke?"

Teen tobacco exposure? Yes_____ No_____ Advice given_____

Teen tobacco use? Yes_____ No_____ Advice given_____

FIGURE 70.4 Tobacco as a vital sign: teen and parent forms (see below).

A FIRM QUIT DATE IS AN IMPORTANT STEP IN QUITTING SMOKING

I agree to quit smoking on the following date: _____.

I understand that quitting smoking is the single best thing I can do for my health.

My signature: _____.

My health care professional's signature: _____.

Today's date: _____.

I understand that my health care professional will contact me on or around my quit date

to see how things are going, and to arrange a follow-up visit at the office.

FIGURE 70.5 A firm quit date is an important step in quitting smoking. Adapted from Ammerman SD. Helping kids kick butts. *Contemp Pediatr* 1998;15(2):64.

TABLE 70.2

Guide for Patients: How to Stop Smoking

Quitting smoking is not easy but millions of people have done it and so can you. These tips will help.

Getting ready to quit
- Set a date for quitting. Try to convince a friend to quit with you, so you will have mutual support. Let your family and friends know that you are trying to quit; they can help you through the harder times and give you ongoing encouragement.
- Notice when, where, and how you smoke—list the times when you usually light up—with morning coffee, after a meal, while driving, or whatever your usual smoking occasions are.
- Change your smoking routines. Keep your cigarettes in a different place, do not hold your cigarette in the hand you are used to using, switch brands, and do not carry on any other activity—such as reading, driving, talking on the phone, or watching television—while you smoke.
- Designate one place to smoke—such as the back porch—and do not smoke anywhere else.
- When you want a cigarette, wait a few minutes before you light up. Try doing something else, such as chewing gum or drinking a glass of water, and see if the urge passes.
- Buy only one pack of cigarettes at a time.
- Ask your doctor about medications that ease withdrawal symptoms and reduce cigarette cravings. You may want to have nicotine patches or gum on hand, ready for quit day.

On quitting day
- Get rid of all your cigarettes and put away your ashtrays.
- Change your morning routines, especially where and when you eat breakfast. Try sitting somewhere else, or going out to eat.
- When you get the urge to smoke, do something else instead.
- Carry substitutes to put in your mouth, such as chewing gum, hard candy, or toothpicks.
- Reward yourself at the end of the day. See a movie, or eat a favorite treat.

Staying smoke free
- Do not be upset if you feel sleepy or short tempered. These are symptoms of nicotine withdrawal and they will go away in a few days.
- Exercise regularly. Go for walks, ride a bike, or take part in sports you enjoy.
- Think about the positive aspects of not smoking: Your self-image as someone who has kicked the habit, the health benefit you and your family get from living in a smoke-free environment, and the example you set for others.
- When you feel tense, think about the problem that causes those feelings and try to solve it. Tell yourself that smoking will not make it better.

(continued)

TABLE 70.2

(Continued)

- Eat regular meals, so you do not have times when you feel hungry and confuse that feeling with the desire to smoke.
- Put the money you would have spent on cigarettes in a money jar every day, and watch it mount up. Plan to buy something special for yourself.
- Let other people know you have stopped smoking. Your friends who still smoke may want to know how you did it.
- If you break down and smoke a cigarette, do not give up. Many former smokers made several attempts to stop before they succeeded. Quit again.

From Ammerman S. Helping kids kick butts. *Contemp Pediatr* 1998;15:71.

smoking half a pack of cigarettes or more per day, smoking the first cigarette of the day within 1 hour after awakening, or having had withdrawal symptoms during a previous quit attempt. Withdrawal symptoms and cravings can make quitting very difficult and may be mitigated in large part with use of pharmacotherapy. Prescribing instructions for these medications can be found in Table 70.3. Note that nicotine patches and the lozenge and gum are now over-the-counter medications. Distraction and relaxation techniques should also be encouraged to help patients deal with withdrawal and craving symptoms.

5. ***Arrange*** follow-up. Cessation rates have been shown to significantly improve with regular follow-up. For example, we usually call the patient on the quit date to congratulate him or her on the effort and then talk with or see the patient every 1 or 2 weeks during the first 3 months of the quit attempt—the time of greatest relapse. If a patient is able to quit for 3 straight months, he or she is more likely to quit for good. It is rare for a patient to relapse after remaining smokefree for an entire year. For smokers with numerous unsuccessful quit attempts, referral to a support group such as Nicotine Anonymous may be helpful.

ADVOCACY ISSUES

The most successful tobacco-control efforts involve a number of concerted actions. These include increasing the cost of tobacco products through higher taxes on the products; litigation against the tobacco industry to hold corporations financially responsible for the disease and death their products cause; ending government subsidies to the tobacco industry; banning advertising of tobacco products in youth-oriented media (see above, concerning the Smoke Free Movies Campaign) and youth-frequented activities such as sporting events; enforcing laws that ban minors from buying tobacco products; banning cigarette vending machines; promoting adoption of clean indoor air laws and smokefree facilities such as schools, day care centers, office buildings, restaurants, and bars; getting pharmacies to stop selling tobacco products;

TABLE 70.3

Pharmacotherapeutic Aids

Type	Indications	Warnings	Adverse Effects	Dosage	Prescribing Instructions	How to Obtain
Patch	Indicated for the relief of nicotine withdrawal symptoms, as part of a comprehensive smoking cessation program	Potential for fetal harm; cardiovascular effects may occur	Local skin reaction, usually mild	Nicoderm CQ and Habitrol: 21 mg (if smoke >10 cigarettes/d; otherwise start with 14 mg) × 6 wk, then 14 mg × 2 wk, then 7 mg × 2 wk; worn 24 hr/d Nicotrol: 15 mg × 6 wk, then 10 mg × 2 wk, then 5 mg × 2 wk, worn either 16 hr while awake, or 24 hr/d	Start the first patch on awakening on quit day Do not smoke while using the patch; if you must smoke, take off the patch Each morning, place a new patch on a relatively hairless spot between the neck and waist Use a different spot each day, to reduce skin irritation	Over the counter
Gum	Appropriate for patients who prefer it, or who have had skin reactions, or failure with the patch	Potential for fetal harm; cardiovascular effects may occur	Mouth soreness, hiccups, dyspepsia, and aching jaws are common, mild, and usually transient	2 mg and 4 mg Use 4 mg if smoking >25 cigarettes/d, use 2 mg if smoking <25 cigarettes/d Preferable to chew at least one piece every 1–2 hr; may chew up to 30 pieces of the 2 mg, or 20 pieces of 4 mg gum/d	Do not smoke while using the gum Chew gum slowly until it tastes minty, peppery, or orange, then park it between the cheek and gum to enhance nicotine absorption Chew slowly and park intermittently for approximately 30 min Reduce number of pieces chewed gradually over time	Over the counter Mint, pepper, or orange flavors

Nasal spray	Same as gum	Not recommended for patients with chronic nasal disorders; keep out of the reach of children	Nasal irritation	1–2 sprays in each nostril/hr, at least 8 times/d, to a maximum of 80 sprays/d; maximum recommended duration of treatment is 3 mo	Use as frequently as needed to counter withdrawal symptoms for approximately 8 wk, then reduce use over the next 4–6 wk	Prescription only
Inhaler	Same as gum	Same as gum	Use with caution in asthma	Up to 20 cartridges/d, up to 6 mo	Insert cartridge into mouthpiece; cartridge lasts approximately 20 min	Prescription only
Nicotine lozenge	Same as gum	Same as gum	Same as gum	2 mg or 4 mg Use 4 mg if smoke first cigarette of day within half hr of awakening Otherwise use 2 mg	Do not chew or swallow the lozenge Allow the lozenge to slowly dissolve over 20 or 30 min There may be a warm or tingly sensation in the mouth Intermittently shift the lozenge around in the mouth Reduce number of lozenges used gradually over time	Over the counter

(continued)

TABLE 70.3

(Continued)

Type	Indications	Warnings	Adverse Effects	Dosage	Prescribing Instructions	How to Obtain
Bupropion	For smokers who have failed to quit using nicotine medications alone	Should not be used in patients already on bupropion, or in patients with anorexia, bulimia, or seizure disorders	Dry mouth, insomnia, headache, rhinitis	150 mg once or twice a d, for up to 6 mo	Start with 150 mg q.o.d for 3 d, increase as needed to a maximum of 300 mg/d Initiate 1 wk q.o.d before quit date, to allow time for blood levels to build up May use in conjunction with nicotine replacement products	Prescription only
Varenicline	For smokers who prefer non-NRT or oral therapy	No studies in patients younger than 18 years, or pregnant women	Nausea, sleep disturbance, constipation, flatulence, vomiting	0.5 mg days 1–3 0.5 mg b.i.d. days 4–7, 1.0 mg b.i.d. day 8—end of treatment May use for up to 6 mo	Initiate 1 wk before quit date, to allow time for blood levels to build up	Prescription only

NRT, nicotine replacement therapy

advocating for divestment of tobacco industry stocks by state and local government investment agencies; shareholder efforts to change tobacco industry behavior; and giving the federal government regulatory oversight of tobacco as a drug. To fight the global epidemic of tobacco-related disease, the WHO (http://www.who.int/tobacco/en/) has developed a treaty on tobacco control, the International Framework Convention on Tobacco Control.

WEB SITES AND REFERENCES

http://www.cdc.gov/tobacco. CDC Web site on tobacco.

http://www.hhs.gov/safety/index.shtml#smoking. Department of Health and Human Services.

http://www.tobaccofreeperiodicals.org. Lists magazines that do not accept tobacco advertising.

http://www.aap.org. American Academy of Pediatrics Web site.

http://www.cancer.org. American Cancer Society Web site.

http://www.lungusa.org/tobacco. American Lung Association tobacco information and materials.

http://www.ahcpr.gov. Agency for Health Care Policy and Research Web site.

Colby SM, Monti PM, O'Leary TT, et al. Brief motivational intervention for adolescents in medical settings. *Addict Behav* 2005;30(5):865.

Killen JD, Robinson TN, Ammerman S, et al. Randomized clinical trial of the efficacy of bupropion combined with nicotine patch in the treatment of adolescent smokers. *Journal of Consulting and Clinical Psychology.* 2004;72(4):729–735.

CHAPTER 71

Psychoactive Substances of Abuse Used by Adolescents

Sharon Levy and Alan D. Woolf

Misuse of drugs, chemicals, plants and herbs, mushrooms, and other agents continues to be a major cause of mortality and morbidity for adolescents and young adults. Adolescents are vulnerable to the direct toxic effects of drugs and chemicals, but they also suffer collateral injury in terms of family and social relationships as well as work or school performance. The loss of a productive life can follow from the long-term adverse effects of drugs on learning, behavior, personality, vocational choices, and psychosocial adjustment.

MARIJUANA

Prevalence/Epidemiology. Marijuana is the most widely abused illicit drug in the United States, with >90.8 million adults (42.9%) aged 18 or older admitting marijuana use at least once. Since marijuana is readily available and perhaps not as stigmatized as other substances, it often serves as the introduction to illicit drug use. Marijuana has negative effects on physical and psychological health and is associated with tolerance, dependence, and a withdrawal syndrome.

Medical Use. The active ingredient, delta-9-tetrahydrocannabinol (THC), has been synthesized and is available in capsule form known as dronabinol (Marinol), a second-line agent for the treatment of anorexia associated with AIDS or for nausea and vomiting associated with chemotherapy.

Preparation and Dose. Marijuana is derived from the resinous oil of the flowering tops and leaves of the plant *Cannabis sativa*. Marijuana joints have a THC content of 0.5% to 5.0%, hashish contains 2% to 20%, and hashish oil may contain 15% to 30%.

Routes of Administration. Marijuana is usually smoked but may be eaten, brewed in tea, or ingested in pill form.

Physiology (Table 71.1)
Effects of Intoxication. Low to moderate doses of marijuana produce euphoria, time distortion, increased talking, and auditory and visual enhancements or distortions, increased heart rate, erythema of the conjunctivae, dry mouth and throat, dilated pupils, and impaired learning and cognitive functions. As acute effects wear off, marijuana users often have increased appetite

TABLE 71.1

Cannabinoid Physiology

Receptors	Pharmacodynamics	Distribution	Metabolism and Excretion
• CB1–brain • CB2–peripheral tissue	Stimulates the dopamine pathway from the ventral tegmental area to the nucleus accumbens	Lipid soluble; accumulates in fat stores	Cytochrome P-450 system • 65% excreted in feces • 35% in urine

(Pertwee, 1997).

and feel sleepy. High doses of marijuana may produce mood fluctuations, depersonalization, and hallucinations. Toxic reactions include anxiety, panic, organic brain syndrome, psychoses, delusions, hallucinations, and paranoia. Marijuana may produce seizures in epileptic individuals or psychotic episodes in schizophrenic individuals. Marijuana use has also been associated with the precipitation of psychotic episodes in patients not previously diagnosed with schizophrenia, which may not resolve with discontinuation.

Adverse Effects. (1) *CNS:* Marijuana causes a decrease in psychomotor functions and reaction times, making driving dangerous. Marijuana can cause lingering effects on memory and coordination. Studies have suggested that regular heavy use of marijuana may lead to long-term adverse neurocognitive effects. Chronic buildup of cannabinoids may affect executive functions such as focus, attention, and ability to filter out irrelevant information, and it may impair memory, learning ability, and perception. (2) *Amotivational syndrome:* Chronic heavy marijuana use may lead to a state of passive withdrawal from usual work and recreational activities. (3) *Pulmonary and cardiovascular:* Marijuana smoking results in a substantially greater respiratory burden of carbon monoxide and tar than does cigarette smoking and causes functional impairment of airway conductance, bronchoconstriction, cellular inflammation and damage, and bronchitis with cough, increased sputum production, wheezing, a decrease in forced expiratory volume in 1 second (FEV_1), a decrease in maximal midexpiratory flow rate (MMFR), and an increase in airway resistance. A link between chronic exposure to marijuana smoke and lung cancer in humans has been postulated. Marijuana use leads to an increase in sympathetic tone and a decrease in parasympathetic activity, producing tachycardia, increased myocardial oxygen consumption, and an increased cardiac output. (4) *Endocrine and immune function effects:* Marijuana lowers testosterone secretion, impairs sperm mobility, impairs menstrual cycles in animals, and may suppress immune function.

Acute Overdose and Emergency Treatment. Large doses can cause delirium, nausea, vomiting, dizziness, and anxiety. It can be contaminated by diarrhea-causing infectious agents (e.g., *Salmonella* species) or mixed with other drugs, which also may cause toxicity.

Withdrawal Syndrome. Including restlessness, irritability, mild agitation, insomnia, nausea, cramping, and sleep electroencephalographic disturbances on cessation.

Drug Interactions. May enhance sedation when used with alcohol, diazepam, antihistamines, phenothiazines, barbiturates, or narcotics and may enhance stimulation when used with cocaine or amphetamines. Antagonistic to the effects of phenytoin, propranolol, and insulin.

COCAINE

Prevalence/Epidemiology. More than 5.9 million Americans aged 12 or older (2.5%) have used cocaine within the past year, with males predominating 2:1 over females as abusers of the drug. Lifetime prevalence rates are down from the peak of the epidemic in the 1980s.

Medical Use. Cocaine is used medically to provide local anesthesia in surgical repairs. It provides hemostasis in the operative field by the vasoconstriction of mucous membranes and is often used topically in otolaryngology, plastic surgery, and emergency medical procedures.

Preparation and Dose. Cocaine (benzoylmethylecgonine, molecular weight 339.81, $C_{17}H_{21}NO_4$) is a stimulant made from an alkaloid contained in the leaves of the coca bush, *Erythroxylon coca*. Nasal insufflation is the most common route of ingestion. The cocaine "high" associated with nasal insufflation lasts about 60 to 90 minutes. "Crack" is a free-base form of cocaine (that can be smoked) made with baking soda, heat, and water. It is inexpensive, safe to produce, and highly addictive. The high associated with crack smoking lasts about 20 minutes.

Routes of Administration. Cocaine is most often insufflated but may also be smoked, injected intravenously, or ingested orally.

Physiology (Table 71.2)
Effects of Intoxication. Cocaine is a stimulant of the central and peripheral nervous systems; it has local anesthetic activity and is a vasoconstrictor. The CNS stimulation produces an intense euphoric "rush" (feelings of extreme pleasure, power, strength, and excitement) and "high" (increased alertness, confidence, and a general sense of well-being) upon ingestion when smoked or injected intravenously. Inhaled cocaine generally produces the high without the rush. Symptoms of cocaine intoxication include a hyperalert state, increased talking, restlessness, elevated temperature, anorexia, nausea, vomiting, dry mouth, dilated pupils, sweating, dizziness, hyperreflective reflexes, tachycardia, hypertension, and arrhythmias. People "coming down" from cocaine experience dysphoria, depression, sadness, crying spells, suicidal ideation, apathy, inability to concentrate, delusions, anorexia, insomnia, and paranoia.

TABLE 71.2

Cocaine Physiology

Receptors	Pharmacodynamics	Distribution	Metabolism and Excretion
D_1 and D_2 dopamine receptors	• Release of dopamine, epinephrine, norepinephrine, and serotonin • Blockade of neurotransmitter reuptake • Increase sensitivity of postsynaptic receptor sites	Plasma and extracellular fluid	• Hepatic esterases (80%) and plasma cholinesterase to form benzoylecgonine and ecgonine methyl ester • Hepatic-N-demethylation to form norcocaine

Adverse Effects. (1) *Psychiatric:* toxic psychosis, hallucinations, delirium, formication (hallucination that insects are creeping on or under the skin), body image changes, agitation, anxiety, or irritability. (2) *Neurologic:* seizures, paresthesias, hyperactive reflexes, tremor, pinprick analgesia, facial grimaces, headache, cerebral hemorrhage, cerebral infractions, cerebral vasculites, or coma. (3) *Skin:* excoriations, rashes, secondary skin infections. (4) *Cardiovascular:* (a) Acute: vasoconstriction, increased myocardial oxygen demand, tachycardia, angina, arrhythmias, chest pain, aortic dissection, hypertension, stroke, myocardial infarction, and cardiovascular collapse. (b) Chronic: accelerated atherosclerosis and thrombosis, endocarditis, myocarditis, cardiomyopathy, coronary artery aneurysms. (5) *Gastrointestinal:* acute ischemia, gastropyloric ulcers, perforation of the small and large bowel, colitis, hepatocellular necrosis. (6) *Respiratory:* pneumothorax, pneumomediastinum, pneumopericardium, pulmonary edema, pulmonary hemorrhage, tracheobronchitis, and respiratory failure. (7) *Musculoskeletal:* rhabdomyolysis. (8) *Obstetric:* low birth weight, prematurity, microcephaly, placental abruption.

Acute Overdose and Treatment. Cocaine is a short-acting drug; treatment of acute intoxication is not usually necessary. Acute cocaine use can result in lethal cardiovascular or respiratory collapse. The primary response to manage cocaine overdose is to support respiratory and cardiovascular functions, monitor vital signs and cardiac rhythm, and establish intravenous access. Cocaine is detectable in urine for up to 72 to 96 hours postexposure, whereas blood levels may fall below detectable thresholds as soon as 60 to 90 minutes after use. All residual cocaine should be removed from the patient's nostrils. If ingestions are suspected, activated charcoal should be administered orally or by gastric tube. If the patient presents with altered mental status, a blood glucose level should be checked and hypoglycemia treated if present. Hyperthermia can be treated with antipyretics, a cooling blanket, and iced saline lavage. Muscle paralysis with a nondepolarizing agent may be necessary to reduce muscle contractions contributing to the hyperthermia. Seizures can be treated with benzodiazepines or other standard anticonvulsants. Ventricular dysrhythmias may require an antiarrhythmic agent such as lidocaine, whereas supraventricular arrhythmias may respond to therapy with calcium channel blockers. Cardioversion may be necessary in some patients.

Cocaine-associated chest pain should be treated with nitroglycerin and benzodiazepines. Thrombolysis should be considered if the symptoms and signs of toxicity, an electrocardiogram, and cardiac enzymes are consistent with acute myocardial infarction. Hypertensive crisis can precipitate cerebrovascular hemorrhage and must be treated emergently. Blood pressure elevations may be the result of direct CNS stimulation (treated with benzodiazepines) or peripheral alpha agonist effects [treated with either vasodilators (e.g., nifedipine, nitroglycerin, nitroprusside) or an alpha-adrenergic antagonist such as phentolamine]. Acutely intoxicated patients should be approached in a subdued manner, with soft voice and slow movements. Agitation and psychosis should be treated with haloperidol or droperidol; chlorpromazine should be avoided because of the possibility of a severe drop in blood pressure, provocation of arrhythmias or seizures, or anticholinergic crisis. Flumazenil should be avoided for fear of unmasking seizure activity.

Chronic Use. Cocaine is irritating to the mucosa, skin, and airways; chronic use is associated with erosion of dental enamel, gingival ulceration, keratitis, chronic rhinitis, perforated nasal septum, midline granuloma, altered olfaction, optic neuropathy, osteolytic sinusitis, burns, and skin infarction. People addicted to cocaine also frequently experience anorexia, weight loss, sexual dysfunction, and hyperprolactinemia.

Tolerance and Withdrawal. Because of cocaine's powerful euphoric effects and its short half-life, repeated use leads to rapid development of tolerance, although no tolerance develops to the cardiovascular side effects. Symptoms of cocaine abstinence or withdrawal include depression, anhedonia, irritability, aches and pains, restless but protracted sleep, tremors, nausea, weakness, intense cravings for more cocaine, slow comprehension, suicidal ideation, lethargy, and hunger. There is currently no widely accepted treatment of cocaine withdrawal. Although many uncontrolled studies have been reported in the literature and some drugs look promising in early trials, no drug has been proven effective in controlled studies. Relapse rates are very high in cocaine-addicted patients who attempt abstinence.

Cocaethylene
When alcohol is used with cocaine, a third substance, cocaethylene, is formed in the liver and increases the toxicity of cocaine, particularly on the heart. It is also able to block dopamine reuptake, thereby extending the period of intoxication and toxicity.

AMPHETAMINE (AMPHETAMINE, METHAMPHETAMINE, METHYLPHENIDATE, KHAT)

Prevalence/Epidemiology. In the 2004 National Survey on Drug Use and Health, 20.8 million Americans aged 12 or older (8.8% of the population) had used prescription-type stimulants nonmedically at least once in their lifetimes and an estimated 378,000 persons met criteria for dependence or abuse within the preceding year. Lifetime use of methamphetamine was reported by 12.3 million; prescription diet pills by 8.7 million; Ritalin or methylphenidate by 4.2 million; and Dexedrine by 2.6 million. Continuing surveillance suggests that methamphetamine use is on the rise. In 2004, an estimated 1.4 million persons aged 12 and older (0.6% of the population) had used methamphetamine within the previous year, with 600,000 reporting use within the preceding month. The average age of first users increased from 18.9 years in 2002 to 20.4 years in 2003 to 22.1 years in 2004.

Medical Use. Amphetamines have been used as a weight loss aid, although their efficacy is questionable. Other uses include treatment of narcolepsy and attention-deficit/hyperactivity disorder (ADHD). The recent increase in the diagnosis and medical management of ADHD has increased the availability of amphetamines to adolescents, who may misuse their prescriptions by taking a higher dose than prescribed or distributing pills to peers, who may misuse them either as study aids or for intoxication. Appropriate treatment of adolescents with ADHD has been shown to decrease the risk of illicit substance use, but it must be carefully supervised. Longer-acting medications may have lower addiction potential than short-acting ones.

Preparation and Dose. The term *amphetamine* refers to a class of drugs containing an amphetamine base, available either in prescription form (such as amphetamine, dextroamphetamine, amphetamine sulfate) or illicitly manufactured (mainly in the form of methamphetamine). Amphetamines are CNS stimulants. Methamphetamine has a stronger effect on the CNS than other forms of amphetamine. Methylphenidate is a nonamphetamine stimulant with similar action available in prescription form. The maximum typically prescribed dose of amphetamine is in the range of 60 to 100 mg, but addicted patients may ingest up to 100 times the daily dose during a binge.

Routes of Administration and Street Names (Table 71.3). Prescription amphetamines are typically ingested orally, or via nasal insufflation. Illicit methamphetamine is usually smoked. Either preparation may be ground up, heated, and injected intravenously. Smoking methamphetamine may be more potent and addictive than snorting or ingesting it.

Physiology. Personality changes, aggressiveness, and psychosis.

Effects of Intoxication. Amphetamines are CNS stimulants. Users experience increased energy, psychological euphoria, and physical well-being. These effects are nearly identical to those of cocaine but last much longer. Smoked methamphetamine results in immediate euphoria resulting from rapid absorption in the lungs and deposition in the brain. Symptoms of amphetamine intoxication include alertness, anxiety, confusion, delirium, dry mouth, tachycardia, hypertension, tachypnea, jaw clenching, bruxism, reduced appetite, sweating, and psychosis. Depletion of neurotransmitters leads to post use dysphoria.

Adverse Effects. (1) *Psychiatric:* aggressiveness, confusion, delirium, psychosis. (2) *Neurologic:* seizures, choreoathetoid movements, cerebrovascular

TABLE 71.3

Chemical Names, Brand Names, and Street Names of Amphetamines

	Prescription Medications	
Chemical	Brand Name	Street Name
Dextroamphetamine	Dexedrine	Dexies, hearts, oranges
	Adderall	
Amphetamine sulfate	Benzedrine sulfate	Hearts, peaches, footballs
Benzphetamine	Didrex	
Methamphetamine	Desoxyn	Speed, crystal, meth

Illicit Methamphetamine	
Street Name	Description
Ice, crystal	Purified methamphetamine ingested by smoking
Yaba	Methamphetamine and caffeine tablet which may be smoked or ingested orally
Croak	Methamphetamine and crack cocaine

accidents cerebral edema, cerebral vasculitis. (3) *Cardiovascular:* tachycardia, hypertension, atrial and ventricular arrhythmias, and myocardial infarction, cardiac ischemia, coronary artery vasospasm, necrotizing angiitis, arterial aneurysms, aortic dissections. (4) *Gastrointestinal:* ulcers, ischemic colitis, hepatocellular damage. (5) *Musculoskeletal:* muscle contractions, rhabdomyolysis. (6) *Respiratory:* pneumomediastinum, pneumothorax, pneumopericardium; acute noncardiogenic pulmonary edema, pulmonary hypertension. (7) *Renal:* acute tubular necrosis. (8) *Dental:* chronic gingivitis, numerous dental caries, severe dental abscesses and necrosis known as "meth mouth."

Overdose and Emergency Treatment. Complications of amphetamine overdose resemble those of cocaine; as with cocaine, emergency treatment is directed toward cardiovascular and respiratory stabilization and control of seizures. Hyperactive or agitated persons should be treated with dopamine-blocking agents such as droperidol or haloperidol, which specifically antagonize the central behavioral effects of methamphetamine. Both drugs produce clinically significant reductions in pulse, systolic blood pressure, respiration rate, and temperature over a 60-minute period. Avoid chlorpromazine (Thorazine) because of the possibility of a severe drop in blood pressure, anticholinergic crisis, or seizure activity. Beyond 5 to 10 mg of haloperidol or droperidol, the sedating benefit is minimal and benzodiazepines should be added.

Chronic Use. Chronic use of amphetamines can produce severe psychiatric as well as physical problems, including delusions, hallucinations, and formication, leading individuals to tear and damage their skin. Some former users seem to have permanent personality changes even after long periods of abstinence from methamphetamine.

Tolerance and Withdrawal. Tolerance does occur with chronic methamphetamine use, and users may escalate their dose or change the route of exposure in order to maintain effect. Symptoms of withdrawal include depression, fatigue, sleep problems, increased appetite, headaches and drug cravings; these symptoms may begin as soon as the high ends and can last up to 7 to 10 days. There is no specific medical treatment for acute amphetamine withdrawal other than supportive care.

"ECSTASY" (METHYLENE DIOXYMETHAMPHETAMINE/MDMA)

Prevalence/Epidemiology. In the 2003 National Survey on Drug Use and Health, 2.1 million persons aged 12 and older reported ecstasy use within the past year, with virtually all of them reporting concomitant use of alcohol and 90% reporting use also of other illicit drugs. The Youth Risk Behavior Survey reported lifetime ecstasy use rates of 11.1% of students nationwide in 2003. According to Monitoring the Future (MTF), reported lifetime use of MDMA by high school students has declined slowly with a peak in 2001 at rates of 5.2% of 8th graders, 8.0% of 10th graders, and 11.7% of 12th graders to the current lower rates of 2.5%, 4.5%, and 6.5% in 2006.

Medical Use. There are no current medical uses for MDMA.

Preparation and Dose. The drug is sold as a tablet or capsule, often with a symbol printed on it. Tablets sold as MDMA may actually contain MDA, MDEA, or something entirely unrelated to the drug such as LSD, caffeine, pseudoephedrine, or dextromethorphan. The typical ecstasy tablet contains 0 to 100 mg of MDMA, although the concentration of MDMA may vary 70-fold or more among tablets sold. Orally ingested doses take approximately 30 minutes for onset of effect, and the duration of action is 1 to 2 hours. Many users begin with a low dose (40 to 70 mg) and gradually add more pills until they experience the desired effect at a common dosage range of 75 to 125 mg, a practice known as "rolling."

Routes of Administration and Street Names. MDMA can be snorted, smoked, or injected, but it is usually taken orally.

Physiology (Table 71.4)
Effects of Intoxication. MDMA has both stimulant and hallucinogen effects. Users describe feelings of enhanced well-being and introspection, empathy, love, affection, and energy.

Adverse Effects. (1) *Psychological:* confusion, depression, fatigue, sleep problems, anxiety, paranoia. (2) *Neurologic:* seizures, muscle spasms, bruxism, hyperthermia, sweating, syndrome of inappropriate secretion of antidiuretic hormone (SIADH), blurred vision, faintness, chills, excessive sweating, hyponatremia, serotonin syndrome (with repeated dosing). (3) *Musculoskeletal:* muscle rigidity, rhabdomyolysis. (4) *Cardiovascular:* tachycardia, hypertension, arrhythmias, cardiovascular failure, and asystole. (5) *Gastrointestinal:* nausea, severe hepatic damage. (6) *Fatalities:* There have been reports of life-threatening toxicity and death associated with ecstasy use. The mechanisms of death appear to be related to fatal hyperthermia, disseminated intravascular

TABLE 71.4

Methylenedioxymethamphetamine Physiology

Receptors	Pharmacodynamics	Distribution	Metabolism and Excretion
• Serotonin 5-HT$_2$ receptors • Central and peripheral catecholamine receptors	• Release of serotonin into the synapse • Release of endogenous catecholamines • Inhibition of serotonin reuptake • Depletion of serotonin stores occurs with repeated dosing, after which no further effect is achieved by taking more drug	• Few pharmacological studies have been performed in humans • Peak concentrations at 2 hours, half-life 8–9 hours	• Metabolized through cytochrome P-450 isoenzyme CYP2D6 into 3,4-methylenedioxyamphetamine (MDA) • 75% excreted in the urine as parent compound

coagulation, rhabdomyolysis, renal failure, cardiac arrhythmias and sudden asystole, hyponatremia, and seizures. Other reports have described deaths from serotonin syndrome, disseminated intravascular coagulation (DIC), hepatic failure, cerebral infarction, and cerebral hemorrhage.

Overdose and Emergency Treatment. The most common severe reaction to toxic MDMA ingestion is a syndrome of altered mental status, tachycardia, tachypnea, profuse sweating, and hyperthermia. This syndrome can appear similar to acute amphetamine overdose. The clinician is cautioned that MDMA may not be detected in routine toxicologic screening of the urine for amphetamines. The most frequent signs related to sympathetic over activity and include agitation or disturbed behavior and increased temperature. Serious complications such as delirium, seizures, and profound coma were more frequent with the combination of MDMA and other substances. Teens and young adults who present late at night on weekends and have clinical manifestations of sympathetic overactivity and increased temperature ("Saturday night fever") should be suspected of using stimulants and MDMA in particular.

The treatment of toxic ingestions of MDMA is supportive and similar to that for amphetamine overdose, including support of airway, breathing, and circulation; assessment and treatment of cardiac arrhythmias, monitoring of vital signs and level of consciousness. Close monitoring of vital signs, serum electrolytes and fluid balance, and urine output is required because of the possibility of SIADH and/or water loading–induced hyponatremia. Hyperthermia should be treated with cooling blankets and intravenous fluids. Muscle relaxants, anticonvulsants, and sedatives may be indicated.

Chronic Use. Research links MDMA to long-term damage to areas of the brain that are critical to thought and memory. Long-lasting impairment of the 5-hydroxytryptamine (5-HT) system has been found in past users of MDMA, which may be more prominent in female patients and may be reversible in some patients.

Withdrawal Syndrome. Ecstasy withdrawal is similar to withdrawal from stimulants; the most common symptoms include depression, anxiety, panic attacks, sleeplessness, paranoia and delusions. Treatment is supportive. While depressed affect may persist, there is no role for psychopharmacologic management.

OPIOIDS: OPIUM, HEROIN, MEPERIDINE, OXYCONTIN, OXYCODONE, FENTANYL, SUFENTANYL

Prevalence/Epidemiology. Opioids, especially the potent oral analgesics such as hydrocodone (Vicodin) and oxycodone (OxyContin) and oxycodone + acetaminophen (Percocet), continue to be attractive to teenagers. The prevalence of nonmedical oxycodone use increased significantly from 2002 to 2003, with an estimated 11 million Americans aged 12 and older reporting nonmedical oxycodone use at least once in their lifetimes. In 2006, 3.0% of 8th graders, 7.0% of 10th graders, and 9.7% of 12th graders reported experimenting with Vicodin at least once within the preceding year. Usage rates of OxyContin in the same year were 2.6%, 3.8%, and 4.3% respectively. Heroin use, which had briefly increased in popularity in the late 1990s, has since dropped off to lifetime usage rates among high school students averaging 1.4% to 1.6% in the past several years, with prevalence rates of annual use averaging 0.8% to 0.9% among 8th, 10th and 12th graders. According to the Drug Abuse Warning Network (DAWN), rates of emergency room visits for heroin overdose among 12- to 17-year-olds increased sharply between 2003 and 2004 and then dropped slightly between 2004 and 2005.

Medical Use. Opioids have several legitimate medical uses; they are potent antitussives, antidiarrheals, and extremely potent pain relievers. Newer oral medications with extended half-lives are a tremendous asset in the field of pain management. Synthetic narcotics, such as fentanyl, are 80 times more potent than morphine and pose an increased danger of death by overdose.

Preparation and Dose. Opium has been known and used for centuries. The term *opioid* refers to all drugs, natural and synthetic, with morphinelike activity as well as to antagonists that bind to opioid receptors, while *opiate* refers to opium, morphine, codeine, and heroin, all derived from the opium poppy, *Papaver somniferum*. The average purity of heroin sold on the street is 38%, up from 18% in 1990, allowing users to snort or smoke heroin. Over the past 10 years, the price of heroin has dropped significantly. The ability to use heroin without needles and the lower prices have made heroin more accessible to adolescents, and the average age of first use dropped from 23 years in 1992 to 19.8 years in 1999. Synthetic opioid pain relievers such as oxycodone, hydrocodone, and oxymorphone are pharmaceutical products that may be diverted and sold on the street. Many teens believe that these products are safer than drugs manufactured in clandestine laboratories, and their popularity has increased dramatically since 2000.

Routes of Administration and Street Names. Opioids can be ingested, insufflated nasally, smoked, or injected intravenously or subcutaneously. Most adolescents first use prescription pain medications either orally or by insufflation. OxyContin was developed as a long-acting pain reliever. It is intended to be swallowed whole so as to prolong its analgesic efficacy over 8 to 12 hours. Crushing the tablet destroys this continuous release property and makes the total dose available for a rapid "rush." Heroin is most potent when injected intravenously. Besides leg and arm veins, the veins between the toes, under the tongue, and the dorsal vein of the penis are often used for injection. Heroin is sometimes injected under the skin ("skin popping"), insufflated in the same manner as cocaine, or smoked; the effect is less intense with any of these methods than with intravenous use. The duration of the effects of intravenously injected heroin is 3 to 6 hours.

Physiology (Table 71.5)
Effects of Intoxication. Opioids produce analgesia, and, in high doses, euphoria. Symptoms of intoxication include anxiety, slow comprehension, euphoria, floating feeling, flushing, hypotonia, pinpoint pupils, skin picking, sleepiness, poor appetite, and constipation.

Adverse Effects. (1) *Psychiatric:* sedation, apathy, dysphoria, psychomotor agitation or retardation, impaired judgment, delirium, stupor. (2) *Neurologic:* diminished reflexes, miosis, pinprick analgesia, ataxia, hypothermia,

TABLE 71.5

Opioid Physiology

Receptors	Pharmacodynamics	Distribution	Metabolism and Excretion
μ, κ, and δ Opioid receptors (primarily μ).	Stimulation of opioid receptors produces euphoria, pain relief, and other effects	• Morphine—low lipid solubility, crosses blood–brain barrier slowly • Heroin—high lipid solubility, crosses blood–brain barrier quickly and then is metabolized, creating a "morphine rush"	• Metabolized by the liver (N-demethylation, N-dealkylation, O-dealkylation, conjugation and hydrolysis) • Primarily excreted in the urine (90%)

hypotonia, coma. (3) *Cardiovascular:* circulatory collapse, hypotension, hypothermia, peripheral vein thrombosis, phlebitis. (4) *Respiratory:* blocked cough reflex, bradypnea, respiratory failure, pulmonary edema. (5) *Gastrointestinal:* constipation. (6) *Skin:* rashes, allergic reactions, secondary bacterial infections, abcesses, cellulitis. (7) *Obstetric:* low birth weight, neonatal withdrawal and respiratory compromise.

Overdose and Emergency Treatment. Opioid overdose results in respiratory depression or failure and circulatory collapse. Treatment begins with support of respiratory and circulatory function, protection of the airway to prevent aspiration, and treatment of hypoglycemia if present. Patients should receive naloxone (0.4 to 2 mg) IV every 5 minutes until response occurs or up to a maximum of 10 mg. Usually if there is no response after three IV doses, this indicates that the individual has not taken an opioid overdose. Repeated doses may be needed in 2 to 3 hours as the naloxone wears off. Naloxone lasts for about 1 or 2 hours, whereas the effects of most opioids last 3 to 6 hours, and methadone lasts 24 to 36 hours, necessitating close observation during the treatment for opioid overdose. Resedation and respiratory failure may recur as the effects of naloxone wear off. Naloxone does not reverse hypotension that is caused by opiate-induced histamine release.

Chronic Use. Problems related to chronic use are primarily secondary to impurities present in the drugs taken, complications of injection or insufflation, and behaviors associated with addiction, such as prostitution, lying, and stealing.

Tolerance and Withdrawal. Tolerance, dependence, and addiction occur very quickly, and patients must increase dose and frequency constantly to avoid withdrawal symptoms. Opioid withdrawal presents with flulike symptoms, which can be extremely unpleasant but are not life-threatening in otherwise healthy individuals. Symptoms include anxiety, irritability, yawning, restlessness, sleep disturbances, muscle aches, chills and sweating, piloerection, hyperthermia, lacrimation and nasal secretions, abdominal cramps with vomiting and diarrhea, paresthesias, tremors, mydriasis, hypertension, and tachycardia. The Clinical Opiate Withdrawal Scale (COWS) (Table 71.6) was developed to quantify the symptoms of opioid withdrawal. Treatment for opioid withdrawal is supportive and includes symptomatic treatment of aches and pains with nonsteroidal anti-inflammatory medications, abdominal cramping with dicyclomine (Bentyl), and reassurance. Clonidine may also be helpful. Withdrawal can also be managed with buprenorphine (see Chapter 74).

Medical Management of Addiction. Methadone and buprenorphine are two medications that can be used as replacement therapy for opioid-dependent patients. Each of these medications has been shown to reduce the relapse rate in patients seeking treatment (see Chapter 74).

NONNARCOTIC CNS DEPRESSANTS

The CNS depressants include the barbiturates, benzodiazepines; nonbarbiturate hypnotic drugs such as glutethimide (Doriden) and methaqualone

T A B L E 7 1 . 6

Clinical Opiate Withdrawal Scale (COWS)

Resting pulse rate: (record beats per minute)
Measured after patient has been sitting or lying for 1 minute
0 Pulse rate 80 or below
1 Pulse rate 81–100
2 Pulse rate 101–120
4 Pulse rate greater than 120

Sweating: *Over past $\frac{1}{2}$ hour not accounted for by room temperature or patient activity*
0 No report of chills or flushing
1 Subjective report of chills or flushing
2 Flushed or observable moistness on face
3 Beads of sweat on brow or face
4 Sweat streaming off face

Restlessness: *Observation during assessment*
0 Able to sit still
1 Reports difficulty sitting still, but is able to do so
3 Frequent shifting or extraneous movements of legs/arms
5 Unable to sit still for more than a few seconds

Pupil size:
0 Pupils pinned or normal size for room light
1 Pupils possibly larger than normal for room light
2 Pupils moderately dilated
5 Pupils so dilated that only the rim of the iris is visible

Bone or joint aches: *If patient was having pain previously, only the additional component attributed to opiates withdrawal is scored*
0 Not present
1 Mild diffuse discomfort
2 Patient reports severe diffuse aching of joints/muscles
4 Patient is rubbing joints or muscles and is unable to sit still because of discomfort

Runny nose or tearing: *Not accounted for by cold symptoms or allergies*
0 Not present
1 Nasal stuffiness or unusually moist eyes
2 Nose running or tearing
4 Nose constantly running or tears streaming down cheeks

Gastrointestinal (GI) upset: *Over last $\frac{1}{2}$ hour*
0 No GI Symptoms
1 Stomach cramps
2 Nausea or loose stool
3 Vomiting or diarrhea
5 Multiple episodes of diarrhea or vomiting

Tremor: *observation of outstretched hands*
0 No tremor
1 Tremor can be felt, but not observed
2 Slight tremor observable
4 Gross tremor or muscle twitching

Yawning: *Observation during assessment*
0 No yawning
1 Yawning once or twice during assessment
2 Yawning three or more times during assessment
4 Yawning several times/minute

Anxiety or irritability
0 None
1 Patient reports increasing irritability or anxiousness
2 Patient obviously irritable/anxious
4 Patient so irritable or anxious that participation in the assessment is difficult

Gooseflesh skin
0 Skin is smooth
3 Piloerection of skin can be felt or hairs standing up on arms
5 Prominent piloerection

Total:

Score:
5–12 = mild; 13–24 = moderate; 25–36 = moderately severe; 36+ = severe withdrawal.

(Quaalude), gamma hydroxyl butyrate, flunitrazepam (Rohypnol), major tranquilizers (phenothiazines), and carbamates such as meprobamate (Equanil and Miltown). Physical symptoms of sedative-hypnotic intoxication include slurred speech, incoordination, unsteady gait, nystagmus, decreased reflexes, impaired attention or memory, and stupor or coma; psychiatric symptoms of intoxication include inappropriate behavior, mood lability, impaired judgment, impaired social functioning, and impaired occupational functioning.

Barbiturates

Prevalence/Epidemiology. Nonmedical use of barbiturate tranquilizers continues to be a problem among adolescents. The 2006 Monitoring the Future study recorded an increased in lifetime use of barbiturates among high school seniors from 8.8% in 2003 to 10.2% in 2006.

Medical Uses. Barbiturates are used as sleep aids, for sedative-hypnotic anesthesia, as anticonvulsants, for the reduction of intracranial pressure and cerebral ischemia after head trauma, for poststroke management, and for preinduction of anesthesia.

Preparation and Dose. Barbiturates are sedative/hypnotic drugs derived from barbituric acid. The most frequently abused barbiturates are secobarbital and pentobarbital. Barbiturates are divided into ultra-short-acting [thiopental (Pentothal) and methohexital (Brevital)], short-acting [secobarbital (Seconal) and pentobarbital (Nembutal)], intermediate-acting [amobarbital (Amytal) and butabarbital (Butisol)], and long-acting types [phenobarbital (Luminal)]. Ultra-short-acting barbiturates are often used for anesthesia, while short-acting barbiturates are used as sleeping pills. Some 75% of phenobarbital is hydroxylated in the liver, with 25% excreted unchanged in urine, whereas secobarbital and butabarbital undergo 99% hepatic metabolism with little if any urinary excretion of the parent compound.

Routes of Administration and Street Names. Barbiturates are usually taken orally, although some users inject them intravenously. Street names include reds, red devils, yellow jackets, rainbows, Mexican reds, nimbies, blue devils, blues, yellows, barbs, goofballs, and stumblers.

Physiology and Metabolism (Table 71.7). Barbiturates are GABA A receptor agonists. GABA is the main inhibitory neurotransmitter of the CNS. Barbiturates bind to a unique location on the GABA receptor (separate from the GABA binding site) and are highly potent, with a narrow window of safety.

Effects of Intoxication. Barbiturates are CNS depressants. Low doses result in mild sedation, higher doses result in hypnosis, and still higher doses result in anesthesia and possible death. Symptoms of intoxication include sleepiness, yawning, slowed comprehension, slurred speech, lateral nystagmus, anorexia, dizziness, and orthostatic hypotension. Allergic reactions that can be caused by barbiturates include bronchospasm, urticaria, dermatitis, fever, and angioneurotic edema. When barbiturates are used in combination with other depressants, such as alcohol or opioids, the effects of both are potentiated and lethal overdoses can occur more easily.

TABLE 71.7

Barbiturate Physiology

Receptors	Pharmacodynamics	Distribution	Metabolism and Excretion
GABA-A agonists	• Enhance GABA binding • Open the chloride ion channel of the GABA receptor	Barbiturates bind to plasma proteins in varying amounts (50%–97%), and cross into the cerebrospinal fluid and the placenta to varying degrees	• Metabolized in the liver, may enhance metabolism of other compounds • Excreted by the kidney

Adverse Effects. These include the following: (1) *Fatigue.* (2) *Neurologic:* ataxia, slowed comprehension, diplopia, dizziness, dysmetria, hypotonia, poor memory, lateral nystagmus and slowed speech. (3) *Psychiatric:* euphoria or depressed mood, irritability, violent behavior, toxic psychosis. (4) *Skin:* cutaneous lesions and bullae.

Overdose and Emergency Treatment. Signs and symptoms of barbiturate overdose include miosis, hypotension, hypothermia, respiratory depression, and decreased gastrointestinal motility. Coma, shock, and death are possible. The presentation is indistinguishable from opiate or other sedative overdose on clinical examination. Urine toxicology can be helpful for diagnosis, but quantitative levels are not predictive of the clinical course.

Treatment of barbiturate overdose is primarily supportive and aimed at supporting airway, breathing, and circulation. Because of the decreased gastrointestinal motility and delayed gastric emptying, drug absorption can continue for a long time after ingestion. Unabsorbed toxins should be removed by gastric lavage, followed by activated charcoal for recent ingestion. Absorbed toxins should be removed by alkaline diuresis or dialysis. CNS stimulants should be avoided. Ingestion of >3 g or a blood level of >2 mg/dL is the lethal dose for short-acting barbiturates; ingestion of >6 to 9 g or a blood level >11 to 12 mg/dL is the lethal dose for long-acting barbiturates.

Tolerance and Withdrawal. Few adolescents use barbiturates with the frequency necessary to develop dependence. However, if dependence is suspected, detoxification must be done under close medical supervision, as withdrawal can be life-threatening. The severity of the withdrawal syndrome parallels the strength of the drug, the dose used, and the duration of prior abuse. Withdrawal symptoms include anxiety, delirium, hallucinations, irritability, sleep disturbance, seizures, headaches, weakness, hyperactive reflexes, tremor, abdominal cramps, flushing, nausea, sweating, and increased temperature. Orthostatic hypotension may also occur. Barbiturate withdrawal is treated with replacement by phenobarbital followed by a slow taper until the patient is drug free.

TABLE 71.8

Major Pharmacological Actions of Various Benzodiazepines

Benzodiazepine	Major Pharmacological Action
Diazepam, chlordiazepoxide, oxazepam, chlorazepate, lorazepam, prazepam, alprazolam, halazepam	Anxiolytic
Flurazepam, temazepam, flunitrazepam, triazolam, midazolam	Sedative–hypnotic
Diazepam, clonazepam	Anticonvulsant
Diazepam	Muscle relaxant

Benzodiazepines

Prevalence/Epidemiology. Use of benzodiazepine tranquilizers by teenagers continues to be disturbingly high. The MTF documents a recent slight drop-off in their lifetime use prevalence rates to 4.1% of 8th graders, 7.1% of 10th graders, and 9.9% of 12th graders in 2005. Annual use rates in 2004 were 2.8%, 4.8%, and 6.8% among 8th, 10th, and 12th graders respectively.

Medical Use (Table 71.8). Medical use of the benzodiazepines became widespread in the 1970s, and drugs of this class continue to be used clinically as anxiolytics, hypnotics, anticonvulsants, and antispasmodics. Benzodiazepines are also used to treat the effects of alcohol withdrawal. Initially benzodiazepines were thought to be free of negative consequences, but it is now known that they carry the risk of dependence, withdrawal, and negative side effects.

Preparation and Dose. Several thousand benzodiazepine formulations have been investigated, but only few have found clinical utility, as listed in Table 71.8, particularly for anxiolysis, treatment of insomnia, chemical restraint and alcohol withdrawal.

Benzodiazepines are sedative-hypnotic medications; many drugs of this class are produced and sold in the United States and are readily available on the street. Nearly all the available benzodiazepines have been abused; those that cross the blood–brain barrier more quickly have a higher abuse potential than those that cross more slowly. Benzodiazepines may be obtained by diverting legitimate prescriptions or by theft from pharmaceutical supplies. Diversion of flunitrazepam tablets across the Mexican border has also been reported. Abuse of benzodiazepines generally occurs within the context of another substance abuse disorder. These drugs are often used to augment the effects of another drug or prevent symptoms of withdrawal. However, benzodiazepines are the drug of choice for a small portion of adolescents with substance abuse problems, and sedative/hypnotic dependence has been described.

Routes of Administration and Street Names. Benzodiazepines are most often taken orally, although some adolescents may snort them or inject them. Benzodiazepines can be divided into long-acting (such as diazepam with an elimination half-life of 18 to 100 hours), short-acting (such as oxazepam and

TABLE 71.9

Benzodiazepine Physiology

Receptors	Pharmacodynamics	Distribution	Metabolism and Excretion
GABA-A receptor agonists	Enhance the binding of GABA to the GABA receptor	• Protein bound • Cross into the central nervous system based on their solubility and lipophilicity	• Metabolized in the liver • Many active metabolites, which accounts for wide variation of half-lives

lorazepam, with elimination half-lives of about 6 hours), and ultra-short-acting (such as triazolam, temazepam, and midazolam) types. Midazolam is an example of an ultra-short-acting benzodiazepine.

Physiology (Table 71.9)
Effects of Intoxication. Benzodiazepines are CNS depressants. They produce drowsiness, dizziness, weakness, sedation, and a sense of calmness.

Adverse Effects. (1) *Psychiatric:* paradoxical aggression, anxiety, delirium, agitation. (2) *Neurologic:* over sedation, ataxia, memory loss, impaired psychomotor function. (3) *Cardiovascular:* mild hypotension.

Overdose and Emergency Treatment. Benzodiazepine overdose typically presents with dizziness, confusion, drowsiness or unresponsiveness, and blurred vision. Some patients may present with anxiety and agitation. Physical exam signs include nystagmus, slurred speech, ataxia, weakness or hypotonia, hypotension, and respiratory depression. Treatment for benzodiazepine overdose is primarily supportive, including securing the airway and cardiovascular and respiratory stabilization. Flumazenil is the first specific benzodiazepine receptor antagonist to become available. To treat severe benzodiazepine overdose, flumazenil is given in incremental doses over a few minutes. If a clinical effect is not seen after 5 doses have been given, it is unlikely that higher doses will be helpful. Patients that have overdosed on a long-acting benzodiazepine may require redosing to prevent return of symptoms.

In mixed overdoses involving tricyclic antidepressants or other seizure-causing agents, flumazenil is contraindicated. In this setting it can cause seizure activity by removing any anticonvulsant protection conferred by the benzodiazepine. It is also contraindicated in individuals who are physically dependent on benzodiazepines. This dependence can occur rapidly and use of flumazenil can precipitate a benzodiazepine withdrawal state (agitation, tremor, flushing).

Chronic Use. Benzodiazepines have a high abuse and dependence potential. Care should be used in prescribing benzodiazepines for management of sleep or anxiety in any patient who has been diagnosed with drug problems.

Benzodiazepines are contraindicated in adolescents with alcohol problems, opioid addiction, or on opioid replacement therapy.

Tolerance and Withdrawal. If benzodiazepine dependence is suspected withdrawal must be carefully supervised. Patients who abruptly stop taking benzodiazepines can develop life-threatening, protracted seizures. Other symptoms of benzodiazepine withdrawal include anxiety, agitation, confusion, sleep disturbance, and flulike symptoms, including fatigue, headache, muscle pain and weakness, sweating, chills, nausea, vomiting, and diarrhea. Detoxification from benzodiazepine dependence is done by replacement with long-acting benzodiazepines followed by a taper. The taper can either be accomplished gradually (over 2 to 3 months) on an outpatient basis by decreasing the dose by one sixth every 10 days or rapidly (over 10 to 14 days) on an inpatient basis.

"Date Rape" Drugs

Flunitrazepam, gamma hydroxybutyrate, and ketamine are often colorless, tasteless, and odorless. These drugs have the reputation of being "date rape" drugs because they have been added to beverages and ingested by individuals unknowingly. They can produce both antegrade and retrograde amnesia in the victims, such that they have no memory of events surrounding their use of the drug. In 1996, federal legislation was passed that increased penalties for the use of any controlled substance to aid in sexual assault. Information and educational materials directed toward college students are available from the Rape Treatment Center at Santa Monica—UCLA Medical Center at 1-800-END-RAPE (1-800-363-7273).

Flunitrazepam

Flunitrazepam (Rohypnol), a benzodiazepine, is predominantly a CNS depressant. Use of flunitrazepam began in Europe in the 1970s and appeared in the United States in the early 1990s. Street names include rophies, roofies, roach, and rope. In the 1996 MTF survey, 1.2% of seniors had used Rohypnol; this figure rose to 3.0% in 1998 and fell to 0.8% in 2006. Flunitrazepam is rapidly absorbed within 30 minutes after oral ingestion. It is highly a lipophilic drug, readily crossing the blood–brain barrier; consequently CNS depression is rapid in onset. Clinical effects are the same as those of other benzodiazepines, but with an exaggerated amnesia effect. If mixed with alcohol, this drug can incapacitate victims and prevent them from resisting sexual assault, hence its reputation as a date rape drug. Victims may also have impaired memory for the events surrounding the drug's use. This drug can be lethal when combined with alcohol and other depressants. This drug is not approved for use in the United States, and it is illegal to import flunitrazepam into the United States. Occasionally clonazepam (Klonopin) is sold as "roofies." Flunitrazepam may not be detected in routine laboratory screening for benzodiazepines, but specific testing can detect flunitrazepam in the urine for up to 72 hours after ingestion. Management of patients with suspected overdoses includes decontamination with oral activated charcoal and supportive care.

Gamma-Hydroxybutyrate (Precursors: 1,4 Butane-Diol, Butyrolactone, Gamma-Valerolactone)

Gamma hydroxyl butyrate (GHB) is a CNS depressant that acts through a metabolite of the inhibitory neurotransmitter gamma-aminobutyric acid

(GABA) and can function as a neurotransmitter itself. GHB triggers the release of an opiate like substance and can mediate sleep cycles, temperature regulation, memory, and emotional control. GHB is a schedule I drug that has not been sold over the counter in the United States since 1992, although products containing precursor chemicals can be found in a number of dietary supplements. The illicit use of GHB has grown in North American among both body builders and ravers; it has also been mentioned as one of the several date rape drugs. It has been sold as a strength enhancer, euphoriant, and aphrodisiac. The drug comes in both liquid and powder form.

Adverse Effects. These include the following: (1) *Cardiac:* bradycardia, increased or decreased blood pressure. (2) *Neurologic:* hypothermia, dizziness, weakness, ataxia, vertigo, nystagmus, short-term amnesia, coma, tonic-clonic seizures. (3) *Psychiatric:* confusion, sedation, aggression, impaired judgment, hallucinations. (4) *Respiratory:* respiratory depression with acidosis. (5) *Gastrointestinal:* vomiting. (6) *Endocrine:* mild hyperglycemia.

Withdrawal effects include insomnia, anxiety, tremors, and sweating. Large doses can lead to coma and respiratory depression (particularly if used with other depressants), which can be exacerbated by the use of alcohol. There is no antidote for GHB overdose; the treatment is supportive care.

Ketamine

Ketamine ("Special K") is an arylcycloalkylamine chemical congener of PCP; it is similar to PCP pharmacologically, but it has a more rapid onset and is less potent. It is known as a rapid-acting dissociative anesthetic that combines sedative-hypnotic, analgesic, and amnesic effects with the maintenance of pharyngeal reflexes and respiratory function. Ketamine may produce unpleasant emergence reactions, anxiety, dysphoria, and hallucinations. Users are attracted to the "dreamy" state of mild hallucinations and "out of body" experiences induced by light ketamine anesthesia. Adverse effects include a cataleptic state, with nystagmus, excessive salivation, involuntary tongue and limb movements, and hypertonia. Laryngospasm, seizures, apnea, and respiratory arrest have all been reported on rare occasions with ketamine-induced anesthesia. Accidents secondary to the loss of physical control are often of greater threat to the individual than toxicity. Treatment of ketamine overdose is primarily supportive, with attention to neurologic, cardiovascular, and respiratory monitoring. Airway control and ventilatory support may be necessary for some patients. Treatment of agitation related to an emergence reaction (i.e. psychotomimetic reactions such as vivid dreaming, extracorporeal experiences and illusions) entails dim lighting, reduction of extraneous external stimuli, and administration of a benzodiazepine. For idiosyncratic dystonic reactions, intravenous diphenhydramine may be of benefit.

Baclofen and Muscle Relaxants

Abuse of prescription drugs such as muscle relaxants has become more common among adolescents. Muscle relaxants are diverse in chemical structure and actions; they include such drugs as baclofen, meprobamate, orphenadrine, and methocarbamol. Baclofen (Lioresal) is chemically related to the inhibitory neurotransmitter, gamma-hydroxybutyric acid (GABA), and can induce drowsiness, coma, muscle flaccidity, cardiac dysrhythmias, and respiratory depression or sudden respiratory arrest. Baclofen and other muscle relaxants are not detected in routine toxicological screens of the blood and urine, and should be ordered specifically if an overdose is suspected. Treatment of patients who overdose on muscle relaxants includes oral decontamination with activated charcoal, close monitoring of neurologic and cardiovascular status, and supportive care. Intubation and mechanical ventilation may be necessary in cases of severe poisoning.

INHALANTS

Prevalence/Epidemiology. In the 2002 and 2003 National Survey on Drug Use and Health, an annual average of 718,000 (8.6%) of youths aged 12 and 13 years had used an inhalant in their lifetimes and about 35% of those had used other illicit drugs. The 2006 MTF survey of high school students found a lifetime prevalence of inhalant use by 16.1% of 8th graders, 13.3% of 10th graders, and 11.1% of 12th graders in 2006; there was a rise in prevalence in 2004 and 2005 over the previous 2 years among the 8th graders. This trend may signal resurgence in student acceptance of inhalants as agents for experimentation.

Preparation (Table 71.10). Inhalants are attractive to adolescents because of their rapid onset of action, low cost, and easy availability. They are typically used by inhaling from a plastic bag containing the substance ("bagging") or by inhaling a cloth saturated with the substance ("huffing"). The initial effect is stimulation and excitation, which then progresses to a CNS depressant. Of the many products and substances abused, toluene is the most common volatile component. It is present in spray paint, airplane glues, rubber cement, cleaning fluids, inks (magic markers), and lacquer thinner.

Circumstances of Abuse. Inhalants are inexpensive, legal products that do not arouse suspicion in most homes; some are listed below. When parents report finding fluid-saturated cloths, empty spray-paint cans, or plastic bags in a bedroom along with other paraphernalia or unusual chemicals, they and the physician should suspect inhalant use and ask about it directly.

TABLE 71.10

Classes of Inhalants, Chemical Examples and Toxicity

Class of Inhalant	Product/Chemical Examples	Toxicity
Volatile products	Glues, gasoline, spray paints, butane, paint thinner	Cardiac arrhythmias, respiratory failure, coma, pneumothorax
Gases	Nitrous oxide	Simple asphyxia
Anesthetics	Ether	Coma, respiratory failure
Nitrates	Amyl nitrate, butyl nitrate	Cardiovascular failure, coma methemoglobin

Physiology. The effects of inhalants are felt within minutes of inhalation owing to the immediate availability of the chemicals crossing the large surface area of lung alveoli into the pulmonary circulation. Their lipophilicity facilitates rapid absorption into the brain and anesthetic effects at the cellular level. Peak effects occur within minutes and excretion is rapid, such that the course of intoxication after one huffing event may last only 15 to 30 minutes.

Effects of Intoxication. Inhalant use results in euphoria, decreased inhibition, and decreased judgment. Symptoms of inhalant use include heavy-lidded, glazed eyes, slurred speech, lacrimation, rhinorrhea, salivation, and irritation of the mucous membranes. Anesthesia is common, with drowsiness, stupor, or even obtundation accompanied by respiratory depression. Users report spinning or floating sensations, with disinhibition, exhilaration, and mild delirium. Feelings of grandiosity and omnipotence impart a sense of control and dominance.

Adverse Effects (Table 71.11). These include GI complaints such as anorexia, vomiting, and abdominal pain associated with gastritis. Neurologic effects accompanying inhalant abuse include sleepiness, headaches, dizziness, ataxia, incoordination, and diplopia. Users may have a distinctive chemical odor to their breath, hair, or clothing. Defatting properties of solvents may lead to perinasal and perioral skin rashes and nosebleeds. Respiratory irritation may cause the user to develop a chronic dry cough, new-onset wheezing, and shortness of breath. Overdose of inhalants can result in life-threatening complications, such as seizures, loss of consciousness, arrhythmias, respiratory failure, or cardiopulmonary arrest. In addition, specific inhalant groups are associated with unique toxicities.

Death is not an uncommon outcome in adolescent inhalant abuse, either directly from respiratory or cardiac toxic causes or as a result of trauma from risk-taking behaviors and poor judgment. Sudden sniffing-death syndrome has occurred after inhalation of fluorocarbons or halogenated hydrocarbons and probably involves sensitization of the myocardium by the solvent to the arrhythmogenic effects of epinephrine and increased sympathetic outflow. Although tolerance to inhalants may develop, withdrawal symptoms do not usually occur. Inhalants are difficult or impossible to detect in drug samples.

TABLE 71.11

Agent-Specific Toxicities of Inhalant Chemicals

Inhalant Chemical	Agent-Specific Toxicity
Toluene	Renal damage, embryopathy
Amyl and butyl nitrites	Methemoglobinemia, hypotension
Gasoline	Lead poisoning, benzene-induced leukemia
Carbon tetrachloride, trichloroethylene	Hepatitis, cirrhosis
Methylene chloride (Paint thinner)	Carbon monoxide poisoning

Chronic Use. Inhalant abuse is notable for escalation in the frequency of use and in binge behaviors owing to the short duration of the "high." Chronic effects include irreversible damage to target organs such as the brain and kidneys. Fatty brain tissues such as myelin and neuronal cell bodies are damaged or destroyed, and white matter degeneration may be evident.

Diagnosis. Many inhalants are so quickly metabolized and/or excreted via pulmonary or other routes that they cannot be detected by the time the patient arrives in the emergency department. Standard blood and urine screening tests do not include such chemicals as hydrocarbons or nitrites.

Treatment. Treatment is supportive, and is aimed at control of arrhythmias, respiratory and circulatory support. Epinephrine should be avoided since it may provoke cardiac irritability in those patients who have inhaled halogenated hydrocarbons. Intubation and mechanical ventilation may be necessary in severely affected patients who present with respiratory depression and blood gas evidence of hypoxia, hypercarbia, and respiratory acidosis.

Nitrous Oxide

Also known as laughing gas, nitrous oxide (N_2O) has long been abused by health care personnel. More recently there has been a resurgence of interest in the adolescent population. It is most commonly sold in small balloons or inhaled from whipped-cream cans, in which it is used as a propellant. Deaths have occurred after prolonged inhalation of 100% N_2O in a closed space.

Nitrites

Amyl, butyl, and isobutyl nitrites are examples of nitrites. They are volatile liquids abused for their vasodilatory action and subjective feeling of lightheadedness (known as the "rush"). Amyl nitrite requires a prescription and is currently indicated in cyanide poisoning to produce methemoglobin. Butyl and isobutyl nitrite are available over the counter (commonly in "head shops") as room deodorizers, colognes, or liquid incense. Individuals abusing nitrites rarely seek medical attention for complications of abuse. The most common side effects are severe headache, dizziness, orthostatic hypotension, and occasionally syncope due to smooth muscle relaxation. Nitrites can be oxidizing agents and as such can cause methemoglobin formation, but this is extremely rare as a significant complication of nitrite abuse.

HALLUCINOGENS

The hallucinogen class of drugs includes LSD (D-lysergic acid diethylamide tartrate), PCP (phencyclidine), psilocybin, peyote, mescaline, dimethyltryptamine (DMT), morning glory seeds, STP, jimsonweed, dextromethorphan, MDMA, MDA, and MDEA. The term *hallucinogen* ("producer of hallucinations") is actually a misnomer, because prototypical hallucinogens such as LSD, mescaline, and psilocybin at typical dosage levels do not cause hallucinations (sensory perception changes without a corresponding environmental stimulus) but rather illusions (perceptual distortion of a real environmental stimulus) or distortions of perceived reality. True hallucinations do occur with the use of volatile solvents such as gasoline. With the exception of the hallucinogenic

TABLE 71.12

Types of Hallucinogens and the Psychoactive Effects They Produce

Category	Psychoactive Effect	Examples
Psychedelics	Prominent hallucinations and synesthesias with mild distortion of time and reality, impaired attention/concentration, mild disruption in ego structure	• Indolealkylamines: LSD, psilocybin, DMT • Phenlyalkylamines: mescaline
Enactogens	Structural similarities to psychedelics (mescaline) and amphetamines; unique psychoactive characteristics include improved communication, empathy with others, and positive mood enhancement	MDMA, MDA, MDEA
Dissociative anesthetics	Causes anesthesia, emergence reactions, and 'out of body' experiences	PCP, ketamine
Other	Mild distortion of time, impaired attention/concentration, mild mood enhancement, euphoria and feelings of well-being	Marijuana

LSD, lysergic acid diethylamide; DMT, dimethyltryptamine; MDMA, methylenedioxymethamphetamine; MDA, methylenedioxyamphetamine; MDEA, methylenedioxy-*N*-ethylamphetamine; PCP, phencyclidine.

amphetamines and marijuana, physical withdrawal does not occur. However, long-term recrudescence of fleeting distortions and illusions, termed "flashbacks," are not uncommon. Table 71.12 contains the subgrouping of hallucinogens based on distinctive psychoactive effects and structure-activity relationship similarities.

Lysergic Acid Diethylamide (LSD)

LSD was initially developed as a circulatory stimulant, when it was incidentally found to cause hallucinations. In the 1950s, LSD was marketed under the name Delsyd as a treatment for mental illness; the military also had interest in developing the drug as an agent for "mind control." By the mid-1960s no significant medical benefits of the drug had been found, and development stopped.

Prevalence/Epidemiology. The abuse of LSD peaked in the 1960s and then drifted lower during the 1970s and 1980s, reaching a low prevalence rate of use (7.2%) by high school seniors by 1986, but experienced a resurgence of popularity among youth in the 1990s. Popularity peaked in 1997 when the lifetime usage rate of LSD among high school seniors, at 13.6% of students, had surpassed the rate of 11.3% recorded in 1975.

TABLE 71.13

Hallucinogen Physiology

Receptors	Pharmacodynamics	Distribution	Metabolism and Excretion
Nonspecific intracellular binding throughout the central nervous system	Inhibition of serotonin release, resulting in: • Increased firing of sensory neurons • Nonspecific stress response	Primarily protein bound	Rapidly absorbed through the gastrointestinal (GI) tract • Onset of action is 30–40 minutes • Half-life is 3 hours

Preparation and Dose. LSD is derived from an alkaloid found in rye fungus. It is made by mixing lysergic acid with diethylamide, freezing the mixture, and then extracting the resulting LSD. The procedure is not easy; therefore, much of the LSD sold on the street is either adulterated or contains no LSD. LSD is an extremely potent drug with doses measured in micrograms. Low doses of LSD (50 to 75 μg) produce euphoria, while higher doses result in typical LSD illusions or "trips." In the 1960s, the typical illicit dose of LSD was 100 to 300 μg; today the usual dose is 20 to 80 μg.

Routes of Administration. Commonly distributed as a soluble powder or liquid that is usually colorless, odorless, and tasteless in its manufactured state, but it is most often colored when sold. It is sold as cylindrical tablets or gelatin squares or applied to small pieces of paper called blotters, or may be sold as decals or stickers. The drug is ingested by placing the blotter on the tongue where it dissolves and absorbed through the mucous membranes. LSD can also be mixed in with foods or liquids for oral consumption; liquid LSD can be absorbed through the mucus membranes of the eyes. LSD cannot be smoked as it is destroyed in heat.

Physiology (Table 71.13)
Effects of Intoxication. Intoxication results in euphoria and sensory illusions which may give rise to hallucinations. Symptoms may include dilated pupils, conjunctival injection, hyperthermia, tachycardia, hypertension, flushing and tremor. The sense of being an observer is frequently reported by users and distinguishes LSD psychosis from schizophrenia.

Adverse Effects. (1) *Psychiatric:* visual and auditory hallucinations, synesthesias, depersonalization, loss of sense of time, loss of ego boundaries, impairment of attention, motivation and concentration, anxiety, depression, paranoia, confusion, flashbacks. (2) *Neurologic:* flushing, hyperthermia, piloerection, dizziness, paresthesia, dilated pupils, blurred vision, conjunctival injection, lacrimation, hyperactive reflexes, ataxia and tremor, loss of muscle coordination and pain perception, restlessness, and sleep disturbances.

(3) *Cardiovascular:* hypertension and tachycardia. (4) *Gastrointestinal:* anorexia, nausea, dry mouth.

Overdose and Emergency Treatment. LSD overdose may result in grand mal seizures, circulatory collapse, coagulopathies and coma. Treatment is supportive. LSD can be readily detected in urine by thin layer chromatography or other analytic techniques. Some LSD users experience "bad trips," which are negative emotional responses triggered both by the circumstances of use as well as feelings within the user. These responses terrify the user and may produce a sense of panic, fragmentation, or fear of "going crazy." LSD users may also experience "flashbacks" or the recurrence of the LSD-induced state after the effects of the drug have worn off. Important components of treatment include providing a peaceful, calm environment (darkened lights, few extraneous stimuli) and helping the patient to restore contact with reality. Clinicians should avoid discussing the reasons for use of the drug or personal problems during a bad trip, and medication use should be avoided if possible. It is important to monitor the cycles of lucidity and periods of intense reactions to the drug. If the cycles are frequent, then the individual is probably early in the course of experiencing effects of the drug; if the cycles are less frequent, the drug effects may have peaked. Chemical and physical restraints are discouraged, but may be necessary if the patient remains agitated.

Chronic Use. Chronic adverse effects may include psychosis, depression, and personality changes. The use of a hallucinogen should be considered in the differential diagnosis of an adolescent who presents with the new onset of psychosis.

Tolerance and Withdrawal. Tolerance to LSD develops rapidly but is short-lived. Some daily users of LSD describe the practice of "doubling up" (doubling the previous day's dose) to counteract tolerance. No withdrawal syndrome is described.

Phencyclidine (PCP)

Prevalence/Epidemiology. The use of PCP ("angel dust") has steadily declined from a high of 12.8% in the late 1970s to a lifetime prevalence of use of only 2% to 4% through the 1990s, dropping further to only 2.2% of 12th graders in 2006. Only 0.7% of high school seniors reported using PCP within the previous 12 months in 2006.

Preparation and Dose. PCP (Sernyl) is an arylamine (1-[1-phenyl(cyclohexyl) piperidine]) introduced in the 1950s as a general anesthetic. It is structurally related to ketamine. Clinical trials revealed PCP to be an effective anesthetic, but during surgical recovery the emergence reactions to PCP were frequent and unpleasant, with excessive agitation, excitement, and disorientation; medical use was discontinued in 1965. Dose ranges vary tremendously, from 0.1 to >150 mg in one survey. In addition, approximately 20% of drug samples sold as PCP contained no PCP. Less than 5 mg is considered a low dose, 5 to 10 mg a moderate dose, and >10 mg a high dose.

Routes of Administration. PCP may be packaged as a liquid, powder, tablet, leaf mixture, or rock crystal. It can be used intravenously (average dose: 10 mg),

TABLE 71.14

Phencyclidine Physiology

Receptors	Pharmacodynamics	Distribution	Metabolism and Excretion
Glutamate-N-methyl-D-aspartate (NMDA) receptors	• Increases the production of dopamine • Inhibits dopamine reuptake	Metabolites are fat soluble, although not physiologically active	• Metabolized by the liver to monopiperidine conjugate • pH dependent urinary excretion

intramuscularly, or orally (average dose: 5 mg), or it can be snorted (average dose: 5 mg) or smoked (average dose: 3 mg).

Physiology (Table 71.14)

Effects of Intoxication (Table 71.15). The clinical symptoms of PCP use vary with the dose, the route of administration, and the experience of the user. Intravenous, intramuscular, and oral routes of administration are more difficult to regulate than the smoking of PCP. In addition, inexperienced users have more side effects than experienced users do. PCP is the only drug of abuse that causes a characteristic vertical nystagmus, but can cause horizontal or rotatory nystagmus. Other symptoms include ataxia, miosis with reactive pupils, hypertension and increased deep tendon reflexes. PCP usually induces one of several clinical states.

The diagnosis of PCP use should be suspected in all adolescents with a distorted thought process, especially when there is evidence of analgesia or nystagmus. Any individual with open-eye coma, horizontal and vertical nystagmus, hypertension, and rigidity should be considered to have taken PCP. PCP

TABLE 71.15

Phencyclidine Intoxication States

Acute intoxication	Delusion, disinhibition, dissociation ("out of body" experience)
Acute or prolonged delirium	Disorientation, clouded consciousness, and abnormal cognition
Schizophreniform psychosis	Hallucinations, thought disorder, and delusions
Mania	Hallucinations, elevated mood, elevated self-attitude, feelings of omnipotence
Depressive reactions	Dysphoria, social withdrawal, paranoia, isolation

can be detected in the blood, urine, and gastrointestinal secretions; the best fluid to sample is the urine. A serum concentration of 25 to 100 ng/mL may be found in patients who are in an acute state of confusion; a level of >100 ng/mL may be found in comatose patients. Excretion in the urine is highly pH-dependent and decreases dramatically as the pH becomes alkaline.

Adverse Effects. Adverse effects associated with PCP use are dose-related (see Table 71.16).

Overdose and Emergency Treatment. PCP use may result in generalized motor seizures either early in the course of intoxication or delayed in appearance. Hypertension is usually mild. Death can occur and is usually caused by injuries sustained during periods of analgesia and aggression directed at self or others. Death also can occur as a result of convulsions and cerebral hemorrhage. When treating patients with PCP overdose, clinicians must use extreme caution. Patients are unpredictable and often have little awareness of the consequences of their behavior. Reducing the levels of light, sound, and other external stimuli can rapidly bring down a PCP user. In an emergency, covering the intoxicated patient with a blanket may be helpful. All hazards should be removed from the environment. Patients should not be touched or cornered. Restraints are not recommended; they may cause the patient to harm himself or herself in an attempt to escape. Treatment for PCP overdose is largely supportive. In addition to basic cardiopulmonary resuscitation, it is essential to check for signs of head, neck, back, and internal injuries, which can occur because of the behavioral effects of the drug. Unconscious victims should be placed on the side so that aspiration does not occur.

Try to avoid administering other medications, but if necessary, intravenous diazepam or lorazepam can be used to treat seizures. Severe agitation and psychosis can be treated with haloperidol. Avoid phenothiazines and neuroleptics because of the risk of excessive orthostatic hypotension and the potential for enhancing the cholinergic imbalance. Intravenous diphenhydramine may be used for dystonias. During the recovery phase, an adolescent may require short-term inpatient psychiatric care to deal with paranoia, regressive behavior, and a slow phase of reintegration. Recovery usually occurs within 24 hours but can proceed for days, depending on the dose and the acidity of the urine. With higher doses the coma can last 5 to 6 days and can be followed by a prolonged recovery period marked by behavioral disorders. Cognitive, memory, and speech disorders may last up to 1 year after the last use of PCP. Flashbacks may occur, as with LSD.

Dextromethorphan

Dextromethorphan, the dextro isomer of the codeine analog, levorphanol, has a chemical structure resembling a synthetic opiate but lacks an opiate's potent analgesic, sedative, or addicting properties. The drug's prominent antitussive properties make it a common ingredient in non-prescription cough and cold syrups, usually in amounts of 10 to 15 mg per teaspoon or per tablespoon. While the use of most hallucinogens is on the decline, the misuse of over-the-counter cold and cough medicines as an inexpensive "high" is one of the fastest growing drugs of abuse. Maximum daily doses range from 30 mg for children to 120 mg for adults. Those engaged in substance abuse may drink 8 to 16 oz of such a cough syrup in an attempt to get high. The volume of cough syrup required

TABLE 71.16

Adverse Effects of Phencyclidine by Dose

Low dose (<5 mg)

Blank stare	Behavioral disorders:
Horizontal and vertical nystagmus	• Disorganized thought processes
Ataxia	• Distortion of body image and of
Hypertension	objects
Increased deep tendon reflexes	• Amnesia
Decreased proprioception and	• Agitated or combative behavior
sensations	• Unresponsive behavior
Miosis or midposition, reactive	• Disinhibition of underlying
pupils	psychopathology
Diaphoresis	• Schizophrenic reactions
Flushing	• Catalepsy, catatonia
	• Illusions
	• Anxiety, excitement

Moderate dose (5–10 mg)

Hypertension	Hypersalivation
Vertical and horizontal nystagmus	Mutism
Myoclonus	Amnesia
Midposition pupil size	Anxiety, excitement
Dysarthria	Delusions
Diaphoresis	Behavior:
Fever	• Stupor or extreme agitation
	• Violent or psychotic behavior can
	occur

High dose (>10 mg)

Unresponsive, immobile state	Spontaneous nystagmus
Eyes that may remain open during	Miosis
coma	Decreased urine output
Hypertension	Dysarthria
Arrhythmias	Diaphoresis and flushing
Increased deep tendon reflexes	Fever
Muscle rigidity	Amnesia
Decerebrate posturing	Mutism
Convulsions	

Extremely high dose (>500 mg)

Prolonged coma	Hypoventilation
Rigidity	Hypertension or hypotension
Extensor (decerebrate) posturing	Prolonged and fluctuating
Seizures	confusional state after recovery
	from coma

to get high has led adolescents to order the pure, highly concentrated powder from Internet sources or to purchase high concentration dextromethorphan-containing tablets such as Coricidin products instead. Dextromethorphan can induce euphoria and produce dissociative effects.

Dextromethorphan in high doses binds to opiate sigma receptors, which may account for some of its sedative and psychomimetic properties. The drug is metabolized via O-demethylation to an active metabolite, dextrorphan, which interacts with the same PCP receptor in NMDA neurotransmitter complex. This primary metabolism is under the control of hepatic cytochrome complex, CYP2D6, whose genetic polymorphisms may explain why some users are more susceptible to adverse effects than others. The dug undergoes secondary conjugation in the liver to inactive glucuronide and sulfate esters, and has an elimination half-life of about 3.3 hours.

Dextromethorphan produces PCP-like symptoms in overdose, including somnolence and ataxia, slurred speech, hallucinations, dysphoria, nystagmus, dystonia, tachycardia, and elevated blood pressure. Dextromethorphan also blocks presynaptic serotonin reuptake and has dopaminergic properties. Dextromethorphan may interact with other drugs, including selective serotonin reuptake inhibitors, MAO inhibitors, tricyclic antidepressants, and lithium, to produce movement disorders or the serotonin syndrome of rigidity and hyperthermia. Routine toxic screening of the blood for opiates may remain negative despite recent use of dextromethorphan. However in some cases, depending on concentration, the test for phencyclidine may be weakly positive in dextromethorphan poisoning. Treatment is supportive; the role of naloxone is not well established although there are case reports of its efficacy. Clinicians should note that dextromethorphan poisonings often involve concomitant intoxications with other ingredients in over-the-counter cold medications—such as acetaminophen, antihistamines, pseudoephedrine, and guaifenesin—for which additional medical therapies may be necessary. Since dextromethorphan is formulated as a hydrobromide salt, an overdose with the drug can also produce toxic effects, such as somnolence, related to bromide poisoning.

Psilocybin

Mushrooms containing psilocybin and psilocin produce effects similar to those of the other hallucinogens. Users reportedly experience euphoria, prominent visual and auditory hallucinations and synesthesias (i.e., perceptual distortions resulting in an apparent ability to visualize sounds or hear colors). The mushrooms are ingested orally, and there is a rapid onset of effects in about 15 minutes. The effects peak at 90 minutes, begin to wear off in 2 to 3 hours, and disappear after about 5 or 6 hours. The average dose is 4 to 10 mg of psilocybin. Street names for psilocybin mushrooms include 'shrooms, mushrooms, Silly Putty, magic Mexican mushrooms, and psychedelic mushrooms. Since many other species can be confused with true *Psilocybe* mushrooms, ingestion of misidentified, toxic non-*Psilocybe* species can pose a special danger.

ANABOLIC STEROIDS

Anabolic steroids are synthetic derivatives of testosterone. Abusers of this class of drug exhibit tolerance, withdrawal, and psychological dependence. Treatment may require detoxification and a rehabilitation phase comparable to traditional drug treatment. The numerous agents fit into two basic categories: the oral agents are 17α-methyl derivatives of testosterone and the injectable agents are esters of testosterone and 19-nortestosterone. The ideal anabolic steroid would have maximal anabolic and minimal androgenic activity and a longer half-life than the parent compound, testosterone. The 17α-alkylated steroids have a half-life of 8 to 10 hours, whereas the injectable forms have half-lives in the range of 21 days. Although these agents have less androgenic activity in lower dosage ranges, this advantage is lost at higher doses. Many abusers use 10 times the usual therapeutic dose and use combinations of oral and injectable agents concurrently in 6- to 12-week cycles ("stacking").

Prevalence and Epidemiology. Use of anabolic steroids by high school students in the MTF survey has remained steady in 2006, with 1.6% of 8th graders, 1.8% of 10th graders, and 2.7% of 12th graders reporting that they have experimented with steroids at least once in their lives. Students using anabolic steroids are also likely to be engaging in other forms of substance abuse. Males outnumber females in steroid use 4:1, but females also reported steroid use for increasing strength and muscle tone.

Adverse Effects. (1) *Psychiatric:* psychosis, mania, mood swings, hyperaggressive behavior, violence. Withdawal may be associated with depression. (2) *Cardiovascular:* decreased high density lipoprotein cholesterol, hypertension, ventricular remodeling, myocardial ischemia, sudden death. (3) *Endocrine:* premature epiphyseal closure and shortened stature, female virilization and hypogonadism, testicular atrophy, reduced libido, infertility. (4) *Other:* acne, hemolysis, enlarged prostate gland, hepatocellualar carcinoma with chronic use.

Treatment of Withdrawal or Dependence. Patients exhibiting psychotic behavior or severe depression require inpatient care. Appropriate pharmacological intervention with antipsychotic, antidepressant, and anxiolytic agents may be indicated, usually for a short period. For the patient meeting the criteria of the *Diagnostic and Statistical Manual of Mental Disorders,* fourth edition (3 of 12 listed), for substance dependence, a traditional drug treatment approach is indicated. Attending 12-step meetings and "working a program" are ideal methods to provide the adolescent with a conceptual framework to work through this problem.

WEB SITES

http://www.oas.samhsa.gov/highlights.htm. Substance Abuse and Mental Health Services Administration (SAMHSA).

http://www.monitoringthefuture.org/. Monitoring the Future.

http://www.nida.nih.gov/MOM/MOMIndex.html. National Institute on Drug Abuse (NIDA).

http://www.nida.nih.gov/DrugAbuse.html. Information from NIDA on many drugs.

CHAPTER 72

Laboratory Testing for Psychoactive Substances of Abuse

Sharon Levy and John R. Knight

Drug Testing in the Primary Care Clinic

Drug testing is a complicated procedure that can be a useful part of an assessment for a substance use disorder when used to complement history and physical findings.

Indications for Urine Drug Testing in the Primary Care Clinic. Urine drug testing may be a useful assessment tool when parents notice nonspecific signs of drug use, yet the teenager denies a problem. A drug test may be unnecessary if the teenager is forthcoming; physicians should interview the patient alone before deciding whether to recommend a drug test. A single negative drug test does not rule out a drug use disorder, nor does a positive drug test confirm a diagnosis of drug abuse or dependence. Most experts agree that drug tests are not a useful screening procedure for general populations, as their sensitivity for detecting drug use in unselected populations is low.

Consent/Assent. Guidelines of the American Academy of Pediatrics state that physicians should obtain assent from competent adolescents prior to ordering a drug test; parental consent alone is not sufficient. If a teenager refuses a drug test that is clearly indicated, the physician should counsel parents to use appropriate limit setting and consequences.

Confidentiality/Sharing Results. Federal regulations provide drug use treatment information and greater confidentiality protection than other information recorded in a medical record. A physician should not share drug test results with anyone without the express written consent of the patient or the parent of a minor patient. Before ordering a drug test, the physician, teenager and parent(s) should discuss who will receive results. Prior to sharing positive results, the physician should conduct a private interview with the teenager, as drug tests may be positive even when a teenager had not used illicit drugs.

Types of Drug Tests

Hair/Breath/Saliva/Sweat. Drugs and their metabolites can be detected in several biological matrices, including hair, saliva, breath, blood, and urine. Hair testing can provide a longer window of detection (up to 180 days) in patients with long hair, although recent drug use can be difficult to distinguish from past use with this testing method. Marijuana use is difficult to confirm by hair testing because of slow deposition into some hair types. Because coarse hair absorbs drugs more readily, the possibility may exist of race/ethnicity inequity in hair testing for drugs. Breath tests are available for alcohol and can give a reliable indication of the blood alcohol level at the time of the test. Saliva tests are also available for alcohol, and newer kits test for a variety of drugs. These tests reflect blood drug levels at the time of testing. Saliva testing has not been nationally standardized and cutoff levels vary from product to product. Sweat wipes and patches that can be worn for up to 14 days are available, although they are used infrequently because of the high rate of false-positive results from external sources of drugs.

Urine. Urine drug testing has been well studied and standardized. Urine drug concentrations are relatively high and drugs and their metabolites are excreted in the urine for a period of time after acute intoxication, making urine the preferred biologic fluid for drug testing in the primary care setting. There are two principal types of urine drug tests: immunoassays and gas chromatography/mass spectrometry (GC/MS). Immunoassays are sensitive but relatively nonspecific, and a number of cross-reacting substances can cause false-positive drug test results (Table 72.1). Therefore, immunoassays are best used as screens; all positive tests should be confirmed with a second test using a different, more specific testing method, such as GC/MS.

Practical Issues in Urine Drug Testing

Test Selection. Substance abuse screening panels vary. Immunoassay screens that detect drug classes, such as opiates or benzodiazepines, may not detect every drug in the class. A test for urinary ethyl glucuronide should be ordered to detect alcohol use, as this metabolite has a longer half-life (up to 5 days) and is more sensitive than tests of urinary alcohol. Standard opiate screens may not detect synthetic opioids, such as oxycodone and hydrocodone, which need to be ordered specifically if indicated.

Specimen Collection. Because of the multitude of methods for falsifying urines, physicians who choose to order urine drug tests from their offices must be diligent. Most experts recommend either a directly observed urine specimen or the National Institute on Drug Abuse (NIDA) protocol (www.drugfreeworkplace.com).

Specimen Validation. Samples with a creatinine <20 mg/dL and a specific gravity of <1.005 are too dilute for proper interpretation (American College of Environmental and Occupational Medicine, 2003).

Interpretation

Negative Tests. A drug screen will be negative whenever the drugs in the test panel are not detected in the sample provided. A screening panel will be

TABLE 72.1

Drugs of Abuse, Common Urine Metabolites, Maximum Window of Detection, Molecules that May Cross-react with Screening Panels and Licit Sources of the Drug

Common Name(s)	Urine Metabolite	Maximum Window of Detection	Included in Standard Panels	Substances that Can Cross-react with ELISA Screens[a]	Sources of Clinical False Positives[b]
Alcohol	• Ethanol • Ethylglucuronide	• 24–36 hr • 80 hr	Not part of NIDA-5, but alcohol included on some standard panels		• OTC cough and cold liquid medications • "Nonalcoholic" beer • Foods prepared with uncooked alcohol (such as rum cake)
Marijuana, "weed"	Tetrahydrocannabinol (THC) and other cannabinols	Infrequent users: 3–4 d Daily users: 4–6 wk	Yes	• NSAIDs (ibuprofen, ketoprofen, naproxen) • Promethazine vitamin B supplements	Prescription Marinol use (uncommon in teenagers)
Cocaine	Cocaine, benzoylecgonine	2–3 days	Yes	Amoxicillin	Decocainized teas, commonly in use in South America

Amphetamine	Several members in class	2–4 days	Yes	• Cold medications that contain ephedrine, pseudoephedrine, propylephedrine, phenylephrine, desoxyephedrine • Phenylpropanolamine (present in OTC diet aids)	Prescription use of stimulants (for ADHD or other conditions) including Adderall and Dexedrine
Methamphetamine	Methamphetamine, p-hydroxymethamphetamine, amphetamine	24–48 hours	Yes, detected on amphetamine panel		• Methamphetamine from OTC medications such as Vicks inhaler[c] • Prescription use of Desoxyn, benzphetamine, dimethylamphetamine, famprofazone, fencamine, furfenorex, selegiline

(continued)

TABLE 72.1

(Continued)

Common Name(s)	Urine Metabolite	Maximum Window of Detection	Included in Standard Panels	Substances that Can Cross-react with ELISA Screens[a]	Sources of Clinical False Positives[b]
Ecstasy, 3,4 methylene-dioxymetham-phetamine (MDMA)	MDMA, methylene-dioxyamphetamine (MDA), mono- and dihydroxy derivatives	24–48 hours	No		
Phencyclidine (PCP), "dust"	Glucuronic conjugates of 4-phenyl-4-piperidinocyclo-hexanol and other metabolites	8–10 days	Yes	Dextromethorphan	
Lysergic acid diethylamide (LSD), "acid"	LSD, n-demethylated, deethylated, and hydroxylated metabolites	24 hours	No		

Drug	Metabolites	Detection window		False positives	Other causes
Opiates	• Codeine: norcodeine, morphine • Heroin: 6-acetylmorphine, morphine • Morphine: morphine glucuronide, normorphine	2–3 days	Yes, but synthetic opioids are detected only in very high doses	Fluoroquinolone antibiotics	• Consumption of a large quantity of poppy seeds (poppy seeds contain trace amounts of morphine; typical poppy seed consumption produce urine metabolite concentrations under standard thresholds) • Prescription use of opiate medication for pain
Benzodiazepines	Oxazepam common metabolite for several, but not all, benzodiazepines	Up to 2 weeks, but varies for individual drugs	Not part of "NIDA 5", but included in many standard panels		Prescription use of benzodiazepines for anxiety or other conditions

(continued)

657

TABLE 72.1

(Continued)

Common Name(s)	Urine Metabolite	Maximum Window of Detection	Included in Standard Panels	Substances that Can Cross-react with ELISA Screens[a]	Sources of Clinical False Positives[b]
Inhalants	Many in class	<24 hours	No		Inhalants are largely excreted by the lungs although some metabolites may be excreted in the urine; special testing required for detection

ELISA, enzyme-linked immunosorbent assay; NIDA, National Institute on Drug Abuse; OTC, over-the-counter; NSAID, nonsteroidal antiinflammatory drug; ADHD, attention deficit hyperactivity disorder; MDA,;

[a]Gas chromatography/mass spectrometry (GC/MS) confirmation will be negative.

[b]May result in positive drug test results in the absence of illicit drug use.

[c]Vicks inhaler contains the inactive isomer L-methamphetamine, but trace amounts of the D-isomer may be present, resulting in a positive drug test result.

negative in the context of drug use in the following circumstances: (1) The patient did not use the substance in question within the window of detection. (2) The patient diluted the urine sample. (3) The patient substituted the urine sample. (4) The patient adulterated the urine sample. (5) The patient used a drug that is not detected by the panel ordered.

Positive Tests. A drug screen will be positive whenever a molecule in the urine specimen reacts. A drug screen will be positive in absence of illicit drug use in the following circumstances: (1) A chemical other than an illicit drug has cross-reacted with the drug test panel (see Table 72.1). (2) The patient has consumed the drug in the context of licit use of a prescription or over-the-counter medication or consumed it in a food. All drug screens should be verified with a confirmatory test such as GC/MS.

Specimens Positive for Cannabis. Cannabis is lipid-soluble and significant stores in fat tissue can accumulate with chronic use. Daily users of cannabis can have detectable urine levels for 1 to 2 months after discontinuation. The absolute level of urinary cannabinoid excretion varies with urine concentration. Once use is discontinued, the ratio of urinary cannabinoids to urinary creatinine will fall, and a decreasing ratio supports a history of discontinued use even in a patient with positive urine tests.

Presenting Drug Test Results to Adolescent Patients. All patients with positive, dilute, adulterated, or substituted urine specimens should have a return appointment. Teens should be interviewed privately to determine whether an explanation other than illicit drug use might account for the laboratory findings. Some teens will acknowledge drug use, and this may provide an opportunity to have an honest conversation. If the teen is willing to abstain from drug use, repeat testing may be useful for monitoring. Some teens will deny drug use and insist that the laboratory is in error or offer another inconsistent explanation. The clinician should avoid arguments but remain firm in interpretation.

Presenting Urine Drug Test Results to Parents. Parental involvement is an important part of intervention for many teens with substance use disorders, and disclosing a teen's drug test results to parents may be therapeutically useful. Helpful approaches to sharing urine drug test results with parents include the following: (1) Obtain assent from the teenager to share drug test results *before* ordering the drug test. (2) When a drug test is positive, dilute, adulterated or substituted, always interview the patient privately in order to interpret drug test results prior to sharing information with parents. (3) Discuss with the teen exactly which information will be shared with parents. Avoid sharing details that do not affect further assessment or treatment. (4) Offer the teen the opportunity to speak with parents first (with the clinician present for support and to confirm that information was correctly conveyed). (5) If the teenager has not acknowledged drug use, discuss the teen's alternative explanation for the positive drug test, but, explain that the explanation offered is inconsistent with laboratory results.

Negative drug tests done with proper collection and validation techniques provide good support for a history of no drug use, at least within the window of detection for the substances included in the panel. Clinicians and parents must recognize, however, that even carefully done urine tests have limitations and cannot completely rule out drug use. Continued monitoring by parents, repeat drug testing, or referral to a mental health or substance abuse expert may be indicated if the teenager continues to demonstrate signs and symptoms consistent with drug use even in the context of a negative drug test.

WEB SITES AND REFERENCES

http://www.helpguide.org/mental/drug_substance_abuse_addiction_signs_effects_treatment.htm. This site lists signs and symptoms of drug use in adolescents.

http://www.drugfreeworkplace.com. Federally mandated workplace testing programs.

http://www.acoem.org/. Medical review officer training.

http://www.hipaa.samhsa.gov/Part2ComparisonClearedTOC.htm. Confidentiality of alcohol and drug abuse patient records and the HIPAA privacy rule.

American Academy of Pediatrics. Testing for drugs of abuse in children and adolescents. *Pediatrics* 1996;98:305.

American College of Occupational and Environmental Medicine. *Medical review officer drug and alcohol testing comprehensive/fast track course syllabus.* Arlington Heights, IL: ACOEM, 2003.

Anonymous. Tests for Drugs of Abuse. *Med Lett Drugs Ther* 2002 44:71.

Drummer O. Review: Pharmacokinetics of illicit drugs in oral fluid. *Forensic Sci Int* 2005;150:133.

Gullberg R. Breath alcohol measurement variability associated with different instrumentation and protocols. *Forensic Sci Int* 2003;131:30.

CHAPTER 73

Office-Based Management of Adolescent Substance Use and Abuse

Sharon Levy and John R. Knight

The Role of the Primary Care Provider. Alcohol and drug use are common among American adolescents and present a major public health problem. Primary care providers should ask every adolescent if he or she has tried tobacco, alcohol, or other drugs during each yearly health maintenance visit and screen those who have done so with a validated tool.

Screening

Asking about Drug and Alcohol Use. Providers should ask questions regarding substance use in private, after explaining the rules of confidentiality. Afford confidentiality unless the teen's behavior poses an acute safety concern. To avoid miscommunication, questions about substance use should be clear and concise. Substance use may present with nonspecific signs and symptoms. Concerns of drug use expressed by parents, school officials, coaches, or other adults should be taken seriously. Laboratory testing may be recommended when parents have reasonable concerns that their child is using drugs and yet the adolescent denies drug use (see Chapter 72).

Screens. All teens that report using alcohol or drugs should receive a structured screening to determine whether their use is low- or high-risk; a variety of written and oral tools have been developed for this purpose. The CAGE questions, which were developed to detect alcohol disorders among adults, are not recommended for screening adolescents. The CRAFFT questions are a valid and reliable tool for screening adolescents for drug and alcohol disorders simultaneously, and their psychometric properties are favorable across age, gender, and race/ethnicity. CRAFFT is a mnemonic acronym: During the past 12 months have you ever (1) Ridden in a **CAR** driven by someone, including yourself, who was high or had been using alcohol or drugs? (2) Used alcohol or drugs to **RELAX,** feel better about yourself, or fit in? (3) Used alcohol or drugs while you are by yourself, **ALONE?** (4) **FORGOTTEN** things you did while using alcohol or drugs? (5) Had your **FAMILY** or **FRIENDS** tell you that you should cut down on your drinking or drug use? (6) Gotten into **TROUBLE** while you were using alcohol or drugs?

A "yes" response = 1 point. A score of 2 or greater is a positive screen and indicates that the adolescent is at high risk for having an alcohol- or drug-related disorder.

Assessment

Interview. Teens who screen positive require further assessment, beginning with a detailed substance use history. Clinicians should use open-ended questions whenever possible with an emphasis on the pattern of drug use over time, including whether drug use has increased in quantity or frequency, whether the teen has made attempts to discontinue drug use and why, and whether such attempts have been successful. After interviewing the adolescent about his or her drug of choice, the clinician should ask about the use of other drugs (Table 73.1) indicating higher risk than the use of a single substance. This information may also guide treatment planning, particularly if laboratory testing will be used for monitoring or if medications are indicated. For each drug, ask the teen (1) If he or she has ever used it and, if so, whether it is still being used. (2) Whether the teen has ever tried to quit and why. (3) Whether he or she has experienced any problems associated with using the drug. The clinician should

TABLE 73.1

Guide to Extended Drug History

Drug or Drug Class	Common Street Names[a]
Cocaine	Cocaine or crack
Amphetamines	ADHD medications: Ritalin, Dexedrine, Adderall
	Methamphetamine: meth, crystal meth
Opioids	Pain medications: OxyContin (o.c., oxy), Percocet (percs), Vicodin (vics), codeine, morphine
	Heroin, opium
Benzodiazepines	Klonopin, Valium, Ativan, Xanax, others
Hallucinogens	Cold medications containing dextromethorphan (DXM), often referred to by brand name (Coricidin Cold and Cough [Triple C], Robitussin, NyQuil)
	Psilocybin (mushrooms)
	LSD (acid)
	PCP (dust or angel dust)
Inhalants	Nitrous (often from whipped cream cans or "whippits")
	Lighter fluid
	Paint
	Gasoline
	Markers
	Cleaning fluid
Ecstasy	E
Ketamine	K

ADHD, attention-deficit hyperactivity disorder; LSD, lysergic acid diethylamide; PCP, phencyclidine.

[a]See also Chapter 71.

ask about the seven criteria for a diagnosis of drug dependence for the drug of choice and about each drug the teen has reported using with associated problems.

Physical. A physical exam should be performed as part of a complete assessment (Table 73.2). Signs of chronic drug use are rare in teens but should be noted if present.

Laboratory Evaluation. Laboratory testing may be a useful part of a full assessment (Chapter 72).

Diagnosis

Substance Use Disorders. Substance use can be viewed as a spectrum varying from experimentation to drug dependence and addiction (Table 73.3).

Co-occurring Disorders. Many adolescents with substance-related disorders will have symptoms of a co-occurring mental health disorder; in some circumstances the question of a co-occurring diagnosis cannot be fully resolved until the adolescent has had a period of complete abstinence. However, severe symptoms, symptoms that antedate drug use, or positive family history of a similar disorder all suggest a co-occurring disorder and warrant concurrent treatment. Symptoms beginning after the onset of drug use may resolve completely with abstinence, and patients should then be reassessed (see Chapter 74).

Primary Care Management. The level of intervention for the management of adolescent substance use is based on the level of drug involvement (see Table 73.3). *Brief advice* is defined as an intervention lasting one to several minutes in which the clinician gives general information regarding substance use to a patient; *brief intervention* is an individual interactive counseling session focusing on details specific to the patient's substance use.

Abstinence (Positive Reinforcement). Adolescents who are abstinent from alcohol and drugs should receive praise and encouragement from their physician, using brief but specific statements. Encourage the adolescent to discuss drug use or ask questions in the future should the need arise.

Low Risk (Brief Advice). Adolescents who have used drugs or alcohol but score 0 or 1 on the CRAFFT questions or are otherwise determined to be "low-risk" may benefit from brief general advice pertinent to the drug they have used. Advice may be targeted at abstinence or risk reduction. Knowledge of the patient can help the physician select the most relevant piece of information to share.

Problem Use and Abuse (Brief Intervention). Adolescents who have problems associated with drugs may benefit from a brief intervention designed to encourage them to move in the direction of positive behavior change according to the model of Prochaska and DiClemente (Table 73.4).

Motivational Interviewing (MI) Principles. MI is an empathetic, patient-focused, directive counseling style that seeks conditions necessary for positive

TABLE 73.2

Physical Signs of Drug Intoxication, Recovery from Intoxication, and Chronic Use[a]

Drug	Acute Intoxication	Recovery from Intoxication/Withdrawal	Chronic Drug Use
Alcohol	Fruity smelling breath, disinhibited or silly, clumsiness, vomiting	Headache, nausea, vomiting, dry mouth	Enlarged liver, increased liver enzymes, hypertension
Marijuana	Erythematous conjunctivae, tachycardia, dry mouth, increased talking, euphoria	Anxiety, nervousness	Chronic cough, wheezing Loss of interest in activities/apathy
Cocaine	Hyperalert state, increased talking, hyperthermia, nausea, dry mouth, dilated pupils, sweating, cardiac arrhythmias	Depression, anhedonia, insomnia, lethargy, mental slowing	Erosion of dental enamel, gingival ulceration, chronic rhinitis, perforated nasal septum, midline granuloma, cardiac arrhythmias, hypertension, paranoia, psychosis
Amphetamines	Similar acute intoxication effects as cocaine	Choreoathetoid movement disorders, skin picking, and ulcerations	
Opioids	Constricted pupils, drowsiness ("nodding"), slowed respirations, bradycardia, slurred speech, slowed comprehension, constipation	Flu-like symptoms, muscle and joint aches, dilated pupils, coryza, lacrimation, sweating, abdominal cramps, nausea, vomiting, diarrhea, hot and cold flashes, piloerection, yawning, tremors, anxiety, irritability	Abscesses, cellulites, phlebitis and scarring (from injection use), chronic constipation, malnutrition

Benzodiazepines	Drowsiness, slowed respirations, slurred speech, slowed comprehension	Seizures (may be life threatening), anxiety, restlessness	Sleep difficulties, anxiety, personality changes
Hallucinogens	Toxic psychosis, paranoia, anxiety, tachycardia, hypertension, dry mouth, nausea, vomiting	Flashbacks, which may occur even after the effects of the drug have worn off, unpredictable or self injurious behavior.	Psychosis, depression, personality changes
Inhalants	Euphoria, slurred speech, ataxia, diplopia, lacrimation, rhinorrhea, salivation, irritation of the mucus membranes, nausea, vomiting, arrhythmias	Headaches, sleepiness, depression	Irritation of mucus membranes, changes in neurological examination
Ecstasy	Euphoria, decreased interpersonal boundaries, tachycardia, hypertension, hyperthermia, sweating, muscle spasms, bruxism, blurred vision, chills, nystagmus	Depression, anxiety, paranoia, dehydration	Cognitive deficits

[a]See also Chapter 71.

TABLE 73.3

Spectrum of Drug Use in Adolescents

Primary abstinence	No history of drug or alcohol use
Experimentation	Initial one or few occasions primarily undertaken to satisfy a curiosity to experience intoxication
Regular use	Regularly recurring drug or alcohol intoxication in social situations without associated problems or consequences
Problematic use	Drug or alcohol use associated with new onset problems with relatively limited consequences such as: Parental punishment School detention or suspension Trouble with the police or risky behavior such as: Driving while intoxicated Overdose or black out
Abuse	Recurrent drug or alcohol use despite problems that interfere with functioning, such as decrease in school performance, decreased performance in sports or hobbies, arrests with legal consequences, or serious medical complications, as defined by DSM-IV criteria (American Psychiatric Association, 1994): A. A maladaptive pattern of substance use leading to clinically significant impairment or distress, as manifested by one (or more) of the following, occurring within a 12-month period: 1. Recurrent substance use resulting in a failure to fulfill major role obligation at work, school, or home (e.g., repeated absences or poor work performance related to substance use; substance-related absences, suspension, or expulsions from school; neglect of children or household) 2. Recurrent substance use in situations where it is physically hazardous (e.g., driving an automobile or operating a machine when impaired by substance use) 3. Recurrent substance-related legal problems (e.g., arrests for substance-related disorderly conduct) 4. Continued substance use despite having persistent or recurrent social or interpersonal problems caused or exacerbated by the effects of the substance (e.g., arguments with spouse about consequences of intoxication, physical fights) B. The symptoms have never met the criteria for substance dependence for this class of substance

(continued)

TABLE 73.3

(Continued)

Dependence	Loss of control over a drug or alcohol, as defined by DSM-IV criteria:
	
	A. A maladaptive pattern of substance use, leading to clinically significant impairment or distress, as manifested by three (or more) of the following, occurring at any time in the same 12-month period:
	  1. Tolerance, as defined by either of the following:
	    a. A need for markedly increased amounts of the substance to achieve intoxication or desired effect
	    b. Markedly diminished effect with continued use of the same amount of the substance
	  2. Withdrawal, as manifested by either of the following:
	    a. The characteristic withdrawal syndrome for the substance (refer to Criteria A and B of the criteria sets for withdrawal from the specific substances)
	    b. The same (or a closely related) substance is taken to relieve or avoid withdrawal symptoms
	  3. The substance is often taken in larger amounts or over a longer period than was intended
	  4. There is a persistent desire or unsuccessful efforts to cut down or control substance use
	  5. A great deal of time is spent in activities necessary to obtain the substance (e.g., visiting multiple doctors or driving long distances), use the substance (e.g., chain-smoking), or recover from its effects
	  6. Important social, occupational, or recreational activities are given up or reduced because of substance use
	  7. The substance use is continued despite knowledge of having a persistent or recurrent physical or psychological problem that is likely to have been caused or exacerbated by the substance (e.g., current cocaine use despite recognition of cocaine-induced depression, or continued drinking despite recognition that an ulcer was made worse by alcohol consumption)

Secondary abstinence	No use and a commitment to abstinence after a period of drug or alcohol use

TABLE 73.4

Prochaska and DiClemente Stages of Change Model

Stage	Description
Precontemplation	The patient does not perceive problems related to behavior and has not considered making a change
Contemplation	The patient is considering a behavior change, but is ambivalent
	Perceived benefits of continued behavior are in a dynamic balance with perceived risks
Determination	The patient has decided to make a change and begins to make a specific plan though no change has occurred yet.
Action	The patient is engaged in an action plan and change has occurred.
Maintenance	The behavior change has become internalized
Relapse	The patient has returned to the original behavior

From Prochaska and DiClemente, 1986, 1992.

change. MI assumes that (1) motivation is a product of interpersonal interaction and not an innate character trait and (2) ambivalence toward change is normal and acceptable. In this model the patient presents the arguments for change, while the counselor helps the patient to use his or her own negative feelings regarding drug use as the fuel for behavior change, supports self-efficacy, acknowledges the difficulties of making changes, and avoids resistance by refraining from lecturing or arguing with the patient.

Motivational Interviewing Techniques. A variety of tools are associated with MI. Table 73.5 describes several of the most common techniques and gives sample situations.

Written Agreements. When an adolescent does decide to make a behavior change, it is useful to make a specific written plan detailing the change attempted and a time frame. Sample drinking and driving contracts are available at the Students Against Destructive Decisions (SADD) web site (www.saddonline.com/).

Dependence (Referral). Most adolescents with a substance dependence diagnosis will need intensive services from an addiction or mental health specialist. Pharmacologic treatment may be a useful adjunct for patients with opioid or alcohol dependence (see Chapter 74).

The Role of Parents. Parents play a vital role in the prevention and treatment of adolescent substance abuse. Providers should encourage parents of preteens to discuss drugs and alcohol and to set clear family rules of no use; they should set a good example by consuming alcohol only in moderation, never driving after drinking, and avoiding drug use. Some adolescents who are misusing drugs or alcohol will not engage in treatment. In these cases family or

TABLE 73.5

Motivational Interviewing Techniques

Tool	Technique	Situation Example
Open-ended questions	Encourages the patient to explore potential consequences of a behavior	Patients who have not yet begun to think about making a change *"What do you think would happen if you were caught smoking marijuana at school?"*
Reflections	Echo back what the patient has said to emphasize the point	May help "tip the balance" for an ambivalent patient *"You don't use marijuana during lacrosse season because you feel it really slows you down and makes you short of breath"*
"Rolling with resistance"	Acknowledge the patient's point of view, even if not agreeing with it	Redirects the conversation when a patient gets "stuck" or angry *"It is surprising that you were expelled from school for a first drug incident. What do you think you will do about it?"*
Reframing	Point out that the "glass is half full"	Supports self-efficacy while the patient is attempting a behavior change *"So you didn't make your goal completely, but you did cut back your drug use quite a bit. Keep going—that's a great first step."*

parent support counseling may be useful. Parents should be advised to set firm limits and avoid enabling substance use. *Enabling* refers to any activity that intentionally or unintentionally helps the adolescent to obtain or use drugs (e.g., providing money, cell phones, e-mail accounts, transportation, etc). If parents are unable to enforce the rules of their home, they may seek assistance from the court system by filing a "Child in Need of Supervision" (CHINS) order (or the equivalent in your state) with the police department and having a probation officer assigned to assist them. In all cases the patient and family should be told that they are welcome to return to the office to discuss drugs and alcohol whenever they are ready. Some patients need more time. A supportive word or two may stay with them, preparing them to return at a later time and engage in treatment.

WEB SITES AND REFERENCES

http://www.health.org/. National Clearinghouse for Alcohol and Drug Information.
http://www.nida.nih.gov/. National Institute on Drug Abuse.
http://www.niaaa.nih.gov/. National Institute on Alcohol Abuse and Alcoholism.

http://www.samhsa.gov/. Substance Abuse & Mental Health Services Administration.

http://www.saddonline.com/. Students Against Destructive Decisions.

American Academy of Pediatrics, Committee on Substance Abuse. *Testing your teen for illicit drugs: information for parents.* [Patient education brochure available from the Academy through the AAP Web site (www.aap.org) or by calling (888/227-1770).]

Knight JR, Sherritt L, Harris SK, et al. Validity of brief alcohol screening tests among adolescents: a comparison of the AUDIT, POSIT, CAGE and CRAFFT. *Alcohol Clin Exp Res* 2002;27:67.

Kulig JW and the Committee on Substance Abuse, American Academy of Pediatrics. Tobacco, alcohol, and other drugs. *Pediatrics* 2005;115(3):816–821.

Prochaska JO, DiClemente CC. Stages of change in the modification of problem behaviors. *Prog Behav Modif* 1992;28:183.

Miller WR, Rollnick S. *Motivational Interviewing: Preparing People for Change.* 2nd ed. New York: Guilford Press, 2002.

Levy S, Vaugh BL, Angulo M, et al. Buprenorphine replacement therapy for adolescents with opioid dependence: early experience from a children's hospital-based outpatient treatment program. *J Adolesc Health* 2007;40:477.

CHAPTER 74

Intensive Drug Treatment

Brigid L. Vaughan and John R. Knight

PRINCIPLES OF DRUG TREATMENT IN ADOLESCENTS

The American Academy of Child and Adolescent Psychiatry's (AACAP) Practice Parameter for the Assessment and Treatment of Children and Adolescents with Substance Use Disorders (AACAP, 2005) sets forth evidence-based recommendations regarding the assessment and care of adolescents with substance use disorders (Table 74.1). Matching of treatment settings, interventions, and services to each patient's problems and needs is critical (*Drug Strategies*, 2003). Intensive treatment of substance use disorders in adolescents may occur in a variety of settings and utilize a wide range of services. Common themes include the need for thorough assessment, comprehensive care involving the entire family, as well as thoughtful continuing care. The primary care clinician caring for adolescents can serve an important role by educating teens and their families about treatment needs and options, guiding families through various stages of care, and supporting them during difficulties that may arise. "Treating Teens: A Guide to Adolescent Drug Programs" (*Drug Strategies*, 2003) includes questions (Table 74.2) meant to help families and providers in assessing the appropriateness of potential programs.

OVERVIEW OF AVAILABLE TREATMENTS

Inpatient Care. Treatment should be provided in the least restrictive setting possible. Safety issues, patient or family motivation, medical or psychiatric complications, treatment availability, and failure of treatment in a less intensive setting all may lead to the need for an intensive treatment setting. This may include the following:

Detoxification. *Detoxification* describes the medical monitoring and treatment of withdrawal symptoms. It can be done on an outpatient basis, but detoxification often requires a 3- to 5-day inpatient medical hospitalization and should be considered for all patients who have symptoms of physical dependence on alcohol or benzodiazepines.

Psychiatric Hospitalization or Acute Residential Treatment. For adolescents whose substance use disorder has caused or been accompanied by severe

TABLE 74.1

Recommendations for the Assessment and Care of Adolescents with Substance Use Disorders (American Academy of Child and Adolescent Psychiatry, 2005)

The adolescent must be assured of an appropriate level of confidentiality.

Assessment must include developmentally appropriate screening questions regarding the use of alcohol and drugs.

A positive screen necessitates a more formal evaluation.

Toxicology, that is, drug testing, is to be a routine part of assessment and ongoing treatment.

Adolescents who have substance use disorders need specific treatment.

Treatment of substance use disorders should be in the least restrictive setting.

Family therapy and/or substantial family involvement should be included in treatment of adolescents with substance use disorders.

Treatment programs should strive to fully engage adolescents and maximize treatment completion.

Medication to manage craving or withdrawal, or for aversion therapy can be used as indicated.

Treatment of adolescents with substance use disorders must help develop peer support.

Involvement with 12-step groups, like Alcoholics Anonymous (AA) or Narcotics Anonymous (NA), should be encouraged.

Programs should provide comprehensive services, including vocational, recreational, medical services as indicated.

Adolescents with substance use disorders require comprehensive psychiatric assessment, in order to check for comorbid disorders.

Co-occurring psychiatric disorders require treatment.

Programs must provide or arrange for aftercare.

behavioral or even frank psychiatric symptoms, inpatient psychiatric hospitalization or acute residential treatment may be needed.

Outpatient Care. For medically and behaviorally stable patients, outpatient treatment is the mainstay of substance abuse treatment (see Chapter 73). Multiple treatment modalities can be used: (1) Cognitive behavioral therapy is a structured, goal-oriented counseling style that has been found to be effective. (2) Group therapy involves meeting with a group of adolescents who share similar difficulties. (3) The 12-step fellowship is a form of peer-based support found in 12-step programs, Alcoholics Anonymous (AA), and/or Narcotics Anonymous (NA). (4) Family therapy has been studied extensively and shown to be more effective than many other outpatient options. (5) Drug court is a juvenile court that uses case management, positive reinforcement, and a more "user-friendly" interface with the adolescent and family. (6) Contingency management relies heavily on reinforcement of desirable behaviors through urine testing and substance abstinence.

TABLE 74.2

Ten Important Questions to Ask of a Treatment Program

1. How does your program address the needs of adolescents?
2. What kind of assessment does the program conduct of the adolescent's problems?
3. How often does the program review and update the treatment plan in light of the adolescent's progress?
4. How is the family involved in the treatment process?
5. How do you engage adolescents so that they stay in treatment?
6. What are the qualifications of program staff and what kind of clinical supervision is provided?
7. Does the program offer separate single sex groups as well as male and female counselors for girls and boys?
8. How does the program follow-up with the adolescent and provide continuing care after treatment is completed?
9. What evidence do you have that your program is effective?
10. What is the cost of the program?

From (Drug Strategies, 2003).

Long-Term Residential Treatment. For youths who have "failed" outpatient treatment for substance use disorders, longer-term treatment may be in order. These programs can accommodate adolescents who may have both psychiatric and substance use disorders. (1) Therapeutic communities generally last 18 to 24 months and provide treatment for adolescents with severe substance and behavioral difficulties. (2) Therapeutic schools can be day schools or boarding schools that address substance and behavioral issues. (3) Wilderness therapy involves group therapy, educational curricula, and group living with the application of outdoor-living skills and physical challenges.

Pharmacotherapy

Alcohol. Disulfiram, naltrexone, and acamprosate are the only medications approved for the treatment of alcohol dependence in adults. Disulfiram is an aversive therapy that causes an unpleasant reaction if the patient uses alcohol while taking it. Naltrexone, an opioid antagonist, limits the rewarding effects of alcohol. Acamprosate alleviates cravings, so is useful as a maintenance medication. None of the above is approved for use in adolescents. Selective serotonin reuptake inhibitors (SSRIs) can be of help to patients with alcohol dependence by treating underlying psychiatric disorders.

Opioids. The treatment of opioid dependence in adults has utilized pharmacotherapy since the mid-1960s, when methadone therapy began. Patients who have been dependent on heroin for more than a year and are at least 18 years old are eligible for methadone maintenance. This clearly restricts access for adolescents.

Newer medications used for opioid dependence—levomethadyl acetate (LAAM) and buprenorphine—are similarly effective. Potential cardiotoxicity with LAAM has limited its use in treating drug dependence. Buprenorphine is a partial opioid agonist and, therefore, may have some advantages, including fewer withdrawal symptoms and a lower risk of overdose. The buprenorphine-naloxone preparation lessens risk of abuse.

TREATMENT OF CO-OCCURRING DISORDERS

Mood Disorders. It can be difficult to discern whether a mood disorder preceded or is the result of substance use. The use of SSRIs to treat depression in youths with substance use disorders appears to be safe and likely effective. A controlled study found that lithium had a good safety profile in treating adolescents with co-occurring bipolar and substance use disorders. Pharmacotherapy for the bipolar disorder did not adequately address the substance use disorder in the absence of specific substance abuse treatment.

Anxiety Disorders. It can be difficult to determine whether anxiety led to or was caused by substance abuse. Preliminary data suggest that adolescents with substance use disorders and anxiety may be helped by cognitive behavioral therapy. Additionally, as previously noted, SSRI medications have been found to be safe in adolescents who continue to use alcohol; therefore, it may be used to treat anxiety as well as depression. Benzodiazepines, because of their abuse potential, should not be used to treat co-occurring anxiety in teens with substance use disorders.

Attention Deficit Hyperactivity Disorder (ADHD). Longitudinal studies have shown that ADHD is associated with an increased risk of substance use disorders. A meta-analysis found that stimulant treatment of ADHD is associated with a lower risk of substance use disorders. Health care providers are sometimes reluctant to prescribe stimulants to patients with ADHD and substance use disorders because the medication can be abused if it is ground up and used intravenously or intranasally. Longer-acting stimulant medications, particularly OROS (Osmotic Release Oral System) and methylphenidate (Concerta), have much less abuse potential. Nonstimulant medications like bupropion and atomoxetine are also effective in treating ADHD. Bupropion, which does not have a formal indication for treating ADHD, may be helpful for adolescents with comorbid ADHD and depression; therefore, it could be considered an option for teens with co-occurring ADHD and substance use disorders.

ACUTE AND CHRONIC PAIN

Pseudoaddiction refers to drug-seeking behavior generated by inadequate pain management. Patients with pseudoaddiction may hoard medication, request specific drugs, or escalate medication dose without informing/asking the treating physician. Adequate pain treatment can prevent pseudoaddiction. If a pain patient who is complaining of needing more medication becomes involved with illicit drugs or illegal acts (e.g., injecting oral medications, prescription forgery, stealing drugs from others) or exhibits a decline in functioning, a substance use disorder must be considered.

Patients with a history of past or recent substance abuse or dependence are not immune to pain-related conditions. It has even been suggested that people with opioid dependence are less tolerant of pain. Patients with both substance use disorders and a pain syndrome (e.g., related to cancer or an injury) require comprehensive assessment. Ongoing care necessitates continued open communication between all involved providers.

WEB SITES AND REFERENCES

http://www.drugstrategies.org. Drug Strategies is a nonprofit research foundation that promotes more effective ways of dealing with the nation's drug and alcohol problems.

http://www.dea.gov/pubs/abuse. This site provides text of *Drugs of Abuse,* which offers straightforward information about drugs.

http://www.buprenorphine.samhsa.gov. This Web site provides information about the use of buprenorphine in treating opioid dependence, as well as a "physician locator."

American Academy of Child and Adolescent Psychiatry (AACAP). Practice parameter for the assessment and treatment of children and adolescents with substance use disorders. *J Am Acad Child Adolesc Psychiatry* 2005;44:609.

Drug Strategies. *Treating teens: a guide to adolescent drug programs.* Adolescent programs and resources. Washington DC: Drug Strategies, 2003.

Greydanus DE, Patel DR. The adolescent and substance abuse: current concepts. *Dis Mon* 2005;51:392.

Pumariega A, Kilgus M, Rodriguez L. Adolescents. In Lowinson, J, Ruiz, P, Millman, R, et al., eds. *Substance abuse: a comprehensive textbook*, 4th ed. Philadelphia: Lippincott Williams & Wilkins, 2005:1021.

Waxmonsky JG, Wilens TE. Pharmacotherapy of adolescent substance use disorders: a review of the literature. *J Child Adoles Psychopharmacol* 2005;15:810.

CHAPTER **75**

Common Concerns of Adolescents and Their Parents

Mari Radzik, Sara Sherer, and Lawrence S. Neinstein

Adolescents and their families face a myriad of issues and concerns. Often these issues resolve on their own, may be helped by friends or family, or never come to the attention of a health care provider. Occasionally, the issue becomes severe enough to create family disruption. In the extreme case, these problems may lead to acting-out behaviors such as truancy, juvenile delinquency, substance abuse, or suicide.

Health care providers should consider the following issues in assessing the concerns of adolescents and/or their families:

1. *The severity of the problem:* Is this behavior usual or is there a marked change?
2. *The chronicity of the problem:* How long has the problem been present?
3. *The teen's emotional development:* Are the behaviors consistent with the adolescent's developmental stage?
4. *Daily functioning:* Are the problems severe enough to interfere with the daily functioning of the adolescent, such as school and social activities?
5. *Family functioning:* Try to understand the adolescent's behavior within the social context of his or her immediate world, especially in terms of relationships with caregivers.

Any concern of an adolescent or parent deserves an assessment. When the problem involves severe or chronic disorders or violent or self-injurious behaviors, a referral is usually indicated. Indications for considering a referral include (1) suicidal or self-injurious behavior, (2) mental health disorders such as mood or anxiety disorders, (3) substance abuse, (4) psychotic or other severe psychiatric symptoms, (5) developmental delay or learning disabilities, (6) long-standing or recent behavioral problems, (7) problems that have persisted despite extensive interventions by the primary caregiver, (8) problems outside the skills of the health care provider, (9) a diagnostic dilemma for the health care provider, (10) severe life stressors or changes in the family, (11) a dramatic change in school behavior and/or performance, (12) runaway behavior or behaviors that lead to legal involvement, (13) frequent fighting among peers and/or family, (14) acute or chronic illness.

REFERRALS

When a referral is necessary, several considerations are important:

1. Are the adolescent and parents motivated to seek treatment? Without motivation, compliance is extremely poor.
2. Do the adolescent and family understand the reason for the referral?
3. Is the referral appropriate for the problem?

Several interventions may help in making the referral:

1. Reassure the adolescent that the primary health care provider will continue to follow the adolescent and be involved in his or her care.
2. Explain that as part of the total evaluation and treatment of the adolescent's problem, a psychological or psychiatric evaluation is important.
3. Explain relevant concerns to the adolescent and family.
4. Reassure the adolescent that often counseling will be arranged for a limited period of time. If the counseling does not work out, the adolescent or family can stop.
5. Describe how counseling can be an opportunity to help the adolescent feel better, build coping skills, and enhance family or interpersonal relations.
6. Distinguish the adolescent from his or her behavior.

CONCERNS OF ADOLESCENTS

Common concerns of adolescents include the following:

1. *Parental conflicts:* Rules (e.g., curfew, driving), privacy, expectations, and peer relationships
2. *Peers:* Interpersonal concerns regarding friendships, relationships and sexuality
3. *Identity:* Who am I? Concerns surrounding body image, sexual and gender identity, culture and ethnicity
4. *School:* Popularity, academic pressures, teachers, and adjustment to a new school
5. *Sibling/family conflicts:* Blended and cross-generational differences
6. *Social situations:* Social connectivity, whether isolated or gregarious
7. *Depression:* Moderate or severe
8. *Medical concerns:* Menstrual disorders, short stature, acne, and weight disorders
9. *Psychosomatic problems:* Headaches, stomach pains, and insomnia

10. *Safety concerns:* Violence in the environment, community, home, school, relationships
11. *Prospects for the future:* Economic realities, employment, education, relationship building, and establishing a solid sense of self

CONCERNS OF PARENTS

Common concerns of parents with regard to their adolescent son or daughter include the following:

1. *Adolescent acting-out behaviors:* This may be an indication of emotional or family dysfunction.
2. *Risk-taking behaviors:* Life-threatening, risk-taking behavior requires family interventions.
3. *Emotional lability:* Assessment of the severity, including detailed description of the moods and changes, is required to determine if a mood disorder is the underlying cause.
4. *Drug and alcohol use:* Evaluation of the type (including steroids and complementary and alternative medication) and degree of use is required.
5. *Academic problems:* Evaluation of the type and severity of the problem
6. *Sexual activity and identity:* Issues of confidentiality between the adolescent and the health care provider should be explained to the parents. When adolescents know that their private and personal information will be kept confidential, they are more likely to trust their health care provider and discuss their problems openly. Adolescents and their parents should be encouraged to discuss issues of sexuality, sexual identity, and sexual activity whenever possible.
7. *Eating disorders:* An evaluation of changes in weight, attitudes toward body image, eating habits and behaviors, psychological and emotional health, family functioning, and self-esteem should be undertaken.
8. *Safety issues:* Violence in the environment and driving safety
9. *Peer influences:* Parents should be aware of the importance of peer influences and should monitor behaviors and activities while understanding that youth need to choose their own friends.
10. *Psychosomatic problems:* Medical evaluation should include an exploration of any sources of stress.
11. *"Wasting time" by the adolescent, especially daydreaming:* Parents should be reassured that this is usually a normal part of adolescent development. However, parents should monitor and help redirect youth who may need more direction.

CONCLUSION

Respectful, consistent, and caring parents and caregivers can facilitate a positive transition for their teenager as he or she moves through adolescence toward adulthood.

WEB SITES

http://www.aacap.org/. Questions and answers from the American Academy on Child and Adolescent Psychiatry.

http://www.aamft.org. The American Association of Marriage and Family Therapists website.

http://www.adolescenthealth.org. Society of Adolescent Medicine.

http://www.apa.org. The American Psychological Association.

http://www.ncfy.com. Supporting Your Adolescent: Tips for Parents, prepared by the National Clearinghouse on Families & Youth.

http://www.pflag.org/. National organization supporting parents of gay, lesbian, bisexual, and transgendered persons.

CHAPTER 76

High-Risk and Delinquent Behavior

Robert E. Morris and Ralph J. DiClemente

Changes in society significantly influence adolescents. Adaptation to psychological developmental triggers occur in an environment of varying drug use, sexual activity, media stimulation, and, in some cases, weakened family structure. Attempts to cope with these pressures may result in behaviors with immediate or long-term negative consequences. In the United States, it is estimated that every 37 seconds a teen becomes pregnant, every 1 minute a teen gives birth, every 78 seconds a teen attempts suicide, every 76 minutes a teen is killed in a car accident, and every 90 minutes a teen is murdered and another commits suicide.

RISK AND RESILIENCE

Risk involves exposure to threats. Opposite risk is resilience, defined as functional behavior that moderates exposure to risk. Resilient youth display good mental health, high functional capacity, and social competence in adversity. Resilience also includes protective mechanisms, enhanced by family factors, contributing to successful adaptation to stress events, or a healthy set of flexible behaviors and coping leading to positive choices despite impoverished life experiences.

EPIDEMIOLOGY OF RISK-TAKING BEHAVIOR

Mortality. In 2000, about 17,944 adolescents between the ages of 10 and 19 died. Injuries caused 75% of deaths (55% involved automobiles) and 25% were due to natural causes. Injury deaths were 47% among 10-year-olds and 81% among 18-year-olds.

Morbidity. About 20% of U.S. teens have great difficulty transitioning from childhood to adulthood, with resulting risk taking.

1. *Pregnancy:* In the United States, more than 800,000 pregnancies are reported per year for females between the ages of 15 and 19, with over 60% of these pregnancies occurring in 18- to 19-year-old women. From 1990 to 2003, the birth rate for females between the ages of 15 and 19 decreased by 33%, to 41.6 per 1,000 females (see Chapter 41).

2. *Sexual activity:* The 2005 Youth Risk Behavior Survey (YRBS) found that 46.8% of high school students reported sexual intercourse and 63% of currently sexually active adolescents used a condom during their last sexual intercourse. Chlamydial infection and, to a lesser extent, gonorrhea are epidemic in teens.
3. *Substance abuse:* In 2005, 43.3% of all high school students (42.8% of girls and 43.8% of boys) reported alcohol use during the previous 30 days. Lifetime marijuana use was reported by 38.4% of high school students (CDC, 2006).
4. *Runaway behavior:* See discussion toward the end of this chapter.
5. *Suicide:* The age-adjusted suicide rate was 10.7 deaths per 100,000 in 2001, compared with 11.5 in 1990. Nationwide, 8.4% of students (10.8% females, 6% males) attempted suicide at least once during the year preceding the 2005 survey.
6. *Education:* Students who drop out of school have fewer opportunities to succeed at work or to be fully functional. In 2000, young adults from families with low incomes were six times more likely to drop out than peers from families in the top 20% of income levels.

FACTORS INVOLVED IN RISK-TAKING BEHAVIOR

Childhood and adolescence are contiguous events in the life cycle. The developmental challenges of adolescence depend on personality traits established during childhood. The physical, psychological, and social maturational forces of development combine to determine behavior at any moment. Behaviors constituting a health risk may be perceived as a problem but, viewed developmentally, they accomplish developmental tasks. For adolescents, risk taking is not seen as a problem but as a solution, while the *health professionals see it as a problem.* This paradox helps explain the difficulty of managing high-risk behaviors.

General characteristics of risk-taking behaviors include the following:

1. Behaviors tried during adolescence (e.g., cigarette smoking, sexual activity, study habits).
2. *The more immediate the health risk the greater likelihood of an effective intervention.*
3. Adolescents acquire and consolidate health-related behaviors.
4. Some problem behaviors tend to occur in combinations, but not invariably.
5. Risk at any developmental period reflects the number of risk factors current and previous.

Biopsychosocial Factors. The timing of puberty and the social environment have dramatically changed, increasing pressure to adapt to new norms. These factors include the following:

1. Menarche occurs earlier (12.5 years), marriage is delayed (average age, 26 years), and societal values have changed regarding premarital sexual intercourse.
2. The U.S. population is more *urbanized,* with a lack of *essential* work for youth.
3. Because of increased family mobility, teens must reestablish social relations when social skills are often poorly developed.

4. Family breakdown results in more single and working parents and no extended family.
5. The educational process to prepare the individual for a high-tech society is longer.
6. A shift has occurred from viewing our young as an economic asset to seeing them as a liability.
7. Western cultures expose adolescents to negative environmental influences rather than protecting them from these.
8. Change occurs rapidly during adolescence, and pressures for adaptation are great.
9. *Immature processing of emotions:* Young, physically mature teens, like children, may process emotions and planning in the amygdala rather than the frontal lobes.

Conditions predisposing youth to difficulties with the transition from childhood to adulthood include being reared in poverty; being physically, sexually, and/or emotionally abused; living in pathologic families including mental illness or substance abuse; having educational handicaps; having a gay or lesbian sexual orientation, and being chronically ill.

The majority of these young people mature successfully. The health professional should be vigilant and offer help but should not automatically label such youngsters as being at high risk.

INCARCERATED YOUTH AND JUVENILE DELINQUENCY

Definitions

A *juvenile delinquent* is one who has committed a criminal offense and is younger than 17 or 18 years old. A judge adjudicates in juvenile or family court, with a goal of rehabilitation. For serious offenses, many states try juveniles in adult court and sentence them to adult prisons that lack rehabilitation.

A *status offender* is a juvenile who commits an offense that is not illegal for an adult.

Epidemiology

1. *Prevalence:* In 1997 and 2003, U.S. law enforcement agencies made 2.8 million and 2.2 million arrests of youth under age 18 respectively. Juvenile crime arrests beginning in the late 1980s grew to a peak in 1994 and decreased yearly through 2003. Juveniles commit crimes in groups and are arrested more often than are adults. As of 2000, there were 73 death row inmates who had committed their crimes before the age of 18, and 17 were executed from 1985 through 2000. Table 76.1 compares the types of offenses for which juveniles were held in correctional facilities on index days in 1997 and 2003.
2. Characteristics
   a. *Gender:* In 2003, males accounted for 71% of juvenile arrests (1,577,300) and 82% of juvenile arrests for violent crimes (75,440). Between 1994 and 2003, arrests of girls for various crimes either increased or decreased at a lower rate compared to those of boys. Table 76.2 compares the gender and ages of juveniles held on index days in 1997 and 2003.
   b. *Race:* In 2003, the federal government reported that black youth accounted for 45% of arrests (black youth were 16% of the population) and

TABLE 76.1

Juveniles in Public or Private Detention, Correctional and Shelter Facilities by Offense, United States, on October 29, 1997 and October 22, 2003

Offense	October 29, 1997		October 22, 2003	
	Number	Percentage	Number	Percentage
Total	105,790	100	96,655	100
Violent offenses	35,357	33.4	33,197	34
Murder/manslaughter	1,927	1.8	878	1
Sexual assault	5,690	5.3	7,452	8
Kidnapping	326	0.3	—	—
Robbery	9,451	8.9	6,230	6
Aggravated assault	9,530	9.0	7,495	8
Simple assault	6,630	6.3	8,106	8
Other violent offense	1,903	1.8	3,036	3
Property offenses	31,991	30.2	26,843	28
Household burglary	12,560	11.9	10,399	11
Motor vehicle theft	6,525	6.2	5,572	6
Arson	915	0.9	735	1
Property damage	1,758	1.7	—	—
Theft	7,294	6.9	5,650	6
Other property offense	2,939	2.8	4,487	5
Drug offenses	9,286	8.8	8,002	8
Drug trafficking	3,045	2.9	1,801	2
Drug possession	5,693	5.4	—	—
Other drug offense	548	0.5	6,192	6
Public order offenses	9,718	9.2	9,654	10
Driving under the influence	260	0.2	—	—
Obstruction of justice	1,754	1.7	—	—
Nonviolent sex offense	1,739	1.6	—	—
Weapons offense	4,191	4.0	3,013	3
Other public order offense	1,774	1.7	6,641	7
Probation or parole violation	12,549	11.9	14,135	15
Other delinquent offenses	12	—	—	—
Status offenses	6,877	6.5	4,824	5
Curfew violation	193	0.2	203	0.2
Incorrigibility	2,849	2.7	1,825	2
Running away	1,497	1.4	997	1
Truancy	1,332	1.3	841	0.8
Underage alcohol offense	320	0.3	405	0.4
Other status offense	686	0.6	553	0.5

Adapted from U.S. Department of Justice, Office of Juvenile Justice and Delinquency Prevention. Juvenile offenders in residential placement 1997. Washington, DC. USDOJ, 1999 FS9996 and U.S. Department of Justice, Office of Juvenile Justice and Delinquency Prevention. Juvenile Offenders and Victims: 2006 National Report. Washington, D.C. USDOJ, 2006, NCJ212906.

TABLE 76.2

Juveniles in Public or Private Detention, Correctional and Shelter Facilities by Age and Sex, United States on October 29, 1997 and October 22, 2003

| | October 29, 1997 | | | | | | October 22, 2003 | | | | | |
| | Total | | Male | | Female | | Total | | Male | | Female | |
Age (yr)	Number	%	Number	%	Number	%	Number	%	Number	%	Number	%
Total	105,790	100	91,471	100	14,319	100	96,655	100	82,157	100	14,498	100
<13	2,164	2.0	1,782	82.3	382	17.7	1,933	2	1,643	85	290	15
13	4,627	4.3	3,639	78.6	988	21.4	3,866	4	3,054	79	811	21
14	11,584	10.9	9,160	79.1	2,424	20.9	9,666	10	7,636	79	2,030	21
15	21,251	20.0	17,568	82.7	3,683	17.3	18,366	19	14,876	81	3,490	19
16	28,284	26.7	24,455	86.5	3,829	13.5	25,132	26	21,111	84	4,021	16
17	24,754	23.3	22,355	90.3	2,399	9.7	24,166	25	21,024	87	3,142	13
≥18	13,126	12.4	12,512	95.3	614	4.7	13,533	14	14,709	92	1,015	8

Adapted from U.S. Department of Justice, Office of Juvenile Justice and Delinquency Prevention.
Juvenile offenders in residential placement 1997. Washington, D.C. USDOJ, 1999, FS9996 and U.S. Department of Justice, Office of Juvenile
Justice and Delinquency Prevention. Juvenile Offenders and Victims: 2006 National Report. Washington, D.C. USDOJ, 2006, NCJ212906.

white youth, including Hispanics, accounted for 53% of arrests. Arrests and incarceration for Hispanic youth are increasing rapidly.

c. *Age:* Juvenile arrests peak for youth aged 15 to 16 years old. Eighteen years is the peak age for arrest for violent crimes (homicide, rape, and assault).

d. *History:* Violent or sexually assaulting adolescents were more violent in childhood.

e. *Recurrence:* In one study, 54% of juvenile delinquents accounted for 85% of crimes, with a subgroup of 6.3% committing 52% of crimes.

f. *Medical precursors:* It is important to realize that an association of precursors to delinquency may be valid, although the incidence for many is low. They include the following: *head trauma, XYY (*Klinefelter's syndrome), *fetal alcohol syndrome and exposure to illicit drugs* (prenatal alcohol exposure may result in difficulty understanding consequences of actions, leading to repeated behaviors), *lead exposure, rare frontal or temporal lobe epilepsy,* and *learning disability and/or attention deficit disorder.*

g. *Social and environmental factors:* Low socioeconomic status; lack of employment; sense of failure; low self-esteem; family conflicts; peer-group of delinquent adolescents; gang involvement; disorganized home and/or community environment; estrangement; no good role models; lack of a caring adult; family history of alcoholism, criminal behavior, or psychiatric conditions.

h. Incarcerated delinquents exhibit depression, suicide attempts, and risk taking.

Legal Rights. (1) Adolescents in a juvenile court have the right to legal counsel and adult safeguards. (2) In the past 20 years, many laws were enacted governing the care of detained adolescents.

Effective Rehabilitation for Delinquent and Violent Youth. Until recently, few interventions to reduce delinquent behavior were rigorously evaluated to determine whether they reduced recidivism. Current successful rehabilitation programs address the criminogenic factors of offenders. The major risk factors that correlate with recidivism risk in order of importance are (1) A history of antisocial behavior and poor self-control. (2) Personal attitudes, values, and beliefs supportive of crime. (3) Procriminal associates and isolation from anticriminal others. (4) Current dysfunctional family features. (5) Callous personality factors. (6) Substance abuse.

Further information about assessment of risk and case management can be accessed at www.Assessments.com. Some interventions that have been shown to be effective are Aggression Replacement Training, Multisystemic Treatment, Functional Family Therapy, and Multidimensional Treatment Foster Care. On the other hand, boot camps and programs of the "scared straight" type are not effective in reducing recidivism, while intensive juvenile probation has a mixed record of success.

Health Problems

Between 40% and 80% of incarcerated adolescents have medical problems:

1. General medical problems often preexisting due to lack of access:
   a. Unmet nutritional needs, obesity and dental problems

b. *Common adolescent problems:* headaches, chest and abdominal pains, asthma, acne, scoliosis, weight problems, peptic ulcers, trauma, short stature, delayed puberty, gynecologic problems, cancers, myopia, and hearing loss

2. Problems related to delinquent behaviors and lifestyle:
   a. *Injuries:* Four to eight times more common compared to high school youth.
   b. Substance abuse and withdrawal affect 70% to 80% of delinquents entering detention.
   c. STDs, pregnancy, pelvic inflammatory disease, and occasionally HIV infection. About 10% of boys and 20% of girls entering detention have *Chlamydia.*
   d. Retained bullets with risk of lead toxicity, especially in healing bone, joints, or lung.
   e. Violence resulting in paraplegia, brain injury, bowel injury, and obstruction.

3. Mental health problems due to social and physical environments are very common. Most institutionalized children have histories of neglect and abuse. They respond to kindness and understanding. Medical personnel should remember that they are caregivers.

Incarcerated youth must undergo health and psychiatric screening during intake and have care available. Guidelines for health care in juvenile detention institutions are available through state boards of correction, from the National Commission on Correctional Health Care (NCCHC), and from the American Correctional Association (ACA).

RUNAWAY BEHAVIOR

Definition
Runaway behavior is an unauthorized absence from home overnight.

A *throwaway episode* is when a child is told to leave the home or prevented from returning by a parent or household adult when there is no alternative care.

Epidemiology
1. *Incidence:* In 1999, a total of 1,682,900 youth had run away or been "throwaway" (Hammer, 2002).
2. *Age:* About 68% of runaways/throwaways in the United States are 15 to 17 years old, 28% are 12 to 14 years old, and 4% are between the ages of 7 and 11. Boys and girls are represented equally.
3. *Race:* Over one half (57%) of the runaway/throwaway youth were white non-Hispanic, 17% were black, 15% were Hispanic, and 11% of another race/ethnicity.
4. *Return behavior:* 50% return home on their own; 30% return home through parental or peer involvement; 14% return home through police intervention; and 6% never return.

Types of Runaways
1. *Abortive:* No actual runaway behavior—just a fantasy
2. *Crisis:* A short stay away from home, <3 days, due to an acute problem
3. *Casual:* The street-wise adolescent with frequent runaway episodes

Reasons for Running Away

Reasons include poor communication with parents, school failure, overly strict or permissive parents, discovery of sexual identity discordant with parental values, experimentation, escaping a hopeless situation, revenge, imitation of peers, the simultaneous crises of adolescence, parental middle-age crisis, elderly grandparents, and depression. Twenty-one percent of runaway and throwaway youth had been physically or sexually abused.

Homeless youth lack access to food, shelter, services, and a social network, thus they create their own networks. During their runaway/throwaway episode, 71% could be endangered because of substance dependency, drug use, sexual or physical abuse, presence around criminal activity, unsafe sexual behavior, or extremely young age.

Suicide. This topic is discussed in Chapter 79.

Substance Abuse. This topic is discussed in Chapters 68 through 74.

Interventions. The contact point with at-risk adolescents is a medical problem. Rather than only treating the medical problem, the physician gathers background information using a brief interview that includes a medical and psychosocial evaluation (HEEADSS) (Chapter 3), plus family, vocational and school assessments. Important considerations include the following:

1. *Identifying the youth's needs:* The adolescent's agenda must be determined and validated.
2. Youth with multiple problems are best dealt with by a *multidisciplinary team.* A comprehensive list of local resources is needed. A successful intervention requires a telephone call to a specific contact person while the adolescent is in the office.
3. Basic needs must be addressed before major psychotherapeutic interventions.
4. The approach to the problem involves the adolescent's resources and must be practical.
5. Family involvement may help the intervention but must be done skillfully.
6. Risk profiles may be modified by direct or indirect interventions.
7. The opportunity to change a system (individual or family) is best when the system is unbalanced or in transition. Staff availability during a crisis is better than appointments.

WEB SITES AND REFERENCES

http://ojjdp.ncjrs.org/. Office of Juvenile Justice and Delinquency Prevention.
http://ncjrs.gov/App/Topics/Topic.aspx?TopicID=122. National Criminal Justice Reference Service.
http://www.runawayteens.org
http://www.ncjj.org/. National Center for Juvenile Justice.
http://www.njda.com. National Juvenile Detention Association.
www.ojp.usdoj.gov/bjs/guide.htm Sourcebook on Criminal Justice Statistics.

Centers for Disease Control and Prevention, Department of Health and Human Services. Youth Risk Behavior Surveillance–United States, 2005. *MMWR Morbidity and Mortality Weekly Report* 2006;53(SS-5):1–108.

National Center for Education Statistics. *Dropout rates in the United States: 2000* (Publication No. NCES 2002-114). Washington, DC: U.S. Department of Education, Office of Educational Research and Improvement, 2001.

National Vital Statistics Reports Oct. 12, 2004;53(5).

CHAPTER 77

Youth and Violence

Heather Champion and Robert Sege

Violence is a pervasive problem in American society. Adolescents are particularly likely to be affected by interpersonal violence as victims, perpetrators, and witnesses. In 2005, 5,686 young Americans between the ages of 10 and 24 were murdered; 82% were firearms deaths. Homicide is the second leading cause of death among these young people and the leading cause of death for African Americans in this age group. Despite popular misconceptions, most violent encounters are impulsive acts occurring among friends or acquaintances and within families. Thus the distinction between victim and perpetrator is not always apparent. The consequences of violent behavior are made vastly more lethal by the presence of a firearm, particularly a handgun.

EPIDEMIOLOGY

Homicide. The United States has the highest homicide rate of all industrialized countries. The homicide rate for youth aged 18 to 24 years dropped from 25.7 per 100,000 in 1993 to 15.8 per 100,000 in 2005 (Web-based Injury Statistics Query and Reporting System [WISQARS- www.cdc.gov/ncipc/wisqars/default.htm]). The United States is the only industrialized nation to have a homicide rate among young men (between the ages of 16 and 24 years) of >5 per 100,000; many countries have a rate <1 per 100,000. The highest-risk group, African American men aged 18 to 24 years, experienced a tragically high death rate of 97.2 per 100,000 in 2005.

Of the 5,686 homicides reported in the 10- to 24-year-old age group in 2005, a total of 86.2% (4,901) were males and 13.7% (785) were females; overall, 81% (4,642) of these deaths resulted from firearm injuries. Young males are more likely to be victims of violent crimes of all categories except sexual assault and intimate partner violence. Ninety-four percent of those younger than 18 years who are convicted of murder are males.

Physical Assault and Other Violent Crime. The CDC's National Youth Risk Behavior Survey (YRBS) has consistently found that one third of male high school students had been in one or more physical fights during the previous 12 months. Fights were more common among adolescent boys than girls (43% versus 28%). Rates were higher among blacks (49%) and Hispanics (50%) than among whites (41%).

Sexual Assault and Dating Violence. The 2005 YRBS found female students (11%) more likely that male students (4%) to have been forced to have sexual intercourse, and 9% had been hit, slapped, or physically hurt on purpose by a boyfriend, girlfriend, or date. The prevalence of dating violence was higher among black (12%) students than among Hispanics (10%) or whites (8%). Rates among males and females were comparable within race/ethnicity.

Suicide. In the 12 months preceding the 2005 YRBS, 13% of students nationwide reported a plan to attempt suicide and 8% reported an attempted suicide. Rates of completed suicide among adolescents are highly correlated with rates of household handgun ownership.

RISK FACTORS ASSOCIATED WITH VIOLENCE

Several necessary risk factors for violence and violence-related injuries have been identified. They are complex, interdependent, and influenced by individual, family, and societal variables, including access to firearms and weapon carrying, gang involvement, exposure to violence in the home (including violent discipline, domestic violence, and child abuse), and exposure to media violence as well as the use of alcohol and other drugs.

Access to Firearms and Weapon Carrying. About 43% of homes have one or more handguns; at least 30% of gun owners with children keep one or more loaded guns in the home. When a teenager fires a gun at home, the most common victim is him or herself, with the second most common victim being a friend. The victim is essentially never an intruder. A gun stored in the home is associated with a fivefold increased risk of completed suicide. *The single most important factor in all sorts of firearm-related injuries is the accessibility of firearms themselves.* Nearly one fifth of high school students (19%) in the 2005 YRBS reported carrying a weapon (i.e., gun, knife, or club) on at least one day during the month before the survey. The carrying of weapons increases the risk of violence-related injury by providing a false sense of security, which contributes to impulsive behavior.

Use of Alcohol and Other Drugs. The contribution of drug and alcohol use to violent behavior is not clear. Although most violent adolescent offenders use drugs and alcohol, the onset of substance use usually occurs after the onset of violent behavior. In one study, >80% of self-reported violent incidents involved no drugs or alcohol. Risk may be in the social setting of substance use and violence and engaging in multiple risky behaviors. Some violence stems from the need to support drug abuse and involvement in illicit drug sales.

Gang Participation. Although gang members represent a relatively small proportion of the adolescent population, they are responsible for much of the serious violence perpetrated by youth. Children and adolescents who participated in gangs are more likely to promote aggressive attitudes, report victimization experiences, be involved in fights, carry weapons to school, and use drugs or alcohol at school. Provision of alternative recreational opportunities for youth appears to successfully divert many who join gangs out of fear for their safety or for the sake of belonging to a popular group.

Exposure to Violence. Exposure to violence includes exposure within one's family, including being a victim of and/or witnessing child abuse and/or domestic violence; violence in the media, including television and video games; and exposure within one's neighborhood or community. Long-term effects of both physical abuse and neglect (but not sexual abuse) increased the likelihood of arrest as a juvenile by more than 50%, arrest as an adult by 38%, and arrest for a violent crime by 38%. The use of violent discipline also has a negative impact on children by teaching them that violence is an appropriate means of shaping behavior and solving problems.

RESILIENCE

Protective factors are individual or environmental factors that buffer or moderate the risk of violence. *The Surgeon General's Report on Youth Violence* reviews several proposed individual-level protective factors. These include an intolerant attitude toward deviance (including violent behavior), high IQ, being born female, a positive social orientation, and perceived sanctions for transgression. Family-level factors include a warm, supportive relationship with parents or other adults and parental monitoring or supervision of activities. School- or community-level protective factors include commitment to school, involvement in school activities, and having friends who behave conventionally. Only two of these factors have been shown to buffer the risk of youth violence: an intolerant attitude toward deviance and a commitment to school.

The National Longitudinal Survey of Youth has demonstrated the importance of protective factors at three levels. At all levels of risk, the effects of these protective factors—described as "connectedness"—strongly reduce the likelihood of violence. In the office setting, parents and providers both have strong preferences for asset- or strength-based counseling and assessment (Sege et al., 2006). The American Academy of Pediatrics (AAP) has recently released a new violence prevention program, Connected Kids: Safe, Strong Secure, based primarily on the promotion of resilience.

ASSESSMENT OF RISK

The mnemonic device FISTS (Fighting Injury Sex Threats Self-Defense) can guide the collection of a violence-related medical history (Table 77.1). Youth at low-risk do not report recent fights, are in school, and do not report use of illicit drugs or alcohol. Moderate-risk youth may report one or two fights in the previous year or associated risk factors on the FISTS screen, as well as occasional drug or alcohol use. High-risk individuals are not in school or report two or more fights in the preceding year. Moderate- and high-risk individuals may need further counseling or referral.

PREVENTION AND INTERVENTION

There has recently been a proliferation of violence prevention programs, often funded for relatively short periods and limited in scope, so that longitudinal effects on participants and broader societal measures of violent incidents

TABLE 77.1

FISTS

FISTS: *F*ighting-*I*njuries-*S*ex-*T*hreats–*S*elf-defense
This mnemonic provides the basis for assessment of an adolescent's risk
  for involvement in violence

Fighting
How many fights have you been in during the past year?
When was your last fight?

Injuries
Have you ever been injured in a fight?
Have you ever injured someone else in a fight?

Sex
Are you scared of disagreeing with your partner?
Does your partner criticize or humiliate you in front of others?
Are you scared by your partner's violent or threatening behaviors?
Has your partner ever forced you to do something sexual you didn't want
  to do?
Every family argues. What are fights like in your family or with people
  you're dating? Do they ever become physical?
Do you think that couples can stay in love when one partner makes the
  other afraid?

Threats
Has someone carrying a weapon ever threatened you? What happened?
Has anything changed since then to make you feel safer?

Self-defense
What do you do if someone tries to pick a fight with you?
Have you ever carried a weapon in self-defense?
Asking about weapons in the context of self-defense facilitates a more
  candid response. In all cases, carrying a firearm indicates high risk.
  Carrying a knife is not as clearly identified with violent behavior. For
  example, a small pocketknife may or may not be considered high risk.

The FISTS mnemonic is adapted with permission from the Association of
American Medical Colleges. Alpert EJ, Bradshaw YS, Sege RD. Interpersonal violence
and the education of physicians. *J Acad Med* 1997;72:S46.

cannot be assessed. Promising approaches begin as early in life as possible, are
sustained over time, and enhance nurturant and nonviolent parenting methods. Resources for successful prevention programs are included at the end of
this chapter.

Primary Prevention Interventions. Primary prevention strategies are approaches directed at the entire population. Violence prevention begins with
young children, when basic values and responses to frustration and conflict

are learned. Particular issues to be addressed include family violence, corporal punishment, child abuse, and early exposure to media violence. Recent research suggests that effective primary prevention programs will be directed toward the promotion of resilience as well as risk reduction.

Effective primary prevention programs must be developmentally appropriate and comprehensive in approach (particularly those involving teenagers) and must include multiple components, reinforcing nonviolent behaviors in various contexts such as the family, school, peer groups, and the media. These approaches provide access to ongoing relationships with nonviolent, caring adult mentors, particularly for teens coming from stressed or single-parent families. Through reducing risk factors, children and adolescents are empowered to resist effects of detrimental life circumstances. While many of these programs are community-based, office-based counseling may also be effective. The AAP Connected Kids program offers clinical resources public education materials to support violence prevention in the primary care setting.

Firearms. Fundamental to a public health approach to prevention is a change in environmental risk factors. Access to firearms is the principal environmental risk factor for *lethal* violence. Removal of firearms from the environment of adolescents through legislation, strict enforcement of existing laws, and removal of firearms from the home environment is essential in the prevention of the grave consequences of violent behavior. Educational interventions alone are unlikely to be successful with many children and adolescents who continue to have access to firearms.

Secondary Prevention Interventions. Children and youth hospitalized for violence-related injuries are at particular risk. Hospital based psychoeducational approaches to risk reduction have not been as effective as once hoped; it appears that long-term improvement in outcome depends on linkages with community resources. Several cities have adopted promising programs that link injured youths with community-based service organizations that offer ongoing programs designed to engage these patients positively and to provide concrete services and support.

Tertiary Intervention. Tertiary intervention takes place after a teen has become embroiled in violent activities; they may occur largely through the juvenile justice system. More than 90% of children involved in the juvenile justice system are nonviolent offenders. On any given day, >90,000 children are in juvenile detention or correctional facilities. The 9,000 adolescents younger than 18 years held in adult jails are eight times more likely than those held in juvenile facilities to commit suicide, five times more likely to be sexually assaulted, and twice as likely to be beaten by prison staff.

There is no direct evidence for the effectiveness of incarceration in reducing later illegal activity. Incarcerated adolescents have a 50% to 70% chance of being arrested within 2 years of release; teens who have participated in boot camps have a higher recidivism rate (75%). Investigations into some of the 50 boot camps operating around the country have revealed widespread abuse and neglect. In contrast, family-focused, community-based, supervised programs involving offending teens have markedly lower recidivism rates. There is much room for continued research and modification of public policy regarding our approach as a society to young people who are apprehended for illegal activities. Latino and African-American teens are disproportionately likely to be incarcerated; this results from actions occurring through the entire juvenile justice system, from the decision to make the initial arrest, the decision to hold a youth in detention, the decision to refer a case to juvenile court, the prosecutor's decision to prosecute a case, to the actual judicial decision and the subsequent penalty.

WEB SITES AND REFERENCES

http://www.aap.org/connectedkids. AAP primary care violence prevention program.

http://www.cdc.gov/HealthyYouth/YRBS. CDC, National Center for Chronic Disease Prevention and Health Promotion, Youth Risk Behavior Surveillance.

http://www.cdc.gov/ncipc/dvp/yvp/default.htm. Centers for Disease Control and Prevention and Health Promotion, Youth Violence Prevention.

http://www.cdc.gov/ncipc/wisqars/default.htm. CDC, National Center for Injury Prevention and Control, Web-based Injury Statistics Query and Reporting System (WISQARS).

http://www.safeyouth.org. National Youth Violence Prevention Resource Center.

http://www.buildingblocksforyouth.org. Building Blocks for Youth, *And Justice for Some, 2000*.

Sege RD, Hatmaker-Flanigan E, De Vos E, et al. Anticipatory guidance and violence prevention: results from family and pediatrician focus groups. *Pediatrics* 2006;117(2):455–463.

CHAPTER 78

Adolescent Depression and Anxiety Disorders

Stan Kutcher and Sonia Chehil

Depression and anxiety disorders are common, contributing to an enormous burden of disease in adolescents. These disorders may occur concurrently or separately. Early diagnosis and effective interventions can significantly modify the potentially lifelong chronic nature of these illnesses.

DEPRESSION

Depression is the prolonged presence of persistent low mood, negative cognition, and withdrawn behavior, leading to significant functional difficulties in many aspects of life (social, interpersonal, family, educational, and vocational). It must be differentiated from the transient mood difficulties that many individuals experience in daily living and from "demoralization," a more prolonged mood disturbance from ongoing negative life experiences.

Epidemiology

1. Some 50% of teens in the United States report having felt depressed within the previous 6 months, with a 20% rate of suicidal ideation. Using the criteria of the *Diagnostic and Statistical Manual of Mental Disorders* (DSM-IV-TR), about 5% to 8% of teens have a major depressive disorder (MDD).
2. *Prevalence:* 1% below the age of prepuberty and 8% to 10% by the end of the teen years.
3. *Gender:* Girls have twice the prevalence rate.

Risk Factors for Adolescent Depression

Highly Predictive Risk Factors. (1) maternal history of MDD; (2) a previous episode of MDD.

Associated Risk Factors. These may occur with adolescent depression but are not necessarily predictive of future adolescent depression. (1) Family conflict with poor affective involvement and significant communication difficulties and (2) exposure to significant negative life events.

Diagnosis

DSM classifies depression into 3 main types; MDD, dysthymic disorder and depression in bipolar disorder.

Criteria for MDD. One or more major depressive episodes (MDEs) without a manic, mixed, or hypomanic episode.

Criteria for a MDE. For at least 2 consecutive weeks, the adolescent has experienced five (or more) of the symptoms listed below. One must be either depressed or irritable mood or markedly diminished interest or pleasure.

1. Depressed or irritable mood most of the day nearly every day
2. Markedly diminished interest or pleasure in all or almost all activities nearly every day
3. Significant weight loss when not dieting or a weight gain of more than 5% of body weight in a month) *or* a decrease/increase in appetite nearly every day
4. Insomnia or hypersomnia nearly every day
5. Psychomotor agitation or retardation nearly every day (this symptom *must* be noticeable to others and not merely subjective feelings)
6. Fatigue or loss of energy nearly every day
7. Feeling of worthlessness or excessive/inappropriate guilt nearly every day (this does *not* include self-reproach or guilt about being sick)
8. Diminished ability to think or concentrate or indecisiveness nearly every day
9. Recurrent thoughts of death, recurrent suicidal ideation, a suicide attempt, or a specific plan for committing suicide

In addition, the following *must* also be present: The symptoms (a) cause *clinically significant* distress or *impairment* in social, occupational, or other important areas of functioning; (b) are not due to the direct physiological effects of a substance or a general medical condition; (c) are not better accounted for by bereavement.

Criteria for Dysthymic Disorder
1. Depressed or irritable mood for most of the day, for most days, for at least 1 year
2. Two or more of the following must be present:
   a. Poor appetite or overeating
   b. Insomnia or hypersomnia
   c. Low energy or fatigue
   d. Low self-esteem
   e. Poor concentration or difficulty making decisions
   f. Feelings of hopelessness

In neither MDD or dysthymic disorder can the symptoms be part of a schizophrenic, schizoaffective, bipolar, or delusional illness.

Identifying the Depressed Adolescent
Underrecognition of clinical depression is common in primary care. This may be due to the different clinical presentations of depression in teens and the hesitancy of teens to self-disclose symptoms.

Screening Tests. Screening tools in the primary care setting are strongly recommended, as depending on self-reports of depression may miss many depressed youth. Screening tests include the Kutcher Adolescent Depression

Scale, the KADS-11 (an 11-item version of the KADS self-report questionnaire), the Beck Depression Inventory, the Reynolds Adolescent Depression Scale, and the Mood and Feelings Questionnaire. Other adolescent health screening tools include the Patient Health Questionnaire for Adolescents and the Safe Times Questionnaire.

BIPOLAR DISORDER (MANIC DEPRESSION)

Manic depression (MD) is a chronic psychiatric disorder characterized by periods of depressed mood (which meet the criteria for MDD) and periods of significantly elevated mood (mania). Mania is characterized by intense energy, hyperactivity, elation, grandiosity, sleeplessness, racing thoughts, pressured speech, excessive risk-taking behaviors, excessive impulsive behaviors, and hypersexuality. In most teens with bipolar disorder, a "classic" MDE may be the first presentation. Antidepressant medication can precipitate the development of a manic episode.

Risk Factors for Bipolar Disorder in a Depressed Teenager. (1) Rapid onset of MDD; (2) psychotic symptoms occurring together with MDD; (3) family history of bipolar disorder.

ANXIETY DISORDERS

The diagnosis is made using the DSM-IV-TR. Teens with anxiety disorders must experience certain clearly demarcated symptoms for a specified amount of time associated with impaired function or significant distress. Anxiety disorders that commonly occur during adolescence include generalized anxiety disorder (GAD), social anxiety disorder (SAD), panic disorder (PD), obsessive compulsive disorder (OCD), and posttraumatic stress disorder (PTSD). Teens may fulfill criteria for both depressive and anxiety disorders. Anxiety disorders can often co-occur.

Generalized Anxiety Disorder
- Uncontrollable, excessive, and unrelenting worry that is inappropriate and not restricted to particular events or situations
- Worrying leading to significant emotional distress and functional impairment
- Irritability, difficulty concentrating, and restlessness
- Physical symptoms (recurrent headaches, stomach upset, muscle tension, fatigue, and sleep disturbance)

Social Anxiety Disorder
- Excessive fears of social situations (e.g., public speaking, going to a party, standing up in class, changing in the locker room) where the teen thinks that he or she is the subject of negative scrutiny by others
- Avoidance (or toleration with extreme difficulty) of the feared situations
- SAD may be associated with school refusal or avoidance.

Panic Disorder
- Recurrent, unexpected, rapid-onset, time-limited, intense episodes of severe anxiety (panic attacks)
- Panic attacks associated with autonomic hyperarousal, respiratory and cardiac distress, and cognitions of dread and fear
- Anticipatory anxiety (the teen fears having an attack) between panic attacks
- Phobic avoidance (the teen avoids locations in which panic attacks occurred)

PD often occurs in mid-to-late adolescence and can lead to agoraphobia.

Obsessive Compulsive Disorder
- *Obsessions:* presence of recurrent, intrusive, unwanted thoughts or images that the teen knows are not true
- *Compulsions:* repetitive physical or mental rituals (e.g., counting, washing)
- Significant emotional distress due to symptoms, leading to functional impairment.

Posttraumatic Stress Disorder
This may occur in teens exposed to severe stressors that violate personal safety (e.g., assault or rape) or in those who have witnessed or experienced a horrific event (traffic accident, murder) or a natural disaster. PTSD is characterized by:

- Persistent reexperiencing of the event (through dreams, flashbacks, vivid memories)
- Avoidance of situations or persons associated with the event
- Increased hyperarousal

PTSD must be distinguished from acute stress reaction, which is a normal response to severe stressors and resolves over a short period of time without intervention.

Epidemiology of Anxiety Disorders
(1) One third of youths may suffer from one of the anxiety disorders. (2) Onset generally begins in childhood or adolescence. (3) Incidence is greater in girls, who also have an earlier age of onset.

Risk Factors for Adolescent Anxiety Disorders
These include (1) a family history of parental anxiety or mood disorder; (2) female gender; (3) inhibited or anxious temperament; (4) anxiety sensitivity; (5) increased startle reflex or autonomic reactivity.

LABORATORY EVALUATION FOR DEPRESSION AND ANXIETY

Depression and anxiety disorders are "clinical diagnoses"; no laboratory tests are diagnostic. A careful medical history and physical examination are needed to rule out an underlying or contributing medical disorder and appropriate laboratory investigations should be done if a medical disorder is suspected.

TABLE 78.1

Clinical Measurement of Functioning in Adolescent
Depression and Anxiety Disorders

Domain of Functioning	Score (0–3)[a]	Comments
Family		
School		
Work		
Peer		
Recreation		
Overall		

[a]See scoring scale in text.
0: Not present
1: Present but mild, tolerable, no impairment
2: Present but moderate, some difficulty tolerating, some impairment may be evident
3: Present and severe, difficult to tolerate, impairment evident

Management

Baseline Evaluation

After the diagnosis is made, a baseline evaluation of the depressed or anxious adolescent should include a measure of symptom severity, functional impairment, and somatic symptoms.

Symptom Severity. Symptom severity is best measured using an observer-rated tool. For the depressed teen, the Clinical Assessment of Adolescent Depression (CAAD) is a useful clinical tool. This can be repeated over time to measure treatment response. Similar tools for anxiety disorders include the Screen for Child Anxiety Related Emotional Disorders (SCARED) or the Pediatric Anxiety Rating Scale.

Functional Impairment. A measure of overall functional impairment should include family, school, work, peer, and recreational functioning. One useful tool is the Clinical Measurement of Functioning in Adolescent Depression and Anxiety Disorders (Table 78.1).

Evaluation of Somatic Symptom Side Effects. Somatic symptoms should be assessed at baseline and appropriate intervals during treatment to determine which complaints are side effects of treatment and which are more likely somatic manifestations of the depressive or anxiety disorder (Table 78.2).

Psychoeducation. Educating the teenager and the parent(s)/guardian(s) about the disorder and its treatment is a necessary part of the baseline evaluation.

TABLE 78.2

Somatic Side Effects Evaluation Scale

Item	Score (0–3)[a]	Item	Score (0–3)
Dry mouth		Headaches	
Drowsiness		Insomnia	
Loss appetite		Nausea	
Agitation		Tremor	
Anxiety/nervousness		Sweating	
Diarrhea		Sexual problems	

Suicidal ideation _____ Suicidal intent _____ Suicide plans _____
[a]See scoring scale in text.
0: Not present
1: Present but mild, tolerable, no impairment
2: Present but moderate, some difficulty tolerating, some impairment may be evident
3: Present and severe, difficult to tolerate, impairment evident

Evidence-Based Treatments for Adolescent Depression and Anxiety Disorders

Few interventions are known to have therapeutic efficacy for adolescent depression and anxiety disorders; they include the selective serotonin reuptake inhibitors (SSRIs, particularly fluoxetine and possibly sertraline or citalopram) and psychological treatments (cognitive behavioral therapy (CBT) and interpersonal therapy.

Adolescent Depression. Fluoxetine is the single best intervention and fluoxetine plus CBT is the best overall intervention.

Anxiety Disorders. SSRIs and CBT have been found effective in the treatment of anxiety disorders including GAD, SAD, and OCD. Fluvoxamine or fluoxetine combined with CBT is superior to either alone for OCD. The benefits of CBT for anxiety disorders are greater than those for depression.

Treatment for Depression and Anxiety Disorders
Mild Symptoms and Minimal Functional Impairment
- A period of watchful monitoring (regular telephone contact, face-to-face visits, supportive problem-based counseling) following psychoeducation.
- Continuous evaluation of suicidality.
- If there is no substantial improvement over 4 to 6 weeks, more intensive medical or psychological intervention is indicated.

Moderate to Severe Depressive Symptoms and Functional Impairment
- Initiation of medication or psychological treatments
- Monitoring of suicidality
- Explore the issue of drug or alcohol use, abuse, or dependence.

Psychotic or Manic Symptoms
- Referral to an appropriate mental health professional for assessment and hospitalization

Suicidal Intent or Suicidal Actions
- Hospitalization to maintain safety and provide immediate evaluation and stabilization

Medication

SSRIs are associated with an increase in suicidal ideation and self-harm behaviors (but not completed suicide), which may occur soon after starting the antidepressant. The FDA has issued a "black box" warning and the potential of adverse affects should be discussed with the patient and family.

Individual Medication Categories

SSRIs. Fluoxetine, sertraline, and citalopram have the best effectiveness in the treatment of adolescent depression and anxiety disorders. Doses for older adolescents parallel adult dosing; younger adolescents require lower starting doses and slower upward titration. Venlafaxine, nefazodone, monoamine oxidase inhibitors, and tricyclic antidepressants (TCAs) are not recommended in adolescents under age 18 or 19. Studies are insufficient in individuals 18 to 25 to adequately assess efficacy and safety. Venlafaxine was most likely to be associated with suicidality in children and adolescents. The TCAs have more cardiotoxicity than the SSRIs.

Bupropion (Wellbutrin). Bupropion is a second-line medication in teenagers with MDD who have comorbid attention deficit hyperactivity disorder (ADHD).

Benzodiazepines. Clinical experience and some open label studies suggest that low doses of clonazepam (0.25 mg to 1.0 mg BID) may help in some anxiety disorders (such as PD). Some adolescents may experience a paradoxical response to a benzodiazepine (e.g., agitation, insomnia, and disinhibition); therefore, clinicians must monitor this and provide information about this possible occurrence. Rapid onset, short acting benzodiazepines should be avoided. Long-term use of benzodiazepines is not recommended. Rapid discontinuation should also be avoided.

Antipsychotic Medications and Mood Stabilizers. Antipsychotic medications or mood stabilizers should not be the first-line treatment for depression or anxiety disorders. The use of these medications should be preceded by appropriate subspecialist consultation.

Prescribing Advice. Choose a couple of antidepressants with demonstrated safety and efficacy and use these medications preferentially. In order of preference, fluoxetine, citalopram, and sertraline would be reasonable SSRIs to choose (Table 78.3). Teens with anxiety disorders may be sensitive to the side effects (i.e., "activation," which generally occurs early) of SSRIs.

Initiation

1. *Lower initiation dose:* Some clinicians choose lower initiation doses for teens with anxiety disorders and may add a low dose of clonazepam (0.25 mg BID)

TABLE 78.3

Examples of Selective Serotonin Reuptake Inhibitor Dosing in
Adolescent Depression and Anxiety Disorders

Medication	Generic Name	Starting Dose	Increments (mg)	Effective Dose (mg)	Maximum Dose (mg)
Fluoxetine	Prozac	5–10 mg q.d./o.d.	10–20	20	60
Citalopram	Celexa	10 mg q.d./o.d.	10	20	60

for a week or two when beginning SSRI treatment to cover anxiety symptoms
until the SSRI's antianxiety properties take effect. Start at a low dose (half the
recommended initiation or lower) and increase gradually over 1 to 2 weeks
until the initial target dose is reached.

2. *Time to improvement:* In adolescent depression and anxiety disorders (apart
   from OCD), significant symptom improvement may require 6 to 8 weeks
   following achievement of the initial target dose (e.g., 20 mg of fluoxetine
   daily) while remission may require 8 to 12 weeks. In OCD, significant improvement may not become evident for 10 to 12 weeks (Table 78.4). Ensure
   that the proper dose is maintained for an appropriate length of time.

TABLE 78.4

Fluoxetine (Prozac) Initiation and Dose Titration in Adolescent
Depression and Anxiety Disorders

Day	Dose (mg)	Monitoring of Response
0	0	Patient assessment and baseline measurement of symptoms, function, and side effects
1	5	Check for side effects (by phone if not possible in person)
3	10	Check for side effects (by phone if not possible in person)
7	20	Check for side effects: If 10 mg is well tolerated increase dose to 20 mg
14–54	20	Check for side effects and monitor symptoms and function
54–75[a]	20	Check for side effects and monitor symptoms and function. Decide on next steps regarding treatment depending on outcome

[a]In adolescent obsessive compulsive disorder (OCD) this period should be
lengthened for 14–21 more days because a longer period of time is needed to
determine therapeutic response at a fixed dose in this disorder.

TABLE 78.5

Symptoms of Antidepressant Withdrawal Syndrome

Dizziness	Headaches
Weakness	Anxiety/nervousness
Nausea	Difficulty sleeping
Tremor	"Electricity sensations"

3. *Stopping treatment:* With the exception of fluoxetine (long half-life), antidepressant medications should not be stopped abruptly so as to avoid a withdrawal syndrome (Table 78.5).

Patient Treatment and Monitoring Model

This model is intended for the primary care practitioner, with ongoing consultation.

Patient Evaluation

1. Ensure that the correct diagnosis of depression or anxiety disorder is made.
2. Conduct a thorough psychiatric assessment addressing other disorders.
3. Conduct a careful patient and family psychiatric history focusing on mood, anxiety, bipolar, and substance abuse disorders.
4. Determine presence or absence of symptoms and assess functional impairment.
5. Provide comprehensive information about the disorder and treatment options.
6. Provide information about somatic and behavioral side effects of the medication and the time to symptomatic improvement.
7. Treat following a proper risk–benefit evaluation.
8. Provide open dialogue regarding treatment.

At Medication Initiation

1. Measure somatic and behavioral "side effects" prior to intervention. Use a clinically useful scale (Table 78.2) at baseline. If there is a history of self-harm behaviors and the teen exhibits significant agitation, monitor closely when starting an SSRI.
2. Check for symptoms of panic and impulsivity that may suggest enhanced sensitivity to adverse behavioral effects of SSRIs. Short-term treatment with a benzodiazepine may be indicated in severe anxiety.
3. Begin treatment with a small test dose (half the recommended dose) and increase gradually over 1 to 2 weeks to target dose.
4. Carefully monitor behavioral and somatic adverse effects.
5. Once the initial therapeutic dose is reached, wait 6 to 8 weeks prior to increasing the dose (10 to 12 weeks for OCD). Continue providing psychotherapeutic interventions, including weekly face-to-face sessions and telephone contact.
6. Conduct appropriate laboratory investigations, including pregnancy testing in all females.

7. Without significant improvement in 6 to 8 weeks of appropriate intervention (10 to 12 weeks for OCD), refer for psychiatric consultation.
8. If there is only partial improvement, the diagnosis, treatment plan, and compliance should be reviewed, with referral for psychiatric consultation.
9. The role of the primary care clinician should continue even with referral to a specialist.
10. Monitor throughout treatment for suicide risk, measuring symptoms, side effects, and functioning.

Other Interventions

- Light therapy may serve as a possible adjunct if depression occurs in the winter months.
- Electroconvulsive therapy may be indicated in psychotic depression.

Adolescent depression and anxiety disorders are significant health problems, which can cause significant morbidity and mortality. Effective treatments are available. Evidence-based interventions should be used with ongoing careful monitoring of effectiveness and adverse events.

WEB SITES

http://www.aacap.org/about/glossary/depress.htm. American Academy of Child and Adolescent Psychiatry.

http://www.nmha.org/infotr/factsheets/24.cfm. National Mental Health Association fact sheet and other information on adolescent depression.

http://www.nimh.nih.gov/HealthInformation/anxietymenu.cfm. National Institutes of Mental Health information on anxiety disorders.

CHAPTER 79

Suicide

Sara Sherer

Suicide is a significant contributor to adolescent mortality. More teenagers and young adults die from suicide than from cancer, heart disease, acquired immunodeficiency syndrome, birth defects, stroke, pneumonia and influenza, and chronic lung disease combined. Suicide is the third leading cause of death in adolescence after unintentional injuries and homicide.

Adolescent suicide rates have varied dramatically over the last 50 years, with a decrease in rates since 1990. Initially, the rate of adolescent suicide was attributed to greater access to firearms and an increase in substance use. However, more recently, the reported decrease is thought to be secondary to a reduction in the availability of firearms and an increase in the use of antidepressant medications.

EPIDEMIOLOGY

1. *Suicide rates:* Efforts to estimate attempted and completed suicides are confounded by the fact that many suicidal behaviors are recorded as accidents. In 2004, the Centers for Disease Control and Prevention (CDC) reported 4,316 suicides among people 15 to 24 years old and 283 suicides among adolescents 10 to 14 years old in the United States. Since 1950, suicide rates have increased three to four times for male adolescents 15 to 24 years old. The suicide rate has also increased by approximately 10% for female adolescents in the same age group.
   a. Suicide rates for adolescent males in the United States are shown in Table 79.1.
   b. Suicide rates for adolescent females in the United States are shown in Table 79.2.
   c. Trends from 1950 to 2004 for adolescents 15 to 24 years old are shown in Figure 79.1.
2. *Suicide attempts:* The 2005 Youth Risk Behavior Surveillance System (YRBSS) (Table 79.3) shows that it is not uncommon for adolescents to consider suicide. Overall, 16.9% of students had seriously considered attempting suicide, 13% had a specific suicide plan, and 8.4% had attempted suicide during the preceding 12 months.
3. Ratios of suicide attempts to completed suicide range from 8:1 to 200:1. Preventing and accurately assessing for suicide attempts is essential, since

TABLE 79.1

Adolescent Male Suicide Rates in the United States

Year	Suicide Rate in 15- to 19-Year-Olds (per 100,000)	Suicide Rate in 20- to 24-Year-Olds (per 100,000)
1950	3.5	9.3
1960	5.6	11.5
1970	8.8	19.3
1980	13.8	26.8
1990	18.1	25.7
2000	13.0	21.4
2001	12.9	20.5
2002	12.2	20.8
2003	11.62	20.25
2004	12.65	20.85

From US Department of Health and Human Services. Center for Disease Control and Prevention. National Center for Health Statistics. Health, United States, 2004 With Chartbook on trends in Health of Americans. Hyattsville, Maryland: 2004 and National Center for Injury Prevention and control: at http://www.cdc.gov/nchs/data/hus/hus04.pdf.

TABLE 79.2

Adolescent Female Suicide Rates in the United States

Year	Suicide Rate in 15- to 19-Year-Olds (per 100,000)	Suicide Rate in 20- to 24-Year-Olds (per 100,000)
1950	1.8	3.3
1960	1.6	2.9
1970	2.9	5.7
1980	3.0	5.5
1990	3.7	4.1
2000	2.7	3.2
2001	2.7	3.1
2002	2.4	3.5
2003	2.66	3.39
2004	3.52	3.59

From US Department of Health and Human Services. Center for Disease Control and Prevention. National Center for Health Statistics. Health, United States, 2004 With Chartbook on trends in Health of Americans. Hyattsville, Maryland: 2004 and National Center for Injury Prevention and control: at http://www.cdc.gov/nchs/data/hus/hus04.pdf.

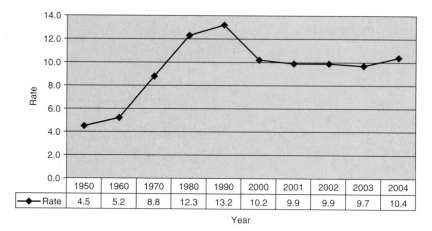

FIGURE 79.1 Suicide rates for adolescents 15 to 24 years old, 1950 to 2004.

one third of all adolescent suicides are committed by youth who were known to have previously attempted suicide.

4. *Gender:* Males outnumber females (6:1) in completed suicides, whereas females outnumber males (4:1) with respect to suicidal ideation and attempts.

5. *Race:* The 2004 suicide rate among Native American male adolescents was significantly higher than the overall suicide rate and the rates reported for white males, African American males, and Latino males. Suicide rates for African American males ages 10 to 19 years old have increased at a higher rate than those for other groups, indicating a higher vulnerability. Hispanic adolescents report more suicide attempts than any other ethnic group.

6. *Age:* The largest increase in suicide rates since 1970 has been in 15- to 19-year-old males.

7. *Psychiatric comorbidity:* A history of a suicide attempt and a history or diagnosis of a mental or addictive disorder is associated with 90% of suicides. The most common psychiatric disorders are mood disorders, alcohol and substance use disorders, conduct disorders, and anxiety disorders.

8. *Method used for completed suicides:* (a) Firearms are the most common method for both males and females. In 2004, firearms accounted for 49% of suicides among 15- to 24-year-olds. (b) Suffocation (especially hanging) is the most common method among adolescents 10 to 14 years old. In 2004, suffocation accounted for 35% of suicides among 15- to 24-years-olds. (c) Poisoning: In 2004, ingested poison was used in 8.4% of adolescent suicides in the 15- to 24-year-old population.

9. *Suicide at college:* Suicide is also the third leading cause of death on college campuses. Approximately 10% of college students contemplate suicide each year; 5% to 6% make a plan and approximately 1.5% attempt.

RISK FACTORS

There are no assessment tools to identify adolescents who will attempt suicide. Risk factors for suicide frequently occur in combination with each other.

TABLE 79.3

Behaviors Related to Attempted Suicide Among High School Students During 12 Months Preceding Survey, 2005

Category	Seriously Considered Attempting Suicide (%)	Made a Suicide Plan (%)	Attempted Suicide (%)	Suicide Attempt Required Medical Attention (%)
Sex				
Female	21.8	16.2	10.85	2.9
Male	12.0	9.9	6.0	1.8
Grade				
9	17.9	13.9	10.4	3.0
10	17.3	14.1	9.1	2.3
11	16.8	12.9	7.8	2.2
12	14.8	10.5	5.4	1.6
Race or ethnicity				
White	16.9	12.5	7.3	2.1
African-American	12.2	9.6	7.6	2.0
Hispanic	17.9	14.5	11.3	3.2
Total	16.9	13.0	8.4	2.3

From Centers for Disease Control and Prevention. Youth risk behaviors surveillance—United States, 2005, *Surveillance Summaries*, June 9, 2006. MMWR 2006;55 (No. SS-5).

Certain risk factors should increase the health care provider's index of suspicion for a potentially suicidal adolescent.

1. *A history of co-occurring psychiatric disorder and substance abuse disorder:* Over 90% of teen suicide victims have a mental disorder (e.g., depression, alcohol or drug abuse).
2. *Prior suicide attempts:* This is one of the strongest predictors of future attempts and death by suicide. About one third of teenage suicide victims have made a previous suicide attempt.
3. *History of suicide in the family:* A history of suicide attempt(s) or completed suicides among first- or second-degree relatives substantially increases the likelihood of attempted and completed suicide in the adolescent.
4. *History of prior physical and sexual abuse:* Adolescents who had been physically or sexually abused are significantly more likely to experience suicidal behaviors. A prior history of physical abuse presents with a five-time greater risk, and a history of sexual abuse presents with a threefold increase of suicidal behaviors.
5. *Family history of psychiatric and substance abuse disorders:* The parents of suicidal adolescents consistently show higher rates of mood disorders, substance abuse, and aggressive and suicidal behaviors.
6. *History of a broken family or family discord including low levels of communication with parents:* Parent–child conflict; history of violence, death, divorce; and lack of family support increase the likelihood of suicidal behaviors.
7. *Stressful life event or loss.*
8. *Gay and bisexual adolescents:* Gay and bisexual adolescents experience higher rates of depression and gay males are four times more likely to attempt suicide.
9. *Easy access to firearms:* In 2004, almost half of the 15- to 24-year-old adolescents who completed suicide used a firearm. The most common location for teen suicide by firearm is in the home. The risk is directly related to the accessibility and number of guns in the home. The presence of firearms in the home is associated with a 31.3- to 107.9-time increase in adolescent suicide even in the absence of clear psychiatric illness.
10. *Suicide contagion:* Suicide clusters account for 1% to 5% of all teen suicides in the United States. They often follow highly publicized suicides of teenagers and popular young adults. It is not necessary for the decedents to know each other or to have direct contact.

WARNING SIGNS

Several signs should alert family, friends, and health care providers to the potential for suicide. They include sadness, hopelessness, emptiness, lack of energy, insomnia, eating problems, loss of interest in social life and school, boredom, loneliness, irritability, truancy, substance abuse, and giving away prized possessions.

ASSESSMENT OF THE SUICIDAL ADOLESCENT

Interview and History

Suicidal adolescents should be interviewed alone as long as they can provide a clear history. Parents or guardians should be involved at some point. Any adolescent with a well-thought-out plan that includes intent, plan for place and time, and access to lethal means should be considered high risk. Based on this screening, the degree of protection and intervention necessary can then be determined.

The following must be assessed in:

1. *All suicidal adolescents:* (a) history of psychiatric disorders and substance abuse; (b) current depressive symptoms; (c) prior self-destructive behavior; (d) history of suicide attempts, psychiatric disorders, or substance abuse in family; (e) history of family, school, or peer problems; (f) history of incest or abuse; (g) sexual orientation; (h) recent experience of loss; (i) available support systems.

2. *Adolescents who present with suicidal ideation:* (a) suicidal ideations (type and frequency); (b) plan and motivation; (c) access to methods; (d) prior suicide attempts; (e) history of psychiatric disorders (i.e., depression) and substance abuse; (f) current life stressors; (g) access to firearms and harmful medications.

3. *Adolescents who have attempted suicide:* Need for medical treatment to address life-threatening medical complications must be assessed. As soon as the medical evaluation and treatment are completed, psychological evaluation should be performed to assess methods, impulsivity of attempt, intent to die, desire to repeat, possibility of rescue, life stressors that precipitated the attempt, access to firearms, and harmful medications. The adolescent should either be hospitalized or sent home with family members who can ensure the youth's safety.

Mental Status

Evaluating the adolescent's mental status is part of the assessment and includes (1) level of depression, hopelessness, helplessness, and self-esteem; (2) feelings of expendability; (3) openness to further interventions; (4) attitude about death.

Disposition

The disposition depends on the resources available to the patient, family, and health care provider. A consultation with a mental health provider is recommended for all suicide assessments. The following guiding principles can be used to determine the most appropriate arrangement for the suicidal adolescent.

1. *Indications for inpatient hospitalization:* (a) medical complications; (b) patient is psychotic; (c) attempt was nearly lethal, premeditated, with clear intent to die; (d) the adolescent is uncommunicative and communicates ambivalence regarding the will to live; (e) there is a history of psychiatric or substance abuse disorders; (f) the adolescent manifests agitation, poor judgment, or refusal of help; (g) there is a lack of family support.

   Adolescents presenting with a strong wish to die and a persistent plan to hurt themselves must remain in a safe and protected environment. Patient and parental consent is highly recommended, but if the adolescent refuses voluntary admission, procedures for involuntary hospitalization should be initiated. Discharge should be considered only once the suicide risk has declined and the youth and family are able to utilize appropriate resources. Following discharge, intense outpatient mental health services are indicated.

2. *Indications for outpatient management:* (a) The adolescent has demonstrated a low suicide risk and has a supportive home environment where appropriate supervision can be established; (b) the adolescent no longer feels actively suicidal; (c) there is no history of a serious suicide attempt; (d) there is no evidence of long-standing psychiatric or substance abuse disorders; (f) appropriate medical and psychosocial follow-up has been arranged.

Follow-up

Every suicidal adolescent should receive follow-up care by a qualified mental health provider. These services should be introduced when the decision is made to discharge the adolescent.

WEB SITES AND REFERENCES

http://www.aap.org/healthtopics/depression.cfm/. Information on suicide from the American Academy of Pediatrics and fact sheets for parents and caregivers on teen depression and preventing youth suicide.

http://www.suicidology.org. American Association of Suicidology, or call 1-800-273-TALK.

American Academy of Child and Adolescent Psychiatry. Practice parameter for the assessment and treatment of children and adolescents with suicidal behavior. *J Am Acad Child Adolesc Psychiatry.* 2001;40(7 Suppl):24S.

Anderson RN, Smith BL. *Deaths: leading causes for 2002.* National Vital Statistics Reports: vol. 53(17). Hyattsville, MD: National Center for Health Statistics, 2005.

Centers for Disease Control and Prevention. *Surveillance Summaries*, May 21, 2004. *MMWR* 2004:53 (No. SS-2). Centers for Disease Control and Prevention. WISQARS. National Center for Health Statistics (NCHS). National Vital Statistics System, 2005.

Douglas J, Brewer M. American Psychiatric Association practice guideline for assessing and treating patients with suicidal behaviors. *Psychiatr Ann* 2004;34(5);373.

CHAPTER 80

School Problems and Attention Deficit Hyperactivity Disorder

Peter R. Loewenson, Howard Schubiner,
Arthur L. Robin, and Lawrence S. Neinstein

School problems, including school phobia, truancy, dropout, academic performance problems, attention deficit hyperactivity disorder (ADHD), and learning disabilities, represent common concerns for adolescents and their families. Evaluation and management includes the following:

1. Evaluating the adolescent for biomedical disorders such as hearing and vision dysfunction, thyroid disorders, subtle cognitive impairments, and seizure disorders
2. Screening the adolescent for emotional disorders such as depression, anxiety, and family conflict and initiating referrals as necessary
3. Assessing the potential impact of chronic illness
4. Assessing the impact of family, school, or community factors on academic performance
5. Initiating and coordinating appropriate referrals for the psychological and psychometric testing necessary to determine the presence of learning disabilities or ADHD
6. Demystifying learning disabilities, ADHD, and related problems, educating the adolescent and family, and encouraging appropriate coping strategies
7. Educating the patient and the family about the legal obligations of public schools to meet the educational needs of youngsters with disabilities
8. Cooperating with public schools in determining eligibility for special education services
9. Contributing to the development and coordination of an overall school-based intervention plan and serving as an advocate for the adolescent
10. Providing short-term counseling for milder school and home-related problems and anticipatory guidance to prevent the development of additional complications
11. Providing medical therapy for anxiety and affective disorders as well as for ADHD
12. Serving as care coordinator to monitor the overall progress of a comprehensive care plan

SCHOOL PHOBIA/AVOIDANCE

School phobia or school avoidance is a persistent and irrational fear of going to school. The problem usually arises either because the adolescent cannot cope with the pressures and challenges at school or as a result of other stresses, usually related to family or peers. Common stress factors include fear of confrontations with teachers or students; fear of poor grades; fears related to participation in athletics; bullying, teasing, or criticism from peers; sexual expression or sexual orientation; or difficulties individuating or separating from parents.

The health care provider must explore with the adolescent his or her fears and reasons for disliking school. A gentle and accepting approach is critical as most adolescent with this disorder are embarrassed or afraid to disclose the nature of their fears or phobia. Depending on the home situation, the practitioner may recommend more parental involvement and an immediate return to school, or in overrestrictive families, the health care provider may wish to lessen parental involvement by working out a contract regarding school attendance between the health care provider and the adolescent. Psychological referral may be advisable, depending on the severity and type of underlying problem (e.g., family dysfunction or clinical phobia). Because anxiety disorders such as social phobia or generalized anxiety disorder are a common cause of school phobia, medications for anxiety disorders can be useful as part of the overall management plan. The selective serotonin reuptake inhibitors (SSRIs) have been shown to be useful for these disorders and are generally very well tolerated. Paroxetine (usual doses of 10 to 40 mg every day), fluoxetine (usual doses of 10 to 40 mg every day), and sertraline (usual doses of 50 to 150 mg every day) have been most often used. The adolescent must be monitored closely for new or worsening symptoms and the emergence of suicidality after starting an SSRI.

SCHOOL TRUANCY AND DROPOUT

Although the adolescent with school phobia has some fear of attending school, the adolescent who is truant or who drops out of school is making a conscious decision to miss school. It is clear that school failure is one of the common precursors to truancy and school dropout. And most importantly, school failure or school dropout often precedes high-risk social behaviors such as involvement in gangs and violence, running away, sexual promiscuity, and excessive drug or alcohol use. Therefore, an educational history that investigates potential causes of poor academic performance is important. Truancy and dropout may also be caused or exacerbated by substance abuse, pregnancy, marriage, or the need to work to support family members.

For those at risk for dropping out (e.g., those with early school failure, high-risk behaviors, poor "fit" within a school system), work with the adolescent and the family to first identify any primary learning disabilities, ADHD, or related conditions and then to establish appropriate goals for academic achievement and define an appropriate placement. Assess the motivation of the adolescent and family for academic performance, their short- and long-term goals, conflicts at home or at school, relationships with peers and teachers, and medical causes of academic difficulties. Identify and support the academic or extracurricular strengths of an adolescent. A behavioral plan of rewards and consequences is often needed to reestablish parental control and motivate the adolescent to attend school and complete homework. Educational options may include work–study programs, vocational programs, independent study programs, early graduation, or adult education programs. Follow-up is essential to determine if the initial plan is working and what further steps need to be taken.

ACADEMIC PERFORMANCE PROBLEMS

During middle school and high school, there is increased dependence on reading and increased need to organize materials, develop appropriate study habits, and use abstract thought processes. Therefore, it is not uncommon for academic problems to arise during these years. An interview with a parent or guardian is crucial in uncovering academic performance problems, because the adolescent may be less concerned with a drop in grades. The specific causes of poor academic performance are often multiple and are not always clear.

Defining the Problem

The identification of academic performance problems is a critical step in the evaluation of every adolescent as school performance may be an important marker of other health risk behaviors. If a potential problem is identified, it is important to clearly define the problem: Has there been a drop in grades, behavior problems, inconsistent performance, emotional issues, or underachievement for the presumed level of intelligence? Who "owns" the problem? Does the adolescent have concerns about his or her progress? Have teachers identified issues that require investigation?

Causes of Poor Academic Performance

1. *Biomedical causes include hearing or vision problems*; subtle forms of mental impairment that may not have been picked up earlier (e.g., patients with fragile X syndrome or Klinefelter syndrome, neurofibromatosis, or fetal alcohol effects); chronic illness (patients with severe asthma, sickle cell anemia, juvenile rheumatoid arthritis, or other disorders may have had sufficient absences or side effects from treatment to cause academic problems); neurologic disorders; or sleep disorders (some adolescents suffer from undiagnosed obstructive sleep apnea, central hypoventilation syndrome, or have poor sleep hygiene, any of which may have adverse effects on learning).
2. *ADHD* not previously diagnosed or not adequately treated.
3. *Learning disabilities*, occurring in approximately 3% to 5% of students.
4. *Psychological and behavioral causes:* school performance may be affected by depression, substance abuse, anxiety disorders, conduct disorder, or abuse.
5. *Family problems* may affect academic performance, including parental depression, drug or alcohol abuse, divorce, or conflict within the family.
6. *School and peer relationships:* adolescents who have poor peer relationships or interact with a peer group that does not value academic achievement.
7. *Cultural or environmental factors:* Adolescents who have lacked opportunity to achieve adequately, received poor teaching, or had cultural or economic disadvantages that interfere with appropriate education may also present with poor academic performance. Children from ethnic or cultural

backgrounds different from that of the prevailing school norm or for whom English is not the primary language may also experience difficulty.

Evaluation

1. **History** (should be collected from the adolescent, the parent, and the school)
   a. *Developmental history:* Prenatal history (use of drugs, alcohol, medications); perinatal history; developmental milestones; speech, vision, or hearing problems
   b. *Medical history:* Chronic illnesses; neurologic disorders; hospitalizations; relevant family history
   c. *Behavioral history:* Peer and family relationships; peer support and influences; suspected drug or alcohol use; psychological symptoms (particularly anxiety and depression); antisocial behaviors; symptoms of ADHD
   d. *School history:* History of prior problems; behaviors reported in school; specific problems (i.e., which classes, which hours, which teachers, missing assignments, missing homework, poor test scores); motivation, goals, future plans; likes and dislikes about school; grades, attendance, suspensions; parents' educational level and their expectations for their adolescent; prior interventions; prior educational or IQ testing
   e. *Specific strengths*: This is a critical area to identify. If an adolescent has one strong area (e.g., art, music, computers, sports), you can often build self-esteem by encouraging development in that area while using it as a "hook" to keep the adolescent motivated to stay in school.
2. **Physical examination:** Height, weight, BMI, and blood pressure; inspection for minor anomalies (e.g., short palpebral fissures, epicanthal folds); ears, nose, and throat; neck for otitis, tonsillar or thyroid enlargement; genital examination for sexual maturity rating, testicular size (large testes in fragile X syndrome, small testes in Klinefelter syndrome); careful neurologic examination.
3. **Testing**
   a. Audiometric and visual acuity testing
   b. *Cognitive testing:* (e.g., Wechsler Intelligence Scale)
   c. Achievement testing (e.g. Woodcock-Johnson III Test of Achievement)
   d. Further educational testing of specific reading, mathematics, writing, and language skills if there is a significant discrepancy between IQ and achievement
   e. Neuropsychological testing is indicated if there is either an unusual pattern of functioning on IQ or achievement tests
   f. ADHD screening
   g. Screening for psychopathology (e.g. Child Behavior Checklist (CBCL)
   h. Adolescents with low or borderline IQ scores should be screened for chromosomal anomalies, such as the fragile X syndrome

ATTENTION DEFICIT HYPERACTIVITY DISORDER

ADHD is a developmental disorder affecting approximately 4% to 12% of children and adolescents with a 3:1 male:female ratio in community samples. ADHD is characterized by developmentally inappropriate degrees of inattention, impulsivity, and hyperactivity. It arises in early childhood, is relatively chronic and pervasive in nature, and is not accounted for on the basis of gross neurologic, sensory, language, or motor impairment, mental retardation, or severe emotional disturbance. As a result of these core symptoms, adolescents with ADHD have difficulty getting their schoolwork done, organizing their personal lives, resolving disputes, communicating with their parents, following rules established by adults, and maintaining good peer relationships. Eventually, such cumulative life failure may thwart them from accomplishing the developmental tasks of adolescence, including independence seeking, identity formation, mature interpersonal relationships, and vocational planning. As a result, many such adolescents develop low self-esteem and depressed affect.

Contemporary follow-up studies have suggested that ADHD is truly a lifespan disorder; 60% to 80% of ADHD children continue to manifest the full clinical syndrome in adolescence, and more than 50% continue to manifest the full clinical syndrome in adulthood. In adolescence, paying attention and controlling impulses remain the greatest problems, whereas motoric hyperactivity usually diminishes and/or transforms into mental restlessness. Adolescents with ADHD alone may exhibit comorbid difficulties such as learning disorders, low self-esteem, depression, or other emotional problems; those with ADHD plus oppositional defiant disorder, conduct disorder, or bipolar disorder are more likely to develop problems with truancy, dropout, substance abuse, and severe family conflict. Although the exact cause of ADHD remains unknown, mounting evidence from neurochemical, brain imaging, genetic, and family studies suggests that in most cases ADHD is an inherited condition with a biochemical basis.

Diagnostic Criteria

The *Diagnostic and Statistical Manual of Mental Disorders, fourth edition* (DSM-IV-TR) includes a list of nine inattention criteria and a list of nine hyperactivity/impulsivity criteria. Subtypes of ADHD are based on various combinations of these lists (1A and 1B), together with criteria 2 through 5:

1. Either inattention (a) or hyperactivity/impulsivity (b)
   a. *Inattention:* At least six of the following symptoms of inattention have persisted for at least 6 months to a degree that is maladaptive and inconsistent with developmental level: (1) often fails to give close attention to details or makes careless mistakes in schoolwork, work, or other activities; (ii) often has difficulty sustaining attention in tasks or play activities; (iii) often does not seem to listen when spoken to directly; (iv) often does not follow through on instructions and fails to finish schoolwork, chores, or duties in the workplace (not due to oppositional behavior or failure to understand instructions); (v) often has difficulty organizing tasks and activities; (vi) often avoids, dislikes, or is reluctant to engage in tasks that require sustained mental effort (such as schoolwork or homework); (vii) often loses things necessary for tasks or activities (e.g., toys, school assignments, pencils, book, tools); (vii) is often easily distracted by extraneous stimuli; and (ix) is often forgetful in daily activities.
   b. *Hyperactivity/impulsivity:* At least six of the following symptoms of hyperactivity/impulsivity have persisted for at least 6 months to a degree that is maladaptive and inconsistent with developmental level: Hyperactivity, including: (i) often fidgets with hands or feet or squirms in seat; (ii) often leaves seat in classroom or in other situations in which remaining

seated is expected; (iii) often runs about or climbs excessively in situations in which it is inappropriate (in adolescents or adults, may be limited to subjective feelings of restlessness); (iv) often has difficulty playing or engaging in leisure activities quietly; (v) is often "on the go" or often acts as if "driven by a motor"; (vi) often talks excessively. (vii) Impulsivity including: often blurts out answers before questions have been completed; (viii) often has difficulty awaiting turn; (ix) often interrupts or intrudes on others (e.g., butts into conversations or games).
2. Some symptoms that caused impairment were present since before 7 years of age.
3. Some impairment from the symptoms is present in two or more settings.
4. There must be clear evidence of clinically significant impairment in social, academic, or occupational functioning.
5. The symptoms do not occur exclusively during the course of another development or mental disorder (e.g., mood disorder, anxiety disorder).

Although the *DSM-IV* criteria capture the core ADHD symptoms of inattention, impulsivity, and restlessness, contemporary conceptualizations of ADHD have placed these symptoms within the broader context of executive functions of the brain. These executive functions include organizing and activating to work, sustaining concentration and attention, sustaining energy and controlling emotions, and utilizing working memory and recall. In ADHD, these executive functions are ineffective.

Comorbidity

Psychosocial and/or psychiatric comorbidity are common in ADHD:

1. Approximately 35% of children with ADHD have oppositional defiant disorder (ODD), a pattern of negativistic, hostile, and defiant behavior lasting at least 6 months.
2. Approximately 26% of children with ADHD have conduct disorder, a repetitive pattern of antisocial behavior violating others' basic rights or societal norms, involving physical aggression, threats, use of weapons, cruelty to people or animals, destruction of property, theft, repeated running away from home, frequent truancy, or sexual assault.
3. At least 20% to 30% of children with ADHD have learning disabilities in at least one area.
4. A coexisting depressive disorder is present in 18% of children with ADHD, which further impairs functioning. Anxiety disorders are present in 26% of children with ADHD.
5. *Substance abuse:* Adolescents with ADHD show more cigarette and alcohol use than matched controls. Effective treatment with stimulant medication, however, has been clearly shown to reduce the risk of subsequent substance use disorder.
6. *Driving behavior:* Adolescents with ADHD show less sound driving skills or habits than matched control groups, Medical treatment for ADHD improves driving performance.
7. *Family relations:* Adolescents with ADHD and their parents display more negative and fewer positive interactions and have more family conflicts than matched controls.
8. *High-risk sexual behaviors:* Adolescents with ADHD have an earlier age at first sexual intercourse, more sexual partners, less use of birth control, more

TABLE 80.1

American Academy of Pediatrics Clinical Guidelines for Attention-Deficit Hyperactivity Disorder Diagnosis and Evaluation

In a child 6- to 12-years-old who presents with inattention, hyperactivity, impulsivity, academic underachievement, or behavior problems primary care clinicians should initiate an evaluation for ADHD

The diagnosis of ADHD requires that a child meet DSM-IV criteria

The assessment of ADHD requires evidence directly obtained from parents or caregivers regarding the core symptoms of ADHD in various settings, age at onset, duration of symptoms, and degree of functional impairment

The assessment of ADHD requires evidence directly obtained from the classroom teacher (or other school professional) regarding the core symptoms of ADHD, duration of symptoms, degree of functional impairment, and associated conditions

Evaluation of the child with ADHD should include assessment for associated (coexisting) conditions

Other diagnostic tests are not routinely indicated to establish the diagnosis of ADHD but may be used for the assessment of other coexisting conditions (e.g., learning disabilities and mental retardation)

ADHD, attention-deficit hyperactivity disorder; DSM-IV, *Diagnostic and Statistical Manual of Mental Disorders, fourth edition.*

sexually transmitted diseases, and more teen pregnancies that their non-ADHD peers.

9. *Sleep disorders:* Sleep disturbances are more common in children with ADHD.

Making a Diagnosis of ADHD: Clinical Guidelines

The American Academy of Pediatrics published evidence-based clinical guidelines for primary care evaluation and diagnosis of ADHD (see Table 80.1). A number of questionnaires and rating scales are available to assess behavioral characteristics. The practitioner should use at least one psychometrically sound parent, teacher, and adolescent self-report rating scale.

Examples of ADHD rating scales include the following:

1. *NICHQ Vanderbilt Parent and Teacher Scales:* These scales are included in the AAP toolkit and may be copied for use in the office or clinic. Screening questions for comorbid conditions and impairment measures are included.

2. *Conners' Rating Scales-Revised (CRS-R):* There are short and long versions of each of the parent, teacher, and adolescent self report scales. Conners' forms are normed for adolescents up to age 17. (Available from Multi-Health Systems, http://www.mhs.com/.)

3. *Brown ADD Scale for Adolescents:* The Brown ADD Scale for Adolescents (Brown, 1996) is a psychometrically sound adolescent self-report measure which can be administered either as a semistructured interview or as a written rating scale.

LEARNING DISABILITIES

Public schools define learning disabilities in accordance with the Individuals with Disabilities Education Act (IDEA). Specific learning disabilities consist of disorders in one or more of the basic psychological processes involved in understanding or in using language, spoken or written, which may manifest itself in an imperfect ability to listen, think, speak, read, write, spell, or do mathematical calculations.

Educators commonly summarize learning disabilities in terms of reading, mathematics, writing, and language disorders. They commonly interpret the presence of a significant discrepancy between actual and expected achievement for a given adolescent's intellectual ability as evidence of a learning disability. Practically, a discrepancy of two standard deviations between scores on an IQ test and scores on an achievement test is often presumptive evidence of a learning disability. Learning disabilities are also often suspected when a significant discrepancy exists between the verbal and performance scores on IQ testing.

A new model, "Response to Intervention," is evolving through educational practice and research. When a student exhibits difficulty with a basic learning process such as reading, the educator locates an evidence-based intervention and applies that intervention to remediate the student's difficulty. If the intervention is successful, it is continued in regular education and no learning disability is diagnosed. If the intervention is not successful, the student is considered to have a learning disability, and special education services are provided. The emphasis within this model is the prevention of later learning problems through the early identification and remediation of deficits using evidence-based interventions.

MANAGEMENT OF LEARNING AND ACHIEVEMENT PROBLEMS

Legal Responsibilities of the Public Schools

Children with disabilities are guaranteed a free and appropriate education by three federal laws:

1. *IDEA:* This special education act requires schools to conduct multidisciplinary evaluations for adolescents suspected of having a disability (including ADHD), and if the disability is confirmed, to provide special education interventions. These interventions are developed in team meetings that include parents and are described in Individualized Education Plans.
2. Section 504 of the Rehabilitation Act of 1973 is a civil rights law that outlaws discrimination against individuals with a disability in federally funded programs in education and the workplace. Schools are required to make reasonable accommodations to educate individuals with disabilities (including ADHD). Children suspected of having a disability must be evaluated, and if confirmed, reasonable accommodations are typically made first in regular education.
3. *Americans with Disabilities Act:* Extends the protections of Section 504 to college students, adults, and the private sector and, therefore, may apply to older adolescents who are working.

Accommodations

Failure to complete or hand in assignments on time is a major deficit of ADHD and learning-disabled teens. Some common accommodations for adolescents with ADHD include: Modifying lessons (e.g., breaking lessons into short segments); adjusting testing procedures (e.g., extended time to complete examinations); and weekly home or school progress reports to assist with task completion.

Special Education. A continuum of alternative placements for students certified as learning disabled or otherwise health impaired includes resource rooms, self-contained rooms, separate schools, residential placements, and even home-bound instruction. Placement is usually in the least restrictive environment to best prepare the disabled individual to live in society. Instructional procedures for reading, mathematics, and writing disabilities emphasize alternative teaching methods that help the learner bypass his or her area of disability.

MANAGEMENT OF ATTENTION DEFICIT HYPERACTIVITY DISORDER

Management of ADHD requires a comprehensive plan that allows the adolescent to participate in setting goals and developing strategies. Comorbid conditions, if present, should be considered in the treatment plan. Management of ADHD includes education, medication, home interventions, counseling, school interventions, and advocacy.

Education

Education about ADHD should be provided for the adolescent, for the parents and family, and for the school. The AAP clinical guidelines for ADHD treatment are in Table 80.2. Adolescents must know that there is hope for improved functional and academic performance.

Medication

Medication (Table 80.3) should not generally be the only treatment received by the adolescent, but it is frequently the cornerstone of treatment for ADHD. Because 75% to 90% of adolescents respond to medical therapy, a medication trial should be undertaken for almost all adolescents diagnosed with ADHD. Results from the large Multimodal Treatment Trial of ADHD (MTA) show that medication therapy was the single most effective intervention and intensive and closely monitored medical therapy was more effective than the usual provision of stimulant medications in the community (The MTA Cooperative Group, 1999).

The stimulants are the most effective of the available medication options and have an excellent record of safety. They have been shown to be effective in improving the core symptoms of ADHD. Long-acting medications are now available in a variety of formulations and are typically the first choice in the treatment of ADHD (see Table 80.3). Short-acting agents are no longer recommended as first-line treatment.

Concerns about cardiovascular risks associated with the use of stimulant medications prompted the requirement of a "black box warning." Significantly

TABLE 80.2

American Academy of Pediatrics Clinical Guidelines for Attention-Deficit Hyperactivity Disorder Treatment

Primary care clinicians should establish a treatment program that recognizes ADHD as a chronic condition

The treating clinician, parents, and child, in collaboration with school personnel, should specify appropriate target outcomes to guide management

The clinician should recommend stimulant medication and/or behavior therapy as appropriate to improve target outcomes in children with ADHD

When the selected management for a child with ADHD has not met target outcomes, clinicians should evaluate the original diagnosis, use of all appropriate treatments, adherence to the treatment plan, and presence of coexisting conditions

The clinician should periodically provide a systematic follow-up for the child with ADHD; monitoring should be directed to target outcomes and adverse effects, with information gathered from parents, teachers, and the child

ADHD, attention-deficit hyperactivity disorder.

increased risks have not been subsequently confirmed; nevertheless, careful screening of patients, including a family history, is essential to rule out the presence of cardiovascular disease or risk factors. Routine ECG screening is not currently recommended.

Intermediate-Release Methylphenidate (Ritalin-SR, Metadate-ER, Methylin-ER)

Immediate-release methylphenidate (Ritalin, Methylin, Focalin) is no longer a recommended first-line choice but is used as an adjunct to longer-acting medications. Sustained-release methylphenidate can be useful because its duration of action is about 4 to 8 hours and it can be given once or twice daily. Ritalin-SR, however, comes only in a 20-mg preparation and is often not as effective as the short-acting tablet. Although it is not commonly used as a single agent, it can be helpful for patients who require lower stimulant doses or those who experience too many "ups and downs" with the short-acting methylphenidate. A good strategy in these situations is to use both short-acting and intermediate-release methylphenidate together as one would use regular and long-acting insulin (e.g., sustained-release 20-mg plus 10- to 20-mg short-acting methylphenidate three times a day).

Timed-Release Methylphenidate Capsule (Concerta, Metadate-CD, Focalin XR, Ritalin LA), and the Methylphenidate patch (Daytrana patch)

Concerta consists of methylphenidate packaged in a medication delivery system similar to that used in the long-acting medications for hypertension and diabetes mellitus. Preliminary studies show good efficacy in the

TABLE 80.3

Stimulant Medications

Generic Name	Trade Name	Available Doses	Length of Action (hr)	Dose Range
Methylphenidate	Ritalin	5, 10, 20 mg	3–5	5–30 mg b.i.d.–t.i.d.
	Methylin	5, 10, 20 mg; 2.5, 5 mg chewable; 5 and 10 mg/5 mL	3–5	5–30 mg b.i.d.–t.i.d.
	Focalin	2.5, 5, 10 mg	3–5	2.5–10 mg b.i.d.
Intermediate-release methylphenidate	Ritalin-SR	20 mg	4–8	20 mg q.d.–b.i.d.
	Metadate-ER, Methylin-ER	10, 20 mg	4–8	10–20 mg q.d.–b.i.d.
Extended-release methylphenidate	Concerta	18, 27, 36, 54 mg	8–12	18–72 mg q.d.
	Metadate-CD	10, 20, 30, 40, 50, 60 mg	8–12	20–60 mg q.d.
	Focalin XR	5, 10, 20 mg	8–12	5–20 mg q.d.
	Ritalin-LA	20, 30, 40 mg	8–12	20–60 mg q.d.
Methylphenidate patch	Daytrana	10, 15, 20, 30 mg	Up to 12	10–30 mg q.d.
Dextroamphetamine tablets	Dexedrine	5 mg	3–4	5–20 mg b.i.d.–t.i.d.
Dextroamphetamine Spansules	Dexedrine, Dextrostat	5, 10, 15 mg	6–8	5–30 mg q.d.–b.i.d.
Amphetamine and dextroamphetamine	Adderall	5, 7.5, 10, 12.5, 15, 20, 30 mg	4–8	5–30 mg b.i.d.–t.i.d.
	Adderall XR	5, 10, 15, 20, 25, 30 mg	10–12	20–60 mg q.d.

treatment of ADHD and most patients do not need a dose during school hours. Concerta is available in 18-, 27-, 36-, and 54-mg capsules, with most patients requiring 36 to 72 mg per dose.

Metadate-CD® consists of beads of methylphenidate with two different release patterns; 30% of the beads are immediately released and absorbed, while the other 70% are released slowly over 8 to 12 hours. Doses of 20 to 60 mg per day in the morning are usually required.

Focalin XR provides an extended release form of D-methylphenidate. It comes in doses of 5, 10, and 20 mg and appears to be effective up to 12 hours.

Ritalin-LA consists of methylphenidate beads in a 1:1 ratio of immediate- and slow-release forms. Half of the dose is released immediately and the rest is released approximately 4 hours later to provide 8 hours of medication effect. Morning doses of 20 to 60 mg are used.

Daytrana, a methylphenidate sustained action transdermal system, is now available. It offers steady-state dosing and variable duration of action with effects continuing for 2 to 3 hours after removing the patch. Skin reactions may occur but are usually mild. It is very difficult to elute the methylphenidate from the patch for purposes of abuse.

Amphetamine and Dextroamphetamine

Dextroamphetamine (Dexedrine Spansules) is an effective long-acting preparation and is also tolerated quite well. It comes in 5-, 10-, and 15-mg Spansules. The duration of action is usually about 8 hours, so it is generally given before and after school with usual doses of 10 to 20 mg twice daily, up to 30 mg twice daily.

Combination Dextroamphetamine and Amphetamine (Adderall and Adderall XR). This is another stimulant for consideration and there is good evidence of its effectiveness and tolerability. Long-acting Adderall XR is effective for 10 to 12 hours with a single morning dose of 10 to 40 mg. Shorter-acting Adderall can be used as an adjunct to Adderall XR. Commonly used doses are 10 to 20 mg two or three times a day, with some patients requiring up to 30 or 40 mg per dose.

Atomoxetine (Strattera) is a nonstimulant selective norepinephrine reuptake inhibitor and is the only medication approved for the treatment of ADHD in adults. The starting dose is 0.5 mg/kg body weight, which may be increased to 1.2 mg/kg/day after 3 to 7 days. The maximum daily dose is 1.4 mg/kg/day or 100 mg/day, whichever is lower. Common side effects include stomach upset, decreased appetite, nausea or vomiting, fatigue, dizziness, mild increase in pulse and blood pressure, and growth delay. There have been several reports of (apparently reversible) severe liver injury associated with atomoxetine use. A recent analysis showed an increased risk of suicidal thinking in children and adolescents during the first few months of treatment with atomoxetine, leading to a black-box FDA warning for this medication. However, the absolute risk of suicidal thinking is quite low.

Antidepressants

Tricyclic antidepressants may be the medication of choice for patients who do not tolerate stimulants. Imipramine (Tofranil) and desipramine (Norpramin) have been used successfully. Electrocardiogram monitoring should be done initially and periodically to look for adverse cardiac effects. The daily dose of imipramine and desipramine is approximately 3 to 5 mg/kg of body weight.

The antidepressant *bupropion (Wellbutrin)* has been shown to be effective for inattention and impulsivity in children and may be beneficial in some adolescents with ADHD, especially those with comorbid depression or anxiety. It is available in sustained-release (Wellbutrin SR) and an extended-release (Wellbutrin XL) formulations at doses of 100 mg to 150 mg twice daily for Wellbutrin SR and 150 to 300 mg daily for Wellbutrin XL. It is contraindicated in patients with seizures or eating disorders. Common side effects include nausea, anorexia, agitation, restlessness, drowsiness, and headaches.

Clonidine (Catapres) is a central-acting alpha$_2$-agonist that has been shown to have limited effectiveness in the treatment of ADHD. However, it can be useful in patients with comorbid conditions such as sleep disturbances, tic disorders, or severe aggressiveness. Clonidine comes in tablets of 0.1, 0.2, and 0.3 mg as well as skin patches of similar strengths. The tablets are taken two to four times a day (or at night only for insomnia) starting with 0.05 mg and then increasing by 0.05 mg/day every 7 days. The maximum daily dose is 0.3 mg/day. The patch is effective for 3 to 7 days. Some experts recommend obtaining a baseline electrocardiogram and blood glucose before starting clonidine. Compliance must be carefully monitored since missed doses or abrupt discontinuation of Clonidine can precipitate hypertensive crisis, even in those with no history of hypertension.

Behavioral or Psychological Interventions

In the large MTA study, a comprehensive behavioral intervention alone was compared with medication alone, a combination of behavioral intervention and medication, and standard community care (MTA Cooperative Group, 1999). Medication was generally found to be more effective in reducing ADHD symptoms than behavioral intervention, and there were few differences between the combined treatment and medication alone in effectively managing ADHD symptoms. However, when it came to other domains of functioning, such as oppositional/aggressive symptoms, internalizing symptoms, teacher-rated social skills, parent-child relations, and reading achievement, there was evidence that the combined treatment was superior to community care, while medication alone was not. In interpreting these results, the health care provider must keep in mind that the study was limited to school-age children, not adolescents.

It is often useful for families with adolescents who are newly diagnosed with ADHD to have a burst of 10 to 15 sessions of behavioral or psychological intervention followed by less frequent checkups. If new problems surface during a follow-up checkup, another burst of therapy may be scheduled. Individual therapy is usually helpful in building self-esteem and reducing anxiety but does not reliably result in behavioral changes in the classroom or at home. Behavioral family system therapy is the treatment of choice for the home-based problems and conflicts between teenagers with ADHD and their parents. External authorities such as the juvenile justice system or mental health inpatient system are used to back up parents when they no longer have the ability to exert any control over the adolescents.

WEB SITES AND REFERENCES

For Teens and Parents
http://www.chadd.org. Official Web site for the support group Children and Adults with ADHD.

http://www.nichq.org/nichq/topics/chronicconditions/ADHD/ADHDhomepage.htm National Initiative for Children's Healthcare Quality (NICHQ) Web site, with link to the ADHD Toolkit.

American Academy of Pediatrics. Clinical practice guideline: diagnosis and evaluation of the child with attention-deficit/hyperactivity disorder. *Pediatrics* 2000; 105:1158.

American Academy of Pediatrics. Clinical practice guideline: Treatment of the school-aged child with attention-deficit/hyperactivity disorder. *Pediatrics* 2001; 108:1033.

American Psychiatric Association. *The diagnostic and statistical manual of mental disorders, text revision,* 4th ed. Washington, DC: American Psychiatric Association, 2000.

Brown RT, Amler RW, Freeman WS, et al. American Academy of Pediatrics Committee on Quality Improvement. American Academy of Pediatrics Subcommittee on Attention-Deficit/Hyperactivity Disorder. Treatment of attention-deficit/hyperactivity disorder: overview of the evidence. *Pediatrics* 2005;115(6):e749.

Brown, TE. *Brown Attention-Deficit Disorder Scales Manual.* San Antonio, TX: The Psychological Corporation, 1996.

The MTA Cooperative Group. A 14-month randomized clinical trial of treatment strategies for attention deficit/hyperactivity disorder. *Arch Gen Psychiatry* 1999; 56:1088.

Robin AL. *ADHD in adolescents: diagnosis and treatment.* New York: Guilford Press, 1998b.

U. S. Food and Drug Administration, Center for Drug Evaluation and Research. (September 29, 2005). *FDA Alert [9/05]: suicidal thinking in children and adolescents* (Alert posted on the World Wide Web). Washington, DC. Retrieved November 1, 2005 from the World Wide Web: http://www.fda.gov/cder/drug/infosheets/hcp/atomoxetinehcp.htm.

Wolraich ML, Wibbelsman CJ, Brown TE, et al. Attention-deficit/hyperactivity disorder among adolescents: a review of the diagnosis, treatment, and clinical implications. *Pediatrics* 2005;115(6):1734.

CHAPTER 81

Sexual Assault and Victimization

Vaughn I. Rickert, Owen Ryan, and Mariam Chacko

The terms used to describe the range of victimizations included in sexual assault are sometimes used interchangeably and some have legal ramifications and reporting requirements. They are as follows:

Sexual Assault. Any act, either physical or verbal, of a sexual nature committed against another person that is accompanied by actual or threatened physical force.

Rape. Nonconsensual sex segmented into two categories: those acts perpetrated by a stranger and those perpetrated by an acquaintance. *Date rape*, nonconsensual sex that occurs between two people in a romantic relationship, is a subset of acquaintance rape. *Rape* is largely a legal term.

Sexual Abuse. Usually refers to the sexual victimization of a minor. In certain contexts, the term can include consensual sex between minors or a minor and an adult (*statutory rape*). Occasionally, the terms *incest* and *intrafamilial sex* become confused with *sexual abuse*. *Sexual abuse*, as with *rape*, is also primarily a legal term.

Female adolescents and young adults 16 to 24 years of age are four times more likely to be sexually assaulted than women in all other age groups; in most instances, the perpetrator is a date or an acquaintance. Male adolescent victimization is underreported, but some studies show a similar frequency of perpetration from individuals known to them. Unfortunately, prevalence of victimization among adolescents and young adults in same-gender relationships is unknown.

Disclosure of sexual assault and victimization requires prompt medical and psychological intervention, but this is rarely forthcoming. Forensic evidence should be collected only by providers willing to devote the time and support needed.

Provider-initiated screening to detect sexual victimization is an important public health strategy to overcome the difficulty that some victims face in disclosing these violent events.

Sexual Assault

1. *Risk factors:* Females (age 16 to 19 years and 20 to 24 years); a history of abuse (sexual or other) as a child or adolescent; for females, younger age of menarche, greater number of dating and/or sexual partners, and a sexually active peer group; for males, homelessness and disability (physical, cognitive, psychiatric); alcohol use by perpetrator or victim, especially in a dating situation; dating relationships that include verbal or physical abuse.
2. *Epidemiology*
   a. Some 11.9% of females and 6.1% of males report that they have had forced sexual intercourse.
   b. About 1 in 12 children and youth (82 per 1,000) aged 2 to 17 years have experienced ≥ 1 sexual victimization during their lives; 32 per 1,000 have experienced a sexual assault; and 22 per 1,000 have experienced a completed or attempted rape.
   c. Adults are responsible for a minority of victimizations (15% of general sexual victimizations and 29% of sexual assault).
   d. Two thirds of sexual assault victimizations reported to the police involve juvenile victims.
   e. Some 17.6% of women stated they had been the victims of a completed or attempted rape at some time in their lives. Of those with a history of rape, 21.6% were below 12 years of age when they were first raped, 32.4% were between the ages of 12 and 17.
   f. Adolescents ≤ 18 years who experience sexual victimization are twice as likely to experience a future assault during their college years.
   g. About 60% of sexual assaults occur at home or at the home of an acquaintance.
   h. The incidence of reported rapes is higher during the summer months and on weekends, and about two thirds of sexual assaults occur between 6 P.M. and 6 A.M. Data suggest an increased vulnerability for adolescents and young adults immediately after school (3 P.M.) and later at night (between 11 P.M. and midnight).
   i. Forceful verbal and physical resistance and fleeing were associated with rape avoidance, and injury rates were no higher in women who used forceful resistance.
3. *Sequelae:* Victimized adolescents experience significantly higher levels of depression and anxiety. Male and female high school–aged victims report decreased life satisfaction coupled with suicidal ideation and attempts. Typically, sexually victimized youth engage in higher-risk sexual behaviors, have poorer attitudes and beliefs regarding sex, and demonstrate a greater prevalence of consequences from sexual activity (i.e., unintended pregnancies and STDs). Several common responses to victimization include phobias, somatic reactions, self-blame, loss of appetite, sleep disturbance, and somatic responses. Sequelae particular to date rape may include self-blame, decreased self-esteem, and a difficult time maintaining relationships. Somatic responses can manifest as chronic pelvic pain or recurrent abdominal pain. The first 2-month period following victimization is a time of particular vulnerability for severe depression.

Sexual Abuse

1. *Incidence:* Unlike other types of child victimization that have seen recent declines, child sexual abuse has remained constant at 1.2 children per every

1,000, with girls being three times as likely as boys to be sexually abused; that vulnerability to sexual abuse has remained consistent after age 3. Adolescents and young adults are most vulnerable to sexual abuse at the hands of those closest to them, with 69% of perpetrators having been a parent, a relative, or a partner to the parent.

2. Situations that should alert the provider to suspect abuse:
   - STD infection in a prepubertal adolescent or teen with no history of sexual intercourse.
   - Recurrent somatic complaints, particularly involving the GI, GU, or pelvic areas.
   - *Behavioral indicators include:* (a) significant change in mood (withdrawal from usual family, school, and social activities); (b) patterns of disordered eating; (c) running away from home; (d) suicidal and self-injurious gestures; (e) rapid escalation of alcohol and/or drug abuse; (f) onset of promiscuous sexual activity; (g) early adolescent pregnancy; (h) onset of sexual activity before age 13 years; (i) sexualized play in the prepubescent child.

3. *Sequelae:* The occurrence of sexual abuse during childhood has been linked to a variety of psychological and emotional problems during adolescence, with some continuing into adulthood. Sequelae include depression, suicidal ideation and attempts, substance abuse, posttraumatic stress disorder, eating disorders, and precocious sexual behaviors (e.g., earlier age at first coitus and greater number of lifetime partners). The relationship between severity/frequency of abuse and mental health disorders remains elusive.

DISCLOSURE AND REPORTING

1. *Screening:* Several useful screening measures that can be easily employed by a clinician and take <15 minutes to complete: Conflict in Adolescent Relationship Inventory, Sexual Experience Survey, the Date and Family Violence and Abuse Scale, or the Sexual Aggression Questionnaire. This examination should take place in a private, quiet space. The concept of limited confidentiality should be introduced to the patient, conveying the legal obligations should any disclosure occur. Following this, a sexual history is important, including sexual partners and experience, any unwanted touch, or previous victimization. If the patient discloses that injuries were sustained, a thorough exam, consented to by the patient, will be required. The adolescent will need to know and consent to the specific purpose and procedures involved in the examination, including the stages of a rape kit. For those who have experienced a recent victimization or are seeking treatment because of assault, the presence of a family member or friend may be important during the exam.

2. *Reporting:* The following professional guidelines have been endorsed:
   - Sexual activity and sexual abuse are not synonymous. It should not be assumed that adolescents who are sexually active are by definition being abused.
   - It is critical that adolescents who are sexually active receive appropriate confidential health care and counseling.
   - Open and confidential communication between the provider and teen, together with careful clinical assessment, can identify the majority of sexual abuse cases.
   - Providers must know their state laws and report cases of sexual abuse to the proper authority after discussion with the adolescent and parent as appropriate.

- Federal and state laws should support physicians and other health care professionals and their role in providing confidential health care to their adolescent patients.
- Federal and state laws should affirm the authority of physicians and other health care professionals to exercise appropriate clinical judgment in reporting cases of sexual activity.

LEGAL ISSUES RELATED TO REPORTING OF SEXUAL ASSAULT AND VICTIMIZATION

Every state has mandatory reporting of a reasonable suspicion of child abuse, including sexual abuse, to a designated authority. Mandated reporters of child abuse include virtually all medical and health professionals involved in the care of adolescents. The abuse does not need to be proven before being reported, and failure to report can result in civil or criminal penalties.

Many states have attempted to increase the reporting of sexually active minors under child abuse reporting laws, either through legislative and policy changes or enforcement of existing laws. These efforts have focused particular attention on younger adolescents who are sexually active. An area of particular confusion is the reporting of statutory rape, defined as consenting sexual contact between two minors or one minor and an adult. The impact of implementing these measures is yet unknown. It is essential that a practitioner consult their local legal and medical authorities regarding laws for their state and be aware of their institution policies as it relates to the screening and reporting of child abuse, sexual abuse, sexual victimization, and violence.

MEDICAL AND FORENSIC ASPECTS OF THE EVALUATION OF SEXUAL ABUSE AND ASSAULT IN ADOLESCENTS

Medical Evaluation

Facilitating an Appropriate Medical Examination with Forensic Procedures

Physicians and nurses have an obligation to provide care to victims; this involves being able to provide a legal defense in all cases including those in which a rape kit may or may not have been completed and as a supportive care provider.

Individual jurisdictions determine the maximum time interval (36 hours to 1 week) in which evidence may be collected. Changing clothes, showering, and brushing teeth can change the yield of the forensic examination. If the adolescent declines a forensic examination, a speculum examination should not be undertaken to obtain STD tests until after 96 hours; a speculum examination conducted prior to forensic work will call into question the accuracy of evidence that may later be collected.

Important Points

- Magnification aids and photography are not absolutely necessary but can be useful in the evaluation and documentation of genital trauma.

- A classification system has been included to assist clinicians in the interpretation of physical and laboratory findings and to provide an opinion as to the likelihood of sexual abuse or assault in children and adolescents (Table 81.1).
- If a rape kit is being completed, consent needs to be obtained from the adolescent for the forensic examination, treatment, collection of evidence, and release of medical records.
- A brief description of the incident, including body parts touched, orifices penetrated, the geographic location of the assault, identity of the assailant or alleged perpetrator (if known), whether a condom was used, whether any bleeding was noted from contact sites at the time of the abuse or assault, and the way in which the assailant left the scene.
- Whether a weapon was used and any injuries sustained at the time of attack
- Whether any illicit drugs or alcohol were used to render the victim helpless
- Date of last menses and use of sanitary pads and/or tampons
- Date and time of last voluntary coitus, other recent sexual experiences
- History of previous STDs
- History of prior pregnancy
- Use of contraception
- Any significant actions after alleged assault, such as showering or douching, rinsing of mouth and brushing of teeth

Physical Examination

- Prior to examining the patient, the medical provider should provide a step-by-step explanation of what he or she will be doing and why.
- Reassure the patient that he or she will be in control.
- Keep personal contact with the patient, both through verbal and eye contact.
- Proceed slowly, allowing the patient to relax.
- During the examination, comment on unremarkable or normal findings. It is crucial to convey a sense of normalcy where appropriate. When physical findings are remarkable and injury is present, the medical provider should stress that these injuries are not the patient's fault.
- The examination must include a thorough physical examination for bruises and healing abrasions followed by a genital examination for evidence of trauma and collection of specimens for STDs.

General Physical Findings

- General appearance, emotional state, and behavior should be recorded.
- Condition of patient's clothing should be observed and documented.
- All areas of the body should be explored for signs of trauma, especially the neck and upper arms, where bruises resulting from forced restraint appear.
- Examine the throat.
- Check for abdominal crepitus.

Genital, Pelvic, and Rectal Examination

- *Position:* An exam on an adolescent girl is performed in the lithotomy position. A very young or petite girl or boy can be examined in the knee-chest position for easier visualization of the anogenital area. The anal area in the larger and older male adolescent should be visualized with the adolescent lying in the lateral position and with one or both knees flexed.

TABLE 81.1

Findings Diagnostic of Trauma and/or Sexual Contact[a]

1. Moderate specificity for abuse
   a. Acute lacerations or extensive bruising of labia, perihymenal tissues, penis, scrotum, or perineum (may be from unwitnessed accidental trauma).
   b. Scar of posterior fourchette (discrete, pale, off the midline). Scars are very difficult to assess unless acute injury at same location was documented.
   c. Fresh laceration of the posterior fourchette, not involving the hymen (must be differentiated from dehisced labial adhesion or failure of midline fusion, or may be caused by accidental injury).
   d. Perianal scar. Discrete, pale, off the midline (rare, difficult to assess unless acute injury at the same location was previously documented; may be due to other medical conditions such as Crohn disease, or previous medical procedures).
2. High specificity for abuse (diagnostic of blunt force penetrating trauma)
   a. Laceration (tear, partial or complete) of the hymen, acute.
   b. Ecchymosis (bruising) on the hymen.
   c. Perianal lacerations extending deep to the external anal sphincter (not to be confused with partial failure of midline fusion).
   d. Hymenal transection (healed). An area where the hymen has been torn through, to or nearly to the base, so there appears to be virtually no hymenal tissue remaining at that location, confirmed using additional examination techniques such as a swab, prone knee-chest position, Foley catheter, water to float the edge of the hymen. This finding has also been referred to as a *complete cleft* in sexually active adolescents and young women.
3. Presence of infection confirms mucosal contact with infected genital secretions; contact most likely to have been sexual in nature
   a. Positive confirmed culture for gonorrhea, from genital area, anus, and throat, in a child outside the neonatal period.
   b. Confirmed diagnosis of syphilis, if perinatal transmission is ruled out.
   c. *Trichomonas vaginalis* infection in a child older than 1 year, with organisms identified (by an experienced technician or clinician) in vaginal secretions by wet mount examination or by culture.
   d. Positive culture from genital or anal tissues for *Chlamydia*. If child is older than 3 years at time of diagnosis, and specimen was tested using cell culture or comparable method approved by the Centers for Disease Control and Prevention. Positive serology for HIV, if neonatal transmission and transmission from blood products has been ruled out.
4. Diagnostic of sexual contact
   a. Pregnancy.
   b. Sperm identified in specimens taken directly from a child's body.

HIV, human immunodeficiency virus.

[a]Findings which in the absence of a clear, timely, plausible history of accidental injury or nonsexual transmission should be reported to child protective services.

Adapted from Adam J, Medical evaluation of suspected sexual abuse. *J Pediatr Adolesc Gynecol* 2004;17:191 (with permission).

- *External genitalia:* Note and record signs of blood secretions and sites of bruising, hematoma, ecchymoses, abrasions, lacerations, and redness and swelling in the external genitalia, including the hymen.
- *Hymen:* The hymen can be observed by using a cotton applicator swab moistened with water or by using a Foley catheter balloon to visualize the edges of the hymen. When manually visualizing the hymen, gently stretch the hymen all around to clearly define any partial or complete fresh hymenal tears and the amount of hymenal tissue present, especially at the 6 o'clock position of the posterior rim, where acute hymenal tears are more likely to be found. Spread apart any areas that appear to be notches or clefts with the swab to define the depth of the notch or cleft. Remember the absence of notches does not rule out previous penetration; therefore, the term *intact* hymen should be avoided.
- *Anus:* The perianal and anal area must be inspected carefully for scars, fissures, sphincter tears, evidence of chronic fissuring, distortion of the anus, skin tags, and localized venous engorgement. Recurrent anal penetration must be suspected when the skin around the anal opening is smooth and thickened and the external sphincter has lost tone and does not contract readily. Loss of tone is assessed by presence of a relaxed external anal sphincter almost to the point of gaping, along with loss of puckering of the mucous membrane. Location of anal findings using the face of a clock must be documented.
- *Internal examination:* An internal pelvic and rectal examination must be performed if there is pain, bleeding, a history of vaginal or rectal penetration, or signs of injury. Physicians should avoid further trauma to these areas by using a warm water-lubricated speculum (small-sized is preferred for peripubertal teens). General anesthesia may be indicated. An anoscopy or a proctoscopy is recommended when internal trauma and pathology (warts) is suspected. Internal trauma should be suspected when rectal bleeding, fever, or signs of an acute abdomen are present.

Collection of Specimens—Rape Kit

- The provider first sees an instruction sheet, a consent form, and numerous sexual assault forensic examination forms. The rape kit also contains a paper sheet, envelopes, slides, and swabs.
- The collection of legally mandated tests for the rape kit must be synchronized with the general physical examination, pelvic examination, and hospital laboratory tests. Remember that the patient's permission is required for photographs of areas of trauma.
- Legally mandated tests for evidence collection may include foreign hair collection, clothing, blood from victim for typing, filter paper disk with saliva from victim, and swabs from perianal area, anal verge, and rectal canal for presence of acid phosphatase. Appropriate specimens for DNA testing should be obtained. The "chain of evidence" must be maintained in collecting forensic specimens by strictly following rape kit protocols; otherwise the evidence will not be of value in criminal prosecution.
- Treatment for significant trauma should precede collection of medicolegal information.
- The Wood's lamp has been shown to be unreliable in screening for the presence of semen, but it may be helpful in identifying foreign debris.

- Evidence for the kit is collected and handed over to a police officer according to legal procedure, with associated specimen analysis cost covered the police.

Hospital Laboratory Tests

- *Cultures:* Gonorrhea cultures should be obtained from the endocervix, rectum, and pharynx. Chlamydial cultures should be obtained from the endocervix and rectum. Noncultural techniques (i.e., FDA-approved nucleic acid amplification tests) should not be used because they have inadequate specificity for criminal prosecution.
- Gram stain of any urethral or anal discharge should be obtained. A Gram stain from the cervix or vagina is not useful.
- If genital ulcers or vesicles suspicious for herpes genitalis are present, a viral culture from the lesions should be sent for herpes simplex virus.
- Wet mount of vaginal secretions should be prepared and examined for evidence of *Trichomonas* and bacterial vaginosis. If sperm are identified, the laboratory technician validates these findings with the examiner and/or a senior pathologist.
- Serum sample for the Reactive Protein Reagin or Venereal Disease Research Laboratory test should be obtained as a baseline test and repeated within 6 to 8 weeks for syphilis.
- Serum sample for hepatitis B surface antigen and antibody should be obtained.
- Discuss possible testing for HIV and provide appropriate pretest counseling. If testing is desired, a serum sample should be obtained and repeated at 6 weeks, 3 months, and 6 months.

Treatment

Clinicians must be sensitive to the likelihood of gastrointestinal side effects from multiple oral medications dispensed or prescribed following a sexual assault evaluation. In this event, treatment should begin with emergency contraception and intramuscular medication for gonorrhea. Medications for other common STDs can begin after the emergency contraception regimen is completed.

- Tetanus toxoid, 0.5 mL intramuscularly (plus tetanus immune globulin if there is a dirty wound) is indicated for severe or penetrating trauma.
- *STD prophylaxis:* Many specialists recommend routine preventive therapy after a sexual assault. Prophylactic treatment for chlamydial infection, gonorrhea, trichomoniasis, and bacterial vaginosis may be provided: Ceftriaxone 125 mg IM in a single dose *plus* metronidazole 2 g orally in a single dose *plus* azithromycin 1 g orally in a single dose or doxycycline 100 mg orally twice a day for 7 days.
- *Hepatitis B infection:* Empiric treatment for hepatitis B with hepatitis B immune globulin (HBIG) following sexual assault is controversial. Its efficacy in adolescents who are already immunized against hepatitis B infection is unknown. The Centers for Disease Control (CDC) recommend postexposure hepatitis B vaccine without HBIG as adequate protection against hepatitis B infection.
- *HIV postexposure prophylaxis (PEP):* It is difficult to discuss PEP issues in the acutely traumatized victim. See Chapter 31 for additional information.

- *Prevention of pregnancy:* Emergency contraception may be provided without speculum examination.
- Sleep aids should be given in small quantities.
- *Medical follow-up:* An appointment with a physician should be scheduled as indicated or within 14 to 21 days after the assault, especially in adolescents with penetration and penetrative injuries. A third visit may be scheduled at 8 to 12 weeks to repeat initial serologic studies, including tests for syphilis, hepatitis B, or HIV. The adolescent should be followed and evaluated for psychological symptoms (i.e., posttraumatic stress disorder, depression). Health care providers should determine the appropriate supports and treatment required.
- *Psychological supports:* Advocates, law enforcement representatives, and other responders can coordinate with the provider to discuss a range of issues prior to discharge from the emergency center. In many cities, rape crisis centers will send a supportive individual to the emergency department if notified. The adolescent victim should ideally see a social worker or counselor trained in this area of work prior to and after the medicolegal evaluation.
- Areas to explore with the adolescent during the initial examination and follow-up:
  a. Feelings during the assault, medical examination, and legal process; feelings regarding perpetrator, family, peers, school, and job.
  b. Concerns regarding physical health, emotional reactions, sexuality, and unusual behaviors.
  c. Willingness to receive crisis intervention services (from professionals, paraprofessionals, peers, religious, and other possible resources).
  d. Issues around safety should be reviewed and patient should be released to a caring friend or family member. Eligibility for protection orders and/or enhanced security measures should be assessed. Telephone numbers of rape hotlines or crisis centers should be provided as well.
  e. A follow-up appointment should be scheduled with a counselor.
- *Written materials:* Written materials regarding victims' rights, the rape experience, reporting rape, feelings about rape, and special reactions (the teenage victim, male victim, and the disabled victim) should be given to the victim before leaving the hospital.

WEB SITES AND REFERENCES

http://www.cdc.gov/ncipc/factsheets/svfacts.htm. CDC Sexual Violence Fact Sheet.

http://www.ncjrs.org/pdffiles1/ovw/206554.pdf. A National Protocol on the Sexual Assault Medical Forensic Examinations, Adults/Adolescents, 2004.

Adams JA. Medical evaluation of suspected child sexual abuse. *J Pediatr Adolesc Gynecol* 2004;17:191.

American Academy of Pediatrics, Committee on Adolescence. Care of the adolescent sexual assault victim. *Pediatrics* 2001;107:1476.

Society for Adolescent Medicine. Protecting adolescents: Ensuring access to care and reporting of sexual activity and abuse. *J Adolesc Health* 2004;35:420.

CHAPTER 82

Chronic Illness in the Adolescent

Susan M. Coupey

With the extraordinary technologic advances in medicine of recent decades, the prevalence of chronic conditions in adolescents has increased dramatically. Developmental, psychosocial, and family factors all feature prominently in the ongoing care of adolescents with chronic conditions.

Definition and Prevalence. In 2001, the Maternal and Child Health Bureau of the National Institutes of Health (NIH) conducted the National Survey of Children with Special Health Care Needs, defining these children as "...those who have or are at increased risk for a chronic physical, developmental, behavioral, or emotional condition and who also require health and related services of a type or amount beyond that required by children generally." This survey found that 12.8% of children under age 18 or about 9.4 million children in the United States had special health care needs, as do 15.8% of adolescents aged 12 through 17. Asthma and other chronic respiratory tract conditions and musculoskeletal disorders account for most of the physical disabilities (Table 82.1). Mental health disorders also are a leading cause of disability.

Interaction of Adolescent Development and Chronic Illness. Early adolescence is a period of accelerated physical growth and pubertal development; in middle and later adolescence, acceleration in cognitive and psychosocial development predominates. The interaction of chronic illness with these different developmental streams is complex and bidirectional; the illness may affect the development and/or the development may affect the illness. For example, some chronic diseases, such as cystic fibrosis or sickle cell disease, can cause delayed puberty; but for other chronic diseases, such as diabetes mellitus, normal puberty can cause exacerbation of the disease. Disabling chronic conditions may impede normal peer interaction. Conversely, features of normal psychosocial development, such as increasing independence from parents or increased risk taking, can lead to poor medication adherence and exacerbation of illnesses such as asthma or chronic renal disease.

Specific psychosocial areas, notably achieving independence and family relationships, have been found to be most vulnerable to dysfunction in adolescents with chronic health conditions. Most studies indicate that the presence of a chronic physical illness, even with its attendant problems and stresses, does not necessarily lead to emotional dysfunction. Adolescents with a chronic

TABLE 82.1

Prevalence of Selected Chronic Conditions in
Adolescents Aged 10–17 Years

Condition	Cases per 1,000 U.S. Adolescents
Impairments	
Musculoskeletal impairments	20.9
Speech defects	18.9
Deafness and hearing loss	17.0
Blindness and visual impairments	16.0
Diseases	
Asthma	46.8
Heart disease	17.4
Arthritis	8.7
Epilepsy and seizures	3.3
Diabetes mellitus	1.5
Sickle cell disease	0.9

From Westbrook LE, Stein RE. Epidemiology of chronic health conditions in adolescents. *Adolesc Med* 1994;5:197–209, with permission. Based on Newacheck PW, McManus MA, Fox HB. Prevalence and impact of chronic illness among adolescents. *Am J Dis Child* 1991;145:1367–1373.

condition who are also disabled, however, are at increased risk for psychosocial and emotional dysfunction.

Another approach is to evaluate the cumulative risk and protective factors borne by each adolescent and to view chronic physical illness as one of several important risk factors for psychosocial and emotional dysfunction. Risk factors other than chronic illness include male sex, severe family discord, and low socioeconomic status. Protective factors include positive temperament, above average intelligence, and family closeness. Using this approach, clinicians can target adolescents with multiple risk factors, in addition to the chronic illness, for enhanced intervention to prevent dysfunction.

Specific Developmental Risks

Independence/Dependence. Because chronic illness may prolong dependence on parents and others, including physicians, the adolescent may become compliant and child-like or noncompliant and rebellious.

Body Image. Delayed puberty or visible markers of the illness may contribute to poor self-image. Body image concerns may lead to poor self-esteem, increased anxiety over sexual function and relations, and eating disorders.

Peer Group. Chronically ill adolescents may experience real or imagined rejection by peers. These problems may lead to social isolation and a fear of peer involvement.

Identity. The adolescent with a chronic illness often has difficulties consolidating a mature identity. Concerns with future vocation, financial resources, separation from parents, marriage, and reproduction may all lead to identity problems.

Modifying Factors

Age at Onset. The stage of development during which the chronic illness appears may have considerable bearing on the psychological impact of the illness. Chronic illness or disability that originates early in life may lead to lowered parental expectations of the adolescent's potential and, in turn, reduced self-expectations by the teen. Chronic illness diagnosed in early adolescence may be particularly likely to provoke deep concerns about body integrity and body image. Such concerns can set the stage for dysfunctional coping; if these issues are not resolved, eating disorders may develop later on. Middle adolescence may be the most devastating time for a chronic illness to strike. During this phase, the adolescent is intensely involved with separation, peers, and sexual development. Poor adherence to medical therapy is a frequent problem during this period, as is depression, sexual acting out, and substance use. Chronic illness with an onset in late adolescence usually causes less upheaval. Concerns are focused on how the disease may disrupt vocational and educational plans, romantic and other relationships, parenthood, and the prospects for living independently.

Characteristics of the Illness. These include duration and course; limitation of age-appropriate activities; visibility of the condition; expected survival; mobility; physiologic functioning; cognitive, emotional, and social functioning; and impairment of communication. For example, a highly visible disease such as psoriasis may cause more emotional disruption than a life-threatening malignancy such as lymphoma. However, as is true for all of these dimensions, there is a complex relationship between visible deformities and adjustment. An exacerbating and remitting course of illness with the accompanying uncertainty and lack of control over when the symptoms will strike seems more likely to be associated with emotional problems.

Coping with Chronic Illness

To cope with chronic illness, the adolescent usually adopts various coping mechanisms that may include insightful acceptance, denial, regression, projection, displacement, acting out, compensation, and/or intellectualization. Over time, the adolescent with a chronic illness or disability likely uses many coping mechanisms, often using different mechanisms to cope with different situations. Many adolescents cope amazingly well with a multitude of stressors and are able to use these situations as emotional growth experiences, especially those who come from psychologically healthy and supportive families. For those adolescents who cannot consistently meet the challenges of chronic illness, breakdown of coping may be manifest behaviorally by poor adherence to treatment recommendations, increased risk-taking behaviors, withdrawal from developmental tasks, or symptoms of depression.

Risk Behaviors. Risk taking, particularly in the areas of sexuality and substance use, contributes substantially to morbidity in healthy adolescents. Risk taking in the setting of chronic illness, however, often has more negative health consequences.

Sexuality. For adolescents with a chronic illness, the health risks of sexual activity may be exacerbated by the illness itself, the medications used to treat it, or a maladaptive emotional response to illness.

1. *Prevalence of sexual activity:* Some physically disabled teens are as sexually active as their nondisabled peers. However, onset of sexual activity may be delayed for adolescents with illnesses that delay puberty, with mobility limitations, and with brain-based conditions that result in fewer opportunities for peer interaction. Sexual assault also is a salient issue, particularly for cognitively impaired adolescent girls, who are uniquely vulnerable to exploitation.
2. *Fertility:* Most chronic illnesses do not impair fertility, and particularly for sexually active girls, effective contraception is extremely important (Table 82.2). Girls with chronic illness should be counseled about the necessity of carefully planning pregnancies so as to minimize teratogenicity from medications and treatments and to ensure the best outcome for both mother and fetus.
3. *Sexually transmitted diseases:* Girls who are immunosuppressed either from their disease (e.g., HIV) or its treatment (e.g., organ transplant) are at risk for a prolonged and more complicated course if infected with a sexually transmitted disease. Genital infection with human papillomavirus (HPV) is particularly virulent in girls who are immunocompromised, and they are also at increased risk of developing cervical cancer.

Substance Use
Substance use by adolescents with chronic illness can contribute significantly to morbidity and mortality.

Prevalence of Substance Use. One study found that fewer teens with cystic fibrosis versus matched controls smoked regularly (2.6% versus 29.6%), were binge drinkers (18.0% versus 35.3%), or had tried marijuana (9.7% versus 29.4%), respectively. Although the proportion of adolescents with chronic illness using substances may be less than that of their healthy peers, the absolute numbers are still quite high and the risk for health complications are greater.

Management of Chronic Illness in the Adolescent
Optimal care of the adolescent's medical condition is of primary importance. However, high-quality treatment often cannot be achieved without consideration and exploration of the adolescent's mental health, developmental progression, and family relationships. Simply prescribing treatment is not enough. The adolescent must cooperate with the health care team, believe that adhering to a complex regimen is better than the alternative, and have family support and assistance in carrying out the treatment plan. Principles for management include involving both the patient and the family in all aspects of care, using a multidisciplinary team, providing continuity of care, considering self-help techniques, and referral to peer and disease support groups.

TABLE 82.2

Choice of Contraceptives for Girls with Selected Chronic Conditions

Condition	Special Considerations	Suggested Contraceptives
Diabetes mellitus	Low-dose OCPs do not affect glucose tolerance. Estrogen-dominant pills promote a favorable lipid profile. Obesity is often a problem in type 2 diabetes.	Second- or third-generation combination OCPs, patch, or ring plus male latex condom. Avoid DMPA in girls with type 2 diabetes.
Heart disease	OCPs, patch, and ring contraindicated with pulmonary vascular disease, thromboembolic disease, and cerebrovascular disease.	Progestin-only injectable or implantable methods plus male latex condom. Consider progestin-releasing IUD (Mirena). May use OCPs if no contraindications.
Immunosuppression	STDs, especially viral pathogens such as HPV, are more virulent and hard to treat.	Male latex condoms preferred. Consider female condom. May use hormonal methods as well if no contraindications.
Mental retardation	Compliance is an issue unless parent will administer pills. Barrier methods difficult to use.	Long-acting injectable or implantable methods are preferred.
Seizure disorder	OCPs, patch, and ring have lowered efficacy with some seizure medications but not with valproic acid.	DMPA or combination OCPs plus male latex condom. Progestin-only OCPs are contraindicated.
Sickle cell disease	Hormonal methods reduce frequency of vasoocclusive crises. OCPs, patch, and ring contraindicated with history of stroke.	DMPA with male latex condoms is preferred. OCPs, patch, or ring may be used if no contraindications.

(continued)

TABLE 82.2

(Continued)

Condition	Special Considerations	Suggested Contraceptives
Spina bifida	May have latex allergy. OCPs have lowered efficacy with some seizure medications. OCPs, patch, and ring may have higher thrombosis risk in immobilized patients. DMPA may exacerbate osteopenia in immobilized patients.	Polyurethane condoms (male or female) plus hormonal methods if no contraindications. DMPA is not advised for those who are wheelchair bound. Consider progestin-releasing IUD (Mirena–reduced uterine bleeding, no osteopenia).

OCP, oral contraceptive pill; DMPA, depot medroxyprogesterone acetate; IUD, intrauterine device; HPV, human papillomavirus; STD, sexually transmitted disease.

Health Care Transition from Pediatric to Adult Services for Young Adults with Chronic Illness

Approximately half a million youth with special health care needs will turn 18 each year in the United States and most will need to be transitioned to the adult health care system. An appropriately timed transition to adult-oriented health care allows youth to optimize their independence and assume adult roles and functioning. A joint consensus statement issued in 2002 by leading pediatric and adult health care societies recommends that a written health care transition plan for adolescents with special health care needs be created by age 14 and that affordable, continuous health insurance coverage be ensured throughout adolescence and adulthood. However, there are several barriers to effecting a successful health care transition, including lack of adequately trained adult-oriented physicians to manage chronic childhood conditions such as congenital heart disease or cystic fibrosis, loss of health insurance coverage when the young adult is no longer covered on the parents' policy, and reluctance of patients, families, and pediatric subspecialists to terminate a long-standing relationship.

In one study, only 50% of youth and parents had discussed transition issues with the adolescent's doctor and only 1 in 6 (16%) had developed a transition plan, suggesting that there is much room for improvement in this area.

WEB SITES AND REFERENCES

http://www.pacer.org/links/national/disability.html. PACER Center (Parent Advocacy Coalition for Educational Rights). This site has up-to-date links and addresses for more than 160 specific disability resources.

http://www.nichcy.org. National Dissemination Center for Children with Disabilities. Information on disabilities in children and youth, special education, and research.

American Academy of Pediatrics, American Academy of Family Physicians, American College of Physicians, American Society of Internal Medicine. A consensus statement on health care transitions for young adults with special health care needs. *Pediatrics* 2002;110:1304.

Rosen DS, Blum RW, Britto, M, et al. Transition to adult health care for adolescents and young adults with chronic conditions: position paper of the Society for Adolescent Medicine. *J Adolesc Health* 2003;33:309.

CHAPTER 83

Complementary and Alternative Medicine in Adolescents

Cora Collette Breuner and Michael Cirigliano

Complementary and alternative medicine (CAM) encompasses a spectrum of healing practices other than those intrinsic to the conventional health system. An open dialogue is important when an adolescent is interested in the use of CAM. The health care provider should provide advice on the use of CAM to their adolescent patients based on the best available evidence that is compatible with the patient's personal needs and in the clinician's best judgment.

HERBAL THERAPIES

Regulation. The Dietary Supplement Health and Education Act (DSHEA) of 1994 defines herbal therapies as supplements. As such, herbal therapies are not tested according to the same scientific standards as conventional drugs. Packaging or marketing information does not need to be approved by the FDA. Guidelines listed in Table 83.1 may ensure that safety standards are met. Herb–drug interactions are listed in Table 83.2.

Adverse events associated with herbal therapies should be reported to FDA's MedWatch program: 1-800-332-1088 or www.fda.gov/medwatch.

Dosing Issues and Active Compounds. Herbs represent complex entities containing hundreds of constituents, making it difficult to find one particular component representing the active agent. Counsel on the use of the specific extract clinically studied in an herbal product.

Long-Term Use. Most studies involving herbal therapies do not evaluate long-term effects. Herbal therapies should be used only on a time-limited basis until more data are available, and patients should be monitored periodically for signs of toxicity and adverse effects.

Contamination. Herbal therapies may be contaminated with heavy metals or bacteria/fungal organisms when being manufactured or stored. Patients and families should be advised to use products from manufacturers which use high regulatory standards.

TABLE 83.1

Guidelines for Use of Herbal Therapies in the Clinical Setting

All patients should be asked about use of alternative/complementary treatments during routine office visits and initial visits.

Care should be exercised when combining herbal therapies with standard pharmaceuticals.

Because herbal contaminants have been documented in a number of products due to poor manufacturing and lack of standardization, use of herbal therapies by reputable manufacturers is advised.

Larger than recommended doses of herbal therapies should be discouraged.

Until safety data exist, herbal therapies should not be used in pregnancy or lactation.

Long-term use of herbal therapies should be done only under the supervision of a knowledgeable health care provider.

Herbal therapies with known toxicity and side effects should not be used in children and adolescents.

Use of herbal stimulants and performance enhancers in the adolescent population should be discouraged.

All proven treatment options should be discussed with patients and their families before entertaining any form of complementary therapies.

From *The review of natural products*. St. Louis, MO: Facts and Comparisons, 1999, with permission.

Use in Pregnancy and Lactation. Women contemplating pregnancy, currently pregnant, or nursing should not use herbal therapies given the lack of evidence on safety.

COMMON HERBAL THERAPIES USED BY ADOLESCENTS

Psychoactive Herbal Therapies
St. John's Wort
Uses. Used for depression.

Mechanism of Action. The two active ingredients, hypericin and hyperforin, inhibit the reuptake of serotonin, norepinephrine, and dopamine.

Clinical Studies. St. John's wort has been found to be superior to placebo and as effective as low-dose tricyclic antidepressants in mild depression. Comparable responses with high doses of St. John's wort and low doses of selective serotonin reuptake inhibitors (SSRIs) in mild depression.

Side Effects. Has a low incidence of side effects, including gastrointestinal (GI) symptoms, dizziness, and confusion. Phototoxicity may occur with ingestion of high doses.

TABLE 83.2

Selected Drug–Herb Interactions Important in Adolescent Health

Herbal Product	Drug or Drug Class	Potential Interaction
Green tea	Warfarin	Decreased anticoagulant activity due to vitamin K content
Kava	Alprazolam	Additive or synergistic effects
St. John's wort	Cyclosporine Digoxin OCP Protease inhibitors TCAs Theophylline Warfarin	Significant metabolism through P-450 system may lead to decreased serum drug levels
	Iron	May lead to decreased absorption or iron
	SSRIs	May lead to increased side effects as well as the serotonin syndrome
	Benzodiazepam	May reduce the effectiveness in reducing anxiety and may increase the risk of side effects such as drowsiness
	Photosensitizing drugs (e.g. lansoprazole, omeprazole, piroxicam, and sulfonamide antibiotics)	Increased risk of sun sensitivity
Valerian	Barbiturates Benzodiazepines	Possible synergistic effects Increased sedation and increased side effects
Yohimbe	TCAs	Hypertension
Panax ginseng Garlic Feverfew Ginkgo	Anticoagulants	Inhibition of platelet aggregation through inhibition of thromboxane synthetase, arachidonic acid production, inhibition of epinephrine, platelet thromboxane synthetase aggregation inhibition of platelet-activating factor
Panax ginseng	Oral hypoglycemics	Enhanced effects
Echinacea	Immunosuppressants	Interference with immunosuppression

OCP, oral contraceptive pill; SSRI, selective serotonin reuptake inhibitor; TCA, tricyclic antidepressant.

Adapted from Drug-herb interactions. In: *The review of natural products*. St. Louis, MO: Facts and Comparisons, 1999, with permission.

Drug Interactions. Is known to interact with cyclosporine, oral anticoagulants, oral contraceptives, and certain antiretroviral agents including indinavir. The concomitant use of St. John's wort with standard antidepressants may increase the risk of serotonin syndrome.

Kava
Uses. Used as a natural alternative to sedatives and anxiolytics.

Mechanism of Action. May inhibit gamma-aminobutyric acid (GABA) receptor binding.

Clinical Studies. Reduces anxiety scores when compared with placebo.

Side Effects. May produce yellowing and flaking of the skin ("kava dermopathy"), has been reported to cause extrapyramidallike dystonic reactions.

Drug Interactions. Sedation associated with combined use of sedatives and alcohol and kava.

Valerian Root
Uses. Sedative agent and treatment for migraine headaches, fatigue, and intestinal cramps.

Mechanism of Action. Binds to GABA receptors, leading to its sedative effects.

Clinical Studies. Several trials confirm a mild sedative effect.

Side Effects. Headache, excitability, uneasiness, and cardiac disturbances.

Drug Interactions. May cause increased sedation if used with other sedative agents.

Chamomile
Uses. Used for GI discomfort, peptic ulcer disease, pediatric colic, and mild anxiety.

Mechanism of Action. Binds to central benzodiazepine receptors.

Clinical Studies. Several small trials noted chamomile to have hypnotic-sedative properties.

Side Effects. The FDA regards chamomile as safe, although allergic reactions have been reported.

Drug Interactions. No drug–herb interactions have been noted.

Herbs for Weight Loss
Ma Huang (Ephedra)
Uses. Used to aid weight loss, enhance sports performance, and increase energy. In 2004, the FDA banned the sale of ephedra-containing products.

Mechanism of Action. Ephedra may increase the levels of norepinephrine, epinephrine, and dopamine by stimulating both alpha and beta adrenoreceptors.

Clinical Studies. One meta-analysis and case reports showed that ephedrine and ephedra promoted modest short-term weight loss (about 0.9 kg per month compared with placebo).

Side Effects. Side effects include increased blood pressure, palpitations, tachycardia, chest pain, coronary vasospasm, cardiomyopathy, and death. The combination of caffeine and ephedra may cause euphoria, neurotic behavior, agitation, depressed mood, giddiness, irritability, anxiety, and physical/psychological dependency.

Guaraná [Paullinia cupana (syn. P. crysan, P. sorbilis)]
Uses. Used as a stimulant owing to its caffeinelike products guaranine, theobromine, theophylline, xanthine, and other xanthine derivatives.

Mechanism of Action. Guarana contains 3.6% to 5.8% caffeine (compared to 1% to 2% in coffee).

Clinical Studies. One study of overweight adults reported that the combination of yerba mate, guarana, and damiana significantly delayed gastric emptying, causing prolonged perceived gastric fullness and weight loss over 45 days.

Side Effects. Similar to those of ephedra and caffeine.

Hydroxycitric Acid (Garcinia cambogia)
Uses. Used as an herbal weight-loss agent.

Mechanism of Action. May increase fat oxidation.

Clinical Studies. No benefit reported over placebo.

Side Effects. May cause abdominal pain and vomiting.

Hoodia Gordonii
Uses. Used as a weight-loss product.

Mechanism of Action. A decrease in hunger associated with an isolated steroidal glycoside termed P57AS3 (P57).

Clinical Studies. In a preliminary study, overweight men who consume P57 had significantly lower calorie intake than those taking a placebo.

Side Effects. None reported.

Herbal Therapies for Sports Enhancement
Ginseng (Panax Ginseng)
Uses. Used to improve both mental and physical performance.

Mechanism of Action. May effect nitric oxide synthesis in lung, heart, and kidney.

Clinical Studies. Studies are inconclusive.

Side Effects. Adverse effects include nervousness, insomnia, and GI disturbance. Owing to the estrogenlike effect, it may cause mastalgia and vaginal bleeding in women.

Drug Interactions. May interact with oral anticoagulants, antiplatelet agents, corticosteroids, and hypoglycemic agents.

Miscellaneous Herbal Therapies
Echinacea (E. angustifola, E. pallida, E. purpurea)
Uses. Used for aches, colds, and as a topical analgesic for snake bites, stings, and burns.

Mechanism of Action. Works by protecting the integrity of the hyaluronic acid matrix and by stimulating the alternate complement pathway. It promotes nonspecific T-cell activation by binding to T cells and increasing interferon production.

Clinical Studies. Preparations were found to be better than placebo for the treatment of upper respiratory symptoms but no better than placebo for the prevention of the common cold.

Side Effects. Adverse effects include skin rash, GI upset, and diarrhea.

Drug Interactions. Should not be used in patients who are immunosuppressed or on immunosuppressant medications.

Feverfew
Uses. Used for the prevention and treatment of migraine headaches.

Mechanism of Action. May inhibit prostaglandin, thromboxane, and leukotriene synthesis.

Clinical Studies. Two randomized trials have shown benefit for migraine prevention.

Side Effects. Adverse effects include occasional mouth ulcerations, contact dermatitis, dizziness, diarrhea, and heartburn.

Drug Interactions. May interact with anticoagulants and antiplatelet agents.

Garlic
Uses. Used as a cholesterol-lowering agent.

Mechanism of Action. May reduce cholesterol synthesis by reducing the activity of beta-hydroxy-beta-methylglutaryl-CoA (HMG-CoA) reductase.

Clinical Studies. Studies are inconclusive.

Side Effects. May cause GI distress.

Drug Interactions. Should not be used with anticoagulant medication.

ACUPUNCTURE

Acupuncture is an ancient Chinese therapy based on the concept that energy (*qi, chi*) flows through the body along channels or meridians connected by acupuncture points. The flow of *qi* is manipulated by insertion of fine needles at acupuncture points.

The history and examination includes the determination of the shape, color, and coating of the tongue and the force, flow, and character of the radial pulse. The specific treatment is based on the diagnosis and may include solid sterile needle placement, moxibustion (the practice of burning dried herbs over the acupuncture needles), acupressure, or cupping.

Evidence of Health Benefits. Dental pain, postoperative nausea and vomiting, nausea and vomiting secondary to chemotherapy.

Possible Health Benefits. Migraine/tension headaches, back pain, dysmenorrhea, acute and chronic pain, substance abuse.

Complications. Pneumothorax, angina, septic sacroiliitis, epidural and temporomandibular abscess.

YOGA

Yoga is widely known for helping to build strength and flexibility through a combination of meditation, controlled breathing, and stretches.

Possible Health Benefits. Relief of anxiety, hypertension, heart disease, depression, low back pain, headaches, cancer.

MASSAGE

Massage therapy is thought to release muscle tension, remove toxic metabolites, and facilitate oxygen transport to cells and tissues.

Evidence of Health Benefits. Preterm infants have shortened hospital stays, improved glucose control in type I and II diabetes mellitus, decreased pain in juvenile rheumatoid arthritis.

Possible Health Benefits. Less need for topical steroids in atopic dermatitis, improved pulmonary function in patients with cystic fibrosis, decreased anxiety in eating disorders, improved mood in depression, improved control in asthma.

Complications. None reported.

CHIROPRACTIC

Chiropractic is based on the theory that all diseases can be traced to malpositioned bones in the spinal column, called "subluxations," which lead to the entrapment of spinal nerves. Physical adjustment of the spine restores proper alignment by relieving nerve entrapments.

Evidence of Health Benefits. Decreased pain in acute low back pain.

Possible Health Benefits. Improvement in symptoms of acute otitis media.

Not Effective. Asthma.

Complications. Strokes, myelopathies, and radiculopathies after cervical manipulation.

Adverse Outcomes. With bleeding dyscrasia, when improper diagnosis is made, in the presence of a herniated disc, or when an improper manipulative method is utilized.

HOMEOPATHIC MEDICINE

Three concepts embody the philosophy of homeopathic medicine: (1) finding the similium or similar substance, (2) treating the totality of symptoms, and (3) using the minimum dose through potentization.

The "principle of similars" is that highly dilute preparations of substances may stimulate healing in ill patients who have similar symptoms. The curative power of the remedy is engrafted into the water molecules and the water retains a "memory" of these changes.

Possible Health Benefits. Recurrent upper respiratory infections, otitis media, attention deficit disorder.

Complications. Aggravation of symptoms, contamination of remedy.

CONCLUSION

Clinicians need to understand and appreciate the variety of health care options available to adolescents and their families. Open, honest, and nonjudgmental discussions with adolescents either using or planning to use CAM will bring about a safe and rational use of those treatments for which there is evidence of efficacy. Further, such an approach will enable adolescents to make informed choices. Improved communication can be addressed by following the recommendations outlined in Table 83.3. Health care providers need to inquire regularly about CAM use, since such insight will help them to provide better care to adolescents.

TABLE 83.3

Talking with Your Patients about Complementary and Alternative Medicine

Be open-minded. Most patients are reluctant to share information about their use of CAM therapies because they are concerned their physicians will disapprove. By remaining open-minded, you can learn a lot about your patients' use of unconventional therapies. These strategies will help foster open communication.

Ask the question. I recommend asking every patient about his or her use of alternative therapies during routine history taking. One approach is simply to inquire, "Are you doing anything else for this condition?" It's an open-ended question that gives the patient the opportunity to tell you about his or her use of other health care providers or therapies. Another approach is to ask, "Are you taking any over-the-counter remedies such as vitamins or herbs?"

Avoid using the words "alternative therapy," at least initially. This will help you to avoid appearing judgmental or biased.

Don't dismiss any therapy as a placebo. If a patient tells you about a therapy that you are unaware of, make a note of it in the patient's record and schedule a follow-up visit after you have learned more—when you'll be in a better position to negotiate the patient's care. If you determine the therapy might be harmful, you'll have to ask the patient to stop using it. If it isn't harmful and the patient feels better using it, you may want to consider incorporating the therapy into your care plan.

Discuss providers as well as therapies. Another way to help your patients negotiate the maze of alternative therapies is by stressing that they see appropriately trained and licensed providers and knowing whom to refer to in your area. Encourage your patients to ask alternative providers about their background and training and the treatment modalities they use. By doing so, your patients will be better equipped to make educated decisions about their health care.

Discuss CAM therapies with your patients at every visit. Charting the details of their use will remind you to raise the issue. It may also help alert you to potential complications before they occur.

CAM, complementary and alternative medicine.
Breuner CC. Complementary medicine in pediatrics: a review of acupuncture, homeopathy, massage and chiropractic therapies. *Current Probs in Pediatric and Adolescent Health Care.* 2002;32(10):347–384.

WEB SITES

http://www.nccam.nih.gov. National Center for Complementary and Alternative Medicine.
http://www.herbmed.org. HerbMed database.
http://www.herbalgram.org. American Botanical Council.

http://www.naturaldatabase.com. Natural Medicines Comprehensive Database.
http://www.cmbm.org. The Center for Mind Body Medicine.
http://www.americanyogaassociation.org/. American Yoga Association.
http://www.aaom.org. American Association of Oriental Medicine.
http://www.medicalacupuncture.org. American Academy of Medical Acupuncture.
http://www.amerchiro.org. American Chiropractic Association.
http://www.chiropractic.org. International Chiropractors Association.
http://www.homeopathic.org. National Center for Homeopathy.
http://www.amtamassage.org. American Massage Therapy Association.
http://www.ncbtmb.com. National Certification Board for Massage Therapy and Bodywork.

CHAPTER 84

Overview of Health Issues for College Students

Lawrence S. Neinstein, Paula Swinford, and James Farrow

Over 17.6 million students were enrolled in 2006 in the nation's 4,392 colleges and universities, with an anticipated 19.5 million by 2014. Some 63% are 14 to 24 years of age. College students of traditional age (18 to 24) comprise a unique population with specific health–related assests and vulnerabilities, while the college campus is a unique health environment that creates both risks and opportunities for preventing or reducing health-risk behaviors and enhancing well being.

The primary mission of college health is to enhance the health of students in support of advancing student academic success. Nationally, there are about 1,600 colleges or universities that provide some level of services to advance the health of students. The most common services are medical or clinical services directed by a physician, nurse, nurse practitioner, or administrator. There are about 10 million students making as many as 30 million visits to these services per year at an approximate cost of $1.4 billion. About 5% to 25% of these visits were made to counseling services.

THE PHILOSOPHY OF A MODEL COLLEGE HEALTH PROGRAM

Services have developed over the past 150 years to maintain the student's health for academic studies, address the public health communicable disease and health care needs, and provide access to care for the many uninsured individuals in this population.

At its best, college health embraces a model that focuses on students' physical, emotional, and social health in the context of their cultural and academic influences. This model includes significant interactions with the campus community and uses available health insurance resources with a strong emphasis on health promotion, including primary and secondary prevention. It also involves treating medical conditions while assessing, intervening, and preventing the student's behavioral and health risks. Optimally, services provided are continually assessed and adjusted based on health status of the student population.

ENROLLMENT

There are almost 4,400 institutions of higher education in the United States, with approximately 17.6 million students in the fall 2006, likely rising to about 18.8 million by the year 2010 and 19.5 million by 2014. Data and extensive tables are available from the National Center for Education Statistics at: http://nces.ed.gov/programs/digest as well as the almanac issues of the *Chronicle of High Education.*

Gender: Approximately 42% are male and 58% female.

Full-Time versus Part-Time: Approximately 62% are full-time and 38% are part-time.

Age Distribution (Fall, 2005, NCES, 2007): Projected distribution of students in 2006 are 14 to 17 years of age (1.0%), 18 to 19 (21.0%), 20 to 21 (21.4%), 22 to 24 (17.4%), 25 to 29 (14.4%), 30 to 34 (7.3%) and over 35 (17.6%). Overall, 60.6% of enrolled students are 24 years of age or younger.

Race/Ethnicity (2005): College enrollment in 2005 was white (65.7%), black (12.6%), Hispanic (10.8%), Asian or Pacific islander (6.5%), American Indian/Alaska Native (1.0%), and nonresident alien (3.3%). Black enrollment increased from 10.3% in 1995 and Hispanic from 7.6%.

Types of Universities: According to the National Center for Education Statistics, 2006, 60% are 4-year institutions, with the majority being private, and 40% are 2-year, with the majority being public.

Level of Student: Undergraduate: 14,780,630/17,272,044 = 85.6%. Postbaccalaureate: 2,491,414/17,272,044 = 14.4%, including first-professional 334,529 (1.9%) and graduate 2,156,885 (12.5%).

CHANGING STUDENT PROFILE

1. Students 25 years old and over increased from 4.9 million in 1987 to 6.89 million in 2005, an increase of 41%. The proportion of students 25 years of age and over increased from 38.0% in 1987 to 43.8% in 1995 and then dropped in 2005 to 39.3%.
2. Female student enrollment increased from 6.4 million in 1982 to over 10 million in 2005, an average annual growth rate of over 2.5% and a 57.5% increase over the period.
3. The number of international college students was back up since 1998, with an increase of almost 14% between 2000 and 2003. Almost two thirds are from Asia.
4. Some 25% of students do not have health insurance coverage and about 18% to 24% have inadequate insurance.
5. Increasing numbers of college students are on financial aid (undergraduate students rising from 58.7% in 1992 to 1993 to 72.5% in 1999 to 2000 to 76.1% in 2003 to 2004).
6. Enrollment as a percent of all 18- to 24-year-olds has increased between 1990 and 2001 from 35.2% to 39.3% for white non-Hispanics; from 25.3% to 31.3% for African Americans; and from 15.8% to 21.7% for Hispanic students.
7. Between 2004 and 2014, enrollment is expected to rise from 17.6 million to 19.5 million. The increase is expected to be 16% for students 18 to 24 years old, with an expected increase of 12% for men and 21% for women.

MORBIDITY AND MORTALITY

Morbidity and mortality data are less available on college students than other populations, as college enrollment data are rarely collected as part of standard demographic data. The Centers for Disease Control (CDC) collected data in 1995: National College Health Risk Behavior Survey (NCHRBS)—United States, 1995, and currently there is a yearly health status data set available from the American College Health Association as the ACHA National College Health Assessment Survey (www.acha-ncha.org) National data are also available on specifically on drug use from several studies, including Monitoring the Future Study (since 1975 at www.monitoringthefuture.org), Core Alcohol and Drug Survey (since 1989), the College Alcohol Study (Wechsler, 1993, 1997, 1999), and the Cooperative Institutional Research Program (CIRP) Freshman Survey.

The ACHA National College Health Assessment suggests that:

- Over one third (37%) of college students reported at least one event of consuming five or more alcoholic drinks at a setting, during the 2-week period preceding the survey.
- Many college student fail to protect themselves against STDs and pregnancy. Some 52% of those who are sexually active used a condom the last time they had vaginal intercourse.
- About 60% of students failed to engage in vigorous or moderate physical activity at recommended levels three times per week or more.

INJURIES (2006)

Unintentional Injuries. Within the previous school year, 5.9% of students rarely or never used a seat belt (of drivers), 67.5% rarely or never wore bicycle helmets (of riders), and, in the previous 30 days 5.0% of drivers drove a car after five or more drinks.

Intentional Injuries (2006). Within the previous school year, 6.2% of students were involved in fights (11.3% males and 3.0% females), 1.4% experienced sexual penetration against their will (1.8% females and 0.7% males), while 2.7% experienced attempted sexual penetration against their will. [See Suicide (2006 ACHA-NCHA data).]

Suicidal Ideation and Attempt within the Last School Year

	Suicidal Ideation	*Suicide Attempt*
Total	9.3%	1.3%

Although lower than among the high school adolescent population, in which almost 12% of female adolescents and 5.6% of boys have attempted suicide, the rates are still significant.

USE OF ALCOHOL, TOBACCO, AND OTHER DRUGS

Yearly updated data are available from Monitoring the Future for college students in volume II of the *National Survey Results on Drug Use, 1975–2006, Monitoring the Future* (Johnston et al., 2006 www.monitoringthefuture.org). Extensive tables and figures are available on lifetime, annual, 30-day, and daily prevalence use of drugs and drug use trends among college students compared to their age matched peers not in college. Trends noticed in this report include the following:

- Use of illicit drugs fell among American college students and young adults between late 1970s and early 1990s. However, there have been increases in the usage rates since 1994 for many drugs among high school seniors and college students.
- In 2006, the rank order for annual prevalence of using any illicit drug was 12th graders (36.5%) college students (33.9%), 19- to 28-year-olds (32.1%), 10th graders (28.7%), and 8th graders (14.8%). In general, the trends for most illicit drugs use among college students paralleled that among noncollege peers in the 1980s. In 2006, for most categories of drugs, college students had rates of use similar to those among their age peers. While college-bound seniors have below-average rates of use in high school for all of the illicit drugs, these students' eventual use of some illicit drugs becomes equal to or exceeding that among those not attending college.
- *Smoking:* In 2006, cigarette smoking showed the greatest difference between age-matched college students and noncollege students (9.2% daily smoking prevalence versus 18.6% for same-aged high school graduates not in college). Since 2001, there is little consistent gender difference in smoking among college students.
- *Alcohol use:* Alcohol has been tried by 86.6% of college students. In 2006, the lifetime and annual use of alcohol among college students was not significantly different from that among age-matched peers not in college. In 2006, the 30-day use was higher (65%) among college students than noncollege age-matched peers (61%), but daily drinking among college students was lower (4.8%) than that among their noncollege peer group (5.7%). However, college students have the highest rate of occasions of heavy drinking (five or more drinks in a row in the previous 2 weeks). Because college-bound seniors in high school are consistently less likely to report occasions of heavy drinking compared to non-college-bound students, it appears that the higher rates of heavy drinking episodes in college indicate a college related increase in binge drinking or what is being called the "college effect." Among college men, 50% reporting five or more drinks in a row over the prior 2 weeks compared with 34.4% of women.
- *Marijuana use:* The annual prevalence decreased markedly from 1981 through 1991 from 51% to 27%. Daily marijuana use rose substantially among college students between 1992 and 2003, but it appears to have decreased since.
- *LSD:* During the early 1980s, one of the largest proportional declines in drug use was in LSD, with annual prevalence rates falling from 6.3% in 1982 to 2.2% in 1985. After peaking at 6.9% in 1995, use among college students and young adults declined through 2005 (0.7%), but it increased in 2006 to 1.4%.
- *Amphetamines:* Between 1982 and 1992, annual use of amphetamine declined among college students, from 21% to 3.6%. However, annual use increased

among college students to 7.2% in 2001, and it has decreased slightly since then to 6.0% in 2006.

- *Cocaine:* Use of cocaine among college students dropped dramatically from 1983 to 1994 (17.3% annual use to 2.0%); however, it later increased to 5.1% in 2006.
- *Other drugs:* The annual prevalence of Vicodin use increased from 6.9% in 2002 to 7.6% in 2006; Rohypnol use decreased from 0.7% to 0.2%; GHB decreased slightly, and ketamine also decreased from 1.3% to 0.9%. Ritalin usage decreased slightly in annual use from 5.7% in 2002 to 3.9% in 2006. Tranquilizers also followed a similar pattern as cocaine usage, with annual prevalences falling from 6.9% in 1980 to 1.8% in 1994 and then reversing to 6.9% in 2003. The rates from 2003 to 2006 have decreased to 5.8%.

Tobacco (2006 ACHA-NCHA)

"Number of Days of Any Cigarette Use in Past 30 Days."[a]

	≥10 Days	1–9 Days
Total	8.4%	9.3%
Female	7.8%	8.7%
Male	9.2%	10.2%

[a]Perception of tobacco use rates was much higher, with reported actual daily use within the previous 30 days of 4.3% compared with a perceived daily use of 32.1%.

Alcohol (2005 ACHA-NCHA)

"How Many Days Did You Consume Any Alcohol in Past 30 Days?"[a]

	≥10 Days	1–9 Days
Total	15.6%	54.0%
Female	13.0%	55.9%
Male	20.0%	51.1%

[a]For all students, 17.2% reported no alcohol use within the previous 30 days, while the perception was that only 3.6% of all students drank no alcohol within the past 30 days.

High-Risk Drinking (Five Drinks or More at a Sitting in Previous 2 Weeks)[a]

Frequency	Total	Female	Male
None	62.9%	68.0%	54%
1–2 times	21.4%	21.0%	25.0%
3–5 times	11.3%	9.0%	15.0%
≥6 times	3.4%	1.0%	6.0%

[a]Consequences of drinking in previous school year for those who drank alcohol included the following: 18.2% had an injury to self, 4.1% injured another person, 35.7% did something they later regretted, 1.3% were involved in forced sexual activity, and 13.9% were involved in unprotected sexual activity.

Marijuana Use (2006 ACHA-NCHA)

"How Many Days Did You Use Marijuana in Past 30 Days?"[a]

	≥ 10 Days	1–9 Days
Total	4.5%	10.0%
Female	3.0%	9.0%
Male	6.0%	11.0%

[a]Reported actual daily use of marijuana for all students within the previous 30 days was 1.2%, compared with the perceived daily use of marijuana by all students of 18.5%.

SEXUALITY

Among sexually transmitted diseases (STDs), human papillomavirus (HPV) infections are the most common among college students, and chlamydial infections are the most common bacterial STDs.

Sexual Behaviors (2006 ACHA-NCHA)

Prevalence of Intercourse

	Ever Had Vaginal Intercourse	Ever Had Anal Intercourse	Ever Had Oral Intercourse
Total	68.6%	25.1%	72.1%
Female	69.0%	23.0%	72.0%
Male	68.0%	29.0%	73.0%

Prevalence Condom Use at Last Sexual Intercourse (excluded if "never did this activity")

	Vaginal Intercourse	Anal Intercourse	Oral Intercourse
Total	52.1%	27.7%	3.8%

Number of Partners (Vaginal, Oral, Anal Intercourse) within the Last School Year

	None	1	2 or 3	≥ 4
Total	29.2%	46.5%	16.7%	7.6%
Female	29.0%	49%	16.0%	5.0%
Male	30.0%	43%	17.0%	11.0%

Emergency Contraception Use and Unintended Pregnancies—Past Year

- 11.2% of sexually active college students reported using (or reported their partner used) emergency contraception within the previous school year (male: 9.7%; female 12.7%)

- 2.1% of college students who had vaginal intercourse within the previous school year reported experiencing an unintentional pregnancy or their partner becoming pregnant.

DIETARY, PHYSICAL ACTIVITY AND SLEEP BEHAVIORS

Dietary Behaviors (2006 ACHA-NCHA)

"In the Past 30 Days, to Lose Weight You ... "

	Dieted	Exercised	Purged	Used Diet Pills
Total	34.5%	55.2%	2.5%	3.6%
Females	42.4%	62.7%	3.6%	4.6%
Males	22.1%	43.7%	0.7%	1.9%

Physical Activity Behaviors (2006 ACHA-NCHA)

"In the Past Week, Participated in Exercise for at Least 20 Minutes ... "

	None	1 or 2 days	3–5 days	6 or 7 days
Total	24.4%	31.4%	35.6%	8.6%
Females	25.7%	31.2%	35.0%	8.0%
Males	22.1%	31.7%	36.6%	9.6%

Sleep Behaviors (2006 ACHA-NCHA)

"In the Past Week, Getting Enough Sleep to Feel Rested in the Morning ... "

	None	1 or 2 days	3–5 days	6 or 7 days
Total	10.4%	28.0%	47.7%	13.9%
Females	10.8%	28.3%	47.1%	13.8%
Males	9.4%	27.4%	49.1%	14.1%

Body Mass Index (2005 ACHA-NCHA)

Estimated Body Mass Index (BMI), Incorporates Reported Gender, Height, and Weight

	<18.5 Underweight	18.5–24.9 Healthy Weight	25–29.9 Overweight	30–34.9 Class I Obesity	35–39.9 Class II Obesity	≥40 Class III Obesity
Total	4.5%	64.1%	21.9%	6.2%	2.1%	1.2%
Females	5.6%	67.6%	17.8%	5.5%	2.0%	1.4%
Males	2.6%	58.2%	28.8%	7.4%	2.1%	0.8%

PREVENTIVE HEALTH CARE, PROBLEMS, AND HEALTH INFORMATION

Preventive Health Care Practices (2006 ACHA-NCHA)

Hepatitis B vaccination	73.4%
Meningococcal vaccination	57.1%
Chickenpox vaccination	50.0%
Flu immunization last year	26.0%
Dental examination last year	77.2%
Testicular self-examination last month	38.8%
Breast self-examination last month	39.4%
Gynecologic examination last year	59.2%
Cholesterol check in past 5 years	45.1%

Health Problems (2005 ACHA-NCHA)

Within the previous year, students reported experiencing back pain (46.6%), allergy problems (45.5%), sinus infections (28.8%), depression (17.8%), strep throat (13.2%), anxiety disorder (12.4%), asthma (11.2%), ear infection (9.3%), seasonal affective disorders (8.1%), bronchitis (7.8%), carpal tunnel syndrome (6.8%), fracture (4.7%), high blood pressure (4.5%), high cholesterol (4.0%), substance abuse (3.4%), chronic fatigue (3.4%), bulimia (2.3%), genital warts (2.2%), mononucleosis (2.2%), anorexia nervosa (1.9%), genital herpes (1.0%), diabetes (0.9%), chlamydial infection (0.8%), hepatitis B or C, (0.4%) and HIV (0.3%).

IMPEDIMENTS TO ACADEMIC SUCCESS (2006 ACHA-NCHA)

Students reported the following factors affecting their individual academic performance within the preceding school year (i.e., received an incomplete, dropped a course, received a lower grade in a class, on an exam, or on an important project). These included stress (32.2%), cold/sore throat (26%), sleep difficulties (23.9%), concern for a troubled friend or family (18%), depression/anxiety (15.7%), relationship difficulty (15.6%), Internet use/computer games (15.4%), death of a friend/family member (8.5%), sinus infection (8.3%), alcohol use (7.3%), allergies (4.2%), injury (3.3%), learning disability (3.2%), chronic pain (2.9%), chronic illness (2.7%), drug use (2.3%), mononucleosis (1.5%), eating disorder (1.3%), pregnancy (0.9%), sexual assault (0.8%), physical assault (0.6%), and STDs (0.4%).

It appears that of the top ten impediments to academic success only two are biomedical, while psychosocial issues—such as depression, relationships, and stress—carry the greatest impact on student learning. Of interest is the high percentage with academic performance problems due to Internet use.

TYPES OF HEALTH PROBLEMS

1. Acute medical problems such as minor infections, musculoskeletal injuries, minor trauma, and skin problems. Occasionally, some of the infections

become life-threatening, such as meningitis and tuberculosis. Reproductive issues are common, including the diagnosis and treatment of STDs, contraception, emergency contraception, routine gynecology, and men's health care.

2. Chronic medical problems, such as asthma, diabetes, seizure disorders, thyroid disorders, hypertension, hyperlipidemia, eating disorders, and malignancies, with higher rates in this age group.
3. Mental health issues, such as stress-related symptoms, eating disorders, anxiety, depression, suicidality, chronic fatigue, and other disorders affecting academic performance, such as attention deficit disorder and sleep disorders.
4. Substance abuse: diagnosis and treatment.
5. Screening programs for STDs.
6. Immunization programs.
7. Tuberculosis screening.
8. Routine screening for other health risks including smoking and hyperlipidemia, excessive alcohol use and unsafe sexual behaviors.

Trends and Challenges. There are numerous challenges facing both student affairs and health care professionals in the college health setting in the 21st century, including stability of finances, continued national accreditation of ambulatory care services, improved information technology for a population raised on technology, and strong supplemental insurance policies. It is critical that college health programs explore adequate supplementary or major medical coverage opportunities for students including coverage for common needs such as contraception, acne treatment, immunizations, mental health, smoking cessation, and substance abuse?

THE PRECOLLEGE MEDICAL VISIT

Information for Providers to Consider When Sending Their Patients off to College

The precollege visit marks the beginning of the transition for the adolescent from health care largely supervised by parents to health care that is a personal responsibility. The precollege medical visit is intended to update the medical history, perform a complete physical examination, screen for health risk behaviors, update immunizations, and provide prevention counseling and education.

Prematriculation Requirements. Most universities require certain immunizations and tuberculosis screening, and others will have a health form that must be completed before the student arrives on campus.

Health History. Health risk behaviors are important to consider before the adolescent leaves for college. Screening questions should cover eating disorders, alcohol and tobacco use, sexual activity and contraceptive use, psychiatric issues, and learning disabilities.

An example of comprehensive screening questions on these topics can be found in the NCHA survey, which is posted on the ACHA Web site (at www.acha.org). Table 84.1 gives examples of a simplified version of these questions.

Examination. If a complete physical examination has been completed in the past 3 years, the assessment during the precollege visit may be limited to determination of the height, weight (and calculation of body mass index), and blood pressure, vision and hearing screen, as well as performance of a focused physical examination based on problems uncovered in the screening history. For sexually active women (3 years after the onset of sexual activity), a pelvic examination with Papanicolaou (Pap) smear and testing for STDs is indicated. If the college-bound student presents for a preparticipation sports physical, a more comprehensive physical assessment is necessary.

Diagnostic Testing. The precollege visit is limited to fasting cholesterol screening if the adolescent has other risk factors for future cardiovascular disease (e.g., smoking, hypertension, obesity, diabetes mellitus, excessive consumption of dietary saturated fats, and cholesterol; screening tests for chlamydial infection, gonorrhea, syphilis, and/or HIV should be based on risk factors. A Pap smear (preferably liquid-based) should be obtained annually on all sexually active women 3 years after the onset of sexual activity. A skin test for tuberculosis should be placed only if there are risk factors for tuberculosis exposure. The ACHA guidelines indicate that students should undergo tuberculin skin testing if they have arrived within the previous 5 years from some regions of the world. Individuals with positive skin test results should have a chest radiograph. If the chest radiograph is negative and there are no contraindications to preventive therapy, isoniazid should be prescribed daily for 9 months.

Immunizations. Most colleges and universities mandate proof of certain immunizations before arrival on campus. Although the ACHA gives guidelines for institutional prematriculation immunizations (www.acha.org/info_resources/guidelines.cfm), the institution may vary these requirements as mandated by state law or institutional policy . Therefore, to minimize disruption in the enrollment process, the health history form provided to the college-bound student by the college or university should be consulted. If proof of immunization cannot be obtained, then titers demonstrating immunity may often be substituted. An alternative is to reimmunize. Many colleges are now requiring or strongly recommending immunization against varicella, hepatitis B, and meningococcal disease with the quadravalent conjugate vaccine. The latter vaccine is now recommended for entering college students by the CDC's Advisory Committee on Immunization Practices (ACIP 2005). These inoculations may be begun at the precollege visit and either completed before leaving for college or after arriving on campus.

Pertussis Vaccination. In recent years, pertussis (whoopingcough) has increased approximately 400% in adolescents and adults. It appears to account for 20% to 30% of cough lasting over 2 weeks in adolescents and adults. It also appears that adolescents and young adults are a significant source vector (76% of cases), leading to the rising infection rates in infants. Recent ACIP recommendations include that a Tdap should replace Td for all 11- and 12-year-olds; those between the ages of 13 and 18 years who have not yet received a Td booster should receive Tdap in place of Td.

TABLE 84.1

Examples of Screening Questions

Eating disorders:
- Do you worry about gaining weight? Do you feel that food controls your life?
- Do you do any of the following (select all that apply)?
  1. Exercise to lose weight
  2. Diet to lose weight
  3. Vomit or take laxatives to lose weight
  4. Take diet pills to lose weight
  5. None of the above
- Have you ever been told that you had anorexia nervosa or bulimia?

Tobacco use:
- Have you ever used any tobacco products (cigarettes, cigars, smokeless tobacco)?

Alcohol and other abusable substances:
- Do you drink alcohol (beer, wine, liquor)?
- Do you use marijuana (pot, hash, hash oil)?
- Do you use cocaine (crack, rock, freebase)?
- Do you use amphetamines (diet pills, speed, meth, crank)?
- Do you use steroids for body building or to improve athletic performance?
- Do you use other drugs such as Rohypnol (roofies), GHB or liquid X?

Sexual behaviors:
- Have you ever been sexually active?
- Are you currently sexually active?
- Have you ever been diagnosed with a sexually transmitted infection (STD) such as chlamydia, gonorrhea, syphilis, pelvic inflammatory disease, genital warts (human papillomavirus), herpes, hepatitis B, or HIV?
- Do you practice safe sex (use a condom or dental dam)?
- Do you use a method of contraception?
- Have you unintentionally become pregnant or gotten someone else pregnant?
- Have you been tested for HIV?

Mental heatlh
- Do you have any mental health disorders?
- Do you feel depressed, sad, or lonely?
- Have you ever seriously considered or attempted suicide?
- Do you have difficulty controlling your temper?

Emotional, physical, or sexual abuse:
- Have you been or are you in a relationship that is emotionally, physically, or sexually abusive?

(continued)

TABLE 84.1

(Continued)

Learning problems
- Have you been told you had a learning disorder or attention deficit disorder?

Risk for tuberculosis infection:
- Have you ever had a positive skin test for tuberculosis?
- Were you born in a country other than the United States? If yes, where?
- Have you ever injected street drugs?
- Have you tested positive for HIV?
- Have you ever resided in, volunteered in, or worked in a prison, nursing home, hospital, residential facility for patients with acquired immunodeficiency syndrome, homeless shelter, or a refugee camp?
- Have you ever been on steriods (prednisone, cortisone) for at least a month?

GHB, gamma-hydroxybutyrate; HIV, human immunodeficiency virus.

Health Guidance. The remainder of the precollege visit should be devoted to the provision of health guidance information. Selected information, based on responses to the screening questionnaire, may be discussed during the office visit and additional information may be given out via handouts or brochures. The American Academy of Pediatrics publishes a brochure entitled *Health Care for College Students*, which covers recommendations for sleep, nutrition, exercise, responsible sexual activity including abstinence, responsible drinking including abstinence, common health problems, mental health, and safety on campus. The ACHA publishes a multitude of brochures on many of these topics as well. *The Healthy Student, A Parent's Guide to Preparing Teens for the College Years,* is available from the Society for Adolescent Medicine. (www.acha.org/info_resources/guidelines.cfm).

For the adolescent with chronic medical conditions, an attempt should be made to arrange for transition of care, either to the health care providers in the college health service or to community providers near the college or university. The parent should sign a release of information (for the minor child) and a copy of the medical record or send an introductory letter summarizing the medical history to the new provider.

Information for Parents to Consider When Sending Their Children off to College

Available College Health Center Services and Costs. Services provided by the college health service are often found on the college's Web site. Services vary from large, multispecialty centers providing all outpatient primary care, specialty, and diagnostic services to those that provide only rudimentary first aid. In general, however, college health services provide high-quality, low-cost accessible primary care and health education services. Parents and students should determine what services are available and what the student health fee (if any) covers. Information about provision of after-hours care and emergency services, pharmacy services, and the location of the referral hospital should be obtained and kept in an accessible location.

Health Insurance. Most colleges have no facilities such as infirmaries for overnight stays. Parents should ensure that the college-bound student has adequate health insurance to cover hospitalization and emergency, specialty, and diagnostic health services. An unexpected medical bill can interrupt or terminate a college career, and it is strongly recommended that students not go without adequate health insurance. Many campuses sponsor a group health insurance plan at reasonable rates.

Consent and Confidentiality
1. *Minor Consent:* If the college-bound student will be an unemancipated minor child on arrival on campus, the parent should sign a generic "consent for treatment" and forward this to the college health service. The parent should be aware that certain disorders or conditions may be treated without parental consent, even if the student is an unemancipated minor. These may include care for STDs, contraception, pregnancy, mental health or emotional disturbance, and/or substance abuse.
2. *Confidentiality:* In most states, once the student is age 18 years, he or she is considered an adult. At this point, the college health service will adopt a policy of strict confidentiality regarding medical records and medical information. Medical information will not be released to anyone (even the parent who is paying the tuition and fees) without the student's written consent or a court order. This often causes anguish and frustration on the part of the parent but is essential if the student is to engage openly in a professional relationship with the health care provider. Furthermore, confidentiality is essential if the college health service is to assist the student in assuming increasing responsibility for personal health care. Counseling services on campus will adopt the same policy of strict confidentiality.

Personal Health Information. The parent should ensure that the student is knowledgeable about his or her personal health information such as medications, allergies, family medical history, prior health problems and records, and precollege exam and immunizations. The student should have a copy of his or her major medical insurance card.

First Aid Supplies. Every student should have basic health care supplies and equipment to deal with minor illnesses and injuries. These include a first aid kit (bandages, antibiotic ointment, elastic wrap such as an Ace wrap, liquid soap, 2 × 2 gauze pads, acetaminophen, ibuprofen, pepto-Bismol, cough and cold medicine, sore throat lozenges or throat spray, and allergy medicine), electronic thermometer, ice pack, or chemical cold pack.

Guidance Regarding Transition. Parents should be aware that entering college marks a transition for the student that reaches far beyond merely leaving home. Parents will no longer be personally responsible for attending to the health care needs of their son or daughter. Rather, the student begins the process of learning self-care and good health practices. Parents can assist with this process by "letting go" and allowing students to engage in their own decision making. The campus health service will assist with this transition by one-on-one counseling and education within the clinic and through programmed health promotion activities on campus. Through these combined efforts, the student will transition toward a state of optimal health, physically, emotionally, socially, intellectually, and spiritually.

WEB SITES AND REFERENCES

http://www.health.gov/healthypeople/. Healthy People 2010 home page.

http://www.nces.ep.gov. National Center Education Statistics.

http://www.acha.org/. ACHA home page, including position papers.

http://www.chronicle.com/. Home page for Chronicle of Higher Education.

American College Health Association. *Guidelines for a college health program.* Baltimore, MD: ACHA, 2001.

Chronicle of Higher Education. Almanac issue 2005–2006, http://chronicle.com/free/almanac/2005/notes/notes.htm

Johnston LD, O'Malley PM, Bachman JG, et al. *Monitoring the Future national survey results on drug use, 1975–2006.* Volume II: College students and adults ages 19–45. NIH Publication No. 07-6206. Bethesda, MD: National Institute on Drug Abuse. Available at: www.monitoringthefuture.org.

National Center for Education Statistics. Available at: http://www.nces.ed.gov.

Hussar WJ. Projections of Education Statistics to 2014 (NCES 2005-074). U.S. Department of Education, National Center for Education Statistics. Washington, DC: U.S. Government Printing Office.

Wechsler H, Davenport AE, Dowdall GW, et al. Binge drinking, tobacco, and illicit drug use and involvement in college athletics: a survey of students at 140 American colleges. *J Am Coll Health* 1997;45:195.

Wachsler H, Molnar BE, Devenport AE, Baer JS. College alcohol use: a full or empty glass? *J Am College Health.* 1999;47(6):247.

Wechsler H, Lee JE, Kuo M, Seibring M, Nelson TF, Lee H. Trends in college binge drinking during a period of increased prevention efforts. Findings from 4 Harvard School of Public Health College Alcohol Study surveys: 1993–2001. *J Am College Health.* 2002;50(5):203.

Working Group Report from the National High Blood Pressure Education Program, Update on the Task Force (1987). *On blood pressure in children and adolescents.* NIH publication no. 96-3790. Washington, DC: National Institutes of Health; September 1996.

INDEX

*Page numbers followed by *f* in italics indicate figures; those followed by *t* indicate tabular material.